The Mental Health of Medical Students

The Mental Health of Medical Students

Supporting Wellbeing in Medical Education

Edited by

Andrew Molodynski

Consultant Psychiatrist, Oxford Health NHS Foundation Trust and Honorary Senior Lecturer, Oxford University, Oxford, UK

Secretary General, World Association of Social Psychiatry

Sarah Marie Farrell

Academic Clinical Fellow in Neurosurgery, Nuffield Department of Surgical Sciences, John Radcliffe Hospital, Oxford, UK

Dinesh Bhugra

Professor Emeritus of Mental Health and Cultural Diversity, Institute of Psychiatry, Psychology and Neuroscience, Kings College London, London, UK

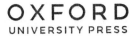

OXFORD
UNIVERSITY PRESS

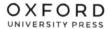

Great Clarendon Street, Oxford, OX2 6DP,
United Kingdom

Oxford University Press is a department of the University of Oxford.
It furthers the University's objective of excellence in research, scholarship,
and education by publishing worldwide. Oxford is a registered trade mark of
Oxford University Press in the UK and in certain other countries

Published in the United States of America by Oxford University Press
198 Madison Avenue, New York, NY 10016, United States of America

British Library Cataloguing in Publication Data

Data available

Library of Congress Control Number: 2023946180

ISBN 978–0–19–286487–1

DOI: 10.1093/oso/9780192864871.001.0001

Printed in the UK by
Ashford Colour Press Ltd, Gosport, Hampshire

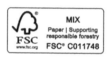

For the medical workforce of the future

Contents

PART 3

List of Contributors

Redouane Abouqal, Professor and Head of the Acute Medical Unit, and Director of the Biostatistics and Epidemiological Research Laboratory, Faculty of Medicine and Pharmacy, Mohammed V University, Rabat, Morocco

Sapna Agrawal, GPST Primary Care, Executive member and secretary. BAPIO GP Forum, Birmingham, United Kingdom

Telma Almeida, Psychiatrist, Department of Psychiatry, CUF Porto Hospital, Porto, Portugal

Olatunde Ayinde, Lecturer in Psychiatry, Department of Psychiatry, College of Medicine, University of Ibadan, Ibadan, Nigeria

Hannah S. Barham-Brown, GP Trainee, Leeds, UK

Jihane Belayachi, Professor of the Acute Medical Unit, and member of Biostatistics and Epidemiological Research Laboratory, Faculty of Medicine and Pharmacy, Mohammed V University, Rabat, Morocco

Ekaterine Berdzenishvili, Invited Lecturer, Department of Psychiatry, American MD Program, Tbilisi State Medical University, Tbilisi, Georgia

Dinesh Bhugra, Professor Emeritus of Mental Health and Cultural Diversity, Institute of Psychiatry, Psychology and Neuroscience, Kings College London, London, UK

Israel Kanaan Blaas, Assistant Psychiatrist, Medical Student Welfare Center (NUBEM), Medical School, FMABC University Center, Santo André, Brazil; and Assistant Psychiatrist and Researcher, Interdisciplinary Group for Studies on Alcohol and Drugs (GREA), Institute of Psychiatry, Clinics Hospital of the Medical School of the University of São Paulo (HCFMUSP), São Paulo, Brazil

Nancy Brager, Professor Emeritus, Department of Psychiatry, Cumming School of Medicine, University of Calgary, Calgary, Canada

Mary Cannon, Professor of Psychiatric Epidemiology and Youth Mental Health, Department of Psychiatry, RCSI University of Medicine and Health Sciences, Dublin, Ireland

João Mauricio Castaldelli-Maia, Associate Professor, Department of Neuroscience, and Postgraduate Sponsor, Department of Psychiatry, Medical School, University of São Paulo, São Paulo, Brazil; and Adjunct Assistant Professor, Department of Epidemiology, Mailman School of Public Health, Columbia University, New York, USA

Linda Chan, Clinical Assistant Professor, Department of Family Medicine and Primary Care/Bau Institute of Medical and Health Sciences Education, LKS Faculty of Medicine, The University of Hong Kong, Hong Kong

Santosh Kumar Chaturvedi, Honorary Consultant Psychiatrist, Jagadguru Kripalu Chikitsalaya, Vrindavan, Uttar Pradesh, India

Maha Lemtiri Chelieh, General Practitioner, Faculty of Medicine and Pharmacy, Mohammed V University, Rabat, Morocco

Julie Chen, Associate Professor of Teaching, Department of Family Medicine and Primary Care/Bau Institute of Medical and Health Sciences Education, Assistant Dean (Learner Wellbeing), LKS Faculty of Medicine, The University of Hong Kong, Hong Kong

Weng Chin, Honorary Assistant Professor, Department of Family Medicine and Primary Care, LKS Faculty of Medicine, The University of Hong Kong, Hong Kong

Eka Chkonia, Associate Professor, Department of Psychiatry, Tbilisi State Medical University, Tbilisi, Georgia

Egor Chumakov, Assistant Professor, Department of Psychiatry and Addictions, St. Petersburg State University, Saint-Petersburg, Russia

Darien Alfa Cipta, Lecturer, Medical Education Unit, Pelita Harapan University, Siloam Hospitals, Indonesia

Theresia Citraningtyas, Lecturer, Faculty of Medicine and Health Sciences, Krida Wacana Christian University, Jakarta, Indonesia

Debbie Cohen, Emeritus Professor, School of Medicine, Cardiff University, Cardiff, UK

Anna Collini, Lecturer in Medical Education, King's College London, London, UK

Dulangi Dahanayake, Consultant Psychiatrist, Child and Youth Mental Health Service, Darling Downs Health Service, Queensland, Australia

Harmani Daler, Medical Student, University of Lancaster, Lancaster, UK

Umakant Dave, Consultant Gastroenterologist, School of Medicine, Swansea University, Swansea, UK

Raymond Effah, Medical Student, University of Southampton, Southampton, UK

Dina Aly El-Gabry, Assistant Professor of Psychiatry, Okasha Institute of Psychiatry, Faculty of Medicine, Ain Shams University, Cairo, Egypt

Caroline Elton, Associate Professor, Norwich Medical School, Norwich, UK

Sarah Marie Farrell, Academic Clinical Fellow in Neurosurgery, Nuffield Department of Surgical Sciences, John Radcliffe Hospital, Oxford, UK

Andrea Fiorillo, Full Professor of Psychiatry at Department of Psychiatry, University of Campania 'L. Vanvitelli', Naples, Italy

Liz Forty, Senior Lecturer, School of Medicine, Cardiff University, Cardiff, UK

Grace W. Gengoux, Clinical Professor, Department of Psychiatry and Behavioural Sciences, Stanford University School of Medicine, Stanford, USA

Israel González, Acting Consultant in Adult Psychiatry, Jane Atkinson Health and Wellbeing Centre, North East London Foundation Trust, London, UK

Andrew Grant, Emeritus Professor, School of Medicine, Swansea University, Swansea, UK

Oye Gureje, Professor of Psychiatry, Department of Psychiatry, College of Medicine, University of Ibadan, Ibadan, Nigeria

Thomas Hewson, Academic Clinical Fellow in Psychiatry (ACFST3), Health Education North West School of Psychiatry and the University of Manchester, Manchester, UK

Johanna Holm, Manager, Student Advocacy and Wellness Hub, Cumming School of Medicine, SAW office, University of Calgary, Calgary, Canada

Chris Horn, GP Tutor, School of Medicine, Swansea University, Swansea, UK

Sara Hunt, Consultant Anaesthetist, School of Medicine, Cardiff University, Cardiff, UK

Kate Irvine, Senior Registar in Child and Adolescent Psychiatry and Consultant Adult Psychiatrist, Saint Vincent's Hospital, Fairview, Dublin, Ireland

Bikram Kafle, Associate Professor, Department of Psychiatry, Devdaha Medical College, Rupandehi, Nepal

Jay Kaplan, Medical Director of Care Transformation, LCMC Health; Clinical Associate Professor of Medicine, Section of Emergency Medicine, LSU Health Sciences Center; Attending Physician, Emergency Department, University Medical Center New Orleans, New Orleans, USA

Evie Kemp, Retired Consultant in Occupational Medicine, Medical Educator and Emeritus Director of Medical Student Wellbeing, Technion American Medical School, Technion Israel Institute of Technology, Haifa, Israel

Almu'atasim Khamees, Surgical Resident, Department of General Surgery, King Hussein Cancer Center, Amman, Jordan

Thomas Kitchen, Consultant Anaesthetist, Cardiff and Vale University Health Board, Honorary Lecturer, Cardiff University, Cardiff, UK

Jesper Nørgaard Kjær, Psychiatrist, Department of Psychosis, Aarhus University Hospital—Psychiatry, Aarhus, Denmark

Nabila Ananda Kloping, Student, Faculty of Medicine, Universitas Airlangga, Surabaya, Indonesia

Hannah Koury, Medical Student, University of Calgary, Calgary, Canada

Rossalina Lili, Member, Community Mental Health Section, Indonesian Psychiatry Association, Jakarta, Indonesia

Eteri Machavariani, Postdoctoral Associate, Section of Infectious Diseases, Department of Internal Diseases, Yale School of Medicine, New Haven, USA

Sridevi Sira Mahalingappa, Consultant Psychiatrist, South London and Maudsley NHS Foundation Trust, London, UK

Yamilka Alsina Martin, Wellness Program Coordinator, Department of Psychiatry and Behavioural Sciences, Stanford University School of Medicine, Stanford, USA

Rawan Masri, Psychiatrist and Lecturer, Faculty of Medicine, Yarmouk University, Irbid, Jordan

Christopher Mohan, Senior Registrar in Liaison Psychiatry, St Vincent's University Hospital, Elm Park, Dublin, Ireland

Fiona Moir, Pastoral Care Chair and Wellbeing Lead, Medical Programme Directorate, and Department of General Practice and Primary Health Care, Faculty of Medical and Health Sciences, The University of Auckland, Auckland, New Zealand

Andrew Molodynski, Consultant Psychiatrist, Oxford Health NHS Foundation Trust, and Honorary Senior Lecturer, Oxford University, Oxford, UK; Secretary General, World Association of Social Psychiatry

Tarek Okasha, Professor of Psychiatry Okasha Institute of Psychiatry, Faculty of Medicine, Ain Shams University, Cairo, Egypt

Eimear O'Neill, Senior Registrar CAMHS, UCC Deanery, Cork, Ireland

Mike Paget, Manager, Academic Technologies, Cumming School of Medicine, University of Calgary, Calgary, Canada

Ivan Pchelin, Associate Professor, Department of Faculty Therapy, St. Petersburg State University, Saint-Petersburg, Russia

Max Pemberton, Specialist Registrar, Camden and Islington NHS Foundation Trust, London, UK

Nataliia Petrova, Head of Department and Professor, Department of Psychiatry and Addictions, St. Petersburg State University, Saint-Petersburg, Russia

Sharad Philip, Assistant Professor, Department of Psychiatry, All India Institutes of Medical Sciences, Guwahati, Assam, India

Daniel Poulter, Specialist Registrar, South London and Maudsley NHS Foundation Trust, London, UK

Roshelle Ramkisson, Child and Adolescent Consultant Psychiatrist, Pennine Care NHS Foundation Trust; and Deputy Director, Institute of Psychiatry, and Reader, School of Medicine, University of Bolton, Manchester, UK

Nyapati R. Rao, Retired, Private practice; Formerly Van Tauber Chair of Psychiatry, and Chief Academic Officer, Nassau University Medical Center, East Meadow, New York; and Professor of Psychiatry, Stonybrook, SUNY, New York, USA

Gaia Sampogna, Associate Professor of Psychiatry, Department of Psychiatry, University of Campania 'L. Vanvitelli', Naples, Italy

Amy Schranz, Medical Student, University College Dublin, Dublin, Ireland

Nermin Shaker, Professor of Psychiatry Okasha Institute of Psychiatry, Faculty of Medicine, Ain Shams University, Cairo, Egypt

Avinash Shekhar, Senior Resident, Father Muller Medical College, Mangalore, India

Gemma Simons, Consultant in Physical and Rehabilitation Medicine, Solent NHS Trust, and Honorary Senior Clinical Lecturer, University of Southampton, Southampton, UK

Julio Torales, Professor of Psychiatry, Department of Psychiatry; and Professor and Head of the Department of Medical Psychology, School of Medical Sciences, National University of Asunción, San Lorenzo, Paraguay

Kristy Usher, Clinical Medical Education Fellow, Medical Programme Directorate, Faculty of Medical and Health Sciences, University of Auckland, Auckland, New Zealand

Antonio Ventriglio, Clinical Researcher, Department of Clinical and Experimental Medicine, University of Foggia, Foggia, Italy

Anuprabha Wickramasinghe, Senior Lecturer, Department of Psychiatry, Faculty of Medicine, University of Colombo, Colombo, Sri Lanka

T. Christopher R. Wilkes, Professor Emeritus, Department of Psychiatry, Cumming School of Medicine, University of Calgary, Calgary, Canada

Hamish Wilson, Associate Professor, Department of General Practice and Rural Health, Otago Medical School, University of Otago, Dunedin, New Zealand

Isheeta Zalpuri, Clinical Associate Professor, Department of Psychiatry and Behavioural Sciences, Stanford University School of Medicine, Stanford, USA

Introduction

Andrew Molodynski, Sarah Marie Farrell, and Dinesh Bhugra

Our decision to put together this volume was made after we developed an increasing understanding of the experience of medical students and the pressures they are subjected to and experience. As doctors in very different stages in our careers and from different backgrounds, we all have different takes on the issues but are all united by our real and growing concerns for the welfare of generations of doctors to come. Because of this we set out on a journey to make links on all five major continents and to collect data on student wellbeing in as many countries as possible. Teams of clinicians, researchers, authors, educators, and students alike all came together to share their findings. We salute them—this was not an easy task and, in some countries, involved hazards for those running projects and for those taking part. Indeed, politics and unrest led to some projects not making it to these pages. We wish we could acknowledge those people by name but cannot—they know who they are, and we wish them well. What we found overall is deeply disturbing. It did not shock us as we were half expecting it, but it does lay bare a real and urgent problem for medical education and thus for healthcare systems worldwide over the coming years.

It is important to recognise that there never was a 'golden era' of medical education—DB was at medical school in the 1970s, AM in the 1990s, and SF in the 2000s—all of us have our scars to bear as well as lifelong friendships and joyous memories too. Medical school has always been an intense and life-defining period, though if you read Chapters 1 and 4 by Bhugra and Rao, respectively, it perhaps lacked intensity of action and learning at least in those very early days described!

It is our belief though that the nature of medical education has fundamentally changed in the last two or three decades as has the nature of the practice of medicine. It would be odd if that were not the case, as education needs to evolve to provide the skills needed by practitioners to function safely and effectively in a changing healthcare environment. The reasons for change are complex and several chapters in the book examine what may be happening and why. What we do know unfortunately is that levels of burnout, emotional distress, and substance misuse are very high amongst medical students wherever one goes in the world. This situation mirrors that found amongst doctors of all grades working in different healthcare systems and cultures. Training for and practising medicine have always been stressful, but increased complexity in investigations, interventions, and management along with societal changes and higher patient expectations have contributed to increasing levels of stress and distress. The big unknown is to what extent this is a developing phenomenon. Attempts to measure and identify distress and burnout in medical students have been fairly limited until recent years so historical comparisons are generally not possible. There has been more research among practising doctors and that does indeed suggest a worsening over time. It seems reasonable to extrapolate that the same will be occurring in students.

Dinesh Bhugra, Daniel Poulter, and Max Pemberton, *Medical Education* In: *The Mental Health of Medical Students.*
Edited by: Andrew Molodynski, Sarah Marie Farrell, and Dinesh Bhugra, Oxford University Press.
© Oxford University Press 2024. DOI: 10.1093/oso/9780192864871.003.0001

While practising doctors can, to some extent, manage their own lives and destinies, especially in some high-income Group countries (and perhaps more so in private practice where one can exert better control over numbers and costs), the same cannot be said for medical students. By virtue of being students, individuals are likely to experience high levels of stress related to frequent and multiple assessments and placements over which they have limited or no control. Most medical students around the world are young adults between 18 and their late 20s—this is well-known to be a time of particular vulnerability for the development of mental health problems in any case. Students are often far from home and accumulating debt, in unfamiliar environments and away from those they love. These stressors are likely to make them even more vulnerable—**that** is why this book exists and **that** is why we believe that urgent action is needed.

We hope that this book will be of benefit to students themselves, those designing and running courses, teachers, those hosting clinical placements, and those making decisions about resource allocation and the structure of teaching both locally and nationally, amongst others too. The combination of wide-ranging discourse on the history and development of training, the measurement of burnout, and the challenges faced by different systems around the world will provide a point of reference in a developing field.

This volume could not have been put together without huge amounts of work from our teams on each chapter and we would like to thank each and every person who took part. We know that in several countries it was especially difficult to gather data, and that it even involved risk in some cases. This latter phenomenon is a very poor reflection on the relevant regimes, who sadly must remain nameless to protect those who helped us. We thank all the students who trusted us, gave their time, and expressed their (often difficult) emotions to allow this work to happen.

AM
SF
DB

Introduction

How to navigate this book

This book has three sections:

The **first section** provides an overview of medical education over time and across different regions of the world. Chapters 1 and 2 outline key aspects of the history and development of medical student teaching around the world, touching on key moments in history and key movements in different countries that altered the course of medical education for ever. The rise of German medical education in the nineteenth century and the Flexner report and its aftermath in early twentieth-century USA are both real landmarks, and both are discussed and explained by Rao in Chapter 2. The following chapters compare and contrast the issues in medical student teaching in countries from different economic groups. Cohen and Kitchen, using the fascinating analogy of agriculture, explore the need for radical reform not just of medical education but of medicine itself ('the soil'). Not only does the analogy hold, but it also allows for a highly original (if sobering) way to think about the system we are in. We expect readers to pick and mix what they read but we believe this chapter forms the bedrock of what we all need to understand to begin the process of fundamental change in ensuring that medical students' mental health and wellbeing are looked after. It provides a precious opportunity to take a step back and see the bigger picture in the context of our ever busier and faster paced but also more complex lives and learning. The following chapter by Hewson and colleagues focuses on the particular challenges for healthcare systems and medical education in low- and middle-income group countries and expands on these ideas and highlights some of the different pressures and stressors that may arise, alongside potential societal strengths. The final chapter in this first section is a systematic analysis of how we measure wellbeing and a great piece of co-production between a seasoned academic and a gifted medical student.

The **second section** includes nineteen reports from countries based upon our three-year project with colleagues from all substantially inhabited continents of the globe. Researching at times of stress in a country's life such as the impact of the Covid-19 pandemic with all hands on deck, civil unrest in Hong Kong, dark times in Russia, and a terrorist atrocity in New Zealand was not easy for many of our groups. Our friends and colleagues across the world persisted through these challenges to jointly accumulate and analyse the broadest set of data on global medical student wellbeing to date. To put it bluntly—they delivered! Though the core methods used were always the same, necessarily so for comparative purposes, the results and the contexts varied enormously. Each chapter is a vivid and individual description of what was done and what is happening in that country for medical students. Very worrying levels of burnout, distress, and help-seeking were found across the board, but rates did vary. Just under half of respondents in Morocco (47%) were cases on the General Health Questionnaire-12 (GHQ12) with the highest rate being 95% of respondents in Paraguay. Burnout rates varied between 61% on one subscale of the Oldenburg Burnout Inventory (OLBI) in Paraguay to 95% in Hong Kong. On the other OLBI measure, Paraguayan students scored extremely highly at 99% and the 'lowest' rates were in Canada and Denmark at 70%.

There were more significant variations in things such as drug and alcohol misuse and sources of stress, perhaps unsurprisingly given their strong cultural determinants. For example, rates of reported cannabis use varied from almost nil in several largely Muslim countries such as Jordan and Indonesia to 50% in Brazil and 79% in Portugal—on reflection, perhaps that latter 79% is a bit of a surprise after all! Various interventions are described in these chapters, from Jasper the therapy dog in Hong Kong to yoga in Wales, and many things in between! Never has there been such detail from so many countries in one place, especially those outside the traditional dominance of a small number of English-speaking High-Income Group (HIG) countries. Indeed, this group of countries is sparsely represented in these pages as the barriers to completing our project were more numerous and more immovable—a fact that did not pass us by and is addressed in Chapter 25 and in our conclusions. Those establishments and countries most able to ask how their students were doing often seemed the least willing to try. In any case, we hope that the wide scope of our group's efforts has resulted in a resource that can be genuinely useful to people undertaking or organizing medical courses, regardless of their region's economy, religion, or prevailing cultural norms.

The **third and final section of the book** gives a broad overview of both personal experiences and the needs of those who have moved between countries to study medicine, an increasingly common phenomenon in this increasingly interconnected world. This brings with it well-known challenges on top of those faced by all medical students, but as the chapter outlines, not enough is generally done in mitigation. The barriers faced by those who have additional challenges, another group of increasing numbers and prominence, are considered in detail the chapter by Hannah Barham-Brown, with a focus on longstanding difficulties and also what we may have learnt during Covid that could help people with different needs long term if (and only if) flexibility is maintained. It then goes on to suggest, with a clear and strong voice, what must be done. Chapter 28 contains moving and uplifting first-hand accounts from students around the world about their experiences and challenges and how they have risen to soar above them. Substance misuse is a known issue amongst young people in general and is a significant problem amongst medical students, despite (or perhaps because of?) their unusual exposure to the vagaries of life at an early age. Whether it be high rates of cannabis use in Portugal, high rates of drinking alcohol in our UK, Russian, and Canadian samples, or the use of stimulants to pass exams, there are troubling themes which need to be addressed urgently by providers and society at large.

Several chapters now provide a forward view. Collini and Elton remind us that, while many of the sources of stress and poor wellbeing are external and systematic, this does not mean that students are powerless and there are many things they can do to protect themselves and flourish. Their use of a framework of four domains of wellness—mental, physical, social, and integrated—feels especially helpful. Kemp focuses with clarity from an occupational health background on what institutions can and should do to support and protect those under their care as students, with a wealth of practical suggestions for those involved in running courses. We finish on a positive note, exploring crucial ideas around fulfilment and how that can be enshrined in both medical education and in medical practice, important to us all because of its association with better wellbeing and longer and more sustainable careers. The final chapter of the book by Kaplan is a whistle-stop tour of some real-life examples of good practice highlighting what has worked in different places.

We conclude the book with a brief and easily accessible medical student wellbeing charter which can be adapted and used globally.

References

Kadhum, M., Ayinde, O.O., Wilkes, C., Chumakov, E., Dahanayake, D., Ashrafi, A., Kafle, B., Lili, R., Farrell, S., Bhugra, D., & Molodysnki, A. (2022). 'Wellbeing, burnout and substance use amongst medical students: a summary of results from nine countries'. *Int J Soc Psychiatry* **68**(6): 1218–1222.

Molodynski, A., Lewis, T., Kadhum, M., Farrell, S.M., Chelieh, M.L., Almeida, T.F. De, Masri, R., Kar, A., Volpe, U., Moir, F., Torales, J., Castaldelli-Maia, J.M., Chau, S.W.H., Wilkes, C., & Bhugra, D. (2021). 'Cultural variations in wellbeing, burnout and substance use amongst medical students in twelve countries'. *Int Rev Psychiatry* **33**(1–2): 37–42.

PART 1

1
Medical Education

History and Challenges

Dinesh Bhugra, Daniel Poulter, and Max Pemberton

Introduction

Societies have always needed doctors to prevent, diagnose, and manage symptoms and diseases that people develop due to a number of reasons and may present with. From simply feeling unwell to identifying that something in their constitution, mind, or body is not right, people follow a certain pathway into help-seeking. This pathway into care is influenced by a number of factors, including cultural factors and influences as well as availability of resources. People will seek help depending on the explanatory models they have. Before going to an allopathic doctor when they may have realized that whatever they are experiencing is probably medical, they may have sought advice and help in the personal, folk, or social sector. They may also have used complementary and alternative medicines from other healthcare systems. They may see an allopathic practitioner as their last resort and may believe that allopathic doctors are interested in drugs only and may not have holistic approaches and may not give enough time for assessment and understanding the context in which symptoms may have emerged.

There is no doubt that progress in medicine has been dramatic in the last 70 years from the development of antibiotics to newer antipsychotics and targeted interventions but also to sophisticated investigations from MRI scans to functional MRI and positron emission tomography (PET) scans to gastroscopies, colonoscopy, and so on, to using cameras in pills for investigations and interventions. There is also an ever-increasing emphasis on using artificial intelligence (AI) and diagnostic and management algorithms. Increasingly people are using smartphones and smartwatches to monitor their blood pressure, blood sugar levels, and cardiac activity amongst other observations. In such a rapidly changing scenario where medicine is becoming increasingly technical, medical school curricula and training need to keep pace.

In this chapter we aim to provide a very brief history of medical education, an overview of its present state, and various ways forward to prepare medical students for clinical practice in the first half of the twenty-first century. This chapter does not aim to compare medical education and training across countries but focuses on a very brief history of medical education taking into account differences in disease and illness, looking at idioms of distress and explanatory models which dictate pathways into healthcare. We recommend some basic general principles that should guide education, training, assessments, and standards.

Dinesh Bhugra, Daniel Poulter, and Max Pemberton, *Medical Education* In: *The Mental Health of Medical Students*.
Edited by: Andrew Molodynski, Sarah Marie Farrell, and Dinesh Bhugra, Oxford University Press. © Oxford University Press 2024.
DOI: 10.1093/oso/9780192864871.003.0001

History

In previous centuries doctors were often 'learned' gentlemen with very few practical skills, and neither competencies nor duration of education were an issue. Often apprenticeship models worked. Over centuries uniform criteria for education at undergraduate and post-graduate levels emerged but their oversight by regulatory bodies followed much later. With increasing costs of healthcare, changes in relationships between patients and doctor and changing patient expectations as well as access to information from the internet, the thera-peutic relationship between the clinician and the patient (as well as their carers and families) has changed and evolved. It is necessary to have a standardized optimal level of education and training, especially as doctors and other healthcare professionals move across national borders. Length of training in different medical specialities has been agreed historically but the actual evidence of suitability of duration is often not very clear. Postgraduate training, for example in psychiatry, varies from 3 to 4 years in many countries, including the USA, to 6 or 7 years in parts of Europe. It is entirely possible that there may be more equivalence in so-called craft specialities rather than art ones. The introduction of competency-based training and workplace-based learning and assessments have introduced a practical dimension.

Fulton highlighted that from the days of early priest-physicians, the teaching (but also learning) of medicine has had a highly personal flavour (Fulton, 1953). He noted that per-sonal ties between the teacher and the pupil were important and varied and then became less so. Mentoring, apprenticeship, and supervision models have continued to change. A major challenge in current times is the use of simulation learning where anecdotally some students felt that they could not bring about empathy as at the back of their minds they knew that actors were not real patients and were being paid to play a role. Fulton cites ancient pre-cepts in Ayurvedic medicine where those students interested in medicine were encouraged to find the right teachers who have sound precepts, but who were also clever, dextrous, patient and kind, among other qualities (Lakshmipathi, 1944). Fulton also noted that the medical literature of Greece and Rome was concerned with the education of medical students, and texts existed (Drabkin, 1944) indicating that there was an ambition to standardize learning. According to Fulton, a medical school existed in southernmost Italy. Not surprisingly per-haps, medical education was focused on experience through practical learning, teaching, and apprenticeship. Books were used as adjuncts. Scientific approaches started to develop and were inevitably incorporated into teaching and learning, although sometimes it took a long time for this to happen.

In medieval times in the medical school in Salerno, students dissected animals to learn about anatomy. Around the same period, examinations and licensure based on examin-ation were introduced during the Mongol dynasty in China. Fulton describes the setting up of medical schools in Europe and the establishment of various teaching posts during the Renaissance and after. In the Renaissance period, medical schools were established in Italy, Spain, France, and England where gradually other subjects were introduced. Between 1100 and 1800, formal medical education in Europe is said to have started in northern Italy (Custers & Cate, 2018). There was a distinction between surgeons who were training on the job and academic doctors who were trained in the skills of drug preparation. Assessment of skills varied. After 1800, the medical education system gradually but profoundly changed. Acquisition of academic degrees became increasingly important and standards (for training and assessments) were being established and students assessed accordingly. Almost 600 years ago, a law was introduced in England that students who had studied in medical schools on the Continent prior to working in England needed to obtain an MD from Oxford or Cambridge. Eventually the very first institution setting formal standards under the Royal Charter, the Royal College of Physicians, was established in London in 1518. Fulton describes the period between 1600 and 1800 as a period of transition during which medical education in England could be obtained in London, Edinburgh, Aberdeen, and also in Dublin. Only a selected number of hospitals provided practical training. During the eighteenth century, the conditions of training in the USA varied both in duration and quality of medical education. The predominant form of medical education in the USA, as in many countries around the world, followed the apprenticeship model. The duration of training in medical schools varied between 2 and 3 years. Many private medical schools opened with a financial aim in mind. The American Medical Association (AMA) in 1847 recommended minimum periods of study (6 months) and practical training (2 years). Medical education in the United States was not regulated and did not originate in universities until much later.

It was only in 1919 that AMA set up rules for the duration of training. The late nineteenth century saw Osler set up training at different levels (more interns, fewer residents. and single chief residents who could stay on for 7–8 years) at Johns Hopkins University. The variation in levels of training was inspected by Abe Flexner who produced the Flexner Report after visiting medical schools in the USA and Canada (Flexner, 1910). The impact of the Flexner Report was indeed significant as its observations and findings led to the closure of some medical schools and standards improved in others through the use of philanthropy. In the 1980s the USA established the Accreditation Council of Graduate Medical Education (ACGME). Around the turn of the twenty-first century, the introduction of competency-based curriculum led to focus on specific competencies.

After 1950, medical education in Europe had become standardized at a number of universities and the European Union of Medical Specialists was set up to set standards of postgraduate training. However, in spite of this, duration and quality vary across various European nations. The range of specialities and sub-specialities also varies.

Fulton (1953) in his conclusions recommends that medical school curricula be liberalized and lightened with elimination of outmoded and unused areas of instruction, thereby reducing their duration. In theory, that observation still rings true. However, the reality is that as medicine advances, regular further additions are made to the curriculum, but nothing ever gets dropped! His second recommendation is that universities should create halls of residences and facilities where students of all faculties including medicine come together to learn from each other. Thus medical students are able to be exposed to various broader humanistic interests and establish contact with them.

Curriculum Changes

Buja (2019) looks at recent changes in medical education and raises questions about the characteristics of today's medical students. There is no doubt that the current generation has different attitudes towards things like work–life balance from earlier generations (Bernstein & Bhugra, 2011). These students have high levels of assertiveness, self-liking and narcissism and score lower on self-reliance (e.g. they show little interest in reading long texts (Twenge, 2009,

2014, 2017)). In his review, Buja (2019) notes that traditional curricula have failed to produce the desired outcome of producing physicians fit for the twenty-first century (Stevens, 2018). Concerns have been raised for a number of years about the contents of curricula and processes of training (see Gutierrez et al., 2016; Ludmerer, 1999; Samarasekara et al., 2018; Shelton et al., 2017).

There is an increasing consensus that major parts of the curriculum need to be repealed or replaced with more up-to-date information and research applications to ensure that the doctors of tomorrow are fully trained (Cooke et al., 2006; Frenk et al., 2010; Irby et al., 2010). Buja (2019) divides the typical undergraduate curriculum into preclinical (or first 2 years), which he argues are the integration of physical, biomedical science and physical examination and history taking. Clinical knowledge is gained from the integration of conceptual knowledge (facts, information), strategic knowledge (how), and conditional (why) knowledge. (2019). Similarly, in the clinical training phase, integration of social, psychological, and spiritual/anthropological factors can help produce more rounded training which will help the doctor of the future to provide appropriate services and care.

Buja (2019) argues persuasively that medical sciences need to be tailored at the right level so that students can learn other skills. In order to become a proper physician in the future, students must embrace science and demonstrate a focus for the public good while demonstrating integrity, honesty, and kindness. They must be fair and respectful, with a clear understanding that no two patients are going to behave in exactly the same way. Medical educators should lead by example and instil passion in students along with an appreciation of individual variability along with a facilitatory learning environment (Cofrancesco et al., 2018). Physicians, on the one hand, also have to contend with personal, professional, and public arenas in their life (Keen, 1900) but on the other there appears to be a broad consensus among teachers and the public as well as regulatory bodies that a good doctor has both humanistic and scientific abilities and attributes (Hurwitz et al., 2013). It can be argued that medicine is an art backed by science.

On the other hand, recent recommendations from the CanMeds (RCPSC, 2015) model place the 'medical expert' at the core with six components of the physician's role:

1. Communicator: The ability to communicate with the patient, carers, and other stakeholders in a language which is easily understandable is important.
2. Collaborator: In this context, the doctor has to be seen as a team player. Often the medically qualified individual, although working in a team, is expected to take on leadership roles.
3. Manager: The medical expert is a manager of resources but also has a role in managing teams, people, and other disciplines. This needs a clear differentiation from management roles in healthcare systems. Managing patients and often holding their anxiety is important. It is worth remembering that there remains considerable ambiguity in medicine and a key responsibility is about managing that ambiguity.
4. Health advocate: Advocating for patients, their families, and their care and carers is an important role, but very often undergraduate or even postgraduate curricula do not teach students how to advocate. This advocacy can be direct with policymakers and indirect advocacy too. Seeing policymakers with patients present can help bring a human dimension to advocacy and also working with local media and communities can help emphasize the importance of advocacy.

5. Scholar: With the rapid advances in medicine it is vital that clinicians are up to date with recent research development but also its application to improve patient care. An ability to study research, interpret findings, and apply them to improve or change one's clinical practice is a crucial skill to have. Patents may appear in the clinic with information from the internet, so the clinician must be able to sift the information. Interpreting research can also enable the clinician to advocate to policymakers.

6. Professional: Professionalism has at its core not only professional standards and values but also ethical practice and an awareness of responsibilities, and an ability to follow the standards set by local regulatory bodies. Accountability in a professional capacity applies to patients, their carers, the profession, and the general public.

These six components bring together medical expertise. Thus, undergraduate medical education must start and continue with these six characteristics in mind. Teaching psychiatry from day one would help integrate physical and mental health and thereby provide holistic care with little stigma.

In the past few years, there has been an increasing focus on the development of competency-based education and learning with assessments. Competency-based education and assessment focus on demonstrating a set and level of competencies. The Accreditation Council for Graduate Medical Education (ACGME) introduced a set of six competencies. It is an interesting theoretical approach and assesses practical skills at a certain level. One problem is that once reached, the level of competencies is often not followed-up to ascertain whether they are maintained or not. ACGME introduced milestones in the assessment of competencies to deal at least in part with that criticism (Byrne et al., 2017; Wagner et al., 2016). Other strategies are being developed for assessment.

What's Next in Training?

A knowledge of how patients see their illnesses and the models they use to explain their distress and idioms that are expressed can help engage patients and their families. Furthermore, such knowledge makes the clinician rooted in the culture within which they are practising. In this context, awareness of three areas is crucial: how people see their distress and symptoms, how they express it, and how they understand and explain it. We shall deal with these very briefly here.

Disease Versus Illness

In the first instance there needs to be a distinction made and focused upon between the concepts of disease and illness. Eisenberg (1977) defined disease as dis-ease which is caused by underlying pathology. Illness on the other hand is a social application where symptoms of disease start to influence social functioning of the individual. Here, as a result of symptoms, the individual may not be able to work, may take to bed, and may need looking after. It is important to recognize that individuals can live with their symptoms more so in certain conditions than others as long as they are able to function and have employment, a roof over their head, relationships, and money to meet their basic needs. Sickness is often defined by the society for things like the time off from work, sickness benefits, and so on.

Medical training and routine clinical practice often focus on the diagnosis of disease and not illness. The challenge is to put together biopsychosocial and anthropological models across all conditions be they physical or mental. Some medical conditions may be caused by biological factors, including genetic factors, but their presentation and the experience of symptoms will be influenced by social, psychological, and cultural factors. Medical students need to be made aware of this disjunction between medical and patient perspectives and be trained to manage illnesses which may need for them to take on more of an advocacy role.

Idioms of Distress

In a similar way, an awareness of what idioms of distress are being used by patients, their carers, and families will help improve therapeutic engagement. These idioms do vary according to a number of factors, of which culture is probably the most important one. When an individual develops distress and recognizes that they may have a problem, their behaviour will be strongly influenced by a number of factors such as educational and socio-economic status and cultural factors. Cultures which do not follow a Cartesian mind-body dichotomy may influence individuals to present symptoms in somatic or physical forms, as these patients and their families may not believe in a separation between physical and psychological symptoms. Some cultures illustrate distress through the use of metaphors. In the past, cultures which used physical symptoms have been criticized as being inferior to those showing psychological symptoms (Leff, 1984). The reality is that these models depend upon how cultures perceive mind–body relationships and no one paradigm is superior to another.

Explanatory Models

These are the explanations people have for their distress. Although primarily explored and discussed in the context of psychiatric disorders in many cultures, these can be equally relevantly applied to physical distress and conditions. These explanations have been divided into:

1. Supra natural: Evil eye, possession, for instance
2. Natural: Weather environment, for example
3. Psychological: Internal or external factors
4. Social: External factors such as poverty
5. A mixture of any of these

In addition, patients and their families in many cultures will have other models, such as seeing their illnesses as hot or cold which will affect their perception of the role of medication. Once again, it is important that clinicians of the future are aware of the explanatory models so that they can be recognized as pathology rather than normalcy where indicated. In Hispanic Americans, among others, for example, *ataque de nervios* is a common presentation of anxiety. An awareness of explanatory models in undergraduate as well as postgraduate training can help improve therapeutic engagement because clinicians can recognize and acknowledge these views.

A key tension in some countries is the generalist versus specialist debate of whether there should be more generalists or more specialists. There is no easy answer to this, as healthcare services require both generalists and specialists. The question arises whether some of the generalist work that doctors do can be managed by others. With the development of specialist nurses and physician associates, urgent debate is required not only about how team working will change and what the doctor of the future will have to deal with in service needs, service development, and service delivery but also which aspects of the doctor's roles can be taken on by others.

Training in undergraduate and postgraduate settings must focus on the social and cultural factors that influence illness and disease. Social determinants play a major role in the development of illnesses. As has been illustrated by the WHO Commission on social determinants led by Sir Michael Marmot, poverty, poor housing, overcrowding, unemployment, poor transport access, lack of green spaces all contribute to physical and mental ill-health and reduce longevity. Social determinants in turn are affected by geopolitical determinants such as natural disasters (e.g. earthquakes, flooding, tsunamis, hurricanes) or manmade ones like wars and conflicts.

An awareness and understanding of the impact of social determinants in a broader context needs to be an integral part of both learning and of assessment at all levels.

It is crucial that modern physicians are aware of mutual learning across nations (Kalra & Bhugra, 2014) particularly as there is an increasing movement of physicians across borders. Furthermore, an awareness of cultural factors and cultural awareness is important so that the patient and the physician can be placed at the core of a cultural assessment. To demonstrate cultural competence, physicians must explore the use of complementary and alternative medicines, some of which may interact with prescribed medication. In addition, cultural attitudes and responses to medicine and other therapies may differ and the physicians must take that into account. Explanatory models may be used to expect different kinds of medication. As Bhugra et al. (2015a, b) have illustrated, some cultures prefer injections whereas others prefer big tablets, and some cultures prefer small pills. The colours of pills may also affect compliance. As part of the core curriculum, the assessment of cultures, models of care, and the role of spirituality must be taken into account in developing and delivering any therapeutic interventions. People often prefer complementary and alternative therapies as they are seen as 'natural' and less toxic but also holistic. Hence, part of the training for doctors needs careful attention, especially with the movement of doctors across countries. A degree of homogeneity in training across countries is needed. Support, mentoring, and appropriate career advice would help. They can be encouraged to change something in their working lives every few years to remain fresh.

Conclusions

With the ongoing rapid advances in investigations and interventions in medicine, it is critical that medical schools play their role in changing patterns of teaching and assessment. Using bio-psycho-socio-anthropological models in all branches of medicine can help. The curricula need urgent refining in many settings, and students must be advised to look after their own mental health and wellbeing. One option is to ensure that their training includes parameters of self-improvement and career planning so they can select the right specialty and get appropriate mentoring when they need it. As there is an increasing movement of doctors across the globe due to globalization and the inter-connectedness of countries, it is important that there are common areas of instruction but it is critical that students and their teachers are aware of cultural relativism. On a more practical note, it is important that doctors look after their own mental health and wellbeing as well as physical health.

References

Bernstein, C.A. & Bhugra, D. (2011). 'Next generation of psychiatrists: What is needed in training?' *Asian J Psychiat* 4(2): 88–91.

Bhugra, D., Ventriglio, A., & Vahia, V. (2014). 'The role of Flexner Report for medical education in India'. *APJ Psych Med* 15: 162–164.

Bhugra, D. & Ventriglio, A. (2015). 'Do cultures influence placebo response?' *Acta Psychiatr Scand* 132(4): 227–320.

Bhugra, D., Ventriglio, A., Till, A., & Malhi, G. (2015). 'Colour, culture and placebo response'. *Int J Soc Psych* 61(6): 615–617.

Buja, L.M. (2019). 'Medical education today: all that glitters is not gold'. *BMC Med Educ* 19, 110.

Byrne, L.M., Miller, R.S., Philibert, I., Ling, L.J., Potts III, J.R., Lieh-Lai, M.W., & Nasca, T.J. (2017). 'Program performance in the next accreditation system (NAS): results of the 2015–2016 annual data review'. *J Grad Med Educ* 9(3): 406–410.

Cofrancesco Jr., J., Ziegelstein, R.C., & Hellmann, D.B. (2018). 'Developing foundational principles for teaching and education for a school of medicine'. *The Pharos/Spring*, pp. 43–46.

Cooke, M., Irby, D.M., Sullivan, W., & Ludmerer, K.M. (2006). 'American medical education 100 years after the Flexner Report'. *N Engl J Med* 355(13): 1339–1344.

Custers, E.J.F.M. & Cate, O.T. (2018). 'The history of medical education in Europe and the United States, with respect to time and proficiency'. *Acad Med* 93(3S Competency-Based, Time-Variable Education in the Health Professions): S49–S54.

Drabkin, I.E. (1944). 'On medical education in Greece and Rome'. *Bull Hist Med* 15(4): 333–351.

Flexner, A. (1910). *Medical Education in the USA and Canada*. New York: Carnegie Foundation.

Frenk, J., Chen, L., Bhutta, Z.A., Cohen, J., Crisp, N., Evans, T., Fineberg, H., Garcia, P., Ke, Y., Kelley, P., Kistnasamy, B., Meleis, A., Naylor, D., Pablos-Mendez, A., Reddy, S., Scrimshaw, S., Sepulveda, J., Serwadda, D., & Zurayk, H. (2010). 'Health professionals for a new century: transforming education to strengthen health systems in an interdependent world'. *The Lancet* 376(9756): 1923–1958.

Fulton, J.F. (1953). 'History of medical education'. *BMJ* 2(4834): 457–461.

Gutierrez, C.M., Cox, S.M., & Dalrymple, J.L. (2016). 'The revolution in medical education'. *Texas Med* 112(2): 58–61.

Hurwitz, S., Kelly, B., Powis, D., Smyth, R., & Lewin, T. (2013). 'The desirable qualities of future doctors—a study of medical student perceptions'. *Med Teach* 35(7): e1332–e1339.

Irby, D.M., Cooke, M., & O'Brien, B.C. (2010). 'Calls for reform of medical education by the Carnegie Foundation for the Advancement of Teaching: 1910 and 2010'. *Acad Med* 85(2): 220–227.

Kalra, G. & Bhugra, D. (2010). 'Mutual learning and research messages: India, UK and Europe'. *Ind J Psych* 52(Suppl): S56–S63.

Keen, W.W. (1900). 'The ideal physician'. *JAMA* 34(25): 1592–1594.

Lakshmipathi, A. (1944). *A Textbook of Ayurveda*. India: Bezwada.

Ludmerer, K.M. (1999). *Time to Heal: American Medical Education From The Turn of The Century To The Era of Managed Care*. New York: Oxford University Press, p. 514.

RCPSC (2015). 'CanMEDS: Better standards, better physicians, better care'. Ottawa: College of Physicians and Surgeons of Canada. http://www.royalcollege.ca/rcsite/canmeds/canmeds-framework-e (Accessed 17 October 2022).

Samarasekera, D.D., Goh, P.S., Lee, S.S., & Gwee, M.C. (2018). 'The clarion call for a third wave in medical education to optimise healthcare in the twenty-first century'. *Med Teach* 40(10): 982–985.

Shelton, P.G., Corral, I., & Kyle, B. (2017). 'Advancements in undergraduate medical education: meeting the challenges of an evolving world of education, healthcare, and technology'. *Psychiatr Q* 88(2): 225–234.

Stevens, C.D. (2018). 'Repeal and replace? A note of caution for medical school curriculum reformers'. *Acad Med* **93**:1425–1427.

Twenge, J.M. (2009), 'Generational changes and their impact in the classroom: teaching Generation Me'. *Med Educ* **43**: 398–405.

Twenge, J.M. (2014). *Generation Me: Why Today's Young Americans Are More Confident, Assertive, Entitled—And More Miserable Than Ever Before*. New York: Simon and Schuster.

Twenge, J.M. (2017). *IGen—Why Today's Super-connected kids are Growing Up Less Rebellious, More Tolerant, Less Happy—And Completely Unprepared For Adulthood*. New York: Simon and Schuster.

Wagner, R., Weiss, K.B., Passiment, M.L., & Nasca, T.J. (2016). 'Pursuing excellence in clinical learning environments'. *J Grad Med Educ* **8**(1): 124–127.

2

Globalization and Medical Education in a Post-Pandemic World

A Historical Review

Nyapati R. Rao

Introduction and Background

Globalization may be defined as a process in which the traditional boundaries separating individuals and societies gradually and increasingly recede, leading to change in the nature of human interaction in economic, political, social, cultural, environmental, and technological spheres (Giddens, 1990). This phenomenon highlights global interconnectedness and encourages innovation. Globalization's use of technology results in the shrinkage of time and space and a rapid flow of information, communication, and travel (Bhattacharya et al., 2010). The rise in international trade and commerce contributes to the increase in the living standards of billions of people and boosts intercontinental and local travel of masses of people, which leads to the rapid spread of diseases (Giddens, 1990).

In addition, globalization contributes to a phenomenon called 'Climate Change', caused by the release of global heat-trapping gases like methane and carbon dioxide into the atmosphere due to the excessive use of fossil fuels, widespread deforestation, destruction of coral reefs, and rapid industrialization worldwide. In turn, the rising temperature of the earth and the oceans results in the melting of polar caps, hurricanes, floods, tsunamis, droughts, forest fires, and pandemics. In the following section, one such event-a pandemic caused by a virus is described. (Golden, 2014; Kumar, 2021; Sullivan, 2022; Mehta, 2022).

The COVID-19 pandemic started as just another upper respiratory tract illness caused by a common coronavirus and rapidly exploded into a pandemic of gargantuan proportions, killing millions of people, disabling millions more and dramatically changing life, work, travel, commerce, and migration of billions of people. This deadly outcome was due to the ability of the COVID-19 virus to infect and quickly morph into more lethal mutants.

The pandemic emphasized the vital contributions made by physicians and medical students from the US and abroad as care providers, researchers, public health experts, vaccine inventors, and elucidators of various aspects of the disease. This pandemic also provided a birds-eye view of the strengths and weaknesses of the current medical students' training and the reforms needed to educate the physician of the future (Brown et al., 2021).

No country can single-handedly face such catastrophes. Nonetheless, successive pandemics have demonstrated the need for efficient international collaboration and fast and

Nyapati R. Rao, *Globalization and Medical Education in a Post-Pandemic World* In: *The Mental Health of Medical Students.*
Edited by: Andrew Molodynski, Sarah Marie Farrell, and Dinesh Bhugra, Oxford University Press. © Oxford University Press 2024.
DOI: 10.1093/oso/9780192864871.003.0002

accurate communication in managing them. When the first wave of COVID-19 cases appeared, public health experts, governments, and the media were caught flat-footed. The authorities offered confusing and conflicting advice because of the unknown mode of virus transmission and the lack of preventive measures at that time. Eventually, in light of swiftly mounting casualties, governments recommended that their citizens use personal protective measures such as masks and frequent hand washing. Also, they advised their citizens to stop the further spread of the virus by avoiding crowds and maintaining a six-foot interpersonal distance. As an ultimate measure, governments locked down entire cities for months at a time causing immense damage to their economies and to people's lives.

The authorities also instructed their scientific communities to find vaccine/s and therapies that would confer immunity or cure to their populations. The researchers responded by finding effective and safe vaccines in less than a year, but it was too late to save the millions who had died and the millions more who had developed a syndrome called long COVID-19.

COVID-19's Impact on Medical Education

Before COVID-19, US medical schools had been working to transform pedagogy by eliminating and reducing lectures, using technology to replace and enhance anatomy and laboratories, implementing team-facilitated, active, self-directed learning, and promoting individualized and interprofessional education. The development of entrusted professional activities and milestones for achievement has transformed assessment. Many schools had decreased the initial pre-clinical science curriculum to 12 or 18 months and revisited the basic sciences later in school. (Rose, 2020).

At the onset of the pandemic, the Association of American Medical Colleges (AAMC) suspended clinical rotations and issued guidance for medical students to avoid all activities involving direct patient contact. This unprecedented fiat caused widespread uncertainty among students and faculty about the sustainability of the existing medical education structure and process.

Challenges and Innovative Responses to COVID-19

The medical education community rose to the challenge and managed the response remarkably by making curricular changes while ensuring the safety, wellbeing, and future viability of the system (Brown et al., 2021; Papapanou, 2021).

Educational Changes

In many schools, medical students meet in small groups for interactive problem-solving or discussion in the first 12–18 months (pre-clinical phase) of their education. They learn through this early didactic experience the importance of the doctor-patient relationship, professionalism, communication, and interviewing skills. This practice provides them with an early immersion in clinical medicine and an opportunity to complete their clerkship curricula. This hands-on, bedside teaching method has been the backbone of medical education all around the world. The last 18 months of medical school are individualized, with students participating in advanced clinical rotations, sub-internships before residency, scholarly projects, or 'Away Rotations'. However, regardless of the phase or specialty of their learning, medical students encounter physical proximity to one another as an unavoidable reality of medical education (Papapapou, 2022).

The new imperative foisted by COVID-19 triggered new methods of learning in medical education. In order not to disrupt the learning process, academic institutions worldwide have accelerated the development of the online environment. As a result, medical schools offer two distance learning formats: Online Distance Education (ODE) can be delivered in two forms: asynchronous distance education, such as recorded videos and podcasts, and (live) synchronous distance learning education (SDE). One of the newer models is a 'flipped classroom', a blended learning mode that offers flexibility in scheduling asynchronous mode and a synchronous component that offers direct contact between students and faculty. Studies have demonstrated a higher overall satisfaction with SDE than with traditional methods (Hilberg et al., 2020; Mukhtar et al., 2020; Rallis et al., 2020; Ooi et al., 2020; Martagy et al., 2021; Tsang et al., 2021).

Online learning in medical education offers flexibility in time and location, resulting in increased convenience. In addition, ODE is available for students in different institutions globally, facilitating the adoption of the web-based curriculum. However, the unintended consequences of these technological innovations could be diminished interpersonal contact that may lead to students' feelings of insecurity and isolation and the development of poor interviewing and empathic skills. These deficiencies might affect the student's performance in clinical rotations and their future career choice.

Furthermore, students and faculty may encounter technical challenges, including problems with video and audio, errors in downloading or streaming, login problems, poor internet quality, and security issues.

Examinations

In many countries, clinical and written examinations were cancelled or replaced by online exams or newer assessment methods such as Open book examinations (OBE) and Closed book (CBE). The OBE fosters medical students' critical thinking, analytic skills, and conceptual understanding of medicine. Anxiety in taking these examinations is reduced. OBEs reinforce evidence-based learning, and using the internet helps make students self-directed learners. Also, OBEs foster deeper processing more effectively and strengthen their long-term memory. However, medical students may prefer CBEs over online OBEs.

Medical students who participated in online OBE had significantly higher mean scorers in both multiple-choice and essay questions but significantly lower—scores in short-answer examinations. At the same time, compared with the traditional written assessments, the online OBE group had a significantly lower correlation between the essay and their grade point average than the conventional groups. Changes enforced by this pandemic offer a rare opportunity to evaluate alternative medical education and assessment models globally (Rafi et al., 2020).

Mental Health

The challenges of going through med school and medical education may contribute to psychological distress, such as anxiety, depression, grief, and burnout among medical students. Medical students typically encounter stressful situations such as high workload, multiple evaluations, career assessments, the pressure of clinical training, numerous responsibilities, anxiety regarding their grades, long study hours, and concern about future opportunities. This structure and knowledge of what to expect were lost during the pandemic (Tsamakis et al., 2020).

The authorities made the situation more stressful through the imposition of unfamiliar public health measures, including wearing masks, social distancing, and lockdowns. In addition, fear of being infected by the virus as first responders, anxiety about their removal from clinical practice, worries about older relatives, and the abrupt shift to a new reality have caused further damage to the psychological wellbeing of students (Chang et al-2021).

Medical students' experience of pre- and post-pandemic anxiety and depression differs based on their cultural backgrounds. The prevalence of depression and anxiety in the US was not significantly higher compared to the pre-pandemic level, while in Turkey, India, Iran, and Malta, the reverse was true. The poor sleep quality of medical students and their decreased appetite were reported. The female gender was frequently associated with higher rates of anxiety and depression. Other predisposing factors leading to higher psychological distress were low families' monthly income, lower GPA, and experience with COVID-19 symptoms (Tsammakis et al., 2020).

Residency Selection

The inability to explore specialties of interest and the loss of electives and core rotations may put significant pressure on medical students' career choices due to the reduced clinical experience and limited access to real-life residency. Medical students have more limited exposure to positive role models among faculty members. Such a development may result in the lack of enthusiastic recommendation letters, adversely influencing their choice of specialty. Finally, the inability to schedule the 'Away Rotations' may affect medical students' ability to get the residency of their choice as well as the geographical location of their residency (Fodje et al., 2020).

Medical Students as Frontline Workers

The new reality triggered the deployment of medical students as frontline workers with their assignments adapted to institutional and national healthcare needs and their knowledge, experiences, and preparedness. This new role as the frontline worker was perceived by many as a possible learning experience in disaster medicine. In addition, the urgency for rapid and novel adaptation to changed circumstances has functioned as a catalyst for remarkable innovations in medical education, including promoting a more evidence-based approach (Hammond et al., 2020; Wang et al., 2020).

The history of medicine informs us that humanity has confronted many pandemics over its 10,000-year history. Lacking modern technological developments, there were even more lives lost or damaged. However, the current pandemic happening on a global stage has demonstrated the success of international collaborative efforts in containing and limiting the further spread of COVID-19. Globalization both caused the spread of the pandemic and its devastating effects and facilitated rapid recovery from the pandemic by creating easy communication tools such as video conferencing, inexpensive connectivity, and international collaborative efforts.

With the previous discussion of the phenomenon of globalization as the backdrop, the author will discuss historical perspectives on the development and evolution of medical education across the globe, starting with the USA's efforts in the development of its system of medical education serving as one model of excellence. However, one must not overlook the impact of various cultural, scientific, social, and economic realities on the evolution of medical education among the nations of the world.

The Evolution of Medical Education in the USA

In the mid-nineteenth century, the pre-Penicillin era, when infectious diseases ravaged America, the only medications available were chloroform, ether for anaesthesia, and quinine to treat malaria. Amputation was the standard treatment for injured limbs, and the poor quality of surgery is reflected in an 87% mortality rate of all amputations conducted during the Civil War. In comparison, there was only a 3% mortality rate for this procedure in World War II—a great measure of progress. Elementary techniques of the physical exam, such as measuring temperature, percussing the chest, or using stethoscopes or ophthalmoscopes, were done by very few physicians.

The preparation of medical students for a career as physicians was more an enterprise of commerce than an enterprise in science (Baron, 2005; Ludmerer KM, 1999).

Against this backdrop, American physicians' exposure to two foreign medical systems, Germany and France, was critical in lifting American medicine from its morass and setting it on the path to excellence (Baron, 2005). In the early 1800s, France was the favourite destination for American physicians eager to work alongside luminaries like Louis Pasteur, Claude Barnard, and Xavier Bichat. The phrase ''*peu lire, beaucoup voir, beaucoup faire, and* '**read little, see much, do much**' embodied the principle of education in France (Baron, 2005; Ludmerer, 1985).

While eschewing grand theories, French medicine emphasized the importance of keen observation of clinical phenomena and letting facts speak for themselves. It also pioneered the study of the natural history of disease and therapeutics using numerical or statistical methods. These influences of French medicine acted as an antidote to 'outlandish theories and speculative abuses' in American medicine. American physicians were greatly influenced by the French methods in that they practised observation and distrusted experimental research and laboratory (Ludmerer, 1985).

In the middle of the nineteenth century, its lack of research basis and its disdain for biological sciences caused French medicine's downfall. Subsequently, Germany became the centre of European medicine. The rise of research laboratories in German universities where disease mechanisms were experimentally examined and confirmed was novel then. In addition, some of the features of German education, such as employment of full-time salaried professors, division of education into undergraduate and postgraduate domains, creation of specialties and subspecialties, and an emphasis on laboratory science, made American students seek their medical education in Germany.

Upon returning to the US with their newfound knowledge and skills, these foreign-trained US physicians found that the US still faced significant challenges due to a lack of standardization in medical education. Medical schools, except for a few, had become a lucrative business. Several systemic issues still plagued the system: a need for uniform standards, minimal requirements for admission, establishing clinical and basic research as a priority, and initiating an effort to foster an academic environment for all medical schools through affiliation with the universities. German-trained American physicians changed the system by applying their new knowledge, thus influencing the transformation of American medical education from a mediocre enterprise into a model of excellence for the rest of the world (Ludmerer, 1985; 1999).

The American Medical Association (AMA) and its medical and educational component, the Council on Medical Education, took the lead in identifying the problems and seeking solutions. In this effort, philanthropies such as Carnegie Endowment and Rockefeller Foundation and universities such as John's Hopkin's, Cornell, and Columbia endorsed the process and put their organizational might behind the success of the reforms.

Flexner's Observations

In 1908, the Carnegie Foundation appointed Abraham Flexner, headmaster at a high school in Louisville, to study the American medical education system and suggest remedies. Flexner had little knowledge of medicine but rose to the challenge and delivered a report that changed the fundamental nature of medical education in the US. After visiting 155 medical schools in the US and Canada, Flexner found an abysmal state of affairs confronting the nation.

Lack of Standardization

Flexner observed, '*A century ago, being a medical student in America was easy. No one worried that admission standards for entrance requirements were lower than for a good high school. Instruction was superficial and brief. The terms only lasted for 18 weeks, and after the second term, the MD degree was automatically given, regardless of a student's academic performance. Teaching was by lecture alone. Thus, students were spared the arduous chores of attending laboratories, clinics, and hospital wards. And students would often graduate without touching a patient*' (Ludmerer, 1996).

Lack of Inquiry

Furthermore, the curriculum consisted of '*received wisdom and practices of physicians*', and there was no connection between the practice of medicine and the science of medicine. Many schools were of poor quality due to a lack of accepted academic standards and accreditation. The emphasis on memorization through rote learning was problematic due to the expansion of medical knowledge and evidence-based practice. In medicine, Flexner felt that there should not be any difference between research and practice. Ideally, the intellectual attitude to research and clinical practice should be identical' Consequently, '*the ward and the labora-tory are logically from the point of the investigation, treatment, and education, inextricably intertwined*'. Finally, all these shifting models in a physician's education led to the recommen-dation that medical education should be located within universities and teaching hospitals where discovery and advancement of knowledge are central to their mission.

Lack of Professional Identity

Flexner believed that students lacked role models in the practice of medical professionalism. In a lecture-dominated curriculum, students had limited opportunities to observe practi-tioners' professional demeanour or actions and thus had no professional role models to emu-late. He suggested that the remedy would lie in a student's immersion in university culture and constant contact with the professor.

Flexner's final recommendations included changes in medical school admission standards and emphasis on basic sciences such as statistics, physics, and chemistry in the curriculum. In addition, medical education should be extended to four years: the initial half for studying pre-clinical subjects in basic sciences; and the latter for studying clinical subjects. Instruction by physician-scientists and student participation in supervised laboratory and clinical re-search would subsequently influence the development of academic and hospital-based clin-ical medicine. (Flexner, 2002).

The Response to Flexner's Report

The AMA's response was to embrace his call for standardization of medical education enthu-siastically. These recommendations (Flexner, 1910) would subsequently include the frame-work for developing American medicine, which would become '*excellent and very expensive*'. Full-time academics (called professors) would teach medical students, and philanthropy would support medical schools. Teaching hospitals provided clinical resources to train med-ical students and the university hospitals conducted advanced research. By the mid-1940s, the physician workforce shortage had begun due to the closure of substandard medical schools. As new specialties were formed in response to scientific progress, Graduate Medical Education (GME) was better organized. The Medical College Admission Test (MCAT) was introduced as an examination to test the readiness of students to seek medical training (Ludmere, 1985; Irby et al., 2010).

A decade after the report, as stated earlier, approximately one-third of medical schools with inadequate instruction, substandard facilities, unscientific faculty members, and poorly prepared students had been closed. These were owned mostly by minorities that educated students exclusively from minority communities and women. Consequently, Flexner was ac-cused of racism. He was also criticized for ignoring the doctor-patient relationship in his zeal for making American medicine scientific. In addition, he was perceived as being an elitist who favoured the Ivy League schools such as Harvard and Chicago. On the positive side, his recommendation to train researchers in biomedical research led to the creation of the

National Institutes of Health (NIH), higher admission and graduating requirements, great scientific advances, pedagogic changes, and the strengthening of GME.

After World War II, the Federal government created the GI bill to improve war veterans' opportunities. To recruit the most talented employees, employers offered free healthcare as an inducement in addition to the usual salary, vacation, and other perks. This development freed millions of Americans from paying for healthcare through their earnings while their employers picked up the expense. As a result, Americans in large numbers sought healthcare due to increased access. The Federal Government, through the launching of Medicare, Medicaid, and Social Security in the creation of the 'Great Society', hastened the expansion of medical care. This rapid infusion of patients and funds resulted in an explosion of research, an expansion of clinical care, and the creation of specialization. Due to the continued workforce shortage in medicine, the US turned to international medical graduates (IMGs) physicians trained in foreign schools- to bolster its healthcare workforce (Rao et al., 2016; Ludmerer, 1999). The primary source countries were India, China, sub-Saharan Africa, and South and Central America.

Globalization's Impact on Medical Education

As stated by Rizwan and others, 'the global healthcare markets are expanding rapidly, and advances in the globalization of education are having an unprecedented impact on medical education worldwide' (Rizwan et al., 2018). The emerging trends due to international education include a rapid increase in the number of medical schools (Cassimatis, 2013; Rao et al., 2016; Rizvzn, 2018) and medical students (Wu, 2020), increased privatization of medical schools (Davey, 2014; Scheffer, 2015), migration of medical students (Mullan, 2005; Rao, 2006, 1989; Stilwell, 2004), the movement towards international standardization of quality (Rao et al., 2016) and the development of new collaborative models between medical schools worldwide (Jones, 2011; Williams, 2008; Bedoll et al., 2021). People worldwide can benefit from the easy availability of state-of-the-art treatments due to globalization (Carrera, 2006). In the following, the author will provide a summary of terms used in the global medical literature.

Internationalization of Medical Education

The internationalization of medical education (IoME) is the purposeful integration of international, intercultural, and/or global dimensions into medical education to enhance its quality and prepare graduates for professional practice in a globalized world (Wu et al., 2020). Public Health (PH) plays a central role in the education of the future global physician, and the term PH is synonymous with Global Health (GH). PH is 'the science and art of preventing disease, prolonging life and promoting health through the organized efforts and informed choices of society, organizations, public and private communities, and individuals ... ' (Winslow, 2020). GH, as its global counterpart, historically evolved from International Health—an area that addresses local, national, and international health concerns on all levels.

GH was defined (Koplan et al., 2009) as 'An area for study, research, and practice that prioritizes improving health and achieving Health Equity for all people worldwide'. GH is frequently conceived as a multidisciplinary field of service, research, and education undertaken as part of an altruistic 'Global North to Global South' collaboration and/or as part of a national/Local health equity programme. Its primary goals—as it oftentimes appears in published work—are to improve the health of underserved individuals and populations and to achieve health equity for all people worldwide, with the primary focus on the resource-poor abroad.

Programmes in low- and middle-income countries (LMICs) are frequently used to report on the internationalization of the medical curriculum—primarily to describe extracurricular activities or projects in LMICs or other underserved populations. Thus, the enactment of GH in medical education programmes appears to be narrower and more limiting than the definition of GH itself suggests. GH includes the vision of the improvement of health for all people worldwide. In contrast, IoME is an area of educational science, an educational concept, a framework, and a means to developing international and intercultural learning outcomes in all students.

IoME encompasses the international collaborative goals and dimensions between nations and does not solely focus on cultural differences. Internationalization of medical education includes, but is not limited to, learning about and understanding differences in international healthcare, education, healthcare delivery systems, health economics, health ethics, and health laws; building an international care network; providing future physicians with skills in intercultural competencies, collaboration, and international leadership.

Evolution of Global Medical Education

This section will highlight the central role of the World Health Organization (WHO) in launching critical reform initiatives and their outcomes in the formation of modern medical education, which is not widely known among international medical educators (Weisz & Nannestad, 2021). This history has much to tell about the evolution of medical training, international and global health, and the relationship between the Global North and the Global South. While the AMA led the Medical Education (ME) reform efforts in the US, the WHO was responsible for the reforms of ME worldwide.

In the following sections, the author will discuss the efforts by the WHO and its principal ally, the World Federation of Medical Education (WFME), to strengthen and standardize global medical education worldwide. The primary focus will be on their global initiatives and not on any individual country. The consideration of the US as a model to emulate is due to the extraordinary progress the US has made in clinical medicine, training of physicians, and medical research. Despite its restrictive immigration laws, the US attracts thousands of physicians worldwide for training in various medical fields. Even though most of these physicians continue their careers in the US upon their training, a sizeable number return to their countries of origin, carrying their new knowledge and skills.

The efforts of the WHO to reform occurred over three distinct periods. In the First Period from 1949 to 1973, the WHO's emphasis was on expanding the number of health personnel, particularly in LMICs, and introducing the compatibility of their diplomas to facilitate the international movement of health workers. Furthermore, transferring the scientific instruction characteristic of medical schools in High-Income Countries (HIC) to LMICs and training health personnel in the tenets of public health and prevention were the WHO's priorities.

The second period from 1973 to the mid-1980s associated these traditional concerns with adapting medical training to the WHO's new orientation, expressed as Primary Health Care (PHC) or Health For All (HFA). The third period from the 1980s onward has been characterized by attempts to operationalize these concerns and improve the quality and safety of medical practice. The WHO has used formal training standards published as guidelines and accreditation procedures for training institutions (Weisz & Beata Nannestad, 2021).

First Phase (1949–1973)

The lack of skilled personnel has always been a major obstacle to the delivery of safe care. The WHO focused its attention on expanding existing schools and starting new ones. There were 533 medical schools in WHO member countries around 1950, and their numbers increased to 717 by 1966. International medical educators have been concerned about the tension between global pressure to standardize models to those in wealthy countries and local healthcare needs. One of the suggestions was that the training of physicians in developing countries should be different from that in HIC. Another approach was to send foreign personnel abroad to train the students.

The WHO sent professors to needy institutions, reorganized departments, taught courses, and initiated research projects to transfer these responsibilities to local professionals. They also provided teaching equipment and medical literature. From 1950 to 1956, the WHO organized 129 courses with 2,500 participants. In addition, an extensive programme of Fellowships was established with financial support. Healthcare professionals participated in training programmes, educational meetings, and conferences. Fellowships were seen as critical to the improvement of healthcare training. Fellows brought back new ideas and techniques to their countries of origin. The WHO published the World Directory of Medical Schools to facilitate this process, which contained worldwide tabular information on medical schools (WHO, 1958).

Second Phase (1973–1980s)

Now the WHO integrated its earlier focus on increasing the number of health personnel and modernizing their training into a broader framework of national health services planning. Under the leadership of its Director General, Halfdoan Mahler, the WHO championed equity among nations, health system planning based on permanent infrastructure rather than foreign-organized disease-based programmes, basic primary care rather than high-tech medicine, and a greater emphasis on socio-economic determinants of health and illness. The new orientation dubbed 'Health for All 'by the year 2000' (HFA) was summarized in the 'The Ama Alta' Declaration of 1978.

The consequence of this Framework was a greater emphasis on adapting medical training to local and national needs. Central to this vision was responsiveness to communities, which could mean anything from specific geographical units to the world outside medical schools and hospitals. The perceived lack of healthcare personnel, particularly physicians, was a significant impediment. A study by the WHO and UNICEF in 1969–1971 in nine countries found severe shortages of health personnel. It also found that career structures, national planning, and training facilities were inadequate, the quality of training was unpredictable, and the curriculum ignored essential topics such as Tropical Medicine that had greater relevance to local conditions. In addition, the study found that these nine countries organized much of the training of physicians in hospitals with no attempt to involve the community. These inadequacies were linked to the increasingly visible migration of healthcare professions from LMIC to HIC.

Since 1969, a comprehensive and long-term programme has been underway to train teachers of medicine and other health sciences in WFME-sponsored institutions such as the Central Institute for Advanced Medical Studies in Moscow and the 'Center for the Study Medical Education at the University of Illinois College of Medicine in Chicago. By the end of 1977, several national centres were training teachers in their settings and languages. By 1974, the programme's objectives had evolved to take into account the WHO's new system-based approach, which meant conceiving training in terms of the personnel needs of the overall healthcare system. Later the WHO expanded the programme to include training auxiliary personnel to retain them in their native countries.

To study the lack of trained personnel, particularly the LMIC, the WHO, in collaboration with UNICEF, undertook a comprehensive assessment of their assistance to education and training programmes in nine countries. This study confirmed the current views about the inadequacy of training personnel and the quality of training. An example, TropicalMedicine was not a priority of many programmes. These inadequacies resulted in the increasing migration of physicians. The WHO asked its member states to involve their universities in educating the communities on the value of Health For All (HFA).

A network of community-oriented educational institutions for the Health Sciences was formed at the instigation of WHO. The goal was for institutions to help each other develop training programmes that prioritized the health problems of local populations outside the hospital setting. In addition, to 'community-oriented' and 'problem-based learning', the newer 'active' pedagogical methods, rather than passive rote learning, produced self-directed independent study and life-long learning. Furthermore, a review of these problem-based and student-oriented programmes found that their graduates chose primary care programmes more than traditional ones (WHO, 1966).

Third Phase: 1980–1990s

A third period from the late 1980s found the WHO intensifying its focus on physician training. It corresponded with the intensified work of an allied organization, the WFME, established in 1972 with the collaboration between the WHO and the World Medical Education (WMA). It sought to introduce international standardization to medical training. The justification for this effort was the multiplication of new medical schools worldwide, many private or for-profit and of unknown quality, that appeared to adversely impact the free international mobility of medical students and physicians. There was unacknowledged tension between the twin goals of getting medical schools to reform themselves and setting up regulatory mechanisms to control the movement of physicians internationally. Two global conferences on medical education were held in Edinburgh. Graduates widely acknowledged that poor training and lack of opportunities in many countries were the catalysts for physician migration from LMIC to HIC.

Also, HFA required action on the social, economic, and political aspects and made the perspectives of non-medical disciplines indispensable. However, universities were not enthusiastic about participating in this initiative due to the fear that 'community-oriented teaching and research will lower standards'—initially, the WHO was the only organization involved in these initiatives. Then, foundations such as the Rockefeller Foundation joined the efforts of the WHO to improve medical education.

In 1978, the Foundation launched the International Clinical Epidemiology Network (INCLEN) in all countries to train these physicians in Clinical Epidemiology and familiarize them with the population-based perspectives necessary to manage limited resources. In addition, in 1979, 19 medical schools formed a network of community-oriented educational institutions.

In the 1980s, the WHO further intensified its focus on physician training. It provided a roadmap for educational reform comprised of twelve actions to guide national and international leaders. These actions stated that the education of health professionals should be relevant to the needs of the population being served and carried out in those environments most healthcare takes place in, i.e., community health facilities. In addition to teaching biomedical science, medical curricula needed to include training in health promotion and to take account of local resources while instilling values of social responsibilities.

The second Edinburgh conference held in 1993 made further recommendations, such as streamlining interactions between medical education and national health systems and promoting curricular changes by introducing medical ethics, communication skills, and population-based medical training. In 1996, the WHO called for collaborative efforts to define the profile of the 'future doctor'. The influence of Primary Health Care and HFA was visible in the strategy's list of the five essential skill sets for physicians: care provider, decision-maker, communicator, community leader, and manager. Biomedical and scientific knowledge were deemphasized in favour of communication and leadership skills (WHO, 1968–1977).

The Era of Global Standards and Accreditation

In 1998, the WFME Executive Council declared its intention to expand the accreditation of medical schools worldwide. As a result, task forces produced global standards for all three levels of training-basic (undergraduate), medical education (BME postgraduate (PME), and continuing professional development (CPD). The trilogy of standards was launched at the WFME World Conference in Copenhagen in 2003. The WFME clarified that these standards were not intended to weaken national authority over health professionals' medical education or to make medical education uniform across the globe.

Global standards were accompanied by pressure to develop accreditation programmes for medical schools as quality improvement. The Guidelines for Accreditation described the essential elements of accreditation: Institutional self-evaluation, evaluation by the external accreditation agency, and the public dissemination of the agency's final report and the accreditation outcome. The guidelines provided a framework for accreditation rather than stipulating the exact content of accreditation. One report observed that although accreditation was voluntary, incentives and professional and market pressures would, over time, make it 'virtually compulsory'. The addition of accreditation to the Directory of Medical Schools was one such incentive. An agreement in 2007 transferred the existing WHO database to the University of Copenhagen, where the headquarters of WFME was located. The new database was called the Avicenna Directory of Medical Schools. The Avicenna Directory was merged with the International Medical Education Directory to form the World Directory of Medical Schools.

The accreditation effort received a boost when the Educational Commission for Foreign Medical Graduates, responsible for certifying foreign graduates to attend postgraduate programmes in the US and Canada, announced that starting in 2023, only graduates of medical schools that had been accredited by an approved agency (ECFMG) would be eligible for its examinations and certifications agency (Cassimatis, 2013).

Concerns Over Accreditation

One common criticism of these proposals was the difficulty of implementing effective educational reforms. A traditional reproach was that these reforms were not relevant to the needs of LMICs, and the HICs were viewed as imposing their agenda on an unwilling clientele. Also, African countries warned against copying accreditation systems from HIC in 'an effort to conform to Western educational imperatives'. Such concerns have been expressed in attempts to develop global curricula for specialties around measurable competencies. Some argued that the standards were too expensive to implement for many countries. Nevertheless, the standardization movement received strong support from academics in HICs.

There were also concerns that wealthy nations that depended on International Medical Graduates to fill their workforce needs would face severe personnel shortages. Others suggested that many of these standards that followed the latest trends in Western medical education were steeped in a particular set of cultures incompatible with cultural values in many nations. Another common argument was that global health itself was rife with the values of colonialism. Some critics identified the 'enterprise of globalizing the medical curriculum' as a new wave of neo-colonialism. It was also suggested that the standardization language was self-contradictory, insisting on the need for local differences and diversity while promoting western standards as core competencies.

Additionally, some critics say that the Problem-based Learning (PBL) interpretation differs from place to place and thus does not represent a single hegemonic discourse, the concerns were expressed that there is little evidence that it improves the quality of medical education. Standardization and accreditation are not the only forms of globalization affecting medical education. Some medical schools in the Caribbean, Eastern Europe, and Asia brand themselves as international schools that train students worldwide to practice medicine anywhere. The move to improve medical education in LMICs has gone through several stages, from providing courses and fellowships to teach western medical science to adapt training to local needs to the current move towards *merging* global standards with local needs. Whether it is about ending practice variation through guidelines measures for life-long learning and periodic recertification for physicians, or new courses in professionalism and bioethics, the goal is to transform medical practice.

The current COVID-19 pandemic has disrupted all walks of life. As the saying goes, every crisis offers an opportunity for progress as was demonstrated in the current pandemic. Healthcare is not a privilege but a fundamental human right. Therefore, in this era of globalization, the nations of the world must strive to provide affordable, competent, high-quality, and appropriate healthcare to their communities. The most effective and productive way of training future physicians is by studying the history of medicine and medical education. The price of not doing so may be is to repeat past mistakes.

References

Kumar, A. & Ayedee, N. (2021). 'An interconnection between COVID-19 and climate change problem'. *J Stat Manag Syst* 24(2): 281–300.

Baron, J.H. (2005). 'American medical students in 19th century Europe'. *Mt Sinai J Med* 72: 270–273.

Bedoll, D., van Zanten, M., & McKinley, D. (2021). 'Global trends in medical education accreditation'. *Hum Resour Health* 19, 70.

Bentley, C.Z. (2021). 'Global health in medical education'. Med.Sci.Educ 31 (Suppl 1): 5–8 ().

Bhattacharya, R., Gupta, S., & Bhugra, D. (2010). 'Globalization and psychiatry'. *Principles of Social Psychiatry*, pp. 141–153. https://lccn.loc.gov/2013039405

Brown, A., Kassam, A., Paget, M., Blades, K., Mercia, M., & Kachra, R. (2021). 'Exploring the global impact of the COVID-19 pandemic on medical education: an international cross-sectional study of medical learners'. *Can Med Educ J* 12(3): 28–43.

Carrera, P.M. & Bridges, J.F.P. (2006). 'Globalization and healthcare: understanding health and medical tourism'. *Exp Rev Pharmacon Outcomes Res* 6(4): 447–454.

Cassimatis, E.G. (2013). 'Globalization of medical education: Educational Commission for Foreign Medical Graduates (ECFMG) concerns and initiatives'. *Innovations in Global Medical and Health Education* 4 http://dx.doi.org/10.5339/igmhe.2013.4

Chang, J., Ji, Y., Li, H., Pan, F., & Su, Y. (2021). 'Prevalence of anxiety symptom and depressive symptom among college students during COVID-19 pandemic: a meta-analysis'. *J Affect Disord* 292: 242–254.

Davey, S., Davey, A., Srivastava, A., & Sharma, P. (2014). 'Privatization of medical education in India: a health system dilemma'. *Int J Med Pub Health* 4:17–22.

Flexner, A. (2002). 'Medical education in the United States and Canada. From the Carnegie Foundation for the Advancement of Teaching, Bulletin Number Four, 1910'. *Bull World Health Organ* 80(7): 594–602.

Flexner, A. (1940). 'I remember: the autobiography of Abraham Flexner'.

Fodje, T. & Choo, E. (2020). 'Applying for residency in the time of COVID-19'. *Lancet* 396:1718.

Golden, I. (2014). *The Butterfly Defect: How Globalization Creates Systemic Risks, and What to Do About It*. Princeton, NJ: Princeton University Press.

Hallock, J.A., McKinley, D.W., & Boulet, J.R. (2007). 'Migration of doctors for undergraduate medical education'. *Med Teach* 29(2–3): 98–105.

Hammoud, M.M., Standiford, T., & Carmody, J.B. (2020). 'Potential implications of COVID-19 for the 2020–2021 residency application cycle'. *JAMA* 324: 29.

Hilburg, R., Patel, N., Ambruso, S., et al. (2020). Medical education during the coronavirus Disease—2019 pandemic: learning from a distance. *Adv Chronic Kidney Dis* 27: 412–417.

Irby, D.M., Cooke, M., & O'Brien, B.C. (2010). 'Calls for reform of medical education by the Carnegie Foundation for the Advancement of Teaching: 1910 and 2010'. *Acad Med* 85(2): 220–227.

Jones, P.D., Seoane, L., Deichmann, R., & Kantrow, C. (2011). Differences and similarities in the practice of medicine between Australia and the United States of America: challenges and opportunities for the University of Queensland and the Ochsner Clinical School. *Ochsner J* 11:253–258

Karle, H., Executive Council, World Federation for Medical Education (2008). International recognition of basic medical education programs. *Med Educ* 42(1): 12–17.

Koplan, J., Bond, T.C., Merson, M., Reddy, K.S., Rodriguez, M.H., & Sewankambo, N.K. (2009). Towards a common definition of global health. *Lancet* 373: 1993–1995.

Kunitz (2000). 'Globalization, states, and the health of Indigenous Peoples'. *Am J Public Health* 90(10): 1531–1539.

Ludmerer, K. (1985). *Learning to Heal: The Development of American Medical Education*. New York, NY: Basic Books.

Ludmerer K. (1999). *Time to Heal: American Medical Education From the Turn of the Century to the Era of Managed Care*. Oxford, UK: Oxford University Press.

Mehta, N. & Isaacson, J.H. (2022). 'Climate change and medical education: an integrative model'. *Acad Med* **97**(2): 188–192.

Mortagy, M., Abdelhameed, A., Sexton, P., Olken, M., Hegazy, M. T., Gawad, M. A., Senna, F., Mahmoud, I. A., Shah, J., & Aiash, H. (2021). 'Online medical education in Egypt during the COVID-19 pandemic: a nationwide assessment of medical students' usage and perceptions'. BMC Med Educ 22. https://doi.org/10.1186/s12909-022-03249-2

Mukhtar, K., Javed, K., Arooj, M., & Sethi, A. (2020). 'Advantages, limitations and recommendations for online learning during COVID-19 pandemic era'. *Pak J Med Sci* **36**: S27–S31.

Mullan, F. (2004). A Legacy of Pushes and Pulls: An Examination of Indian Physician Immigration. Report prepared for World Health Organization Geneva.

Mullan, F. Quantifying the Brain Drain; International Medical Graduates in the United States, the United Kingdom, Canada, and Australia. Under review, NEJM

Mullan, F. (2005). 'The metrics of the physician brain drain'. *N Engl J Med* **353**: 1810–1818.

Mullan F. (2005). 'The metrics of the physician brain drain'. *N Engl J Med* **353**(17): 1810–1818.

Ooi, S.Z.Y. & Ooi, R. (2020). 'Impact of SARS-CoV-2 virus pandemic on the future of cadaveric dissection anatomical teaching'. *Med Educ Online* **25**: 1823089.

Papapanou, M., Routsi, E., Tsamakis, K., Fotis, L., Marinos, G., Lidoriki, I., Karamanou, M., Papaioannou, T.G., Tsiptsios, D., Smyrnis, N., Rizos, E., & Schizas, D. (2022). 'Medical education challenges and innovations during COVID-19 pandemic'. *Postgrad Med J* **98**(1159): 321–327.

Pinsky WW. Benefits of the ECFMG 2023 Accreditation Requirement. *Acad. Med.* 2020;95(1):7. doi: 10.1097/ACM.0000000000003029.

Rafi, A.M., Varghese, P.R., & Kuttichira, P. (2020). 'The pedagogical shift during COVID 19 pandemic: online medical education, barriers and perceptions in central Kerala'. *J Med Educ Curric Dev* **7**: 238212052095179.

Rallis, K.S. & Allen-Tejerina, A.M. (2020). 'Tele-oncology in the COVID-19 era: are medical students left behind?' *Trends Cancer* **6**: 811–812.

Rao, N.R., Meinzer, A.E., Manley, M., & Chagwedera, I. (1998). 'International Medical Students' Career Choice, Attitudes Toward Psychiatry, and Emigration to the United States, Examples from India and Zimbabwe'. *Acad Psychiatry* **22**: 117–126.

Rao, N.R., Kramer, M., & Mehra, A. (2016). The history of international medical graduate physicians in psychiatry and medicine in the United States: a perspective. In: Rao, N., Roberts, L. (eds) *International Medical Graduate Physicians*. Springer, Cham. https://doi.org/10.1007/978-3-319-39460-2_1

Rao, N.R., Uttam, K., & Cooper, R.A. (2006). 'Indian medical students' views on immigration for training and practice'. *Acad Med* **81**(2), 185–188.

Rizwan, M., Rosson, N., Tackett, S., & Hassoun, H. (2018). Globalization of Medical Education: Current Trends and Opportunities for Medical Students.

Rose, S. (2020). Medical student education in the time of COVID-19. *JAMA* **323**(21): 2131–2132.

Scheffer, M. & Dal Poz, M. (2015). The privatization of medical education in Brazil: trends and challenges. Human Resources for Health **13**: 96.

Stevens, RA. International Medical Education and the Concept of Quality: Historical Reflections. Acad Med. (1995): S11–S18

Stilwell B, Diallo K, Pascal Z, Vujici M, Adams O, Dal Poz M. Migration of health- care workers from developing countries: strategic approached to its management. Bulletin of the World of the Health Organization. 2004; 82:595–600.

Sullivan JK, Lowe KE, Gordon IO, Colbert CY, Salas RN, Bernstein A, Utech J, Natowicz MR,Tsamakis K, Rizos E, Manolis AJ, et al . COVID-19 pandemic and its impact on mental health of healthcare professionals. Exp Ther Med 2020;19:3451–3.doi:10.3892/etm.2020.8646 pmid:http://www.ncbi.nlm.nih.gov/pubmed/32346406

Tsang ACO, Shih KC, Chen JY . Clinical skills education at the bedside, web-side and lab-side. Med Educ 2021;55:112–4.doi:10.1111/medu.14394 pmid:http://www.ncbi.nlm.nih.gov/pubmed/33047370

Turner, B. S. (1992). Weber, Giddens, and Modernity. Theory, Culture & Society, 9(2), 141–146. https://doi.org/10.1177/026327692009002008

Van Zanten M, Boulet JR, Greaves I. The importance of medical education accreditation standards. *Med Teach*. 2012;34(2):136–145. doi: 10.3109/0142159X.2012.643261.

Wang JH-S, Tan S, Raubenheimer K . Rethinking the role of senior medical students in the COVID-19 response. Med J Aust 2020;212:e1:490–490.doi:10.5694/mja2.50601 pmid:http://www.ncbi.nlm.nih.gov/pubmed/32368797

Weisz and Nannestad Globalization and Health (2021) 17:96

Weisz, G., Nannestad, B. The World Health Organization and the global standardization of medical training, a history. Global Health 17, 96 (2021). https://doi.org/10.1186/s12992-021-00733-0

Wijnen-Meijer M, Burdick W, Alofs L, Burgers C, ten Cate O. Stages and transitions in medical education around the world: clarifying structures and terminology. Med Teach. 2013 Apr;35(4):301–317.

Williams RS, Casey PJ, Kamei RK, Buckley EG, Soo KC, Merson MH, Krishnan RK, Dzau VJ. A global partnership in medical education between Duke University and the National University of Singapore. Acad Med. 2008 Feb;83(2):122–127. doi: 10.1097/ACM.0b013e318160b8bc. PMID: 18303355.

Winslow, C. Introduction to Public Health: Center for Disease Control; 2020 [Available from: https://www.cdc.gov/publichealth101/public-health.html. Accessed 29 May 2020.

World Health Organization. The first ten years of the World Health Organization. Geneva: WHO; 1958.

World Health Organization. The second ten years of the World Health Organization, 93; Pan American Health Organization. Migration of health personnel, scientists and engineers from Latin America (Scientific Publications No. 142). Washington, D.C.: PAHO; 1966. https://iris.paho.org/handle/10665.2/1185

World Health Organization. The third ten years of the World Health Organization, 1968–1977, vol. 159. Geneva: WHO; 2008. https://apps.who.int/iris/handle/10665/43924

Wu, A., Leask, B., Choi, E. *et al*. Internationalization of Medical Education—a Scoping Review of the Current Status in the United States. *Med.Sci.Educ*. 30, 1693–1705 (2020). https://doi.org/10.1007/s40670-020-01034-8

The author would like to thank the research associate Meera Rao, M.Sc, Ph.D., for her assistance in writing this chapter.

3

Future Perspectives in Medical Education

Debbie Cohen and Thomas Kitchen

Introduction

Medical education is a complex system of interactions, processes, relationships, and outcomes. It is a complex system of fundamental importance, being a foundational component of the wider systems of medicine and health; systems that are focused on improving the quality and duration of our very lives.

As such, the importance of medical education cannot be limited to the individual interactions between a teacher and pupil, a trainer and a trainee, a lecturer and the student. Rather medical education affects the nature of medical practice and vice versa. It drives the culture of medicine and the future health security of populations and humanity.

Set in this context, the wellbeing and sustainability of all the components that are encompassed by medical education, beyond just the individuals that work or study within it, must be considered in order for medicine to create positive environments for students, teachers, patients, and healthcare providers to thrive and flourish.

Our premise for this chapter is that medical education across the globe is a failing system. It is failing because it is propping up failing healthcare systems. Both systems need regeneration.

We will argue that current experiences worldwide suggest we have moved past the point where simply looking to reverse individual components of the system will be sufficient to alter the direction of the whole. This is known as a *hysteresis effect*. This hysteresis is amplified by the current consumptive and target focused systems approach found in medical education and medical practice that has contributed to the creation of a toxic environment.

Within the current toxic environment, there are many initiatives that have made and continue to make positive changes at local, regional, and even national levels. However, they have not been able to create a sustained shift in the culture of medical practice towards creating sustainable and regenerative environments which bring a focus on the 'people' of the system alongside other organizational constraints of process and productivity (Magnani et al., 2019). The challenge we set is to ask how might we look at the issues we face in supporting wellbeing in medical education differently, such that we can effect a whole system-level change?

Taking a systems level approach gives licence to look out from our own system and consider systems of other sectors and industries. What can we learn from business, agriculture, ecology, and/or psychology that can be useful? What have they learnt about the principles of sustainability, biodiversity, regenerative agriculture (even rewilding) and wellbeing that we need to or could translate into medicine? Is 'productivity and efficiency' a mantra that has taken us to a place of such vulnerability?

Debbie Cohen and Thomas Kitchen, *Future Perspectives in Medical Education* In: *The Mental Health of Medical Students*. Edited by: Andrew Molodynski, Sarah Marie Farrell, and Dinesh Bhugra, Oxford University Press. © Oxford University Press 2024. DOI: 10.1093/oso/9780192864871.003.0003

In considering a new way forward, we must resist the urge to reinvent the wheel for medicine and rather be courageous, admit vulnerability, and learn from others. We must learn from other systems that have demonstrated that it is possible to shift away from a model where time, resources, environments, people, and energy are considered as commodities to be depleted and move towards a holistic model of regeneration and sustainability that supports both individual and collective growth.

It is hoped that by taking such an approach we may offer the reader, in this short chapter, an opportunity to consider generalized principles that in turn may be transformed into practices that can inspire system-level shifts across cultural, political and geographical boundaries, independent of their socioeconomic status.

When Was It Last Okay?

It is apparent in 2023 that many medical graduates across the world are taught by and work in stressed, unsustainable, or broken healthcare systems.

Calls for impactful changes to the approaches taken to improve wellbeing and mental health support have been made for decades.

Following her suicide in October 2000, the report into the tragic death of Dr Daksha Emson and her daughter Freya (North East London Strategic Health Authority. 2003) brought into focus the real and climactic challenges facing medicine and medical education in its approach to managing mental health among professionals, mental health stigma, and access to mental health wellbeing support services.

This event created and stimulated positive change in perinatal mental health services, exposed the difficulties relating to stigma and the disclosure of ill health across medicine, and ignited a field of research into the provision of specialized confidential support services for health professionals in the UK (Casanova Dias, 2022).

These services were borne from international collaboration, and while similar services have been developed in varying forms worldwide, sadly it is clear that no one service seems to have provided the answer to the very nature and reason for their existence. Stress and distress continue to be a serious and growing problem for healthcare across the globe.

The trajectory of the wellbeing and mental health challenges experienced across medical practice has so far changed very little despite the increased awareness, uptake to, and funding of physician health programmes and other wellbeing initiatives.

These challenges are not limited to doctors or to any other single professional group. They are not bound by country or socioeconomic status.

Healthcare professionals are exposed to multiple stress factors within their education and work, which although not unique to healthcare are influential in impacting individuals' physical, mental, and emotional wellbeing in negative ways. The current system has made the healthcare sector an unhealthy and unattractive place to work, a fact evidenced by the World Health Organization report, Working for Health and Growth, which estimates a projected shortfall of 18 million health workers across the world by 2030 (WHO, 2016).

The National Health Service (NHS) was established in the United Kingdom in 1948 and is a national provider of healthcare that is free at the point of use. It is one of the largest employers in the world with over 1.4 million employees (NHS Digital, 2021). Since its conception, the

NHS has continued to grow and now exists as a complex system of political, management and care delivery models.

Amid the success of the NHS in creating a national, accessible, healthcare system for the population of the UK, the model has become unsustainable. Some evidence for this is:

- Many studies, referencing various professional and interprofessional groups have highlighted the apparent rise in the levels of burnout. Burnout has become a term often incorrectly and incompletely used as a broad descriptor of 'things not being right'. The significant crescendo in publications and proportions of the workforce purportedly affected points to a system-level problem (House of Commons Health and Social Care Committee, 2021).
- Often to the absolution of system-level and cultural responsibilities, the term 'resilience' is harmfully used to describe something that is lacking in individuals who fail to keep pace with the ever-shifting sands of an unrelentingly increasing workload (McCain et al., 2018).
- The cost of delivering healthcare continues to increase, with efficiency falling and the quality of care enjoying variation by region, by hospital, by team, by wealth and socio-economic status (Office for National Statistics, 2021).
- Systems are supported by altruism, benevolence, and goodwill. Individuals, whose values, ethical responsibilities, and personalities have supported the NHS for many years, have been used as commodities to be tapped and consumed in abundance to sustain a system. Yet the hard-to-measure individual costs of these insidious targets to provide ever-increasing 'productivity' of work are not counted.

These challenges in service delivery, education, employment, and retention, which cross political and geographical boundaries, all point towards a system-level problem—that of a non-sustainable consumptive system. Medical education exists as an integral part, and arguably the foundation of, our healthcare services. It will deliver the next generations of medical professionals. Yet we persist in deploying our newly educated and trained doctors into this broken system.

Allow us to draw the analogy of our new doctors being like new seeds planted into a field that is a health service. They will exist and grow and form part of that complex healthcare system—as soil is itself a complex system.

We would argue that these new seeds (the new doctors) who have been carefully selected and cultivated at significant expense, are currently being planted into the soil of an unsustainable system. They are expected by their colleagues, and the wider health systems and societal cultures to deliver a high-quality, empathetic, no-mistake service. Yet the soil (the system) they are planted into is toxic and not fit for purpose.

What is required is a system-level shift. A shift that is not about 'sustaining' the current model but regenerating it into one that allows people, practice, and culture to flourish rather than just grow.

A COVID-19 perspective

All systems have thresholds. Complex systems have multiple, interdependent, and often hard-to-identify thresholds. When thresholds of complex systems are breached, it is almost impossible to simply turn back by reversing the most recent apparent change. Instead, the consequences of breaching such a threshold usually result in a deterioration across the whole system. This in turn leads to an increased risk of uncertainty until the whole system collapses.

The effects of the bankruptcy of Lehman Brothers Holdings Inc in 2008, or the war in Ukraine in 2022 stand as examples of this phenomenon as they have affected complex systems. Medical education and healthcare provision are (obviously) interrelated and complex systems.

The global coronavirus pandemic of 2019 challenged individuals, communities, and systems to consider the status quo that had come to exist in our societies. The normality of education, relationships, community, health, and economic drivers was turned upside down. Some things changed overnight, with others transitioning over weeks and months. The COVID-19 pandemic thus challenged our system thresholds.

The impact of some of these changes are positive, with new opportunities for change and innovation accompanied by shifts in expectations and demands. However, the pandemic also demonstrated that the challenges around training, sustaining, and delivering a healthy and engaged workforce across healthcare are even bigger than we had thought or measured before.

It is yet to be seen whether the pandemic will in retrospect prove to be the event that caused health systems across the world to breach a threshold that leads to system-chaos. But reflecting on the apparent cost, whether measured in money, human life, trust, or relational terms, that the pandemic has levied across the world we need to ask the question—How much worse will it need to be before we are ready to embrace a system-level shift in the way we consider and promote the wellbeing of a sustainable healthcare workforce?

What Might a Future in Medical Education Look Like?

We invite the reader to consider the following perspectives and principles to help bring about a holistic system-level change that can regenerate the complex systems of healthcare across the globe. How might we develop a sustainable, diverse healthcare system so that healthcare does not just grow but flourishes and provides a safe, empathic, workplace with high-quality care that supports both patients and all those working within?

How can medical education discharge its duty as part of a system change that can deliver a sustainable future for medicine in its entirety?

We propose three areas for consideration when designing, preparing, delivering, and assessing educational initiatives of the future.

Shifting the Desired Knowledge Focus

The art of medical practice encompasses more than a purely scientific approach. Yet, as medicine has advanced, the scientific component of our search for the best possible medical practice has created an ever-expanding pool of evidence. This evidence forms the basis for the scientific underpinning of the 'knowledge' of medicine. The drive for conceptual knowledge (facts and figures) has created a situation where there is too much information for any one person to ever know. For example, there were over 1 million MeSH (Medical Subject Headlines) Medline citations in 2021 (National Library of Medicine, 2022).

While it has been long understood that conceptual knowledge on its own is insufficient to support professional medical practice, the medical profession itself is prone to overstressing the importance of this type of knowledge, over that of other types, as it endeavours to fulfil its scientific curiosity.

It could be argued that the professions' unbalanced pursuit of this approach has become detrimental to medical training. Multiple publications cite a measured decrease in levels of empathy in individual students following entry into medical training (Neumann et al., 2011).

Consider this reality against the context of current developments in artificial intelligence algorithms and improvements in the interface between big data and the individual user. Does this provide an opportunity to change the way we approach teaching and learning around conceptual knowledge?

Our founding apprenticeship model of medical education brought conceptual knowledge and married it to experiential learning. This created a foundation around which a relationship between teacher, pupil, and patient was developed—a connected, empathic relationship. This is something students worldwide found and continue to find empowering and motivating for their studies (Schei et al., 2019).

Medical educators in the UK have embedded the concepts and mechanisms of a biopsychosocial approach to medicine into curricula—the holistic approach to medicine. They are challenged as to how to embed other so-called softer subjects, such as what is building inner resilience and empathy or emotional competence. Where attempted, these elements are crammed into an already full medical curriculum. Maybe it is time to consider how and when students must access conceptual knowledge and allow more space in order to concentrate on interpersonal emotion-based skills and metacognitive approaches? It is these skills that are at the very core of good medical practice. They underpin and allow us to improve our communication, connectedness, and understanding of our patients, ourselves, and our colleagues.

Build Sustainability and Resilience

We are living in an era that demands each and every sector to consider sustainability at its core; sustainability of the environment and its people.

A typical business constraint model presents the triad of time, cost, and project scope as the three components of a project. Each project will have a cost, a time for delivery, and a scope. Each of these three things are constrained by the other two (Figure 3.1).

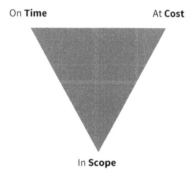

Figure 3.1 A simple constraint triangle.

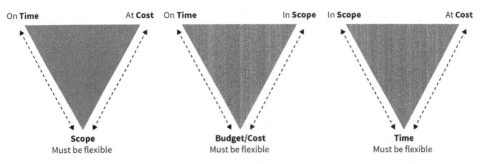

Figure 3.2 Constraint modelling.

The model suggests that by increasing the demand on any one of the three constraints you will be required to limit one or both of the other two other components. For example, if you must deliver the project on time, at a specified cost then the scope of the project must be flexible to suit these constraints. If you have a set project scope, and require it to be delivered at a set time, then the cost of the project will be required to match. Finally, if you require a project to have a defined scope and a fixed budget, then the time over which it is completed will have to be flexible (Figure 3.2).

The same model can be applied to the delivery of a national service or the provision of a single school-based educational programme. In fact, the same constraints can be applied to model any project.

This model doesn't however require its users to consider the concept of sustainability. The model as it is reflects a culture of consumption. If we believe regeneration and sustainability are core principles in the future development of our systems, then sustainability must be built into every concept at a policy, system, and individual level, creating a pyramid rather than a triangular structure (Figure 3.3).

How might this model apply to medical education?

Sustainability is not only about the environment. The concept of sustainability crosses all sector boundaries: ecological, population, financial, and workforce. Thus, if medical education is to be part of the wider system of healthcare, the culture of medicine, and the development of working environments, then it must become sustainable and regenerative rather than consumptive.

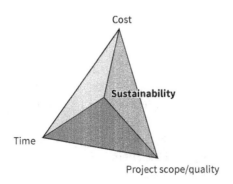

Figure 3.3 A constraint pyramid, adding a fourth component.

This model recognizes the individual's value in contributing across the cost, timeliness, scope, and quality of a project. Understanding that without the individual there would be no project requires us to identify ways to maximize their value at a systems level. This shift towards understanding and supporting the individual in the construct of a business-based model has been described from a quality improvement lens as the quadruple aim (Sikka et al., 2015).

When we apply this model to the individual then we can appreciate how a move from a model of consumption to one constrained by sustainability becomes even more important and recognize that the principle of sustainability must be inbuilt into every aspect of medical education.

First Do No Harm—Develop a Regenerative System and Culture

As systems develop in complexity and grow in size, they face the risk of becoming increasingly disconnected from, in competition with, and eventually consumptive of the environment around them.

We present the reader with an agricultural model as an example. The hunter-gatherer model of survival required the individual unit or family to understand its surroundings and work with and within the limitations of the environment in which it existed; using what was available to them and then moving on before causing an irreversible level of impact. The people and the system relied on each other and existed in a state of continual regeneration that used (in a sustainable way) the right amount of resource to allow a cycle of new and continual growth.

With the transformation towards farming and agricultural industrialization came the disconnect between the system and the environment. The flora, insects, mammals, and plants that used to exist in a regenerative equilibrium under the hunter-gatherer model now become increasingly regarded as competition, a threat to the success of the farmed produce. Walls and fences are constructed, and pesticides and chemical fertilizers utilized to maximize production and profitability. These practices become a learnt and shared technique and become entrenched in culture established over generations (McDonald, 2021).

We use this model as a lens to consider the delivery of healthcare and medical education.

The Hippocratic oath is perhaps the most famous presentation of the foundation ethical principles of care in medicine and is thought to date from between the fifth and third centuries BC. The phrase 'primum non nocere'—first do no harm—although introduced in later iterations of the oath, is a principle that has guided medical practice since it was coined.

This foundation principle pervades through into modern codes of professional, medical ethics. The Declaration of Geneva famously states that 'the health and wellbeing of my patient will be my first consideration', a phrase closely mapped against the General Medical Council's (GMC's) opening statement in its publication *Good Medical Practice* (2013) 'Good doctors make the care of their patients their first concern'.

We can appreciate the hunter-gatherer approach in the concept of 'first do no harm'. In the same way that the hunter (as provider) cannot cause irreversible harm to the community or the environment it relies upon for food, neither should the system cause harm to the provider. If 'you' as a health service look after 'me' as a provider of healthcare, then 'we' as part of 'your' community will look after 'you'. This sense of connectedness serves to promote sustainability without overconsumption.

However, as a health service grows, relationships between the community and care providers become more complex and increasingly fragmented and specialized. Then the connection between the system and the environment, the community, and the care providers becomes increasingly difficult to maintain. The sense of competition between provider, community, and patients grows until the system becomes unsustainable and overconsumptive.

It is into this unsustainable and overconsumptive environment that we introduce medical undergraduate and postgraduate doctors. As part of the system of medical education they become exposed to the expectations and practices of the wider system and quickly assume its cultural norms.

Disconnect from our natural environment has been shown to be unhealthy. There is growing evidence that shows that engagement with natural environments supports wellbeing (Maxwell, 2017). Exposure to green space has been linked with positive outcomes for both mental and physical health. Contact with nature is associated with lower heart rate and blood pressure, lower negative emotions, higher self-esteem, and better mood (van Dillen et al., 2012).

While these benefits can be partly ascribed to higher levels of physical activity and increases in social interactions through engagement with greener areas, activity in natural outdoor spaces rather than indoor ones appears especially therapeutic and is associated with feelings of revitalization, positive engagement, and increased energy.

Yet almost universally, we confine learning and working environments to indoor, 'safer', and more predictable environments. From where does this cultural norm arise?

The NHS in the UK was initially conceived as a mechanism by which individuals belonging to community-based primary care practices, could pay into a nationalized scheme that would provide them with access to healthcare. The scheme was built of three principles:

- That it meets the needs of everyone
- That it be free at the point of delivery
- That it be based on clinical need, not the ability to pay

As this service and complex system has grown it has transformed. Like the agricultural industry that grew out of the hunter-gatherer approach, healthcare has been searching for increased efficiency and capacity. This has transformed an outward-facing, community-based system into one that has become fragmented with barriers, walls, processes, and cultural norms that have disconnected the needs of the system from the needs of the people working in it and the needs of the communities it serves. It has become overconsumptive and competitive.

This competitive approach pervades into the student and training experience. Students in the UK are required to achieve top A-level grades to enter medical school and are ranked against each other as they graduate from medical school. Training programmes apply points-based systems for selection. The drive for success, extensive and growing tick-box training requirements all promote competition. These are processes that break down team-based communities and instil hostile cultural norms.

Turning back to the example of agriculture. It has been recognized that pursuing excessive productivity through overfarming, or using apparent quick-fix solutions in the overuse of fertilizers, pest and weed control are eventually detrimental processes. When soil has been harmed by too much fertilizer, pesticides, or fungicides, excessive ploughing or crushing by heavy machinery, the very nature of the substance of the system starts to deconstruct into less well-performing, less connected, unsustainable parts. This is a process of dysbiosis, a process that can deconstruct any complex ecosystem (Monbiot, 2022). Is medicine immune from such processes?

While for many years it seemed that there was no other way to farm and increase productivity, agriculture has demonstrated that there is another way. While small interventions struggled to alter the direction of the whole industry, we can now appreciate the impact of system-level shifts supporting the introduction of organic, sustainable processes; the use of rewilding natural and farmed landscapes continues to show that it is possible. These approaches aim to restore ecosystem structure and function to achieve a self-sustaining, autonomous, and regenerative system.

Could we consider medicine in the same way? We have a system, a soil, sustained only by every increasing cost and a reliance on altruistic patterns of behaviour. This overconsumptive and competitive environment is unsustainable and destructive. It is in this environment that we introduce medical undergraduates and postgraduates as they enter professional practice and complete their training. The example of agriculture has shown that there is no benefit in trying to prop up small parcels of soil with isolated interventions in the hope that it will affect the whole. The only way to create sustainable regeneration is to shift the entire system.

The Challenge

The challenge to all involved in the design, delivery, and evaluation of our system of medical education is to consider how we can:

1. Shift our focus away from conceptual, fact-based knowledge. Accepting that very soon computer systems will be better than all of us at amassing, sorting, and synthesizing data in a hyperintelligent way. Our role and relationship with knowledge is changing, and so we must equip future generations of doctors with the most valuable of skills—to understand and become masters in the art of being a medical professional—of building emotional connections, knowing *how* to learn and share their understanding.
2. To teach, educate, deliver, and build programmes, systems, and processes that have an inbuilt constraint that considers sustainability alongside cost, scope, and time.
3. But before we try to create a sustainable system, consider how we need to first create a healthier, more nourishing system into which we can sow new seeds. How can we develop a system that is not just sustainable, but is regenerative? Systems of medical education and healthcare that offer individuals the hope to flourish by being intrinsically connected with their environment, their communities, and people.

Shifting our system-level **principles** to support the health and wellbeing of individuals, of a workforce, and an entire system is not a simple task, however it is evident that we are not able to continue in our present state. We concede that there will be no quick fixes and that concerted and sustained efforts are required to reverse the hysteresis and establish a holistic approach to regenerating a sustainable system. But we should never underestimate the power for change encompassed within the foundation system that is medical education.

Into what environment will we sow the next generation of medical professionals?

References

Casanova Dias, M., Sönmez Güngör, E. Dolman, C. De Picker, L. & Jones, I. (2022). '20 years on: the legacy of Daksha Emson for perinatal psychiatry'. *Arch Womens Ment Health* 25(2): 507–510.

GMC (2013). General Medical Council, Good Medical Practice. https://www.gmc-uk.org/-/media/documents/good-medical-practice---english-20200128_pdf-51527435.pdf (Accessed 30 September 2022).

House of Commons Health and Social Care Committee (2021). Second Report of Session 2021–22, Workforce Burnout and Resilience in the NHS and Social Care. HC 22. https://committees.parliament.uk/publications/6158/documents/68766/default/. (Accessed 4 October 2022).

McCain, R.S., McKinley, N., & Dempster, M. (2018). 'A study of the relationship between resilience, burnout and coping strategies in doctors'. *Postgrad Med J* 94: 43–47.

Magnani, F., Carbone, V., & Moatti, V. (2019). 'The human dimension of lean: a literature review'. *Supply Chain Forum* 20:2, 132–144.

Maxwell, S. (2017). Evidence statement on the links between natural environments and human health. Defra and University of Exeter Medical School. https://beyondgreenspace.files.wordpress.com/2017/03/evidence-statement-on-the-links-between-natural-environments-and-human-health1.pdf (Accessed 8 September 2022).

McDonald, M. (2021). *Emergent*. Winchester: Earth Books.

Monbiot, G. (2022). *Regenesis: Feeding the World without Devouring the Planet*. London: Allen Lane.

National Library of Medicine (2022). Citations Added to MEDLINE® by Fiscal Year. https://www.nlm.nih.gov/bsd/stats/cit_added.html (Accessed 4 October 2022).

NHS Digital (2021). NHS Workforce Statistics—January 2021 (including selected provisional statistics for February 2021) https://digital.nhs.uk/data-and-information/publications/statistical/nhs-workforce-statistics/january-2021 (Accessed 10 August 2022).

Neumann, M., Edelhäuser, F., Tauschel, D., Fischer, M.R., Wirtz, M., Woopen, C., Haramati, A., & Scheffer, C. (2011). 'Empathy decline and its reasons: a systematic review of studies with medical students and residents'. *Acad Med* 86(8):996–1009.

North East London Strategic Health Authority (2003). Report of an Independent Inquiry into the care and treatment of Daksha Emson MBBS, MRCPsych, MSc and her daughter Freya. http://www.simplypsychiatry.co.uk/sitebuildercontent/sitebuilderfiles/deinquiryreport.pdf (Accessed 8 August 2022).

Office for National Statistics (2021). Healthcare expenditure, UK Health Accounts provisional estimates: 2021 Provisional high-level estimates of healthcare expenditure in 2021 by financing scheme. https://www.ons.gov.uk/peoplepopulationandcommunity/healthandsocialcare/healthcaresystem/bulletins/healthcareexpenditureukhealthaccountsprovisionalestimates/2021 (Accessed 1 October 2021)

Schei, E., Knoop, H.S., Gismervik, M.N., Mylopoulos, M., & Boudreau, J.D. (2019). 'Stretching the comfort zone: using early clinical contact to influence professional identity formation in medical students'. *J Med Educ Curric Dev* 26(6): 2382120519843875.

Sikka, R., Morath, J.M., & Leape, L. (2015). 'The quadruple aim: care, health, cost and meaning in work'. *BMJ Quality & Safety* 24: 608–610.

van Dillen, S.M.E. de Vries, S., & Groenewegen, P.P. (2012). 'Greenspace in urban neighbourhoods and residents' health: adding quality to quantity'. *J Epidemiol Community Health* 66: e8.

WHO (2016). Working for health and growth: investing in the health workforce—High-Level Commission on Health Employment and Economic Growth. World Health Organization. https://www.who.int/publications/i/item/9789241511308 (Accessed 10 August 2022).

4

Healthcare Systems in Low- and Middle-Income Countries, Future Directions, and Anticipated Medical Workforce Needs

Thomas Hewson, Sridevi Sira Mahalingappa, Roshelle Ramkisson, and Santosh Kumar Chaturvedi

Overview

Numerous differences exist between mental healthcare systems in different world regions. This chapter explores mental healthcare delivery in low- and middle-income countries (LMICs), including the challenges patients, healthcare students, and professionals face in such settings. The critical role of undergraduate medical education in building the workforce, improving the skills and wellbeing of healthcare workers, and promoting international collaboration between high- and low-income countries (LMICs) is discussed.

Defining LMICs

Low-income countries (LICs) have the lowest gross national income (GNI) per capita, which reflects the average income of citizens in each country. For the fiscal year 2022, the World Bank defined LICs as those with a GNI per capita of $1,045 or less; meanwhile, the GNI per capita of lower-middle-income countries was up to $4,095 (World Population Review, 2022). In 2022, 27 countries were defined as LICs and 110 classified as 'middle income' (World Population Review, 2022).

Mental Health in LMICs

Over 70% of the global mental health burden exists in LMICs (Rathod et al., 2017) (Alloh et al., 2018). Depression, schizophrenia, bipolar affective disorder, and alcohol-use disorders represent some of the leading causes of disability, contributing 19.1% of all disability-related health conditions in LMICs (Rathod et al., 2017; World Health Organization, 2003). Worldwide, affective disorders are the most prevalent mental illness, with depression impacting over 260 million people globally (Alloh et al., 2018; Dattani et al., 2021).

Thomas Hewson, Sridevi Sira Mahalingappa, Roshelle Ramkisson, and Santosh Kumar Chaturvedi, *Healthcare Systems in Low- and Middle-income Countries, Future Directions, and Anticipated Medical Workforce Needs* In: *The Mental Health of Medical Students*. Edited by: Andrew Molodynski, Sarah Marie Farrell, and Dinesh Bhugra, Oxford University Press. © Oxford University Press 2024. DOI: 10.1093/oso/9780192864871.003.0004

Major risk factors for mental illness in LMICs include poverty, low socioeconomic status, gender, stigma, discrimination, abuse, and trauma (Maselko, 2017; Rathod et al., 2017). Artificial and natural disasters in LMICs also contribute considerably to mental morbidity, such as the 2010 and 2015 earthquakes in Nepal and Haiti, disease epidemics, and armed conflict (Rathod et al., 2017). For example, high rates of depression, anxiety, and PTSD have been demonstrated among survivors of Ebola disease in the Democratic Republic of the Congo (Kaputu-Kalala-Malu et al., 2021).

Although several risk factors for mental illness exist in LMICs, there are also some protective factors. There is a high prevalence of multigenerational family households, which generally result in greater social support and more caring responsibilities being undertaken by family members in LMICS (Maselko, 2017). This can protect against mental illness, depending on individual family dynamics, attitudes, and relationships. For example, studies have demonstrated an association between the presence of a grandmother in family households and improved mental health outcomes among women and children (Maselko et al., 2015; Rahman et al., 2003). There may also be a greater focus on community support and an enhanced sense of belonging to local communities in some cultures, with positive effects on mental wellbeing.

Health System Challenges in LMICs

A significant treatment gap exists in the world's poorest countries, whereby the number of people with mental illness far exceeds the resources available to treat them (Alloh et al., 2018). Inevitably, this results in many people with mental illness being excluded from treatment, raising important questions relating to medical ethics and social justice. Estimates indicate that treatment rates for various mental disorders in LMICs fall in the region of 35-50% (Bruckner et al., 2011); however, in 2003, the World Health Organization estimated a treatment gap of up to 90% in developing countries (WHO, 2003).

One of the biggest barriers to mental healthcare delivery in LMICs is insufficient healthcare staff. A global deficit of healthcare workers is projected to reach 15 million by 2030 (WHO, 2022). In 2015, the WHO estimated that, on average, there are 50 mental healthcare staff per 100,000 of the population in HICs compared to just 1 per 100,000 people in LMICs (WHO, 2014a). Furthermore, in a study of 58 LMICs, Bruckner et al. estimated that these countries would need to increase their mental health workforce by 239,000 full-time equivalent professionals to rectify current deficits (Bruckner et al., 2011). This shortage of mental health workers is largely due to a lack of specialist training to create more psychiatrists, mental health nurses, and clinical psychologists (Okechukwu, 2022). Staffing problems are also exacerbated by the migration of doctors from LMICs to HICs, which commonly occurs in pursuit of greater pay, working conditions, and career opportunities (Hill et al., 2021; Saluja et al., 2020).

The development of mental health services in LMICs is also limited by inadequate funding, especially compared to HICs. In 2007, the USA possessed 50% of the worldwide expenditure for health and 10% of the global disease burden (Anyangwe & Mtonga, 2007). In contrast, South Africa received 1% of global health expenditure whilst contributing 24% of the global disease burden (Anyangwe & Mtonga, 2007). The proportion of overall health funding attributed to mental healthcare is also generally low within LMICS. For example, Ethiopia and Nepal spend below 2% of their overall health budgets on mental health (Petersen et al., 2017).

The Importance of Undergraduate Medical Education

The aforementioned mental health system challenges highlight the need for effective undergraduate medical education to build and transform the workforce in LMICs. There are several aspects of the design of undergraduate medical education that have important implications for health service delivery. Firstly, the capacity of medical schools and numbers of students admitted directly determines the size of the future medical profession. The types of students admitted into medical school, including their characteristics and locations, may affect the future geographical distribution and specialty choices of healthcare workers. Academic institutions can target evolving deficits in the workforce by selecting and teaching students according to the attributes required by their healthcare systems. Mapping medical curricula to local health needs can ensure that health professionals are equipped to manage the illnesses that they will encounter. Similarly, assessments in undergraduate medical education determine the standards of future healthcare staff, including expected knowledge, skills, and attitudes. The wellbeing of medical students is additionally crucial to maximising their potential and retention of the healthcare workforce. The remainder of this chapter will explore all these aspects of undergraduate medical education and their pivotal role in improving mental healthcare in LMICs.

Medical Student Admissions in LMICs

Recruiting more students into undergraduate healthcare courses is paramount, given the depleted health workforce in the world's poorest countries. This requires scaling up of psychiatric education and training, which demands capital investment to expand infrastructure and purchase more teaching resources and equipment. Recurrent costs are also needed for the remuneration of medical educators, operational costs, and the employment of a growing health workforce. These recurrent costs pose the greatest challenge in LMICs due to the significant proportion of their healthcare financing that is dependent on external aid (WHO, 2013). The WHO highlights that donors will often avoid committing to sustaining financial investments in the long term and that political input is needed to determine the affordability of scaling up measures in LMICs (WHO, 2013).

Besides increasing medical student numbers, admissions processes must be carefully considered to ensure that the future workforce meets the needs of LMIC populations. At present, the limited psychiatric workforce within LMICs is unevenly distributed, with most professionals working in large urban centres (Rathod et al., 2017). This results in significantly poorer access to mental healthcare for rural populations. International evidence demonstrates that medical students recruited from marginalized and rural areas more commonly deliver healthcare in these localities post-qualification, especially in the longer term (Laven & Wilkinson, 2003). For example, the Walter Sisulu Medical School in South Africa recruits students from local communities and delivers health curricula tailored to local priority health needs (Celletti et al., 2011; WHO, 2009). Out of 835 doctors who have graduated from this medical school, approximately 70% continue working in the rural communities from which they were recruited (WHO, 2009). Students admitted from rural areas may also better understand the socioeconomic determinants of health faced by local populations and possess a greater ability to relate to and engage them in care (Briggs & Mantini-Briggs, 2009; Celletti et al., 2011). However, a potential barrier to these recruitment methods is the lower levels of secondary education that exist in LICS in rural areas (WHO, 2010). This means that medical admissions processes risk favouring students from urban areas if they focus solely on prior academic achievement. To overcome this difficulty, some countries, such as China, Thailand, and Vietnam, have created specific quotas for admitting students from rural backgrounds (WHO, 2010). Academic bridging programmes can also be utilized to increase the accessibility of medical schools for less privileged students (WHO, 2010). These programmes teach students who fall short of standard admissions requirements the skills and knowledge needed to participate effectively in undergraduate medical training. In the longer term, the WHO suggests governments should improve primary and secondary education quality in remote areas (WHO, 2010).

Recruiting students with high intrinsic, rather than extrinsic, motivation for studying medicine has also been suggested to improve healthcare systems in LMICs (Tumlinson et al., 2019). The rationale is that students who are passionate about reducing health inequalities and providing care to under-served populations are likely to contribute more to improving health services in rural and less developed regions. Admissions processes that require medical students to pay large fees risk excluding talented applicants from lower socio-economic backgrounds; for this reason, Tumlinson et al. (2019) suggests that admission slots for government-sponsored students should be protected in LMICs.

It is essential to support students beyond recruitment processes to enable them to reach their full potential during medical training and to improve the retention of future doctors. The WHO highlights that financial assistance may be needed for students admitted from lower socioeconomic backgrounds and that students from remote areas may need additional social support, especially if training institutions are urban-centric and require students to relocate (WHO, 2010).

Medical Curricula—Exposure to Psychiatry

In LMICS, increasing mental health treatment provision in primary care has been suggested to improve healthcare delivery for persons with mental illness (Esponda et al., 2020). This requires specialist training of general practitioners to equip them with increased psychiatric knowledge and skills (Esponda et al., 2020). Consequently, it is important that all medical graduates receive adequate training in psychiatry if such approaches are to succeed (Isaac et al., 2018). Currently, there is wide variation in the delivery of medical education around the globe. Within Asia, for example, undergraduate teaching varies widely between countries, from 20 to 260 hours of lectures (Isaac et al., 2018). The duration of clinical rotations in psychiatry is similarly subject to significant national and international variation (Isaac et al., 2018). It is vital that all medical schools provide sufficient psychiatric exposure for future medical workers given the high prevalence of mental health problems internationally.

Ensuring early exposure to psychiatry within medical curricula is also important for promoting mental health awareness and supporting students to develop positive attitudes towards mental illness. In some LMICs, mental illness is viewed as punishment or karma for previous wrongdoing (Okpalauwaekwe et al., 2017) or due to supernatural causes and 'evil spirits' (Muhorakeye & Biracyaza, 2021). These beliefs can cause shame, guilt, and worry among persons with mental illness, preventing them from disclosing their symptoms to others (Rathod et al., 2017). Reducing stigma related to mental illness could reduce the treatment burden by increasing the number of people seeking professional help at earlier rather than later stages of illness (Alloh et al., 2018; Henderson et al., 2013). To achieve this, medical students and healthcare staff should be taught how to effectively communicate with community members about mental health topics, including those who might hold stigmatizing attitudes. This could involve learning how to facilitate healthy discussions about mental illness amongst local citizens and patients' families, culturally adapting psychiatric interventions, and outreaching into communities that traditionally disengage with the medical model of healthcare. For example, in Thailand, some psychiatric providers have incorporated Buddha's teachings into community mental health services, aiming to engage people who believe in the spiritual aspects of health and recovery (Rathod et al., 2017). The National Institute of Mental Health and Neurosciences in Bangalore, as well as the Christian Medical College in Vellore, have maximized the therapeutic input of families by creating facilities for relatives to live with patients undergoing psychiatric treatment (Rathod et al., 2017; Thara et al., 2004).

Medical Curricula—Exposure to Rural Health

The integration of rural health into medical curricula and providing rotations and internships in rural areas have been implemented in Various LMICs, including Afghanistan, Pakistan, Somalia, and Jordan, have integrated rural health into their medical curricula and/or provide medical students with rotations and internships in rural areas. (Khalil & Alameddine, 2020; Khatatbeh et al., 2015; Safi et al., 2018; Suhail & Azhar, 2016). These initiatives aim to increase medical students' exposure to rural mental health and their later recruitment into underserved areas of LMICs. Similarly, in the Philippines, increasing community placements and mandating students to undertake community development and public health activities has been associated with more medical graduates opting to work in rural and/or economically disadvantages areas (Woolley et al., 2018). Some countries have also implemented 1-year mandatory national service postgraduation from healthcare education to address workforce shortages. However, these policies must be more consistently regulated and produce more evaluation data (Khalil & Alameddine, 2020).

Medical Curricula—Exposure to Psychotherapy

The delivery of psychotherapeutic interventions is limited in LMICs, despite the strong evidence supporting their role in numerous mental disorders. Many factors contribute to their low availability, including insufficient resources, staff training, and certain religious, cultural, and political beliefs (Rathod et al., 2017). Medical education plays an essential role in educating students about the evidence for and applications of psychotherapy in treating mental disorders. A survey in India demonstrated that 82% of students perceived a conflict between cognitive behavioural therapy (CBT) principles and their values and beliefs, including their family values and religion (Scorzelli & Reinke-Scorzelli, 1994). Beliefs that are prevalent in some LMICS and which may conflict with CBT include believing that destiny is fixed and that a higher power controls us (Rathod et al., 2017). There is evidence of psychological therapies being adapted to ensure cultural sensitivity and appropriateness in some countries through the work of organizations such as the Pakistan Association of CBT and Indian Association of CBT; however, it is unclear how the current evidence-base for psychotherapy, which is predominantly Western-centric, translates to culturally adapted models of care (Rathod & Kingdon, 2014; Rathod et al., 2017). As such, academic institutions should research the effectiveness of culturally adapted psychological therapies in LMICs and methods for successfully teaching therapeutic modalities to students from different cultures. As described by Erna Hoch and Desai et al., single-session psychotherapies or counselling may be useful for illiterate persons and the overcrowded clinics in LMICs (Desai et al., 2015; Hoch, 1977).

Medial Curricula—Interprofessional and Transprofessional Education

In psychiatry, multiple professionals often interact to provide treatment for patients, including psychiatrists, mental health nurses, psychologists, occupational therapists, and social workers. Each health professional must understand the roles and responsibilities of their colleagues in order to provide effective continuity of care. Interprofessional medical education can achieve this whilst fostering attitudes and teamwork capabilities that support patient care in clinical practice (WHO, 2013). The importance of this training method transcends geographical boundaries since numerous healthcare roles exist in each country, although workforce numbers and proportions may vary.

Transprofessional education involves teaching health professionals how to successfully work with and lead non-professionals in healthcare services, thus supporting a diverse workforce (Frenk et al., 2010). This is particularly relevant to LMICs where auxiliary health workers and community members are often trained to deliver mental health support and rehabilitation to increase treatment coverage for mental illness (Frenk et al., 2010). For example, in Southern Nepal, auxiliary nurse midwives (people with midwifery competencies who assist in maternal and newborn healthcare but who are not qualified midwives or nurses) have received training on mental health issues from UK health staff (WHO, 2014b). This training was helpful for the auxiliary nurse midwives, increasing their capacity to deliver mental health counselling, recognize, and understand mental illness, and address negative family attitudes towards women with mental health problems (Mahato et al., 2018). 'Community champions' have also been utilized to promote mental health awareness and provide low-level community support for citizens in Nigeria with mental illness (Eaton et al., 2018). In India, community health workers known as Accredited Social Health Activists (ASHAs) have been trained to recognize mental disorders, deliver basic counselling, and refer people to treatment (Armstrong et al., 2011; Rahul et al., 2021). The District Mental Health Programme of Ramanagara in India additionally trains paramedical personnel, teachers, firefighters, and workers in childcare centres (known as Anganwadi workers) about mental illness to enhance knowledge and awareness in the region (Rahul et al., 2021). Appropriate support from trained health professionals is paramount to ensure the effectiveness and sustainability of these non-professional health worker initiatives (Frenk et al., 2010). This means that healthcare professionals must develop skills for supervising persons with less extensive training, placing a strong emphasis on teamwork and leadership skills development in medical curricula. They must also learn how to recognize and manage mental illness presentations that exceed the competencies of other staff members.

Medical Curricula—Clinical Attachments Abroad

International clinical rotations, frequently termed 'medical electives', are often undertaken by medical students, especially in HICs. These provide opportunities to experience healthcare systems and challenges in other countries. This can increase students' skills and confidence, awareness of global public health, and cross-cultural communication skills (Drain et al., 2007; Frenk et al., 2010). It may also provide exposure to presentations of illness rarely encountered in the individual's home country. Drain et al. (2007) suggest that direct partnerships between medical schools and hospitals in HICs and LMICs could improve the accessibility of international clinical rotations in both directions (e.g. students from HICs visiting LMICs and vice versa) (Drain et al., 2007). This exchange of resources and training opportunities could improve healthcare delivery in both settings and pave the way for further international collaboration. Despite their benefits, overseas clinical rotations may not be accessible for all students, especially those from lower socioeconomic backgrounds due to international travel and accommodation costs (Wu et al., 2022). Scholarships and bursaries can improve the equitability of such training opportunities, requiring financial investments from institutions or external agencies (Drain et al., 2007).

E-learning in LMICs

E-learning refers to the delivery of educational materials through digital resources, such as the internet, online learning platforms, and video-conferencing software. A key advantage of e-learning is that it does not rely on physical infrastructure, which is limited in low-resource settings (Frenk et al., 2010). Instead, e-learning allows educational content to be distributed to large populations of health students and professionals whilst avoiding significant costs associated with upscaling academic institutions (Barteit et al., 2020). This could address workforce shortages in LMICs by allowing more health professionals to be trained more quickly with fewer demands on physical and financial resources. An example of the scalability of e-learning comes from a distance IT programme in public health created by South Africa's National School of Public Health; this programme, which utilized flexible e-learning components and four two-week blocks of compulsory classroom teaching, produced more graduates over five years than all other schools in the country summed together and attracted students from 16 African countries (Frenk et al., 2010; Mokwena, 2007). Digital educational approaches could also mitigate the shortage of medical educators in LMICs by eliminating requirements for them to travel to deliver pedagogy (Barteit et al., 2020). This could improve access to health education in rural areas and help to train more healthcare staff in underserved communities, resulting in a more equitable distribution of the workforce. Opportunities for international collaborations are also enhanced through the internet, making it possible for international speakers and HICs to contribute to healthcare education in LMICs.

Although e-learning has many advantages, there are several challenges to its implementation in LMICs. In many low-income environments, access to internet connectivity is limited, especially that with adequate broadband widths (Barteit et al., 2020). Furthermore, electricity supplies and electronic devices for accessing digital content may not be accessible for all students. To overcome some of these difficulties, digital educational methods must be flexible and allow materials to be accessed asynchronously and offline, as well as holding synchronous online teaching (Cecilio-Fernandes et al., 2020). Asynchronous and offline teaching methods, such as downloadable text files, allow learners to read relevant information at any time and place. Synchronous student-student and student-educator discussions can also be replaced by asynchronous communication methods, including email and social media, to reduce requirements for higher broadband width demanded by videoconferencing (Cecilio-Fernandes et al., 2020). Due to a shortage of medical educators, some LMICs may have difficulties creating online content for e-learning for health professionals (Frenk et al., 2010). Students themselves can contribute to creating digital learning resources in LMICs, with the added benefit of students' learning skills to become the educators of tomorrow (Barteit et al., 2020).

A recent systematic review of e-learning for medical education in LMICs found that most interventions were pilot studies and lacked methodological rigour (Barteit et al., 2020). Significant heterogeneity existed regarding study designs, evaluation methods, and selected outcome measures, although most outcome data was subjective in nature. Although the limitations of this literature must be acknowledged, many studies demonstrated the effectiveness of e-learning interventions in LMICs (Barteit et al., 2020). More robust evaluations of e-learning interventions in LMICs are needed to better understand their effectiveness and if and how they should be implemented on a larger scale. Future evaluations should explore beyond the immediate effects of e-learning on learners' knowledge and perceptions, instead exploring the longer-term effects on participants' skills, assessment scores, and workplace performance (Barteit et al., 2020). Randomized controlled trials would enhance the strength of current research evidence and permit an understanding of the optimal design and implementation of e-learning approaches.

Recently, blended learning approaches are becoming increasingly common to teach mental health. These approaches combine online distance education with face-to-face educational content and aim to maximize the advantages of both teaching methods whilst reducing their respective limitations. In a systematic review of medical e-learning in resource-constrained LMICs in 2013, blended e-learning methods produced favourable or neutral results relative to traditional instructional methods in most studies (Frehywot et al., 2013). Blended teaching methods were also viewed positively by students, who generally believed that these improved the quality of education (Frehywot et al., 2013). Pre- and post-test evaluations of learner competence demonstrated the effectiveness of blended e-learning in teaching medical curricula (Frehywot et al., 2013). Similarly, a meta-analysis of blended learning methods found that this approach had neutral to positive effects on the acquisition of knowledge by health workers when compared to pure e-learning (Liu et al., 2016).

Collaboration Between HICs and LMICs

Collaboration between medical education departments in HICs and LMICs is an important aspect of reducing global health inequalities and strengthening health systems worldwide. This may involve working together to deliver global health curricula, sharing health knowledge and resources, and delivering large-scale teaching initiatives. Hill et al. (2021) recommend several principles for effective collaboration between HICs and LMICs (Hill et al., 2021). Firstly, international educational partnerships should be mutually beneficial with opportunities for bi-directional learning. HICs are well-placed to contribute professional capabilities and resources, whilst LMICs can share rich contextual knowledge about disease patterns and presentations in different population profiles. Secondly, such collaborations require careful planning and supportive discussions to ensure that educational content is tailored to the specific needs, resources, and contexts of LMICs. For example, access to specialist equipment and electronic devices may be limited in LMICs, requiring educational approaches to be adapted. This may provide opportunities for HICs and LMICs to mutually explore low-cost alternative options for delivering teaching and healthcare, with potential benefits for both parties. Thirdly, organizations should consider 'train the trainer' initiatives to ensure the sustainability of international collaborations; these initiatives involve teaching people how to lead and deliver educational collaboratives so that they can continue to evolve and take place in the future. Maintaining contact between educational organizations in HICs and LMICs also strengthens partnerships over time, with each organization building familiarity with different ways of working and increasing its capacity to support others.

In a systematic review of international health education collaborations between HICs and LMICs, most educational programmes met the specific needs of LMICs and accounted for their social, political, and economic contexts; furthermore, most programmes considered sustainability through increasing educational capacity, skills, and knowledge to deliver health training in LMICs (Hill et al., 2021). A minority of programmes, however, treated HICs and LMICs as equal contributors in the design and delivery of education, representing an area for further development.

Sharing Educational Resources Between Organizations

Sharing educational resources between academic institutions, particularly between HICs and LMICs, could improve the quality of medical education on a global scale (Frenk et al., 2010). This would allow best educational practices to be adopted across diverse geographical regions, reducing the teaching burden on individual educators. As previously mentioned, there is a shortage of medical teachers in LMICS, particularly in rural areas, who may have difficulty balancing the creation of educational content with clinical responsibilities; therefore, sharing educational resources could help to address this problem. In 2001, the Massachusetts Institute of Technology became the first institution to propose this idea and developed 'OpenCourseWare'. This allows universities to digitally share their curriculum, lectures, assignments, and examinations free-of-charge for others to access. Since its inception, OpenCourseWare has been accessed in numerous countries, and regional networks have been established to translate course content into local languages (Frenk et al., 2010) (Carson, 2009). Institutions may choose to replicate materials or adapt them to suit their individual contexts, with the latter allowing educators to account for differing population health needs and sociocultural contexts in different parts of the world.

Medical Research in LMICs

Academic research plays a pivotal role in advancing mental healthcare and medical education. In order to provide the most up-to-date treatments for patients, health professionals must remain abreast of research developments, requiring undergraduate and postgraduate education to evolve continually. At the same time, medical education underpins effective research by building academic competence and research capacity within the medical workforce. International research collaborations can support the development of research capabilities in LMICs where funding and resources for research may be limited (Hill et al., 2021). These collaborations allow individuals and institutions to work together to learn new skills and deliver large-scale studies. Including diverse patient populations in international research also improves the generalisability of research findings globally.

GlobalSurg is an example of a global academic network providing surgical research exposure and skills development for healthcare students and professionals worldwide. This network includes over 5,000 clinicians in more than 100 countries and has collected data on surgical outcomes from over 40,000 patients (GlobalSurg, 2020). Critical features of GlobalSurg that promote inclusivity include the translation of study documents into several languages and the careful design of research studies to ensure their delivery in diverse conditions (Dawidziuk et al., 2021; GlobalSurg, 2020). International research collaborations in psychiatry, similar to GlobalSurg, could accelerate our understanding of global mental health and increase the pace of new research developments in the field. Other methods of increasing research capacity in LMICs include designated funding opportunities and delivering academic skills workshops, such as teaching academic writing skills, to medical students and health professionals overseas (Hill et al., 2021). These measures could increase the visibility of LMICs within the published literature, reducing Western bias and promoting greater awareness of global health (Hill et al., 2021).

Medical Student Wellbeing

Several studies have demonstrated high rates of mental illness and psychological symptoms amongst medical students. Most of these studies have taken place in high income settings, although several studies have also demonstrated high rates of mental morbidity amongst medical students in LMICs. For example, a meta-analysis of 183 studies across 43 countries demonstrated a pooled crude prevalence rate of depression or depressive symptoms of 27.2% amongst medical students (Rosenstein et al., 2016). A further meta-analysis restricted to 24 LMICs reported a pooled prevalence rate of burnout of 12.1% amongst medical students in these countries (Kaggwa et al., 2021). Various factors have been attributed to poor mental wellbeing amongst medical students, including high work intensity, the complexity of medical curricula, perceived lack of control over educational experiences, and exposure to stressful events such as witnessing patient distress and death (Kihumuro et al., 2022).

The aforementioned information highlights a need for strong support systems for medical students in all countries, including monitoring students' wellbeing and providing access to confidential mental health treatment. This has important implications for the future health of the medical and psychiatric workforce in all countries. Various interventions have been described in the literature to successfully promote medical student wellbeing including implementing pass/fail grading systems, collaborative learning approaches, longitudinal clinical rotations, peer mentoring, teaching resilience, promoting socialization amongst students, and encouraging students to maintain their hobbies (Klein & McCarthy, 2022). Low-cost interventions for improving the mental wellbeing of medical students in LMICs may also include mindfulness, yoga, and supportive group discussions between peers, with online guides being available for many such interventions (Kaggwa et al., 2021).

Evidence suggests that the uptake of mental health services by medical students is often impeded by several barriers, including perceived stigma and lack of knowledge about the support available (Kihumuro et al., 2022). These barriers may be particularly prominent in LMICs, where beliefs about mental illness arising from supernatural causes and 'evil spirits' are more common, as mentioned earlier in the chapter. In a meta-analysis, only 15.7% of medical students screening positive for depression were reported to have sought psychiatric treatment (Rosenstein et al., 2016). This demonstrates a need for anti-stigma interventions within medical training. 'The Wounded Healer' is an example of an innovative anti-stigma intervention blending science and art to eliminate myths about mental illness and promote help-seeking behaviour (Hankir & Zaman, 2016). This intervention has been delivered in several countries, and uses storytelling, performing arts, and digital media to convey a health professional's lived experience of mental illness. This intervention has been found to improve medical students' attitudes towards mental illness, reducing stigma and encouraging medics to seek support for their health issues (Hankir et al., 2015; Hankir & Zaman, 2016).

Summary

In summary, addressing the workforce challenges in LMICs is central to lowering global health inequalities. Medical education is a powerful tool that can help to improve mental healthcare delivery in low-resource settings. Medical curricula must be tailored to the healthcare needs of local populations and equip people for working in both current and future healthcare systems. Building and expanding international collaborations and embracing new technologies offer promise for the upscaling of medical education in LMICs in the future.

References

Alloh, F.T., Regmi, P., Onche, I., Teijlingen, E.V., & Trenoweth, S. (2018). 'Mental health in low-and middle income countries (LMICs): going beyond the need for funding'. *Health Prospect* 17(1): 12–17.

Anyangwe, S., & Mtonga, C. (2007). 'Inequities in the global health workforce: the greatest impediment to health in Sub-Saharan Africa'. *J Environ Res Public Health* 4(2): 93–100.

Armstrong, G., Kermode, M., Raja, S., Suja, S., Chandra, P., & Jorm, A.F. (2011). 'A mental health training program for community health workers in India: impact on knowledge and attitudes'. *Int J Ment Health Syst* 5(1): 17.

Barteit, S., Guzek, D., Jahn, A., Bärnighausen, T., Jorge, M.M., & Neuhann, F. (2020). 'Evaluation of e-learning for medical education in low- and middle-income countries: a systematic review'. *Comput Educ* 145: 103726.

Briggs, C.L., & Mantini-Briggs, C. (2009). 'Confronting health disparities: Latin American social medicine in Venezuela'. *Am J Public Health* 99(3): 549–555.

Bruckner, T.A., Scheffler, R.M., Shen, G., Yoon, J., Chisholm, D., Morris, J., Fulton, B.D., Dal Poz, M.R., & Saxena, S. (2011). 'The mental health workforce gap in low- and middle-income countries: a needs-based approach'. *Bull World Health Organ* 89(3): 184–194.

Carson S. (2009). 'The unwalled garden: growth of the OpenCourseWareConsortium, 2001–2008. *Open Learning* 24(1): 23–29.

Cecilio-Fernandes, D., Parisi, M.C.R., Santos, T.M., & Sandars, J. (2020). 'The COVID-19 pandemic and the challenge of using technology for medical education in low and middle income countries'. *MedEdPublish* 9: 74.

Celletti, F., Reynolds, T.A., Wright, A., Stoertz, A., & Dayrit, M. (2011). 'Educating a new generation of doctors to improve the health of populations in low- and middle-income countries'. *PLoS Med* 8(10): e1001108.

Dattani, S., Ritchie, H., & Roser, M. (2021). Mental Health, Our World in Data. https://ourworldindata.org/mental-health (Accessed: 1 November 2022).

Dawidziuk, A., Kawka, M., Szyszka, B., Wadunde, I., & Ghimire, A. (2021). 'Global access to technology-enhanced medical education during the COVID-19 pandemic: the role of students in narrowing the gap'. *Global Health: Science and Practice* 9(1): 10–14.

Desai, G., Thanapal, S., Gandhi, S., Berigai, N.P., & Chaturvedi, S.K. (2015). 'Single session rehabilitation counseling: a session in hand, may be worth many in oblivion!' *J Psychosoc Rehabil Mental Health* 2(1): 75–77.

Drain, P.K., Primack, A., Hunt, D.D., Fawzi, W.W., Holmes, K.K., & Gardner, P. (2007). 'Global health in medical education: a call for more training and opportunities'. *Acad Med* 82(3): 226–230.

Eaton, J., Gureje, O., De Silva, M., Sheikh, T.L., Ekpe, E.E., Abdulaziz, M., Muhammad, A., Akande, Y., Onukogu, U., Onyuku, T., Abdulmalik, J., Fadahunsi, W., Nwefoh, E., & Cohen, A. (2018). 'A structured approach to integrating mental health services into primary care: development of the Mental Health Scale Up Nigeria intervention (mhSUN)'. *Int J Ment Health Syst* 12: 11.

Esponda, G.M., Hartman, S., Qureshi, O., Sadler, E., Cohen, A., & Kakuma, R. (2020). 'Barriers and facilitators of mental health programmes in primary care in low-income and middle-income countries'. *Lancet Psychiatry* 7(1): 78–92.

Frehywot, S., Vovides, Y., Talib, Z., Mikhail, N., Ross, H., Wohltjen, H., Bedada, S., Korhumel, K., et al. (2013). 'E-learning in medical education in resource constrained low- and middle-income countries'. *Human Resources for Health* 11: 4.

Frenk, J., Chen, L., Bhutta, Z. A., Cohen, J., Crisp, N., Evans, T., Fineberg, H., Garcia, P., Ke, Y., Kelley, P., Kistnasam, B., Meleis, A., Naylor, D., Pablos-Mendez, A., Reddy, S., Scrimshaw, S., Sepulveda, J., Serwadda, D., & Zurayk, H. (2010). 'Health professionals for a new century: Transforming education to strengthen health systems in an interdependent world'. *Lancet* 376(9756): 1923–1958.

GlobalSurg (2020). About GlobalSurg. https://globalsurg.org/who-we-are/ (Accessed: 1 November 2022).

Hankir, A., Zaman, R., & Evans-Lacko, S. (2015). '"The Wounded Healer": an effective anti-stigma intervention targeted at the medical profession?' *Eur Psychiatry* 30: 1396.

Hankir, A. & Zaman, R. (2016). '"The wounded healer" challenging the stigma attached to mental health conditions in medical students and doctors'. *Eur Psychiatry* 33: S648.

Henderson, C., Evans-Lacko, S., & Thornicroft, G. (2013). 'Mental illness stigma, help seeking, and public health programs'. *Am J Public Health* 103(5): 777–780.

Hill, E., Gurbutt, D., Makuloluwa, T., Gordon, M., Georgiou, R., Roddam, H., Seneviratne, S., Byrom, A., Pollard, K., Abhayasinghe, K., & Chance-Larsen, K. (2021). 'Collaborative healthcare education programmes for continuing professional education in low and middle-income countries: a best evidence medical education (BEME) systematic review'. BEME Guide No. 65. *Med Teach* 43(11): 1228–1241.

Hoch, M.E. (1977). Psychotherapy for the illiterate In: Arieti S, Chrzanowski G (eds) *A New Dimension in Psychiatry: A World View*. New York: Wiley; 1977, pp 75–92.

Isaac, M., Ahmed, H.U., Chaturvedi, S.K., Hopwood, M.J., Javeed, A., Kanba, S., Mufti, A. A., Maramis, A., Samaniego, R.M., Udomratn, P., Yanling, H., Zainal, N.Z., & Sartorius, N. (2018). 'Postgraduate training in psychiatry in Asia'. *Curr Opin Psychiatry* 31(5): 396–402.

Kaggwa, M.M., Kajjimu, J., Sserunkuma, J., Najjuka, S.M., Atim, L.M., Olum, R., Tagg, A., & Bongomin, F. (2021). 'Prevalence of burnout among university students in low- and middle-income countries: a systematic review and meta-analysis'. *PLoS One* 16(8): e0256402.

Kaputu-Kalala-Malu, C., Musalu, E.M., Walker, T., Ntumba-Tshitenge, O., & Ahuka-Mundeke, S. (2021). 'PTSD, depression and anxiety in Ebola virus disease survivors in Beni Town, Democratic Republic of the Congo'. *BMC Psychiatry* 21(1): 342.

Khatatbeh, M., Alkhaldi, S., Al-Omari, O., & Khader, Y. (2015). 'Factors impact on turnover of physicians in rural Jordan'. *Health Syst Policy Res* **2**(1): 3.

Khalil, M., & Alameddine, M. (2020). 'Recruitment and retention strategies, policies, and their barriers: a narrative review in the Eastern Mediterranean Region'. *Health Sci Rep* **3**(4): e192.

Klein, H.J., & McCarthy, S.M. (2022). 'Student wellness trends and interventions in medical education: a narrative review'. *Human Soc Sci Commun* **9**: 92.

Kihumuro, R.B., Kaggwa, M.M., Nakandi, R.M., Kintu, T.M., Muwanga, D.R., Muganzi, D.J., Atwau, P., Ayesiga, I., Acai, A., Najjuka, S.M., Najjuma, J.N., Frazier-Koussai, S., Ashaba, S., & Harms, S. (2022). 'Perspectives on mental health services for medical students at a Ugandan medical school'. *BMC Med Educ* **22**(1): 734.

Laven, G., & Wilkinson, D. (2003). 'Rural doctors and rural backgrounds: How strong is the evidence? A systematic review'. *Aust J Rural Health* **11**(6): 277–284.

Liu, Q., Peng, W., Zhang, F., Hu, R., Li, Y., & Yan, W. (2016). 'The effectiveness of blended learning in health professions: systematic review and meta-analysis'. *J Med Internet Res* **18**(1): e2.

Mahato, P. K., van Teijlingen, E., Simkhada, P., Angell, C., Ireland, J., van Teijlingen, E., THET team (2018). 'Qualitative evaluation of mental health training of auxiliary nurse midwives in rural Nepal'. *Nurse Educ Today* **66**: 44–50.

Maselko, J. (2017). 'Social epidemiology and global mental health: expanding the evidence from high-income to low- and middle-income countries'. *Curr Epidemiol Rep* **4**(2): 166–173.

Maselko, J., Sikander, S., Bhalotra, S., Bangash, O., Ganga, N., Mukherjee, S., Egger, H., Franz, L., Bibi, A., Liaqat, R., Kanwal, M., Abbasi, T., Noor, M., Ameen, N., & Rahman, A. (2015). 'Effect of an early perinatal depression intervention on long-term child development outcomes: follow-up of the Thinking Healthy Programme randomised controlled trial'. *Lancet Psych* **2**(7): 609–617.

Mokwena, K. (2007). 'Training of public health workforce at the National School of Public Health: meeting Africa's needs'. *Bull World Health Organ* **85**(12): 949–954.

Muhorakeye, O. & Biracyaza, E. (2021). 'Exploring barriers to mental health services utilization at Kabutare District Hospital of Rwanda: perspectives from patients'. *Front Psychol* **12**: 638377.

Okechukwu, C.E. (2022). 'A call for improved mental health workforce in low-income countries'. *Int J Soc Psychiatry* **68**(2): 465–467.

Okpalauwaekwe, U., Mela, M., & Oji, C. (2017). Knowledge of and attitude to mental illnesses in Nigeria: a scoping review. *Integr J Glob Health* **1**: 1.

Petersen, I., Marais, D., Abdulmalik, J., Ahuja, S., Alem, A., Chisholm, D., Egbe, C., Gureje, O., Hanlon, C., Lund, C., Shidhaye, R., Jordans, M., Kigozi, F., Mugisha, J., Upadhaya, N., & Thornicroft, G. (2017). 'Strengthening mental health system governance in six low- and middle-income countries in Africa and South Asia: challenges, needs and potential strategies'. *Health Policy Plan* **32**(5): 699–709.

Rahman, A., Iqbal, Z., & Harrington, R. (2003). 'Life events, social support and depression in childbirth: perspectives from a rural community in the developing world'. *Psychol Med* **33**(7): 1161–1167.

Rahul, P., Chander, K.R., Murugesan, M., Anjappa, A.A., Parthasarathy, R., Manjunatha, N., Kumar, C.N., & Math, S.B. (2021). 'Accredited social health activist (ASHA) and her role in district mental health program: learnings from the COVID-19 pandemic'. *Community Ment Health J* **57**(3): 442–445.

Rathod, S. & Kingdon, D. (2014). 'Case for cultural adaptation of psychological interventions for mental healthcare in low and middle income countries'. *BMJ* **349**(dec16 24): g7636–g7636.

Rathod, S., Pinninti, N., Irfan, M., Gorczynski, P., Rathod, P., Gega, L., & Naeem, F. (2017). 'Mental health service provision in low- and middle-income countries'. *Health Serv Insights* **10**: 1178632917694350.

Rosenstein, L.S., Ramos, M.A., Torre, M., Segal, J.B., Peluso, M.J., Guille, C., Sen, S., Mata, D.A. (2016). 'Prevalence of depression, depressive symptoms, and suicidal ideation among medical students: a systematic review and meta-analysis'. *JAMA* **316**(21): 2214–2236.

Safi, N., Naeem, A., Khalil, M., Anwari, P., & Gedik, G. (2018). 'Addressing health workforce shortages and maldistribution in Afghanistan'. *East Mediterr Health J* **24**(09): 951–958.

Saluja, S., Rudolfson, N., Massenburg, B.B., Meara, J.G., & Shrime, M.G. (2020). 'The impact of physician migration on mortality in low and middle-income countries: an economic modelling study'. *BMJ Glob Health* **5**(1): e001535.

Scorzelli, J.F. & Reinke-Scorzelli, M. (1994). 'Cultural sensitivity and cognitive therapy in India'. *Couns Psychol* **22**(4): 603–610.

Suhail, A. & Azhar, A. (2016). 'Managing human resources in public health care system in South Asia: case study of Pakistan'. *SAJHRM* 3(1): 75–83.

Thara, R., Padmavati, R., & Srinivasan, T.N. (2004). 'Focus on psychiatry in India'. *Br J Psychiatry* 184(4): 366–373.

Tumlinson, K., Jaff, D., Stilwell, B., Onyango, D.O., & Leonard, K.L. (2019). 'Reforming medical education admission and training in low- and middle-income countries: who gets admitted and why it matters'. *Human Resources for Health* 17: 91.

Woolley, T., Cristobal, F., Siega-Sur, J.J., Ross, S., Neusy, A., Halili, S.D., & Reeve, C. (2018). 'Positive implications from socially accountable, community-engaged medical education across two Philippines regions'. *Rural Remote Health* 18: 4264.

World Health Organization (WHO) (2003). 'Investing in mental health'. https://apps.who.int/iris/bitstream/handle/10665/42823/9241562579.pdf?sequence=1&isAllowed=y (Accessed 1 November 2022).

World Health Organization (WHO) (2009). *Report on the WHO/PEPFAR Planning Meeting On Scaling Up Nursing And Medical Education*. Geneva: WHO. https://www.aspeninstitute.org/wp-content/uploads/files/content/images/WHO.PEPFAR_ScalingUpPlanningRept.pdf (Accessed 1 November 2022).

World Health Organization (WHO)\ (2010). 'Increasing access to health workers in remote and rural areas through improved retention: global policy recommendations'. https://apps.who.int/iris/bitstream/handle/10665/44369/9789241564014_eng.pdf?sequence=1&isAllowed=y (Accessed 1 November 2022).

World Health Organization (WHO) (2013). 'Transforming and scaling up health professionals' education and training: World Health Organisation Guidelines 2013'. https://apps.who.int/iris/bitstream/handle/10665/93635/9789241506502_eng.pdf?sequence=1&isAllowed=y (Accessed 1 November 2022).

World Health Organization (WHO) (2014a). 'Mental health atlas'. https://apps.who.int/iris/bitstream/handle/10665/178879/9789241565011_?sequence=1 (Accessed 1 November 2022).

World Health Organization (WHO) (2014b). 'Using auxiliary nurse midwives to improve access to key maternal and newborn health interventions'. https://apps.who.int/iris/bitstream/handle/10665/128037/WHO_RHR_14.22_eng.pdf?sequence=1 (Accessed 1 November 2022).

World Health Organization (WHO) (2022). 'Health workforce'. https://www.who.int/health-topics/health-workforce#tab=tab_1 (Accessed 1 November 2022).

Wu, A., Choi, E., Diderich, M., Shamim, A., Rahhal, Z., Mitchell, M., Leask, B., & DeWit, H. (2022). 'Internationalisation of medical education—motivations and formats of current practices'. *Med Sci Educ* 32(3): 733–745.

5

Measuring Wellbeing

A Methodological Systematic Review of the Challenges and Controversies

Gemma Simons and Raymond Effah

Background

Why Medical Student Wellbeing is Important

The wellbeing of university students was a hot topic even before the COVID-19 pandemic. In UK universities declarations of mental health issues increased 5-fold over a 10-year period (Thorley, 2017) and medical students' wellbeing has been shown to be poorer than those in other undergraduate courses (Firth, 1986; Stecker, 2004). Two studies found that almost a 1/3rd of medical students may be suffering from a common mental health problem, such as anxiety and depression (Farrell et al., 2019; Plominski & Burns, 2017), compared to 1/6th of people in the general population (McManus et al., 2016). The causes of decreased wellbeing in medical students are multifactorial.

Medicine has the highest in person contact hours of all courses (Neves & Hillman, 2016). It is a 4–6-year course and due to the current financial shape of higher education, an expensive one. Medical students can expect to graduate with a minimum debt of £37,000 (Cohen et al., 2013; Health Education England, 2019). Increasingly, students from low socioeconomic status (SES) backgrounds are entering medicine courses. Financial stressors, such as the reduced possibility of getting a part time job, must be endured for more years than with other degree courses and with the added stress of receiving a disproportionately smaller loan in the final year of study, due to the NHS bursary.

Whilst all students face the obstacle of transitioning from college or sixth form to university, this transition can be more problematic in medicine. Those studying medicine are traditionally high achievers, due to the high entry requirements. Thus, students go from being the big fish in a small pond, to one big fish in a shoal of big fish. This can lead to decreased academic self-concept (Cadime et al., 2016; Mendaglio, 2012, Wang & Neihart, 2015) and feelings of inadequacy, also referred to as imposter syndrome. One study showed a ¼ of male and a ½ of female students experienced imposter syndrome in medical school (Villwock et al., 2016).

The consequences of poor wellbeing in medical students present in different ways. Many adopt unhealthy coping behaviours, with 1/10th of medical students exceeding weekly alcohol consumption guidance, and a ¼ exhibiting concerning drinking habits (Farrell et al., 2019; Munn, 2017). Students with poor wellbeing tend to have worse grades (Boulton et al.,

Gemma Simons and Raymond Effah, *Measuring Wellbeing* In: *The Mental Health of Medical Students*. Edited by: Andrew Molodynski, Sarah Marie Farrell, and Dinesh Bhugra, Oxford University Press. © Oxford University Press 2024. DOI: 10.1093/oso/9780192864871.003.0005

2019; Plominski & Burns, 2017). This may partly be explained by these students tending to also to have lower engagement (Boulton et al., 2019; Plominski & Burns, 2017). Sadly, medical students report feeling under-supported and have poor perceptions of the quality of support that is offered to them at university, when they do seek help (Billingsley, 2015; Cohen et al., 2013).

Upon graduation, poor wellbeing has important correlates, with studies demonstrating the frequency of medical errors increasing in line with decreasing wellbeing (West & Coia, 2019; West et al., 2009). It is vital, therefore, for patients, that we understand what medical student wellbeing is, and how it can be measured so that we can identify the contexts and mechanism that improve it and aim to provide them for all medical students. Proactively, addressing wellbeing from the beginning of training through course and support design that is evaluated and quality assured has been suggested (Simons et al., 2022), rather than waiting for problems and pathology, to occur, such as failed assessments, or mental health diagnoses (Bert et al., 2020; Dyrbye et al., 2006).

The Definition of Wellbeing

The definition of wellbeing has been critically reviewed (Simons & Baldwin, 2021) and two key components of a definition were identified. The first was a hedonist component, the experience of positive feelings, and the second was a eudemonic component, meeting full potential (Simons & Baldwin, 2021). Although there is no consensus definition for wellbeing, there are definitions used by respected organizations and all include a hedonist and eudemonic component. The Office for National Statistics (ONS) uses the following definition:

'Wellbeing is "how we are doing" as individuals, as communities and as a nation, and how sustainable this is for the future. It includes an individual's feelings of satisfaction with life, whether they feel the things they do in their life are worthwhile and their positive and negative emotions.' (Office for National Statistics, 2011b)

Interestingly, when measuring the nations' wellbeing, three of these four items included are used; 'negative emotions' is replaced with anxiety. The Office for National Statistics began to measure wellbeing in the UK in 2011 and each year since have asked the same four questions:

1. Overall, how satisfied are you with your life nowadays?
2. Overall, to what extent do you feel the things you do in your life are worthwhile?
3. Overall, how happy did you feel yesterday?
4. Overall, how anxious did you feel yesterday?' (Office for National Statistics, 2011a)

The replacement of 'negative emotions' with 'anxiety' may be symptomatic of the fact that a negative component does not fit well when operationalizing the positively loaded noun wellbeing (Simons, 2022). Approaching wellbeing pathogenically, like a disease, means the best an individual, or population, can achieve is an absence of illness. Wellbeing, should be able to be measured in a positive direction and should, therefore, be approached in a salutogenic way, a way that looks at the resources and capacity for health and wellbeing.

The Department of Health (DOH) also has a definition of wellbeing in the document: Wellbeing, Why it matters to health policy:

'Wellbeing is about feeling good and functioning well and comprises an individual's experience of their life; and a comparison of life circumstances with social norms and values.' (Department of Health, 2014)

This definition, again, only mentions subjective measurement 'an individual's experience' explicitly. The terms 'sustainability' and 'functioning' in these two definitions are of interest as they imply that function, activity, and participation are also ways of assessing wellbeing and these can be measured objectively, by a third party.

The Human Development Index, created by the United Nations Development Programme and based on work in the social sciences (rather than psychology), defines wellbeing with three functional components that can be measured objectively: longevity and health, access to knowledge and standard of living (United Nations Development Programme, 1990). This approach leads to industrialized nations clumping together, limiting the value of using it to define medical student wellbeing.

The Department for the Environment, Food and Rural Affairs (DEFRA) uses the definition:

'Wellbeing is a positive physical, and mental state; it is not just the absence of pain, discomfort and incapacity. It requires that basic needs are met, that individuals have a sense of purpose, that they feel able to achieve important personal goals and participate in society.' (Dolan & Peasgood, 2006; Department for Environment Food and Rural Affairs and National Statistics, 2009)

This definition again has hedonist and eudemonic components and although it does not overtly mention objective measurement, positive physical and social states, and basic needs, can be measured this way. The hedonist and eudemonic components vary in the definitions discussed, but are consistently present, as is the potential for wellbeing to be measured objectively, and not just through self-report. The definition proposed in a recent critical review of the operational definition for wellbeing includes hedonist and eudemonic components, allows for subjective, objective and salutogenic measurement and is therefore used in this review:

'Wellbeing is a state of positive feelings and meeting full potential in the world. It can be measured subjectively and objectively using a salutogenic approach.' (Simons & Baldwin, 2021).

The Measurement of Wellbeing

There are six main variables to consider when thinking of measuring medical student wellbeing.

1) **Why are we measuring?**
   - Screening for pathology
   - Epidemiology
   - Efficacy of an intervention

2) **Who should do the measuring?**
   - An independent, impartial third party, who could be verified by another independent, impartial third party because they can be standardized; objective.
   - The individual themselves, cannot be verified, or standardized, the answers can be ranked with numbers to make ordinal data; subjective.

3) **Where are we measuring, what is the context?**
   - Nationally (General Medical Council, British Medical Association), or locally (University)
   - At University only, or life in general

4) **How should we measure?**
   - Qualitatively: exploratory and descriptive, cannot be quantified, but can be categorized.
   - Quantitatively: conclusive, numerical, and can therefore be counted. This can include yes, no answers (nominal data), where 'Yes' can be assigned 1 and 'No' 2, and a frequency counted.

5) **When should we measure?**
   - In an evaluative way: ask a person what they think about their life in general, over an undefined period
   - In an experienced way: ask a person how they feel now, a specified a short period of less than 2 weeks

6) **What are we measuring?**
   - Determinants
   - Consequences/Outcomes

In addition to this variety of variables there are also multiple outcome measurement instruments that measure the same concept in slightly different ways: different items, different valence, different types of scale. A systematic review of wellbeing measurement scales identified 60 different subjective wellbeing measurement tools (Lindert et al., 2015) and a more recent systematic review identified 99 (Linton et al., 2016). To answer how we should measure medical student wellbeing a methodological systematic review that looks at how we have done this until now was conducted. A systematic review was chosen as it is standardized, rigorous, and repeatable.

Research Questions

1. How was medical student wellbeing operationalized?
2. How was medical student wellbeing measured?

Methods

Protocol and Registration

A methodological systematic review protocol was created and registered on the Prospero website (https://www.crd.york.ac.uk/prospero/display_record.php?ID=CRD42021213606), to answer the research questions. This methodology has been rereported using the PRISMA guidelines (Page et al., 2021).

Eligibility Criteria

This review considered all studies conducted in medical students. Interventional, observational, and review studies were included as well as editorials and letters if wellbeing measurement was discussed. Studies from any country were included.

   PICO Concepts used in the Systematic Review:

   Participants: All years of medical student on any type of medical degree programme (including graduate-entry)

   Intervention: For the research questions posed in this review no intervention needed to be captured, but the measurement of wellbeing was the process that needed to be captured

   Comparison: No control or comparative measure was required

   Outcome: Wellbeing was the outcome of interest

Information Sources

The following bibliographic and subject specific databases were searched: Embase, Medline, Central, PsychInfo, and International Bibliography of social science.

Search Strategy

The search was applied with no defined time-period or language. The search terms used were: (medical student' or 'student doctor' or 'student of medicine', or 'studying medicine") and (wellbeing or well-being or well being). Abstract and title (ab, ti).

Selection Process

Articles identified via title and abstract were screened independently by two reviewers (RE and GS) against the inclusion criteria. Discrepancies and disputes were settled by a meeting between the two reviewers. A third reviewer (AO) was available to resolve disagreements. Full text versions of studies were retrieved and screened independently by two reviewers (RE and GS).

Data Collection Process

Data was extracted, collated, and assessed in Microsoft Excel using a data extraction form designed prior to extraction. If needed, authors were contacted for any data missing.

Data Items

The context of the studies:

- study type
- year of publication
- country conducted in

The sample studied:

- undergraduate/ postgraduate
- average age
- gender
- ethnicity
- religion
- socioeconomic status

Study bias:

- number approached
- number responded
- number at follow up

The mechanism of measurement of wellbeing:

- wellbeing in the title
- operationalization of wellbeing, how it was described as an outcome (as an aim, in the methods, or in the results)
- delivery method for surveys
- outcomes used to capture wellbeing
- measurement instruments used to capture outcomes

Risk of Bias

It was not necessary to assess individual studies for risk of bias as this was a methodological systematic review. To reduce study risk of bias results from running the search strategies in the bibliographic databases were exported into Endnote (Alfasoft, 2021). Search results were merged using Endnote (Alfasoft, 2021), and duplicate records of the same report removed using the Endnote 'Find duplicates' function (year, title, volume, issue, pages). However, the Endnote function did not identify every duplicate, and more were identified manually and removed. Multiple reports of the same study were linked. Two reviewers screened the studies and used the search function in EndNote Click (Clarivate, 2021) to identify where wellbeing was operationalized.

Synthesis of Results

Due to the varied methodology, interventions, and outcome measures used, a narrative synthesis was conducted. The operationalization of wellbeing was conceptualized in three categories:

1) Studies that published wellbeing as an explicit outcome in the results section,
2) Studies that published wellbeing as an explicit outcome in the methods section (but did not use the word wellbeing in the results),
3) Studies that published wellbeing as a measurement aim in the introduction or background (with no explicit mention of wellbeing in the methods or results).

Outcomes and outcome measurement instruments were identified using the criteria shown:

- Outcomes and measurement instruments that captured wellbeing, as defined in the background
- Outcomes and measurement tools that did not

There were many outcomes, and measurement instruments that did not measure wellbeing, but other positive concepts. They were either general, or specific to the context of being a student, and therefore the conceptual model of context was used:

- General positive concepts
- Student-specific

The outcomes and measurement instruments that were not constructed to capture positive concepts were further categorized into:

- Pathologies
- Symptoms of pathologies

Results

Study Selection

One hundred and eighty-three studies were included in the review. Reasons for exclusion are provided in Figure 5.1.

Study Characteristics

The majority of studies were undertaken in the USA (70/183), with the second most frequent country for studies included being the UK (13/183). Before 2008 there were fewer than 5 studies published on medical student wellbeing per year, but from 2008 this number grew

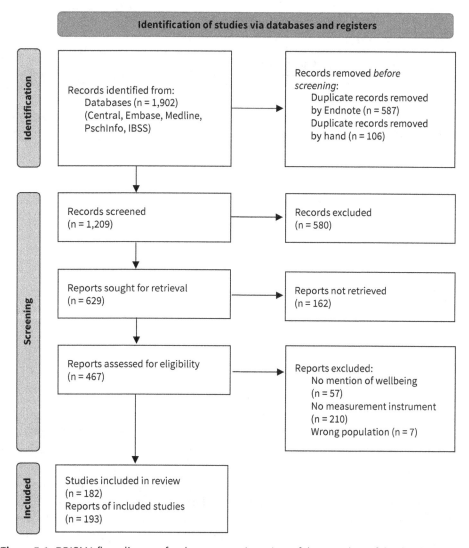

Figure 5.1 PRISMA flow diagram for the systematic review of the searches of the databases.

exponentially reaching 30 studies in the year 2020. The search identified 2 randomized controlled trials, 4 controlled trials, 30 interventional studies with no control, 7 cohort studies, 16 qualitative studies, 5 systematic reviews, and 3 other reviews. The vast majority of studies (120) were cross-sectional surveys.

Out of the cross-sectional surveys that provided a mode of delivery, 80% administered surveys in a digital format, rather than on paper.

Results of Synthesis

Of the studies included 146 (80.2%) recorded the gender of participants, 118 (64.8%) the average age, 51 (28%) the ethnicity, 34 (18.7%) the SES, and 6 (3.3%) the religion. The

Table 5.1 Summary of findings table, the way in which well-being was operationalized and measured

Number of:	Operationalization of well-being			Totals
	In the Aims	In the Methods	In the Results	
Number of:	20	37	125	182
Studies with well-being in the title	12	11	51	74
General well-being outcomes	0	14	71	85
Positive concept outcomes	8	4	39	51
Student-specific outcomes	2	1	12	15
Symptom of pathology outcomes	10	13	19	42
Pathology outcomes	22	22	24	68

postgraduate or undergraduate status of the students was reported in 160 (87.9%) of the studies. The mean and median age of medical students studied was 23 (range 19-35 years old).

Less than half (40.6%) of the included studies had wellbeing in the title, but 68.7% of included studies explicitly had wellbeing as an outcome in the results section (Table 5.1). However, 31.3% of studies while listing wellbeing as either an aim of measurement, or as an intended outcome in the methods, captured a different concept as an outcome in the results section, with no mention of the word 'wellbeing' in the results section (Table 5.1).

Studies could contain more than one wellbeing outcome (range 1–8 outcomes). General wellbeing was an outcome captured in 46.7% of the included studies, and 52% of the outcomes used to measure wellbeing were a positive concept, whether general wellbeing, or another positive concept (Table 5.1). However, 42% of the outcomes used to capture wellbeing were pathogenic outcomes, measuring either a symptom of pathology or pathology itself, with the remaining 6% of outcomes being neutral student-specific outcomes (Table 5.1).

To capture the wellbeing outcomes 85 previously developed outcome measurement instruments were used in the studies, with the GHQ-12 being used most frequently (Table 5.2). Thirty-seven self-created, unique to the study, outcome measurement instruments were used in individual studies. Qualitative methods of outcome measurement were used in 27 of the studies.

Reporting Bias

The purposes of the majority of the studies were establishing correlations between determinants of wellbeing and measuring the prevalence of poor wellbeing. Most eligible studies in this review were cross-sectional surveys capturing epidemiological data at one time point

Table 5.2 Outcome measurement instruments used in three or more studies

Outcome measurement instrument	Number of studies
General Health Questionnaire (GHQ-12)	16
Oldenburg Burnout Inventory (OLBI)	10
Perceived Stress Scale (PSS)	9
Maslach Burnout Inventory (MBI)	8
WHO-5 (General Well-being Index)	8
CAGE Questionnaire	5
Satisfaction with life scale (SWLS)	5
PROMIS Anxiety SF	4
Mental Health Continuum Short Form (MHC-SF)	4
General well-being schedule (GWB) (Dupuy 1977)	4
Warwick-Edinburgh Mental Well-being Scale	4
Depression Anxiety and Stress scale (DASS 21)	3
Medical Outcomes Study Short Form (SF-8)	3
PROMIS Depression SF	3
Medical Student Well-being Index (MSWBI)	3
Short Form Health Survey (SF-36)	3

making the majority of studies unable to comment on causality. Only 19 (10.4%) studies included a second time point measurement.

Selection Bias

Between 32–12,500 (median 493) students were approached in studies and 3–4,764 (median 183) took part in studies. The median response rate reported for the cross-sectional survey studies was 68% (range 10–100%).

Performance Bias

Of the 36 studies that were interventional 16.7% used a control and 5.5% used randomization. All the interventional studies were unable to blind participants, as medical students would be aware of the interventions through their training.

Detection Bias

Given the knowledge of medical students and the role model status of doctors there is potential for medical students to answer self-report outcomes more 'correctly' than the general population to conform with social desirability. Whether this conformity bias would lead to medical students choosing answers that would give them a pathology, or give them good wellbeing, is less clear.

Attrition Bias

For 19 of the interventional studies, and cohort studies the percentage of participants lost to follow up could be calculated with a median attrition rate of 23.5% (range 3.4-87.2%)

Discussion

General Interpretation

No study has been conducted before that synthesizes how medical student wellbeing has been operationalized and measured. This systematic review revealed the heterogeneity of the operationalization of medical student wellbeing in studies. It also highlighted a problem with reporting when it comes to wellbeing studies, with only 68.7% of the studies that set out to measure wellbeing in the aims, or methods, reporting the measurement of wellbeing in the results section. The lack of reporting in the results is most likely a consequence of no operational definition of wellbeing being used in these studies and separate concepts such as quality of life, wellness and even pathologies, such as burnout, being used interchangeably with the concept wellbeing.

The lack of appropriate wellbeing measurement in medical students was highlighted by the General Medical Council (GMC), which found that there was a need to improve the quality of measurements of wellbeing across the United Kingdom (West & Coia, 2019). The GMC commented on the inadequacy of some measures, and other important factors not being measured at all, including the demographics of medical students.

Less than a third of the studies included in this review collected ethnicity, or SES data. The components of SES are income, occupation, and education. Increasingly, students from low SES, and Black and minority ethnic (BAME), communities are being accepted into medicine (General Medical Council, 2017). Studies have shown that low SES is associated with a higher likelihood of developing mental health problems and suffering from poorer wellbeing (Barger et al., 2009; Jokela et al., 2013; WHO & Calouste Gulbenkian Foundation, 2014). Surely, it should be a priority, therefore, to capture these demographics to ensure that the sample studied includes a representative number of students from low SES and BAME communities.

This systematic review identified that 52% of the outcomes used to capture wellbeing were positive and 42% were pathogenic. This is important as it means that when we measure medical student wellbeing the most medical students can achieve is an absence of pathology. The 122 different outcome measurement instruments used to measure wellbeing demonstrated why meta-analysis cannot yet be undertaken. The three outcome measurement instruments used most were the General Health Questionnaire 12 (Jackson, 2007), the Oldenburg Burnout Inventory (Demerouti, 2008)) and the Maslach Burnout Inventory (Maslach et al., 1997)) and these capture risk of mental health pathology. This demonstrates the tendency for wellbeing to be overmedicalized in the context of medical students. All the national definitions explored in the background to this work, would suggest wellbeing is more than this, and we should not limit the potential wellbeing of our future doctors before they have even qualified by the way we define and measure their wellbeing.

There are wellbeing measurement instruments available that measure in a positive direction, as demonstrated by the systematic review of wellbeing measurement scales that identified 60 different subjective wellbeing measurement tools (Lindert et al., 2015) and a more recent systematic review that identified 99 (Linton et al., 2016).

Limitations of the Evidence in the Review

The number of medical students included in studies ranged from 3 to 4,764 (median 183), making the statistical and clinical relevance of the data questionable. Ethnicity, SES, and religion were poorly reported in the studies. The majority of studies used cross-sectional survey methodology and were, therefore, unable to comment on causation.

Limitations of the Review Processes

This systematic review included a wide array of studies of varying types, published over forty years, internationally. The inclusivity of the search for this review provides a representative view of the published research in medical student wellbeing. Due to the large number of studies identified through bibliographic databases it was not possible to search the grey-literature, or citation search the publications found. Studies that have not been published were not, therefore, captured.

Implications for Practice, Policy, and Future Research

Future research into the wellbeing of medical students needs to include an operational definition of wellbeing. A core outcome set is an agreed, standardized group of outcomes to be reported by all trials within a research field (Williamson et al., 2012) and use of a core outcome set in this field would improve the quality of individual studies and the comparability between studies. This would pave the way for wellbeing, or pastoral, support to become quality assured, as the rest of medical education must be (Evans & Elkington, 2012).

Conclusion

Whilst research into medical student wellbeing has been conducted, the differences in outcomes and measurement instruments from study to study create barriers to comparison. Using an operational definition of wellbeing, a core outcome set with valid, reliable, and practical measurement instruments, alongside standards of reporting would seem a great place to start a new era of wellbeing research. An era that moves away from repeatedly measuring what is wrong, but instead identifies and develops the contexts and mechanisms that are right for medical student wellbeing.

References

Alfasoft 2021. Endnote 9.2. UK: Alfasoft.

Barger, S.D., Donoho, C.J., & Wayment, H.A. (2009). 'The relative contributions of race/ethnicity, socioeconomic status, health, and social relationships to life satisfaction in the United States'. *Qual Life Res* [Online] **18**. Available: https://doi.org/10.1007/s11136-008-9426-2 (Accessed 14 October 2022).

Bert, F., LO Moro, G., Corradi, A., Acampora, A., Agodi, A., Brunelli, L., Chironna, M., Cocchio, S., Cofini, V., D'Errico, M. M., Marzuillo, C., Pasquarella, C., Pavia, M., Restivo, V., Gualano, M.R., Leombruni, P. & Siliquini, R. (2020). 'Prevalence of depressive symptoms among Italian medical students: The multicentre cross-sectional 'PRIMES' study'. *PLoS One* [Online] **15**. https://doi.org/10.1371/journal.pone.0231845 (Accessed 14 October 2022).

Billingsley, M. (2015). 'More than 80% of medical students with mental health issues feel under-supported, says <em>Student Bmj</em> survey'. *BMJ* [Online] **351**. Available: http://www.bmj.com/content/351/sbmj.h4521.abstract (Accessed 14 October 2022).

Boulton, C.A., Hughes, E., Kent, C., Smith, J.R., & Williams, H.T.P. (2019). 'Student engagement and wellbeing over time at a higher education institution'. *PLoS One* [Online], **14**. Available: https://doi.org/10.1371%2Fjournal.pone.0225770 (Accessed 14 October 2022).

Cadime, I., Pinto, A. M., Lima, S., Rego, S., Pereira, J., & Ribeiro, I. (2016). 'Well-being and academic achievement in secondary school pupils: the unique effects of burnout and engagement'. *J Adolesc* [Online] **53**. https://doi.org/10.1016/j.adolescence.2016.10.003 [Accessed 14 October 2022].

Clarivate (2021). EndNote Click Plugin v2.3.2. US: Clarivate.

Cohen, D., Winstanley, S., Palmer, P., Allen, J., Howels, S., Greene, G. & Rhydderch, M. (2013). *Factors that Impact on Medical Student Wellbeing—Perspectives of Risks* [Online]. General Medical Council. https://www.gmc-uk.org/-/media/documents/Factors_that_impact_on_medical_student_wellbeing_____Perspectives_of_risks_53959480.pdf [Accessed 14 October 2022].

Demerouti, E. (2008). 'The Oldenburg Burnout Inventory: A good alternative to measure burnout and engagement'. *Handbook of Stress and Burnout in Health Care*.

Department For Environment Food and Rural Affairs and National Statistics (2009). *Sustainable Development Indicators in Your Pocket 2009. An Update of the UK Government Strategy Indicators.* [Online]. https://assets.publishing.service.gov.uk/government/uploads/system/uploads/attachment_data/file/69414/pb13265-sdiyp-2009-a9-090821.pdf [Accessed 17 January 2022].

Department of Health (2014). *Wellbeing: Why It Matters to Health Policy* [Online]. Department of Health. https://assets.publishing.service.gov.uk/government/uploads/system/uploads/attachment_data/file/277566/Narrative__January_2014_.pdf [Accessed 2 August 2019].

Dolan, P. & Peasgood, T. (2006). *Research on the Relationship Between Well-Being and Sustainable Development. Final Report for DEFRA.* [Online]. http://eprints.chi.ac.uk/id/eprint/1168/1/WellbeingProject3A.pdf [Accessed 17 January 2022].

Dyrbye, L.N., Thomas, M.R., Huntington, J.L., Lawson, K.L., Novotny, P.J., Sloan, J.A., & Shanafelt, T.D. (2006). 'Personal life events and medical student burnout: a multicenter study'. *Acad Med* [Online], **81**. https://doi.org/10.1097/00001888-200604000-00010 (Accessed 14 October 2022).

Evans, C. & Elkington, S. (2012). *A Marked Improvement. Transforming Assessment in Higher Education* [Online]. The Higher Education Academy. https://www.heacademy.ac.uk/system/files/A_Marked_Improvement.pdf (Accessed 14 October 2022).

Farrell, S.M., Molodynski, A., Cohen, D., Grant, A.J., Rees, S., Wullshleger, A., Lewis, T., & Kadhum, M. (2019). 'Wellbeing and burnout among medical students in Wales'. *Int Rev Psychiatry* [Online], **31**. https://doi.org/10.1080/09540261.2019.1678251 (Accessed 14 October 2022).

Firth, J. (1986). 'Levels and sources of stress in medical students'. *Br Med J (Clin Res Ed)* [Online], **292**. https://doi.org/10.1136%2Fbmj.292.6529.1177 (Accessed 14 October 2022).

General Medical Council (2017). *The State of Medical Education and Practice in the UK* [Online]. General Medical Council. https://www.gmc-uk.org/-/media/gmc-site-images/about/what-we-do-and-why/data-and-research/somep-2017/somep-2017-final-executive-summary.pdf?la=en&hash=CA9Bcd1BC8C1F20A002E8000262E3F98F12Ffd42 (Accessed 14 October 2022).

Health Education England (2019). *NHS Staff and Learners Mental Wellbeing Commission Report* [Online]. Health Education England. https://www.hee.nhs.uk/sites/default/files/documents/Nhs%20%28Hee%29%20-%20Mental%20Wellbeing%20Commission%20Report.pdf (Accessed 14 October 2022).

Jackson, C. (2007). The General Health Questionnaire. *Occupational Medicine* [Online], 57. https://doi.org/10.1093/occmed/kql169 (Accessed 14 October 2022).

Jokela, M., Batty, G.D., Vahtera, J., Elovainio, M., & Kivimäki, M. (2013). Socioeconomic inequalities in common mental disorders and psychotherapy treatment in the UK between 1991 and 2009. *Br J Psychiatry* [Online], 202. https://doi.org/10.1192/bjp.bp.111.098863 (Accessed 14 October 2022).

Lindert, J., Bain, P.A., Kubzansky, L.D., & Stein, C. (2015). Well-being measurement and the Who health policy Health 2010: systematic review of measurement scales. *Eur J Public Health* [Online], 25. https://doi.org/10.1093/eurpub/cku193 (Accessed 14 October 2022).

Linton, M. J., Dieppe, P. & Medina-Lara, A. (2016). Review of 99 self-report measures for assessing well-being in adults: exploring dimensions of well-being and developments over time. *BMJ Open* [Online], 6. http://dx.doi.org/10.1136/bmjopen-2015-010641 (Accessed 14 October 2022).

Maslach, C., Jackson, S.E., & Leiter, M.P. (1997). *Maslach Burnout Inventory: Third edition. Evaluating Stress: A Book of Resources.* Lanham, MD: Scarecrow Education.

Mcmanus, S., Bebbington, P.E., Jenkins, R. & Brugha, T. (2016). *Mental Health and Wellbeing in England: The Adult Psychiatric Morbidity Survey 2014* [Online]. NHS Digital. https://assets.publishing.service.gov.uk/government/uploads/system/uploads/attachment_data/file/556596/apms-2014-full-rpt.pdf (Accessed 14 October 2022).

Mendaglio, S. (2012). Gifted students' transition to university. *Gifted Education International* [Online], 29. https://doi.org/10.1177/0261429412440646 (Accessed 14 October 2022).

Munn, F. (2017). One in 10 medical students exceeds weekly alcohol consumption guidance, a Student BMJ survey finds. *BMJ* [Online], 358. https://doi.org/10.1136/sbmj.j3707 (Accessed 14 October 2022).

Neves, J. & Hillman, N. (2016). *The 2016 Student Academic Experience Survey* [Online]. Higher Education Academy. https://www.hepi.ac.uk/wp-content/uploads/2016/06/Student-Academic-Experience-Survey-2016.pdf (Accessed 14 October 2022).

Office For National Statistics (2011a). *2011 Census Data* [Online]. Office for National Statistics. https://www.ons.gov.uk/census/2011census/2011censusdata (Accessed 14 October 2022).

Office For National Statistics (2011b). *What Matters to You? Measuring What Matters. National Statisticians' Reflections On The National Debate On Measuring National Well-Being* [Online]. Office for National Statistics. https://www.gov.uk/government/collections/national-wellbeing (Accessed 14 October 2022).

Page, M. J., Mckenzie, J. E., Bossuyt, P. M., Boutron, I., Hoffmann, T. C., Mulrow, C. D., Shamseer, L., Tetzlaff, J. M., Akl, E. A., Brennan, S. E., Chou, R., Glanville, J., Grimshaw, J. M., Hróbjartsson, A., Lalu, M. M., LI, T., Loder, E. W., Mayo-Wilson, E., Mcdonald, S., Mcguinness, L. A., Stewart, L. A., Thomas, J., Tricco, A. C., Welch, V. A., Whiting, P. & Moher, D. 2021. The Prisma 2020 statement: an updated guideline for reporting systematic reviews. *Bmj* [Online], 372. Available: http://www.bmj.com/content/372/bmj.n71.abstract [Accessed 14/10/2022].

Plominski, A. P. & Burns, L. R. 2017. An Investigation of Student Psychological Wellbeing: Honors Versus Nonhonors Undergraduate Education. *Journal of Advanced Academics* [Online], 29. Available: https://doi.org/10.1177/1932202X17735358 [Accessed 14/10/2022].

Simons, G. 2022. *How should wellbeing be measured in UK doctors? A salutogenic, consensus approach, towards a Core Outcome set for doctor wellbeing measurement.*, University of Southampton.

Simons, G. & Baldwin, D. S. 2021. A critical review of the definition of 'wellbeing' for doctors and their patients in a post Covid-19 era. *International Journal of Social Psychiatry* [Online], 67. Available: https://doi.org/10.1177%2F00207640211032259 [Accessed 14/10/2022].

Simons, G., Effah, R. & Baldwin, D. S. 2022. What medical students think about measurement of their well-being: cross-sectional survey and qualitative interviews. *Bmj Open* [Online], 12. Available: https://doi.org/10.1136/bmjopen-2021-056749 [Accessed 14/10/2022].

Stecker, T. 2004. Well-being in an academic environment. *Med Educ* [Online], 38. Available: https://doi.org/10.1046/j.1365-2929.2004.01812.x [Accessed 14/10/2022].

Thorley, C. 2017. *Not by degrees: Improving student mental health in the UK's universities* [Online]. Institute for public policy research. Available: https://www.ippr.org/publications/not-by-degrees [Accessed 14/10/2022].

United Nations Development Programme. 1990. *Human Development Report 1990: Concept and Measurement of Human Development.* [Online]. Available: http://hdr.undp.org/en/reports/global/hdr1990 [Accessed 17/01/2021].

Villwock, J. A., Sobin, L. B., Koester, L. A. & Harris, T. M. 2016. Impostor syndrome and burnout among American medical students: a pilot study. *Int J Med Educ* [Online], 7. Available: https://doi.org/10.5116/ijme.5801.eac4 [Accessed 14/10/2022].

Wang, C. W. & Neihart, M. 2015. Academic self-concept and academic self-efficacy: Self-beliefs enable academic achievement of twice-exceptional students. *Roeper Review: A Journal on Gifted Education* [Online], 37. Available: https://doi.org/10.1080/02783193.2015.1008660 [Accessed 14/10/2022].

West, C. P., Tan, A. D., Habermann, T. M., Sloan, J. A. & Shanafelt, T. D. 2009. Association of resident fatigue and distress with perceived medical errors. *Jama* [Online], 302. Available: https://doi.org/10.1001/jama.2009.1389 [Accessed 14/10/2022].

West, M. & Coia, D. 2019. *Caring for doctors caring for patients* [Online]. General Medical Council. Available: https://www.gmc-uk.org/-/media/documents/caring-for-doctors-caring-for-patients_pdf-80706341.pdf [Accessed 14/10/2022].

Who & Calouste Gulbenkian Foundation. 2014. *Social determinants of mental health* [Online]. Who Geneva. Available: https://www.who.int/social_determinants/sdh_definition/en/ [Accessed 13/10 2018].

Williamson, P. R., Altman, D. G., Blazeby, J. M., Clarke, M., Devane, D., Gargon, E. & Tugwell, P. 2012. Developing core outcome sets for clinical trials: issues to consider. *Trials* [Online], 13. Available: https://doi.org/10.1186/1745-6215-13-132 [Accessed 14/10/2022].

The systematic review included the following studies:

Abe, K., Evans, P., Austin, E. J., Suzuki, Y., Fujisaki, K., Niwa, M. & Aomatsu, M. 2013. Expressing one's feelings and listening to others increases emotional intelligence: a pilot study of Asian medical students. *Bmc medical education*, 13, 82.

Aboalshamat, K., Hou, X. Y. & Strodl, E. 2015. Psychological well-being status among medical and dental students in Makkah, Saudi Arabia: a cross-sectional study. *Medical teacher*, 37, S75–S81.

Abrams, M. P., Eckert, T., Topping, D. & Daly, K. D. 2020. Reflective writing on the cadaveric dissection experience: An effective tool to assess the impact of dissection on learning of anatomy, humanism, empathy, well-being, and professional identity formation in medical students. *Anatomical sciences education*.

AL Breiki, M. H. & AL Muqbali, M. 2019. Well-being among medical students in clinical years at a private college in Oman: Cross sectional study (7526). *Swiss Archives of Neurology, Psychiatry and Psychotherapy*, 70, 50S.

Almeida, T., Kadhum, M., Farrell, S. M., Ventriglio, A. & Molodynski, A. 2019. A descriptive study of mental health and wellbeing among medical students in Portugal. *International review of psychiatry (Abingdon, England)*, 31, 574–578.

Almeneessier, A.S., Al Saadi, M.M., Nooh, R. M. & AL Ansary, L. A. 2015. Family violence among female medical students: Its prevalence and impact on their mental health status—a cross-sectional study. *Journal of Taibah University Medical Sciences*, 10, 33–39.

Ambuel, B., Butler, D., Hamberger, L. K., Lawrence, S. & Guse, C. E. 2003. Female and male medical students' exposure to violence: Impact on well being and perceived capacity to help battered women. *Journal of Comparative Family Studies*, 34.

Amr, M., EL Gilany, A. H. & EL-Hawary, A. 2008. Does gender predict medical students' stress in Mansoura, Egypt? *Medical Education Online*, 13.

Apte, G. M., Pranita, A., Joshi, A. R. & Kharche, J. 2011. Assessment of who-5 well being index in 1st Mbbs medical students. *Indian Journal of Physiology and Pharmacology*, 55, 246.

Arora, S., Russ, S., Petrides, K. V., Sirimanna, P., Aggarwal, R., Darzi, A. & Sevdalis, N. 2011. Emotional intelligence and stress in medical students performing surgical tasks. *Academic medicine: journal of the Association of American Medical Colleges*, 86, 1311–1137.

Aung, M. N., Somboonwong, J., Jaroonvanichkul, V. & Wannakrairot, P. 2016. Possible link between medical students' motivation for academic work and time engaged in physical exercise. *Mind, Brain, and Education*, 10, 264–271.

Awad, F., Awad, M., Mattick, K. & Dieppe, P. 2019. Mental health in medical students: time to act. *The clinical teacher*, 16, 312–316.

Ayala, E. E., Omorodion, A. M., Nmecha, D., Winseman, J. S. & Mason, H. R. C. 2017. What Do Medical Students Do for Self-Care? A Student-Centered Approach to Well-Being. *Teaching and learning in medicine*, 29, 237–246.

Babenko, O. & Mosewich, A. 2017. In sport and now in medical school: examining students' well-being and motivations for learning. *International journal of medical education*, 8, 336–342.

Bhugra, D., Sauerteig, S. O., Bland, D., Lloyd-Kendall, A., Wijesuriya, J., Singh, G., Kochhar, A., Molodynski, A. & Ventriglio, A. 2019. A descriptive study of mental health and wellbeing of doctors and medical students in the UK. *International Review of Psychiatry*, 31, 563–568.

Bíró, É., Balajti, I., Ádány, R. & Kósa, K. 2010. Determinants of mental well-being in medical students. *Social Psychiatry and Psychiatric Epidemiology: The International Journal for Research in Social and Genetic Epidemiology and Mental Health Services*, 45, 253–258.

Bloodgood, R. A., Short, J. G., Jackson, J. M. & Martindale, J. R. 2009. A change to pass/fail grading in the first two years at one medical school results in improved psychological well-being. *Academic medicine: journal of the Association of American Medical Colleges*, 84, 655–662.

Bond, A. R., Mason, H. F., Lemaster, C. M., Shaw, S. E., Mullin, C. S., Holick, E. A. & Saper, R. B. 2014. Embodied health: The effects of a mind-body course for medical students. *Medical Education Online*, 18.

Broukhim, M., Yuen, F., Mcdermott, H., Miller, K., Merrill, L., Kennedy, R. & Wilkes, M. 2019. Interprofessional conflict and conflict management in an educational setting. *Medical teacher*, 41, 408–416.

Brubaker, J. R., Swan, A. & Beverly, E. A. 2020. A brief intervention to reduce burnout and improve sleep quality in medical students. *Bmc medical education*, 20, 345.

Bughi, S. A., Lie, D. A., Zia, S. K. & Rosenthal, J. 2017. Using a personality inventory to identify risk of distress and burnout among early stage medical students. *Education for health (Abingdon, England)*, 30, 26–30.

Bughi, S. A., Sumcad, J. & Bughu, S. 2006. Effect of brief behavioral intervention program in managing stress in medical students from two Southern California universities. *Medical Education Online*, 11, 1–8.

Burris, L. C. 2018. *Insights from narrative reflections of first year medical students on their professional formation*. 79, ProQuest Information & Learning.

Bursch, B., Fried, J. M., Wimmers, P. F., Cook, I. A., Baillie, S., Zackson, H. & Stuber, M. L. 2013. Relationship between medical student perceptions of mistreatment and mistreatment sensitivity. *Medical teacher*, 35, e998–1002.

Byrnes, C., Ganapathy, V. A., Lam, M., Mogensen, L. & HU, W. 2020. Medical student perceptions of curricular influences on their wellbeing: a qualitative study. *Bmc medical education*, 20, 288.

Cameron, D., Katch, E., Anderson, P. & Furlong, M. A. 2004. Healthy doctors, healthy communities. *The Journal of ambulatory care management*, 27, 328–338.

Carla, C., Andrea, O., Dana, H. & Bogdan, N. 2017. Perceived stress and well-being among international first year medical students in romania. *Clujul Medical*, 90, S108.

Carrieri, D., Mattick, K., Pearson, M., Papoutsi, C., Briscoe, S., Wong, G. & Jackson, M. 2020. Optimising strategies to address mental ill-health in doctors and medical students: 'Care Under Pressure' realist review and implementation guidance. *Bmc medicine*, 18, 76.

Chandla, S. S., Sood, S., Dogra, R., Das, S., Shukla, S. K. & Gupta, S. 2013. Effect of short-term practice of pranayamic breathing exercises on cognition, anxiety, general well being and heart rate variability. *J Indian Med Assoc*, 111, 662–665.

Chau, S. W. H., Lewis, T., NG, R., Chen, J. Y., Farrell, S. M., Molodynski, A. & Bhugra, D. 2019. Wellbeing and mental health amongst medical students from Hong Kong. *International review of psychiatry (Abingdon, England)*, 31, 626–629.

Coates, W. C., Spector, T. S. & Uijtdehaage, S. 2012. Transition to life--a sendoff to the real world for graduating medical students. *Teaching and learning in medicine*, 24, 36–41.

Cox, S. M., Brett-Maclean, P. & Courneya, C. A. 2016. 'My turbinado sugar': Art-making, well-being and professional identity in medical education. *Arts & Health: An International Journal of Research, Policy and Practice*, 8, 65–81.

Coyle, C., Ghazi, H. & Georgiou, I. 2020. The mental health and well-being benefits of exercise during the Covid-19 pandemic: a cross-sectional study of medical students and newly qualified doctors in the UK. *Irish Journal of Medical Science*.

Cuschieri, S. & Calleja Agius, J. 2020. Spotlight on the shift to remote anatomical teaching during Covid-19 pandemic: Perspectives and Experiences from the University of Malta. *Anatomical sciences education*.

Cvejic, E., Huang, S. & Vollmer-Conna, U. 2018. Can you snooze your way to an 'A'? Exploring the complex relationship between sleep, autonomic activity, wellbeing and performance in medical students. *The Australian and New Zealand journal of psychiatry*, 52, 39–46.

Daud, S., Shaikh, R. Z., Ahmad, M. & Awan, Z. U. H. 2014. Stress in medical students. *Pakistan Journal of Medical and Health Sciences*, 8, 503–507.

Dayalan, H., Subramanian, S. & Elango, T. 2010. Psychological well-being in medical students during exam stress-influence of short-term practice of mind sound technology. *Indian journal of medical sciences*, 64, 501–5/7.

DE Jonge, P. & Slaets, J. P. J. 2005. Response sets in self-report data and their associations with personality traits. *European Journal of Psychiatry*, 19, 209–214.

DE Oliveira E Sousa Leao, P. B., Martins, L. A. N., Menezes, P. R. & Bellodi, P. L. 2011. Well-being and help-seeking: An exploratory study among final-year medical students. *Revista da Associacao Medica Brasileira*, 57, 379–386.

DE Vries-Erich, J. M., Dornan, T., Boerboom, T. B. B., Jaarsma, A. D. C. & Helmich, E. 2016. Dealing with emotions: medical undergraduates' preferences in sharing their experiences. *Medical education*, 50, 817–28.

Dinyane Szabo, M. & Pusztai, G. 2016. [Use of the short (5-item) version of the Who well-being questionnaire in first year students of Semmelweis University]. *Az Egeszsegugyi Vilagszervezet otteteles jol-let kerdoivenek vizsgalata a Semmelweis Egyetem elsoeves hallgatoinak koreben.*, 157, 1762–1768.

Donohoe, J., O'Rourke, M., Hammond, S., Stoyanov, S. & O'Tuathaigh, C. 2020. Strategies for Enhancing Resilience in Medical Students: a Group Concept Mapping Analysis. *Academic psychiatry: the journal of the American Association of Directors of Psychiatric Residency Training and the Association for Academic Psychiatry*, 44, 427–431.

Dossett, M. L., Kohatsu, W., Nunley, W., Mehta, D., Davis, R. B., Phillips, R. S. & Yeh, G. 2013. A medical student elective promoting humanism, communication skills, complementary and alternative medicine and physician self-care: an evaluation of the Heart program. *Explore (New York, N.Y.)*, 9, 292–298.

Drolet, B. C. & Rodgers, S. 2010. A comprehensive medical student wellness program--design and implementation at Vanderbilt School of Medicine. *Academic medicine: journal of the Association of American Medical Colleges*, 85, 103–110.

Duffy, R. D., Manuel, R. S., Borges, N. J. & Bott, E. M. 2011. Calling, vocational development, and well being: A longitudinal study of medical students. *Journal of Vocational Behavior*, 79, 361–366.

Dyrbye, L., Schwartz, A., Downing, S., Sloan, J. & Shanafelt, T. 2011. Effectiveness of a brief screening tool to identify medical students in severe distress. *Journal of General Internal Medicine*, 26, S49–S50.

Dyrbye, L. N., Satele, D. & Shanafelt, T. D. 2017. Healthy Exercise Habits Are Associated With Lower Risk of Burnout and Higher Quality of Life Among U.S. Medical Students. *Academic medicine: journal of the Association of American Medical Colleges*, 92, 1006–1011.

Dyrbye, L. N., Thomas, M. R., Harper, W., Massie, F. S., JR., Power, D. V., Eacker, A., Szydlo, D. W., Novotny, P. J., Sloan, J. A. & Shanafelt, T. D. 2009. The learning environment and medical student burnout: a multicentre study. *Med Educ*, 43, 274–282.

Dyrbye, L. N., Thomas, M. R., Huntington, J. L., Lawson, K. L., Novotny, P. J., Sloan, J. A. & Shanafelt, T. D. 2006. Personal life events and medical student burnout: a multicenter study. *Acad Med* [Online], 81. Available: https://doi.org/10.1097/00001888-200604000-00010 [Accessed 14/10/22].

Encandela, J., Gibson, C., Angoff, N., Leydon, G. & Green, M. 2014. Characteristics of test anxiety among medical students and congruence of strategies to address it. *Med Educ Online*, 19, 25211.

Farrell, S. M., Kadhum, M., Lewis, T., Singh, G., Penzenstadler, L. & Molodynski, A. 2019a. Wellbeing and burnout amongst medical students in England. *Int Rev Psychiatry*, 31, 579–583.

Farrell, S. M., Kar, A., Valsraj, K., Mukherjee, S., Kunheri, B., Molodynski, A. & George, S. 2019b. Wellbeing and burnout in medical students in India; a large scale survey. *Int Rev Psychiatry*, 31, 555–562.

Farrell, S. M., Moir, F., Molodynski, A. & Bhugra, D. 2019c. Psychological wellbeing, burnout and substance use amongst medical students in New Zealand. *Int Rev Psychiatry*, 31, 630–636.

Farrell, S. M., Molodynski, A., Cohen, D., Grant, A. J., Rees, S., Wullshleger, A., Lewis, T. & Kadhum, M. 2019d. Wellbeing and burnout among medical students in Wales. *Int Rev Psychiatry* [Online], 31. Available: https://doi.org/10.1080/09540261.2019.1678251 [Accessed 14/10/2022].

Finset, K. B., Gude, T., Hem, E., Tyssen, R., Ekeberg, O. & Vaglum, P. 2005. Which young physicians are satisfied with their work? A prospective nationwide study in Norway. *Bmc Med Educ*, 5, 19.

Garrusi, B., Safizadeh, H. & Pourhosseini, O. 2008. A study on the lifestyle of the Iranian University Students. *Iranian Journal of Psychiatry and Behavioral Sciences*, 2, 41–45.

Gates, R., Musick, D., Greenawald, M., Carter, K., Bogue, R. & Penwell-Waines, L. 2019. Evaluating the Burnout-Thriving Index in a Multidisciplinary Cohort at a Large Academic Medical Center. *South Med J*, 112, 199–204.

Gold, J. A., Bentzley, J. P., Franciscus, A. M., Forte, C. & DE Golia, S. G. 2019. An Intervention in Social Connection: Medical Student Reflection Groups. *Acad Psychiatry*, 43, 375–380.

Goswami, G. & Salvi, S. 2020. Video gaming, physiological responses, and well-being in medical students: An essence of intrigue way of learning. *National Journal of Physiology, Pharmacy and Pharmacology*, 10, 468–472.

Greenhill, J., Fielke, K. R., Richards, J. N., Walker, L. J. & Walters, L. K. 2015. Towards an understanding of medical student resilience in longitudinal integrated clerkships. *Bmc Med Educ*, 15, 137.

Guerrasio, J., Garrity, M. J. & Aagaard, E. M. 2014. Learner deficits and academic outcomes of medical students, residents, fellows, and attending physicians referred to a remediation program, 2006-2012. *Acad Med*, 89, 352–358.

Haglund, M. E., Aan Het Rot, M., Cooper, N. S., Nestadt, P. S., Muller, D., Southwick, S. M. & Charney, D. S. 2009. Resilience in the third year of medical school: a prospective study of the associations between stressful events occurring during clinical rotations and student well-being. *Acad Med*, 84, 258–268.

Hamidia, A., Amiri, P., Faramarzi, M., Yadollahpour, M. H. & Khafri, S. 2020. Predictors of Physician's Empathy: The Role of Spiritual Well-being, Dispositional Perspectives, and Psychological Well-being. *Oman Med J*, 35, e138.

Hanáková, M., Sovová, E. & Zapletalová, J. 2015. Psychological health and stress among Czech medical students. *International Journal of Health Promotion and Education*, 53, 328–337.

Hancock, J. & Mattick, K. 2020. Tolerance of ambiguity and psychological well-being in medical training: A systematic review. *Med Educ*, 54, 125–137.

Hansell, M. W., Ungerleider, R. M., Brooks, C. A., Knudson, M. P., Kirk, J. K. & Ungerleider, J. D. 2019. Temporal Trends in Medical Student Burnout. *Fam Med*, 51, 399–404.

Hardeman, R. R. 2014. *Reconstructing Research: Exploring the Intersections of Race, Gender and Socioeconomic Status in Medical Education*. Ph.D., University of Minnesota.

Harth, S. C., Bavanandan, S., Thomas, K. E., Lai, M. Y. & Thong, Y. H. 1992. The quality of student-tutor interactions in the clinical learning environment. *Med Educ*, 26, 321–326.

Hausler, M., Strecker, C., Huber, A., Brenner, M., Höge, T. & Höfer, S. 2017. Associations between the Application of Signature Character Strengths, Health and Well-being of Health Professionals. *Front Psychol*, 8, 1307.

HE, B., Prasad, S., Higashi, R. T. & Goff, H. W. 2019. The art of observation: a qualitative analysis of medical students' experiences. *Bmc Medical Education*, 19, 234.

Helou, M. A., Keiser, V., Feldman, M., Santen, S., Cyrus, J. W. & Ryan, M. S. 2019. Student well-being and the learning environment. *Clin Teach*, 16, 362–366.

Henry, D. S., Wessinger, W. D., Meena, N. K., Payakachat, N., Gardner, J. M. & Rhee, S. W. 2020. Using a Facebook group to facilitate faculty-student interactions during preclinical medical education: a retrospective survey analysis. *Bmc Medical Education*, 20, 87.

Hillis, J. M., Perry, W. R., Carroll, E. Y., Hibble, B. A., Davies, M. J. & Yousef, J. 2010. Painting the picture: Australasian medical student views on wellbeing teaching and support services. *Med J Aust*, 192, 188–190.

Hobfoll, S. E., Anson, O. & Antonovsky, A. 1982. Personality factors as predictors of medical students performance. *Med Educ*, 16, 251–258.

Hojat, M., Gonnella, J., Erdmann, J. & Vogel, W. 2003. Medical students' cognitive appraisal of stressful life events as related to personality, physical well-being, and academic performance: A longitudinal study. *Personality and Individual Differences*, 35, 219–235.

Houpy, J. C., Lee, W. W., Woodruff, J. N. & Pincavage, A. T. 2017. Medical student resilience and stressful clinical events during clinical training. *Med Educ Online*, 22, 1320187.

Imran, N., Tariq, K. F., Pervez, M. I., Jawaid, M. & Haider, II 2016. Medical Students' Stress, Psychological Morbidity, and Coping Strategies: a Cross-Sectional Study from Pakistan. *Acad Psychiatry*, 40, 92–96.

Iqbal, M. Z., Alradhi, H. I., Alhumaidi, A. A., Alshaikh, K. H., Alobaid, A. M., Alhashim, M. T. & Alsheikh, M. H. 2020. Telegram as a Tool to Supplement Online Medical Education During Covid-19 Crisis. *Acta Inform Med*, 28, 94–97.

Isaac, V., Pit, S. W. & Mclachlan, C. S. 2018. Self-efficacy reduces the impact of social isolation on medical student's rural career intent. *Bmc Med Educ*, 18, 42.

Jacob, R., LI, T.-Y., Martin, Z., Burren, A., Watson, P., Kant, R., Davies, R. & Wood, D. F. 2020. Taking care of our future doctors: a service evaluation of a medical student mental health service. *Bmc Medical Education*, 20, 172.

Jafari, N., Loghmani, A. & Montazeri, A. 2012. Mental health of Medical Students in Different Levels of Training. *Int J Prev Med*, 3, S107–S112.

James, J. E., Bruce, M. S., Lader, M. H. & Scott, N. R. 1989. Self-report reliability and symptomatology of habitual caffeine consumption. *Br J Clin Pharmacol*, 27, 507–514.

Jenkins, T. M., Kim, J., HU, C., Hickernell, J. C., Watanaskul, S. & Yoon, J. D. 2018. Stressing the journey: using life stories to study medical student wellbeing. *Adv Health Sci Educ Theory Pract*, 23, 767–782.

Kachel, T., Huber, A., Strecker, C., Höge, T. & Höfer, S. 2020. Development of Cynicism in Medical Students: Exploring the Role of Signature Character Strengths and Well-Being. *Front Psychol*, 11, 328.

Katpar, S., Rana, Z., Hussain, M., Khan, R. & Rehman, R. 2017. Impact of social interdependence on emotional well-being of medical students. *J Pak Med Assoc*, 67, 992–997.

Kattimani, S., Sarkar, S., Bharadwaj, B. & Rajkumar, R. P. 2015. An Exploration of the Relationship Between Spirituality and State and Trait Anger Among Medical Students. *J Relig Health*, 54, 2134–2141.

Kaye-Kauderer, H. P., Levine, J., Takeguchi, Y., Machida, M., Sekine, H., Taku, K., Yanagisawa, R. & Katz, C. 2019. Post-Traumatic Growth and Resilience Among Medical Students After the March 2011 Disaster in Fukushima, Japan. *Psychiatr Q*, 90, 507–518.

Keng, S.-L., Phang, C. K. & Oei, T. P. 2015. Effects of a Brief Mindfulness-Based Intervention Program on Psychological Symptoms and Well-Being Among Medical Students in Malaysia: A Controlled Study. *International Journal of Cognitive Therapy*, 8, 335–s350.

Khan, H., Shafi, M. & Masud, S. 2017. Psychosocial well being of undergraduate medical students of king edward medical university lahore using Dass 21 scoring system-a cross sectional survey. *Pakistan Journal of Medical and Health Sciences*, 11, 764–s766.

King, K. R., Purcell, R. A., Quinn, S. J., Schoo, A. M. & Walters, L. K. 2016. Supports for medical students during rural clinical placements: factors associated with intention to practise in rural locations. *Rural Remote Health*, 16, 3791.

Kjeldstadli, K., Tyssen, R., Finset, A., Hem, E., Gude, T., Gronvold, N. T., Ekeberg, O. & Vaglum, P. 2006. Life satisfaction and resilience in medical school--a six-year longitudinal, nationwide and comparative study. *Bmc Med Educ*, 6, 48.

Knipe, D., Maughan, C., Gilbert, J., Dymock, D., Moran, P. & Gunnell, D. 2018. Mental health in medical, dentistry and veterinary students: cross-sectional online survey. *Bjpsych Open*, 4, 441–446.

Kraemer, K. M., Luberto, C. M., O'Bryan, E. M., Mysinger, E. & Cotton, S. 2016. Mind-Body Skills Training to Improve Distress Tolerance in Medical Students: A Pilot Study. *Teach Learn Med*, 28, 219–228.

Kroska, E. B., Calarge, C., O'Hara, M. W., Deumic, E. & Dindo, L. 2017. Burnout and depression in medical students: Relations with avoidance and disengagement. *Journal of Contextual Behavioral Science*, 6, 404–408.

Lee, J. & Graham, A. V. 2001. Students' perception of medical school stress and their evaluation of a wellness elective. *Med Educ*, 35, 652–659.

Leffel, G. M., Oakes Mueller, R. A., Ham, S. A., Karches, K. E., Curlin, F. A. & Yoon, J. D. 2018. Project on the Good Physician: Further Evidence for the Validity of a Moral Intuitionist Model of Virtuous Caring. *Teach Learn Med*, 30, 303–316.

Lemtiri Chelieh, M., Kadhum, M., Lewis, T., Molodynski, A., Abouqal, R., Belayachi, J. & Bhugra, D. 2019. Mental health and wellbeing among Moroccan medical students: a descriptive study. *Int Rev Psychiatry*, 31, 608–612.

Lin, Y. K., Chen, D. Y. & Lin, B. Y. 2017. Determinants and effects of medical students' core self-evaluation tendencies on clinical competence and workplace well-being in clerkship. *PLoS One*, 12, e0188651.

Lin, Y. K., Yen-JU Lin, B. & Chen, D.-Y. 2020. Do teaching strategies matter? Relationships between various teaching strategies and medical students' wellbeing during clinical workplace training. *Medical Teacher*, 42, 39–45.

Liu, R., Carrese, J., Colbert-Getz, J., Geller, G. & Shochet, R. 2015. "Am I cut out for this?" Understanding the experience of doubt among first-year medical students. *Med Teach*, 37, 1083–1089.

Lonka, K., Sharafi, P., Karlgren, K., Masiello, I., Nieminen, J., Birgegård, G. & Josephson, A. 2008. Med Nord--A tool for measuring medical students' well-being and study orientations. *Med Teach*, 30, 72–79.

Lyons, Z., Wilcox, H., Leung, L. & Dearsley, O. 2020. Covid-19 and the mental well-being of Australian medical students: impact, concerns and coping strategies used. *Australas Psychiatry*, 28, 649–652.

Machado, L., DE Oliveira, I. R., Peregrino, A. & Cantilino, A. 2019. Common mental disorders and subjective well-being: Emotional training among medical students based on positive psychology. *PLoS One*, 14, e0211926.

Machado, L., Souza, C. T. N., Nunes, R. O., DE Santana, C. N., Araujo, C. F. & Cantilino, A. 2018. Subjective well-being, religiosity and anxiety: a cross-sectional study applied to a sample of Brazilian medical students. *Trends Psychiatry Psychother*, 40, 185–192.

Malathi, A. & Damodaran, A. 1999. Stress due to exams in medical students--role of yoga. *Indian J Physiol Pharmacol*, 43, 218–224.

Mascaro, J. S., Kelley, S., Darcher, A., Negi, L. T., Worthman, C., Miller, A. & Raison, C. 2018. Meditation buffers medical student compassion from the deleterious effects of depression. *The Journal of Positive Psychology*, 13, 133–142.

Masri, R., Kadhum, M., Farrell, S. M., Khamees, A., AL-Taiar, H. & Molodynski, A. 2019. Wellbeing and mental health amongst medical students in Jordan: a descriptive study. *Int Rev Psychiatry*, 31, 619–625.

Mcfadden, T., Fortier, M., Sweet, S. N. & Tomasone, J. R. 2021. Physical activity participation and mental health profiles in Canadian medical students: latent profile analysis using continuous latent profile indicators. *Psychol Health Med*, 26, 671–683.

Meo, S. A., Abukhalaf, A. A., Alomar, A. A., Sattar, K. & Klonoff, D. C. 2020. Covid-19 Pandemic: Impact of Quarantine on Medical Students' Mental Wellbeing and Learning Behaviors. *Pak J Med Sci*, 36, S43–s48.

Merlo, L. J., Curran, J. S. & Watson, R. 2017. Gender differences in substance use and psychiatric distress among medical students: A comprehensive statewide evaluation. *Subst Abus*, 38, 401–406.

Michalec, B. & Keyes, C. L. 2013. A multidimensional perspective of the mental health of preclinical medical students. *Psychol Health Med*, 18, 89–97.

Millard, M. L. 2011. *Psychological net worth: Finding the balance between psychological capital and psychological debt*. 72, ProQuest Information & Learning.

Modell, H. I., Demiero, F. G. & Rose, L. 2009. In pursuit of a holistic learning environment: the impact of music in the medical physiology classroom. *Adv Physiol Educ*, 33, 37–45.

Monrad, S. U., Zaidi, N. L. B., Gruppen, L. D., Gelb, D. J., Grum, C., Morgan, H. K., Daniel, M., Mangrulkar, R. S. & Santen, S. A. 2018. Does Reducing Clerkship Lengths by 25% Affect Medical Student Performance and Perceptions? *Acad Med*, 93, 1833–1840.

Morgan, T. L., Mcfadden, T., Fortier, M. S., Tomasone, J. R. & Sweet, S. N. 2020. Positive mental health and burnout in first to fourth year medical students. *Health Education Journal*, 79, 948–962.

Morra, D. J., Regehr, G. & Ginsburg, S. 2008. Anticipated debt and financial stress in medical students. *Med Teach*, 30, 313–315.

Morris, A., DO, D., Gottlieb-Smith, R., NG, J., Jain, A., Wright, S. & Shochet, R. 2012. Impact of a fitness intervention on medical students. *South Med J*, 105, 630–634.

Mosley, T. H., JR., Perrin, S. G., Neral, S. M., Dubbert, P. M., Grothues, C. A. & Pinto, B. M. 1994. Stress, coping, and well-being among third-year medical students. *Acad Med*, 69, 765–767.

Nagji, A., Brett-Maclean, P. & Breault, L. 2013. Exploring the Benefits of an Optional Theatre Module on Medical Student Well-Being. *Teaching and Learning in Medicine*, 25, 201–206.

Nakashima, E. N., Sutton, C. X. Y., Yamamoto, L. G. & Len, K. A. 2020. Wellness Curriculum in the Pediatric Clerkship. *Hawaii J Health Soc Welf*, 79, 50–54.

Nandi, M., Hazra, A., Sarkar, S., Mondal, R. & Ghosal, M. K. 2012. Stress and its risk factors in medical students: an observational study from a medical college in India. *Indian J Med Sci*, 66, 1–12.

Neufeld, A. & Malin, G. 2019. Exploring the relationship between medical student basic psychological need satisfaction, resilience, and well-being: a quantitative study. *Bmc Medical Education*, 19, 405.

Neufeld, A., Mossière, A. & Malin, G. 2020. Basic psychological needs, more than mindfulness and resilience, relate to medical student stress: A case for shifting the focus of wellness curricula. *Med Teach*, 42, 1401–1412.

Nisar, N., Zehra, N., Haider, G., Munir, A. A. & Sohoo, N. A. 2008. Frequency, intensity and impact of premenstrual syndrome in medical students. *J Coll Physicians Surg Pak*, 18, 481–484.

Pagnin, D. & DE Queiroz, V. 2015. Comparison of quality of life between medical students and young general populations. *Educ Health (Abingdon)*, 28, 209–212.

Pankey, T. L. 2019. *Risk and Resilience: A Preliminary Examination of the Race-Based Disparities in Stress and Sleep in Context Model among Black Medical Students*. Ph.D., The University of Wisconsin, Madison.

Park, C. & Adler, N. 2003. Coping Style as a Predictor of Health and Well-Being Across the First Year of Medical School. *Health psychology: official journal of the Division of Health Psychology, American Psychological Association*, 22, 627–631.

Patel, R. S., Tarrant, C., Bonas, S. & Shaw, R. L. 2015. Medical students' personal experience of high-stakes failure: Case studies using interpretative phenomenological analysis. Bmc medical education. *Bmc medical education* [Online]. Available: https://doi.org/10.1186/s12909-015-0371-9 [Accessed 14/10/2022].

Perry, S. P., Hardeman, R., Burke, S. E., Cunningham, B., Burgess, D. J. & Van Ryn, M. 2016. The Impact of Everyday Discrimination and Racial Identity Centrality on African American Medical Student Well-Being: a Report from the Medical Student Change Study. *J Racial Ethn Health Disparities*, 3, 519–526.

Phelan, S. M., Burgess, D. J., Puhl, R., Dyrbye, L. N., Dovidio, J. F., Yeazel, M., Ridgeway, J. L., Nelson, D., Perry, S., Przedworski, J. M., Burke, S. E., Hardeman, R. R. & Van Ryn, M. 2015. The Adverse Effect of Weight Stigma on the Well-Being of Medical Students with Overweight or Obesity: Findings from a National Survey. *J Gen Intern Med*, 30, 1251–1258.

Pisaniello, M. S., Asahina, A. T., Bacchi, S., Wagner, M., Perry, S. W., Wong, M.-L. & Licinio, J. 2019. Effect of medical student debt on mental health, academic performance and specialty choice: a systematic review. *Bmj Open*, 9, e029980.

Pontell, M. E., Makhoul, A. T., Ganesh Kumar, N. & Drolet, B. C. 2021. The Change of Usmle Step 1 to Pass/Fail: Perspectives of the Surgery Program Director. *J Surg Educ*, 78, 91–98.

Potash, J. S., Chen, J. Y. & Tsang, J. P. 2016. Medical student mandala making for holistic well-being. *Med Humanit*, 42, 17–25.

Przedworski, J. 2019. *Medical Socialization & Its Discontents: Heteronormativity in US Medical Schools & Its Impact on Student Psychological Distress*. Ph.D., University of Minnesota.

Rashid, A. A., Shariff Ghazali, S., Mohamad, I., Mawardi, M., Roslan, D. & Musa, H. 2019. Quasi-experimental study on the effectiveness of a house officer preparatory course for medical graduates on self-perceived confidence and readiness: a study protocol. *Bmj Open*, 9, e024488.

Reed, D. A., Shanafelt, T. D., Satele, D. W., Power, D. V., Eacker, A., Harper, W., Moutier, C., Durning, S., Massie, F. S., JR., Thomas, M. R., Sloan, J. A. & Dyrbye, L. N. 2011. Relationship of pass/fail grading and curriculum structure with well-being among preclinical medical students: a multi-institutional study. *Acad Med*, 86, 1367–1373.

Rogers, M., Searle, J., Creed, P. & NG, S. K. A. 2010. A multivariate analysis of personality, values and expectations as correlates of career aspirations of final year medical students. *International Journal for Educational and Vocational Guidance*, 10, 177–189.

Rogers, M. E., Creed, P. A. & Searle, J. 2012. Person and environmental factors associated with well-being in medical students. *Personality and Individual Differences*, 52, 472–477.

Roling, G., Lutz, G., Edelhäuser, F., Hofmann, M., Valk-Draad, M. P., Wack, C., Haramati, A., Tauschel, D. & Scheffer, C. 2020. Empathy, well-being and stressful experiences in the clinical learning environment. *Patient Educ Couns*, 103, 2320–2327.

Rutledge, C. M., Davies, S. M. & Davies, T. C. 1994. Family dysfunction and the well-being of medical students. *Family Systems Medicine*, 12, 197–204.

Ryan, G., Marley, I., Still, M., Lyons, Z. & Hood, S. 2017. Use of mental-health services by Australian medical students: a cross-sectional survey. *Australas Psychiatry*, 25, 407–410.

Saikal, A., Pit, S. W. & Mccarthy, L. 2020. Medical student well-being during rural clinical placement: A cross-sectional national survey. *Medical Education*, 54, 547–558.

Saleem, S. & Saleem, T. 2017. Role of Religiosity in Psychological Well-Being Among Medical and Non-medical Students. *J Relig Health*, 56, 1180–1190.

Salehi, A., Marzban, M. & Imanieh, M. H. 2017. Spiritual Well-Being and Related Factors in Iranian Medical Students. *Journal of Spirituality in Mental Health*, 19, 306–317.

Sankoh, V. 2019. *Mindfulness in medicine: Modified Mindfulness-Based Stress Reduction (Mbsr) program among future doctors* [Online]. Cuny Academic Works. Available: https://academicworks.cuny.edu/gc_etds/3081 [Accessed 14/10/2022].

Shapiro, J., Kasman, D. & Shafer, A. 2006. Words and Wards: A Model of Reflective Writing and Its Uses in Medical Education. *Journal of Medical Humanities*, 27, 231–244.

Simard, A. A. & Henry, M. 2009. Impact of a short yoga intervention on medical students' health: a pilot study. *Med Teach*, 31, 950–952.

Simon, C. R. & Durand-Bush, N. 2009. Learning to self-regulate multi-dimensional felt experiences: The cases of four female medical students. *International Journal of Qualitative Studies on Health and Well-being*, 4, 228–244.

Skokou, M., Sakellaropoulos, G., Zairi, N.-A., Gourzis, P. & Andreopoulou, O. 2021. An Exploratory Study of Trait Emotional Intelligence and Mental Health in Freshmen Greek Medical Students. *Current Psychology*, 40, 6057–6066.

Sletta, C., Tyssen, R. & Løvseth, L. T. 2019. Change in subjective well-being over 20 years at two Norwegian medical schools and factors linked to well-being today: a survey. *Bmc Med Educ*, 19, 45.

Spring, L., Robillard, D., Gehlbach, L. & Simas, T. A. 2011. Impact of pass/fail grading on medical students' well-being and academic outcomes. *Med Educ*, 45, 867–877.

Strayhorn, G. & Frierson, H. 1989. Assessing correlations between Black and white students' perceptions of the medical school learning environment, their academic performances, and their well-being. *Acad Med*, 64, 468–473.

Suárez, D. E., Cardozo, A. C., Villarreal, M. E. & Trujillo, E. M. 2021. Non-Heterosexual Medical Students Are Critically Vulnerable to Mental Health Risks: The Need to Account for Sexual Diversity in Wellness Initiatives. *Teach Learn Med*, 33, 1–9.

Tackett, S., Wright, S., Colbert-Getz, J. & Shochet, R. 2018. Associations between learning community engagement and burnout, quality of life, and empathy among medical students. *Int J Med Educ*, 9, 316–322.

Tackett, S., Wright, S., Lubin, R., LI, J. & Pan, H. 2017. International study of medical school learning environments and their relationship with student well-being and empathy. *Med Educ*, 51, 280–289.

Terebessy, A., Czeglédi, E., Balla, B. C., Horváth, F. & Balázs, P. 2016. Medical students' health behaviour and self-reported mental health status by their country of origin: a cross-sectional study. *Bmc Psychiatry*, 16, 171.

Thomas, M. R., Dyrbye, L. N., Huntington, J. L., Lawson, K. L., Novotny, P. J., Sloan, J. A. & Shanafelt, T. D. 2007. How do distress and well-being relate to medical student empathy? A multicenter study. *J Gen Intern Med*, 22, 177–183.

Torales, J., Kadhum, M., Zárate, G., Barrios, I., González, I., Farrell, S. M., Ventriglio, A. & Arce, A. 2019. Wellbeing and mental health among medical students in Paraguay. *Int Rev Psychiatry*, 31, 598–602.

Trucchia, S. M., Lucchese, M. S., Enders, J. E. & Fernández, A. R. 2013. Relationship between academic performance, psychological well-being, and coping strategies in medical students. *Rev Fac Cien Med Univ Nac Cordoba*, 70, 144–152.

Tucker, P., Jeon-Slaughter, H., Sener, U., Arvidson, M. & Khalafian, A. 2015. Do medical student stress, health, or quality of life foretell step 1 scores? A comparison of students in traditional and revised preclinical curricula. *Teach Learn Med*, 27, 63–70.

Turner, T., Tee, Q. X., Hasimoglu, G., Hewitt, J., Trinh, D., Shachar, J., Sekhar, P. & Green, S. 2020. Mindfulness-based psychological interventions for improving mental well-being in medical students and junior doctors. *Cochrane Database of Systematic Reviews*.

Van Dijk, I., Lucassen, P. L. B. J., Van Weel, C. & Speckens, A. E. M. 2017. A cross-sectional examination of psychological distress, positive mental health and their predictors in medical students in their clinical clerkships. *Bmc Medical Education*, 17, 219.

Van Remortel, B., Dolan, E., Cipriano, D. & Mcbride, P. 2018. Medical Student Wellness in Wisconsin: Current Trends and Future Directions. *Wmj*, 117, 211–213.

Volpe, U., Ventriglio, A., Bellomo, A., Kadhum, M., Lewis, T., Molodynski, A., Sampogna, G. & Fiorillo, A. 2019. Mental health and wellbeing among Italian medical students: a descriptive study. *Int Rev Psychiatry*, 31, 569–573.

Voltmer, E., Kieschke, U., Schwappach, D. L. B., Wirsching, M. & Spahn, C. 2008. Psychosocial health risk factors and resources of medical students and physicians: a cross-sectional study. *Bmc Medical Education*, 8, 46.

Wasson, L. T., Cusmano, A., Meli, L., Louh, I., Falzon, L., Hampsey, M., Young, G., Shaffer, J. & Davidson, K. W. 2016. Association Between Learning Environment Interventions and Medical Student Well-being: A Systematic Review. *Jama*, 316, 2237–2252.

Welcome, M. O., Razvodovsky, Y. E., Pereverzeva, E. V. & Pereverzev, V. A. 2014. Cognitive functions and neuropsychological status of medical students with different attitudes to alcohol use: a study conducted at the Belarusian State Medical University, Minsk, Belarus. *Physiol Behav*, 128, 108–113.

Wilkes, C., Lewis, T., Brager, N., Bulloch, A., Macmaster, F., Paget, M., Holm, J., Farrell, S. M. & Ventriglio, A. 2019. Wellbeing and mental health amongst medical students in Canada. *Int Rev Psychiatry*, 31, 584–587.

Williams, M. K., Estores, I. M. & Merlo, L. J. 2020. Promoting Resilience in Medicine: The Effects of a Mind-Body Medicine Elective to Improve Medical Student Well-being. *Glob Adv Health Med*, 9, 2164956120927367.

Winter, R. I., Patel, R. & Norman, R. I. 2017. A Qualitative Exploration of the Help-Seeking Behaviors of Students Who Experience Psychological Distress Around Assessment at Medical School. *Acad Psychiatry*, 41, 477–485.

Worobetz, A., Retief, P. J., Loughran, S., Walsh, J., Casey, M., Hayes, P., Bengoechea, E. G., O'Regan, A., Woods, C., Kelly, D., Connor, R. O., Grath, D. M. & Glynn, L. G. 2020. A feasibility study of an exercise intervention to educate and promote health and well-being among medical students: the 'Med-Well' programme. *Bmc Medical Education*, 20, 183.

XU, Y.-Y., WU, T., YU, Y.-J. & LI, M. 2019. A randomized controlled trial of well-being therapy to promote adaptation and alleviate emotional distress among medical freshmen. *Bmc Medical Education*, 19, 182.

XU, Y. Y., Feng, Z. Q., Xie, Y. J., Zhang, J., Peng, S. H., YU, Y. J. & LI, M. 2018. Frontal Alpha Eeg Asymmetry Before and After Positive Psychological Interventions for Medical Students. *Front Psychiatry*, 9, 432.

Yamada, Y., Klugar, M., Ivanova, K. & Oborna, I. 2014. Psychological distress and academic self-perception among international medical students: the role of peer social support. *Bmc Med Educ*, 14, 256.

Yen-JU Lin, B., Liu, P. C., KU, K. T. & Lee, C. C. 2019. Adaptation of Medical Students During Clinical Training: Effects of Holistic Preclinical Education on Clerkship Performance. *Teach Learn Med*, 31, 65–75.

Yielder, J., Wearn, A., Chen, Y., Henning, M. A., Weller, J., Lillis, S., Mogol, V. & Bagg, W. 2017. A qualitative exploration of student perceptions of the impact of progress tests on learning and emotional wellbeing. *Bmc Medical Education*, 17, 148.

Yousafzai, A. W., Ahmer, S., Syed, E., Bhutto, N., Iqbal, S., Siddiqi, M. N. & Zaman, M. 2009. Well-being of medical students and their awareness on substance misuse: a cross-sectional survey in Pakistan. *Ann Gen Psychiatry*, 8, 8.

Yusoff, M. S., Yaacob, M. J., Naing, N. N. & Esa, A. R. 2013. Psychometric properties of the Medical Student Well-Being Index among medical students in a Malaysian medical school. *Asian J Psychiatr*, 6, 60–65.

Yusoff, M. S.B. & Fuad, A. 2010. Impact Of Medical Student Well-Being Workshop On The Medical Students' Stress Level: A Preliminary Study. *Asean Journal of Psychiatry*, 11, 6.

Zanardelli, G., Sim, W., Borges, N., & Roman, B. 2015. Well-being in first year medical students. *Acad Psychiatry*, 39, 31–36.

PART 2

6

Brazil

Mental Health of Brazilian Medical Students

Israel Kanaan Blaas and João Mauricio Castaldelli-Maia

Introduction

Because of their contributions throughout history, universities can be considered one of the primary engines of human development. The university environment, on the other hand, can be characterized by a wide range of negative outcomes, such as an excessive workload and high levels of stress, competitiveness, and sleep deprivation. Furthermore, university admission usually occurs in early adulthood, a time when people are more vulnerable to developing mental health problems. These factors may provide a plausible explanation for why college students have higher rates of mental disorders than their non-college counterparts and the general population, and why medical students have more disorders than their non-medical college student counterparts.

This chapter will discuss the major aspects of depression, anxiety, burnout, and alcohol and drug use among Brazilian medical students.

Depression and Anxiety

According to Brazilian studies, medical students have high rates of depression and anxiety, with the prevalence of depression and anxiety in this subpopulation being around 30%. These findings show a high prevalence of anxiety, depression, and stress among medical students, with statistically significant differences across semesters, as well as the impact of several factors such as gender and religiosity on students' emotional states (Brenneisen Mayer et al., 2016). Stress in this group may stem from the nature and workload inherent in the medical course, as well as the academic structure and its teaching methods. Indeed, the start of a medical degree is fraught with difficulties from the very beginning with the selection process, which is undeniably competitive and has a high cut-off point, particularly in public institutions. There is a certain kudos bestowed upon medical students by society, based on the implicit dream of economic success, which may lead to excessive expectations and frustration (Moutinho et al., 2017; Rotenstein et al., 2016).

In Brazil, medical students typically prepare for graduation and commit to beginning their career during the twelfth semester, the final semester before graduation (i.e. six-year course). This period is distinguished by reparation for medical residency tests in the chosen area of specialization, where selection processes are extremely competitive and residency vacancies

Israel Kanaan Blaas and João Mauricio Castaldelli-Maia, *Brazil* In: *The Mental Health of Medical Students*.
Edited by: Andrew Molodynski, Sarah Marie Farrell, and Dinesh Bhugra, Oxford University Press. © Oxford University Press 2024.
DOI: 10.1093/oso/9780192864871.003.0006

are scarce. The increase in stress and lack of time, as well as conflicts in selecting a specialty, probably explain why candidates in their final semesters of college are stressed (Moutinho et al., 2017). Female medical students experience more depressive and anxious symptoms than their male counterparts. This prevalence is also found in the general population when comparing men to women (Rotenstein et al., 2016).

It has also been established that sleep disorders are very common in the overall Brazilian population, with medical students being a particularly vulnerable group. Sleep disorders are more common in medical students than in non-medical students. Many factors contribute to the high prevalence of sleep problems among medical students, including long hours of class and study, night work, emotional stress, lifestyle choices, and extensive use of virtual social networks. Sleep deprivation can make medical students more susceptible to depressive and anxiety disorders. There is robust evidence that getting enough sleep is important for long-term learning, neurocognitive, and psychomotor performance, physical and mental health, and preventing mood and anxiety symptoms (Perotta et al., 2021).

Burnout

A three-dimensional notion known as burnout syndrome is defined as a response to persistent emotional suffering related to working circumstances. It is distinguished among students studying medicine by:

1) fatigue in relation to academic activities
2) disbelief and distancing from studies and patients
3) feeling of incompetence.

The frequency of burnout is almost 50% in the population of medical students (Abreu et al., 2022). This number has grown over the past decade and is notably increasing in residency programmes, reaching 60%, and suggesting that physicians have possibly carried a burden of burnout symptoms since graduation (Abreu et al., 2022).

Several studies have found that Brazilian medical students, on average, have a higher rate of burnout than students from other fields. This raises the possibility that, throughout medical education, factors related to the academic context are combined with individual predispositions, resulting in the emergence of high levels of burnout throughout the medical course. Support from family, friends, and colleagues, as well as high levels of religious observance/spirituality, have been found to be inversely related to the frequency of burnout in medical students, making them protective factors against burnout (Dias et al., 2022).

The protective effect of resilience in this population is illustrated by the finding that students with low or moderate levels of it experience burnout at a rate that is four times greater than that of students with high levels of resilience (Dias et al., 2022). In this way, it seems logical to draw the conclusion that pupils who are better at coping with stress are also better at adjusting to challenging circumstances. Brazilian medical students are more vulnerable than the general population due to their lower levels of resilience, which may be a result of a lack of psychological resources to deal with or lessen the impact of stressors (Solis & Lotufo-Neto, 2019).

Male medical students are more prone to burnout in Brazil. When compared to being married, being single is associated with a fivefold increase in the likelihood of burnout. Furthermore, marital status is a separate predictor of protection. It's possible that factors related to relationship stability, like emotional support from a partner, are linked to lower levels of burnout. Students with lower family incomes (from $250 to $749 per month) had a higher prevalence of burnout, which may be explained by the stress caused by the inability to help support the family, as only a minority of students would be able to coordinate work. As well as the research (Abreu et al., 2022).

When compared to internship and basic cycle students, clinical cycle students (7th to 12th semester) have a higher rate of burnout. This could be related to the gap between students' expectations and reality when it comes to their first contact with patients and the public health system. When the limitations of medical treatment are perceived in the face of chronic, incurable, or often fatal conditions, this moment can be frustrating. We can also imagine that during the basic cycle, students' satisfaction with their recent college entrance exam approval would be dominant, whereas the internship period would be marked by excitement about the impending graduation. On the contrary, the clinical cycle would be an intermediate stage in which the anxiety accumulated up to this point is combined even more with future concerns. Finally, contact with the patient in a context of inexperience, as is typical of the clinical cycle, may predispose students to increased anxiety and an increased risk of burnout (Abreu et al., 2022; Dias et al., 2022).

Alcohol and Drugs

Academic students are a vulnerable population when it comes to substance abuse. The consumption of alcohol, legal, and illegal drugs among university students is increasing, a real cause of concern in many countries. It is even more troubling when we consider that medical students will soon be the professionals in charge of identifying and treating this condition. Furthermore, many physicians are still known to regard substance abuse as a social or moral issue rather than a medical one (Mesquita et al., 1997).

Alcohol consumption is a major public health issue and a major cause of global suffering. Health issues and the social consequences of different patterns of alcohol consumption across continents and countries are of particular concern. According to the most recent World Health Organization (WHO) report (2019), approximately three million people died per year as a result of harmful alcohol use (5.13% of all deaths). Binge drinking is lower in adolescents (15–19 years old) than in the general population, but it is highest in those 20–24 years old worldwide. University students deserve special consideration among this age group. College students are more likely to engage in substance abuse behaviours as a result of lifestyle changes, decreased parental support, and stress. Another growing concern is the dangers of combining alcohol and energy drinks (i.e. substance interactions). According to epidemiological studies, consumers who consume energy drinks are more likely to have a higher concentration of alcohol on their breath than those who do not; are more likely to consume alcohol in larger quantities, engage in aggressive behaviour, suffer injuries, and exhibit symptoms of alcohol dependence, in addition to being at a higher risk of cardiovascular disease (Nasui et al., 2021).

Medical students are known to suffer from high levels of stress and psychological morbidity, such as depression, anxiety, and burnout. They are more likely to use substances to cope with stress, such as alcohol or other drugs, and this stress leads to lower academic success (Rotenstein et al., 2016).

Except for alcohol, tranquilizers, and psychedelics, which are common in medical students, studies show that drug use by medical students is not particularly high when compared to drug use by other young adults of the same age (Lambert Passos et al., 2006; Newbury-Birch et al., 2000). 49% of male and 43% of female medical students reported drinking above the 'low risk' level of alcohol, compared to 41% of men and only 24% of women in the 18–24-year age group in the general population. However, their level of drug use becomes a serious issue when we consider that medical students are a population that should be better informed about and understand the risks and consequences of drug abuse (Mesquita et al., 1998).

According to several Brazilian studies, alcohol and tobacco are usually the first drugs that adolescents try, and they may be the two drugs with the highest prevalence of consumption throughout life in most countries. According to studies, the most common sequence of drug use in this population of medical students is as follows: alcohol and/or tobacco consumption in the first stage, cannabis and/or inhalants consumption in the second stage, and other drugs consumption in the third stage, with inhalants such as 'lança' being closely linked to the combined consumption of alcohol and cannabis (Castaldelli-Maia et al., 2014). Because 'lança' use is toxic and potentially fatal, the observed association between lance perfume, alcohol, and cannabis use should be considered when designing education and other prevention programmes for the medical student population. Students who drink are more likely to smoke tobacco, and those who are already dependent on tobacco smoke even more when they drink alcohol (Castaldelli-Maia et al., 2015; Di Pietro et al., 2007; Mesquita et al., 1998).

Many factors contribute to gender differences in legal and illegal drug abuse. Women frequently report using legal and illegal drugs as a coping mechanism, whereas men have more positive attitudes towards illicit drug use. For example, the nature of the individual's relationship with his or her social environment may be particularly relevant to the phenomenon of alcohol consumption in college, as the college years are typically a time of increased alcohol consumption. Interaction with others. While men are more likely to use inhalants and cannabis, women are more likely to use amphetamines and tranquilizers, with alcohol showing a similar prevalence. However, females are increasingly using it (Wanger et al., 2007).

The lower prevalence of cocaine use among Brazilian medical students may be due to their exposure to the harmful effects of this substance during their training (Lambert Passos et al., 2006). Although this subpopulation is increasingly using tranquilizers and amphetamines, their greater understanding of the effects and properties of the drugs appears to give them a false sense of control over their own use of these substances. This, combined with easier access to medicines, raises the likelihood that medical students will select them as their preferred drug (Kanwal et al., 2018; Silveira et al., 2014).

Several Brazilian studies show higher levels of illicit drug use in the first academic years, particularly among students who live far from home and have higher levels of clinical stress symptoms, particularly when attempting to manage their lifestyle (academic stress). Illicit drug use (particularly inhalants) is more common among students in their early academic years. Thus, experimenting with drugs and regularly using them can be understood as a way for students in their first academic years to relieve psychological stress. Living with parents as opposed to living alone or with friends, is thus a protective factor against cannabis and other illicit drug use. Furthermore, as studies in other populations have shown, participation in some religious practices is a protective factor against the use of cannabis and other illicit drugs (Lambert Passos et al., 2006).

In Brazil, higher levels of abuse in the use of psychostimulants, alcohol, and psychedelics among students in the final period when compared to those in the first period, which can also be explained by greater knowledge of the subject, anxiety at higher levels due to the proximity of medical residency tests, as demonstrated by several studies in which final year medical students resort to non-prescription use of methylphenidate to increase their efficiency in studying (Oliveira et al., 2009).

Drug use by medical students can result in a variety of issues, depending on the student's level of involvement with the drug. The effects of occasional drug use are heavily dependent on the circumstances under which he uses the drug, and may not be noticeable until he suffers from severe impairment in concentration and performance difficulties. There is also an increased risk of abuse or dependence later in life, which has personal and social consequences. Any drug prevention/intervention programme should prioritize early detection of drug problems in this population, ideally while the student is still in medical school. Students must master principles of ethics and professional behaviour at the start of medical school, and because these principles apply to the illicit use of drugs and other potent psychoactive medications, this must be included in the curriculum. Interventions aimed at preventing the negative consequences of academic stress in medical students and improving their lifestyle/wellbeing (i.e. by promoting individual and social skills) can significantly alter their drug use patterns (Candido et al., 2018).

Conclusion

Several studies in Brazil have found equal or higher rates of anxiety, depression, alcohol and other drug use, and burnout than in other parts of the world in medical students (Baldassin et al., 2008; Baldasssin et al., 2013; Castaldelli-Maia et al., 2012). Hence, Brazilian medical schools should assist depressed and anxious students, especially those whose depression is persistent or whose anxiety prevents them from following the course normally, by establishing a system that identifies and supports them as early as possible, because studies show that students are hesitant to seek help. All intervention measures must be tailored to the specific needs of this important group of students, which necessitates the removal of barriers such as the stigma associated with seeking mental health treatment. Medical schools should also encourage students to seek anonymous mental healthcare from outside sources. Student wellness programmes that provide opportunities and resources for healthy living must be implemented in medical schools. These programmes may encourage students to cultivate empathy, stress management, professionalism, frustration tolerance, and active depression coping strategies, self-care based on depression self-diagnosis, knowledge of life contexts, academic and personal practices, maintenance, and the development of interests that are not related to medicine, such as regular physical activity. Its interventions, which include cognitive restructuring and problem-solving strategies, life skills and mindfulness therapy, individual counselling, adaptive and communication skills training, physical activity, and social training, can all be included in the curriculum.

In the FMABC Medical School, there have been changes in the curriculum during the last decade, such as the reduction of workload through the optimization of time with more efficient classes and the exclusion of non-essential content, the removal of Saturday activities and the creation of a period of free time one afternoon a week, as well as the great encouragement of sports practice within the university campus. The medical students confirmed the changes, especially acknowledging the introduction of new electives as part of the changed curriculum. These changes occurred in the clinical and internal placements. These changes were seen as a positive change, along with an increase in scholarship and faculty support (Baldassin et al., 2008; Baldasssin et al., 2013; Castaldelli-Maia et al., 2012).

Medical schools can promote mental health by recognizing and appreciating the individual characteristics and psychological function of the medical student. This will benefit the medical education sector, the medical industry, medical professionals' resilience and satisfaction, and the quality of patient care. Therefore, Brazilian medical schools should prioritize interventions with the potential to increase resilience, such as encouraging physical activity in the curriculum, extracurricular activities, and social life, to reduce burnout among their students, in addition to providing reception mental health services. Finally, the detection of trends in alcohol and drug use by Brazilian medical students over time is a critical step in prevention and treatment programming, allowing you to choose what future actions should be taken through conferences, the implementation of drug use policies in colleges, and preventive programmes.

References

Abreu Alves, S., Sinval, J., Lucas Neto, L., Marôco, J., Gonçalves Ferreira, A., & Oliveira, P. (2022). 'Burnout and dropout intention in medical students: the protective role of academic engagement'. *BMC Med Educ* **22**(1): 83.

Baldassin, S., Silva, N., de Toledo Ferraz Alves, T.C., Castaldelli-Maia, J.M., Bhugra, D., Nogueira-Martins, M.C., de Andrade, A.G., & Nogueira-Martins, L.A. (2013). 'Depression in medical students: cluster symptoms and management'. *J Affect Disord* **150**(1): 110–114.

Baldassin, S., Alves, T.C., Andrade, A.G., & Nogueira-Martins, L.A. (2008). 'The characteristics of depressive symptoms in medical students during medical education and training: a cross-sectional study'. *BMC Med Educ* **8**: 60.

Brenneisen Mayer, F., Souza Santos, I., Silveira, P.S.P., Itaqui Lopes, M.H., de Souza, A.R., Campos, E.P., de Abreu, B.A., Hoffman Ii, I., Magalhães, C.R., Lima, M.C., Almeida, R., Spinardi, M., & Tempski, P. (2016). 'Factors associated to depression and anxiety in medical students: a multicenter study'. *BMC Med Educ* **16**: 282.

Candido, F.J., Souza, R., Stumpf, M.A., Fernandes, L.G., Veiga, R., Santin, M., & Kluthcovsky, A. (2018). 'The use of drugs and medical students: a literature review'. *Rev Assoc Med Bras (1992)* **64**(5): 462–468.

Castaldelli-Maia, J.M., Martins, S.S., Bhugra, D., Machado, M.P., Andrade, A.G., Alexandrino-Silva, C., Baldassin, S., & de Toledo Ferraz Alves, T.C. (2012). 'Does ragging play a role in medical student depression—cause or effect?' *J Affect Disord* **139**(3): 291–297.

Castaldelli-Maia, J.M., Martins, S.S., de Oliveira, L.G., de Andrade, A.G., & Nicastri S. (2015). 'The role of drug use sequencing pattern in further problematic use of alcohol, tobacco, cannabis, and other drugs'. *J Ment Health* **24**(1): 9–14.

Castaldelli-Maia, J.M., Nicastri, S., Garcia de Oliveira, L., Guerra de Andrade, A., & Martins, S.S. (2014). 'The role of first use of inhalants within sequencing pattern of first use of drugs among Brazilian university students'. *Exp Clin Psychopharmacol* **22**(6): 530–540.

Dias, A.R, Fernandes, S.M., Fialho-Silva, I., Cerqueira-Silva, T., Miranda-Scippa, Â., & Almeida, A.G. (2022). 'Burnout syndrome and resilience in medical students from a Brazilian public college in Salvador, Brazil'. *Trends Psychiatry Psychother* 44: e20200187.

Di Pietro, M.C., Doering-Silveira, E.B., Oliveira, M.P., Rosa-Oliveira, L.Q., & Da Silveira, D.X. (2007). 'Factors associated with the use of solvents and cannabis by medical students'. *Addict Behav* 32(8): 1740–1744.

Kanwal, Z.G., Fatima, N., Azhar, S., Chohan, O., Jabeen, M., & Yameen, M.A. (2018). 'Implications of self-medication among medical students-A dilemma'. *J Pak Med Assoc* 68(9): 1363–1367.

Lambert Passos, S.R., Alvarenga Americano do Brasil, P.E., Borges dos Santos, M.A., & Costa de Aquino, M.T. (2006). 'Prevalence of psychoactive drug use among medical students in Rio de Janeiro'. *Soc Psychiatry Psychiatr Epidemiol* 41(12): 989–996.

Mesquita, A.M., de Andrade, A.G., & Anthony, J.C. (1998). 'Use of the inhalant lança by Brazilian medical students'. *Subst Use Misuse* 33(8): 1667–1680.

Mesquita, A.M., Laranjeira, R., & Dunn, J. (1997). 'Psychoactive drug use by medical students: a review of the national and international literature'. *Sao Paulo Med J* 115(1): 1356–1365.

Moutinho, I.L., Maddalena, N.C., Roland, R.K., Lucchetti, A.L., Tibiriçá, S.H., Ezequiel, O.D., & Lucchetti, G. (2017). 'Depression, stress and anxiety in medical students: a cross-sectional comparison between students from different semesters'. *Rev Assoc Med Bras (1992)* 63(1): 21–28.

Nasui, B.A., Popa, M., Buzoianu, A.D., Pop, A.L., Varlas, V.N., Armean, S.M., & Popescu, C.A. (2021). 'Alcohol consumption and behavioral consequences in Romanian medical university students'. *Int J Environ Res Public Health* 18(14): 7531.

Newbury-Birch, D., White, M., & Kamali, F. (2000). 'Factors influencing alcohol and illicit drug use amongst medical students'. *Drug Alcohol Depend* 59: 125–130.

Oliveira, L.G., Barroso, L.P., Wagner, G.A., Ponce Jde, C., Malbergier, A., Stempliuk Vde, A., & Andrade, A.G. (2009). 'Drug consumption among medical students in São Paulo, Brazil: influences of gender and academic year'. *Braz J Psychiatry* 31(3): 227–239.

Perotta, B., Arantes-Costa, F.M., Enns, S.C., Figueiro-Filho, E.A., Paro, H., Santos, I.S., Lorenzi-Filho, G., Martins, M.A., & Tempski, P.Z. (2021). 'Sleepiness, sleep deprivation, quality of life, mental symptoms and perception of academic environment in medical students'. *BMC Med Educ* 21: 111.

Rotenstein, L.S., Ramos, M.A., Torre, M., Segal, J.B., Peluso, M.J., Guille, C., Sen, S., & Mata, D.A. (2016). 'Prevalence of depression, depressive symptoms, and suicidal ideation among medical students: a systematic review and meta-analysis'. *JAMA* 316(21): 2214–2236.

Silveira, R. da R., Lejderman, B., Ferreira, P.E., & Rocha, G.M. (2014). 'Patterns of non-medical use of methylphenidate among 5th and 6th year students in a medical school in southern Brazil'. *Trends Psychiatry Psychother* 36(2): 101–106.

Solis, Ana C. & Lotufo-Neto, F. (2019). 'Predictors of quality of life in Brazilian medical students: a systematic review and meta-analysis'. *Braz J Psychiatry* 41(6): 556–567.

Wagner, G.A., Stempliuk Vde, A., Zilberman, M.L., Barroso, L.P., & Andrade, A.G. (2007). 'Alcohol and drug use among university students: gender differences'. *Braz J Psychiatry* 29(2): 123–129.

World Health Organization (2019). *Global Status Report on Alcohol And Health 2018*. Geneva: World Health Organization.

7

Canada

A Review of Canadian Medical Student Wellbeing

Nancy Brager, Mike Paget, Johanna Holm, and T. Christopher R. Wilkes

Introduction

Canada is a vast and rugged land, stretching almost 4,700 miles (7,560 kilometres) across six time zones. It is the second-largest country in the world, but it has only one-half of 1% of the world's population. Canada is a wealthy nation dominated by the service industry and rich in various resources such as petroleum and natural gases.

The population of Canada is approximately 38 million. Ethnic origins include 72.9% European, Asian 4.9%, Indigenous 3.1%, African 1.3%, and Latin American 0.2%. Canada also led the world in 2020 in the percentage of the adult population that had tertiary education (a bachelor's degree or higher) with around 64% of those aged 25 to 34 having completed tertiary education. Application to medical school is popular and fiercely competitive and students need a good Grade Point Average (GPA) for medical school in Canada, usually 3.8 to 4. See Table 7.1 (then published in MacLean, 2016).

There are 17 medical schools across Canada with over 11,000 medical students. Canada graduates over 2,700 MDs per year. The Canadian medical schools are accredited by the Committee on Accreditation of Canadian Medical Schools (CACMS).

Previously Canadian schools were accredited by the Liaison Committee on Medical Education (LCME), which accredited both American and Canadian schools according to 12 standards. Both accrediting bodies emphasized, according to their standards, that schools must provide environments conducive to learning and appropriate student support services to promote academic, physical, and mental health. Providers of healthcare must not be involved in the student's academic decision-making in order for the student to proceed through their studies.

In 2020, 96.5% of Canadian medical school graduates (CMGs) successfully matched into a medical residency in Canada, compared to only 59.5 % of US medical school graduates (USMGs) and 29.2% of international medical school graduates (IMGs) who applied to Canadian medical residency programmes. However, this is no reason for complacency and final year medical students are very aware that there is considerable distress, pain, and suffering for medical students if they do not match. The tragic case of 25-year-old Robert Chu illustrates this well. He took his own life in September 2016 having been unsuccessful twice in landing a residency spot after medical school. The Canadian Resident Matching Service (CaRMS) process, with its personal letters and numerous interviews with programme directors, leads medical students into an impossible position to understand their status. Robert Chu used freedom of information laws to try and get details, feedback, and insight about his

Nancy Brager, Mike Paget, Johanna Holm, and T. Christopher R. Wilkes, *Canada* In: *The Mental Health of Medical Students*. Edited by: Andrew Molodynski, Sarah Marie Farrell, and Dinesh Bhugra, Oxford University Press. © Oxford University Press 2024. DOI: 10.1093/oso/9780192864871.003.0007

Table 7.1 Average GPA score for Canadian medical students

School	Total applicants	Total admitted	Average GPA (4.0 scale)	Average mCAT
Alberta	1,441	162	3.8	10.95
UBC	2,322	287	3.83*	10.9
Calgary	1,638	147	3.73	10.2
Dalhousie	1,181	115	3.8	9.67
Laval	2,391	233	N/A	Not required
Manitoba	971	110	N/A	10.98
McGill (5-Yr)	750	75	N/A	Not required
(4-yr)	2,005	122	N/A	N/A
McMaster	5,270	206	3.84	Not required
Memorial	710	80	3.85	9.53
Montréal (5-yr)	2,153	214	N/A	Not required
(4-yr)	656	89	N/A	Not required
Ottawa	4,298	163	3.93	Not required
Northern Ontario**	2,132	61	3.8	Not required
Queen's	4,683	100	N/A	N/A
Saskatchewan	694	98	N/A	10.21
Sherbrooke	2,697	208	N/A	Not required
Toronto	3,488	260	3.95	11.03
Western	2,479	170	N/A	11.79

*GPA is from fall 2014.

Reproduced with permission from 'Medical school in Canada: What does it take to get in?'

Comparing admission statistics from medical schools across the country'. Maclean's Universities Guidebook. Available at https://macleans.ca/education/medical-school-in-canada-what-does-it-take-to-get-in/

case. He was told during his first round of interviews that he was too broad with his electives at the expense of his choice of radiology. In his second round of interviews, Roberts's sincere interest in Psychiatry was questioned because of his publications in radiology.

In Canada each year there are a number of medical students who do not get matched. This puts hundreds of thousands of dollars that provincial government invest in education and tutoring future doctors at risk. The head of the association of faculties of medicine of Canada, Dr Genevieve Moineau was quoted in the Toronto Star in 2017 as saying, the unmatched students are victims of a system that no longer meets their needs. Growing numbers of graduates find themselves denied access to residency because they are caught in a regulated system where provincial governments limit the number of residency slots based on the assessed needs of the population. However, we must also recognize that there is also a burden on the postgraduate medical offices to ensure a correct fit for the newly graduated doctor.

In addition to the CaRMS stress, the pandemic added more stressors for students and programmes. Different schools pose unique stressors for students. The University of Calgary and McMaster University are the only 3-year medical schools in Canada and these shorter courses make interruptions in clinical education additionally stressful such as happened during the pandemic lockdown. The geography of Canada may isolate some schools from each other, as well as the student support systems from the student. This was amplified by the pandemic travel restrictions. Nationally, all visiting electives were cancelled. These electives were one of the most important means by which students and schools could evaluate other school's postgraduate training programmes.

Across Canada, students were pulled from clinical rotations and in-person classroom teaching according to pandemic protocols, impacting relationships with faculty mentors and peers, as well as clinical education and experience. The impact on student mental health is an obvious concern for all in the medical community. Across the 17 medical schools, there are provisions to provide a variety of resources for students to seek and receive mental healthcare as is appropriate.

The Canadian Medical Association (CMA) published a paper on medical schools addressing student anxiety, burnout, and depression in 2017 (Glauser, 2017). They found that 37% of medical students met the criteria for burnout. Consequently, there were calls for action to address cultural factors such as normalizing a 70hr work week, a culture of denial, and the persistence of the status quo. Interestingly the CMA released preliminary data recently from a repeat survey done in November 2021, the middle of the COVID-19 pandemic. This included 4,000 responses and revealed that 59% of physicians reported worsening of their mental health during the pandemic, attributed to loss of work-life balance and rapidly changing policies. Nearly half of the Physicians 47% reported low levels of social wellbeing, which has increased from 29% in2017. Emotional and psychological wellbeing had also suffered compared to pre-pandemic levels.

Survey Findings at the University of Calgary Cummings Medical School

A core study group in the UK collaborated with 12 countries around the world to review medical student wellness. In this context, we surveyed 101 medical students in 2021 at the Cummings medical school, Calgary during the height of the COVID-19 pandemic regarding their wellbeing and mental health. We surveyed a smaller group in 2019, 69 medical students, and these two surveys are remarkably consistent despite the COVID-19 pandemic.

Students at the Cumming School of Medicine in Calgary, Alberta, were asked to complete a one-off survey, which formed part of an international collaboration looking at mental health and wellbeing in medical students around the globe.

The survey aimed to quantify and characterize difficulties medical students face concerning stressors, psychological distress, and psychiatric morbidity using standardized, reliable, and valid instruments. In the process of the survey, we aimed to encourage students to self-reflect on wellbeing and self-care.

The survey included:

1. Demographic information including a year of study, age, gender, educational level Of parents.

2. Previous mental health issues prior to medical school entry, if any.
3. Short-form general health questionnaire (GHQ-12) to identify minor Psychiatric disorders.
4. The Oldenburg Burnout Inventory (OLBI).

Access to the survey was emailed to all current medical students at the 3-year Cumming School of Medicine in Canada. Information was provided to students regarding the nature of the study and that data collected would be anonymous. Data was stored anonymously and password protected, with only the study team having access. The students were not required to give personal identifiers as part of the survey. We used an independent, University of Calgary provisioned survey mechanism and stripped the data of any network or electronic metadata before being sent to Europe.

Pre-selected scores were used to indicate 'caseness' for each of the questionnaires embedded within the survey. For the CAGE (Cut, Annoyed, Guilty, and Eye) questionnaire, an answer of 'yes' to two or more questions was used to demonstrate a likelihood of problematic alcohol use. A total score above 2 was selected for the GHQ-12 in line with the commonly utilized cut-off for this survey (Goldberg et al., 1997). Answers to the OLBI were scored against the dimensions of disengagement (mean >2.1) and exhaustion (mean >2.25)—thresholds shown to correspond with Maslach Burnout Inventory predictions for physician-diagnosed burnout (Peterson et al., 2008).

Additionally, we planned to compare the results of the first survey to the second survey, using Chi-square tests to determine if key responses differed.

The results of the second survey will be presented according to the demographics, mental health findings, alcohol, and substance use, and finally the GHQ and OLBI. This survey was larger than its predecessor and exceeded the sample size of 80, necessary to reach 10% of the margin of error. Any major difference with the first survey will be pointed out and discussed later.

Demographics

1. There were 101 respondents, all attended Cumming School of Medicine.
2. 36 (36%) reported being in Clerkship, 39 (38%) in Year 1, 26 (25%) in Year 2.
3. 72 (71%) reported their gender as female, 28 (27%) as male, and one (1%) as other.

The most common highest education status achieved by their parents was Postgraduate degree (44, 43%), followed by Undergraduate Degree (33, 32%).
83 (82%) reported not currently working, 12 (11%) <8 hours a week, 5 (5%) 8-20 hours per week, and one (1%) more than 20 hours per week.

Mental Health

Prior to medical school, 50 (49%) had visited a professional regarding their mental health, and 27 (26%) reported a diagnosis with a mental health condition. 11 reported a previous diagnosis of a depressive disorder, 16 had an anxiety disorder (including OCD), four had an eating disorder, one had Tourette's, and two had PTSD.

15 reported a previous diagnosis of ADHD. None reported a diagnosis of Autistic Spectrum Disorder. 37 (36%) reported having been previously prescribed medication for their mental health. 25 reported having previously been prescribed an antidepressant, 12 an ADHD medication, and 4 a benzodiazepine.

Whilst at medical school, 21 (20%) reported a diagnosis of a mental health condition. Nine reported a diagnosis of a depressive disorder, 12 an anxiety disorder (including OCD), 1 eating disorder, and 1 PTSD. 37 (36%) reported they were currently seeing a professional for their mental health.

27 (26%) reported currently taking medication for their mental health. 18 reported being prescribed an antidepressant, six an ADHD medication, two a benzodiazepine, and one a mood stabilizer

The most commonly reported source of significant stress was studies (82, 81%), the second being relationships (63, 62%). 35 (34%) reported money as a significant source of stress, and 10 (9%) reported housing.

Alcohol and Substance Use

1. 14 (13%) tested as CAGE positive.
2. 19 (18%) reported having taken a non-prescription substance to feel better or uplift their mood on at least one occasion. Six students reported weekly use and two reported daily use.
3. 10 (9%) reported having used a medication to enhance concentration, study, or academic performance. Eight reported using ADHD medications. Two people used these medications daily.
4. 40 (39%) reported having previously used cannabis, Eight (8%) ecstasy, Five (5%) amphetamines, one (1%) ketamine, three (3%) cocaine, two (2%) opiates, and nine (9%) another substance.
5. Three students (3%) reported someone else had been worried about their substance use, while five (5%) reported concern about substance use.

GHQ and OLBI

A total of 75 (74%) met specified case criteria for the GHQ questionnaire.

For the OLBI questionnaire, 62 (61%) met specified case criteria for disengagement, and 76 (75%) met specified case criteria for exhaustion.

See Table 7.2.

University Student Health and COUPE Policies for Medical Student Wellbeing

The National College Health Assessment Group (NCHA) 2013, 2016, 2019 studied self-reports from 58 postsecondary institutions. From this, we can clearly see that even before the COVID-19 pandemic there was almost a doubling of the numbers of students who had been

Table 7.2 Average results for GHQ and OLBI by year of study

Year of study	Average of GHQ	Average of OLBI
1	2.335586	2.484797
2	2.282051	2.480769
3	2.293011	2.4375

diagnosed and treated for anxiety, 12.3% to 23.7%, depression 10% to 19%, and attempted suicide 1.3% to 2.8% from 2013 to 2019. This may represent success on a personal level of the anti-stigma campaigners, like Bells 'let's talk about it', the Zero Tolerance for bullying in schools on 23 February in Canada, or the World Mental Health Day on 10 October. All of which have contributed to a greater willingness to discuss mental health issues such as vulnerabilities to anxiety, depression, and suicide.

However, there may be organizational and cultural factors further complicating the rise in student mental health utilization of services at wellness centres across Canada. It is also well known that since the 1980s universities have admitted proportionately many more women. The top conditions for which students seek treatment are anxiety and depression, and these are known to be more common on women than men. Additionally, a generational effect has been suggested by Jean Twenge and colleagues emphasizing the I GEN (those students born in and after 1995) demonstrates higher rates of anxiety, depression, and suicide. Some of the variance for this may be due to the success of handheld devices, Facebook, and access to social media in that generation. Haidt and Lukianoff in The Coddling of the American Mind have emphasized how good intentions and bad ideas are setting up a generation for failure. They blame three dysfunctional core beliefs: What doesn't kill you makes you weaker: Always trusting your feelings: Life is a battle between good and evil people. When assessing student wellness and service planning Haidt and Lukianoff go on to discuss how six other variables come together and must be taken into account; increasing prevalence rates of anxiety and depression due to the digital age, increasing polarization of society, decreased free play time, paranoid parenting, a huge safety culture impacting the size of university bureaucracy, and greater interest in equity, inclusion, and social justice.

They suggest that these have promoted a 'victimhood' culture in universities with its attendant emotional reasoning, microaggressions, and there has been significant concept creep with the term violence being applied to contradictory views to the orthodox political views of social justice. Now freedom of speech is challenged on the grounds it can make people uncomfortable and the telos of some universities is social justice rather than the pursuit of truth through reflective inquiry. They emphasized that students should be taught cognitive behavioural therapy to promote critical thinking and cultivate a stoic attitude. Further qualitative exploration is clearly needed to understand the sociocultural and political pressures medical students face at university.

After the COVID-19 pandemic hit Canadian Universities, MacLean's magazine in October 2020 reported there was a mental health crisis at Canadian Universities. The difficulty campuses felt when faced with these problems was highlighted by the example of a student in Ontario struggling with academic demands. The day before exams and a critical lecture she felt depressed and suicidal but when she came for help the Campus Police were called and she was handcuffed and taken to a nearby hospital. Most mental health professionals would agree this incident gave the wrong impression to students. This has pushed universities to address the demand for counselling and increase in mental health literacy with a reduction in stigma in a humane and culturally sensitive manner. Research and practice on campuses now focus on mental practice networks which will decrease stigma and promote resilience in a compassionate approach (Szeto et al., 2021).

The Canadian Organization of Undergraduate Psychiatric Educators (COUPE) meets regularly to address medical education but also support student wellness. All university programmes have a student affairs website and can offer personal counselling. Some have ready access to mindfulness, apps, and interactive resources. There is generally low-cost crisis counselling including suicide prevention programmes and wellness resources separate from the universities. One example is the University of British Columbia (UBC) which has a wellness initiative network and a group and peer support programme for medical students. The medical school at the University of Western Ontario, through innovative funding, are able to provide a variety of supports such as training new faculty on how to identify students in distress, improved access to student health services with counsellors on campus, use of an electronic medical record isolated from the academic record, peer mentoring, and culturally matching students with an appropriate support. Generally, each medical school can access a Physician health programme that are often available 24/7 for Physicians and medical learners. Some programmes have access to safe spaces. However, most medical students are advised to access the student affairs services first which can then advise on access to other services.

Relevant to our study of the University of Calgary medical student wellness during the COVID-19 pandemic is another recently published study by Stephana Cherak et al from the University of Calgary. This explored the impact of the COVID-19 pandemic on 20% (540) of the 2,741 enrolled learners at the Faculty of Medicine using a cross-sectional, internet-based survey that collected quantitative and qualitative data. This included 22% of medical students and 23% of postgraduate medical residents as well as 25% of undergraduate students and 27% of graduate students. They demonstrated that learner wellness across all stages of training was negatively impacted. The importance of acknowledging equity, diversity, and inclusion, fostering psychological safety while also engaging learners as active participants are key in developing wellness interventions.

Innovative Research and Initiatives for Student Wellbeing

At the Cumming School of Medicine, there have been efforts since 2017 to reinvent the delivery of education (Kachra et al., 2020). There has been an overhaul of our pre-clerkship programme based on the fact that didactic lecturing is a demonstrably ineffective method for content delivery. Despite this, many medical schools rely on the lecture format due to a lack of obvious alternatives. However, design thinking principles can be implanted to create such alternatives. At Cumming a design-centred approach placed the student at the centre of the design process and several initiatives came up from the observations of lectures, small groups, and student focus discussions. The school has adopted large-scale changes to dismantle the system-driven courses, synchronize the rhythm around the delivery of the programme, and establish clear opportunities for career exploration before CaRMS.

Additionally, the Cumming School of Medicine (CSM) through the Student Wellness Office, the Well-Doc project, and the Physician Family Support Programme (PFSP) are attempting to address mental health issues and enhance resiliency. Students are involved in STRIVE sessions (Simulated Training for Resilience in Various Environments), in conjunction with the Canadian Federation of Medical Students and the Canadian Armed Forces. STRIVE was developed as a road to mental readiness programme training and reinforced with experiential learning through practical simulation training. This focused on the big four: smart goal setting, visualization, positive self-talk, and box breathing with progressive muscle relaxation.

There is a considerable burden of stress for all Canadian medical students in their final year of undergraduate training when they are required to participate in the Canadian Resident Matching Service (CaRMS). This is an extremely stressful, time-consuming, and competitive process involving the creation of individualized applications to specific residency programmes, personal letters, medical CVs, and interviewing for various programmes. An absence of CaRMS support was identified by the Student Advocacy and Wellness Hub (SAW) in the CSM at the University of Calgary. Students were not being coached with the practical skills required to create strong CaRMS applications or opportunities to prepare for interviews. SAW thus developed a series of supportive CaRMS workshops and resources to provide students with the tools needed for the process and to educate them on the process in its entirety, including the unmatched process.

SAW identified the need to address with students the possibility of an unsuccessful CaRMS match and remove the stigma surrounding an undesired match outcome. Research also suggests students feel there is a lack of information regarding the process surrounding an unsuccessful match. A session that occurs prior to CaRMS match results titled 'What's next?—Review of the Unmatched Process' was introduced. In this session, SAW discusses the unmatched process including rules surrounding the second iteration and the extension of clerkship. Students find this session reduces their anxiety about the possibility of going unmatched.

SAW, in collaboration with current residents that have previously experienced going unmatched, host a supportive 'Fire Side Chat—Supporting Unmatched Students' the week match results are released. The purpose of this session is to provide a safe space to allow students to share their experiences with each other and reduce the feelings of isolation and failure. This provides an opportunity for struggling students to hear from residents with a similar shared experience and to strategize for 'what's next'. The students are also provided with many resources, including mentorship from previous unmatched residents and psychological resources.

Medical Student Wellness Representatives have collaborated with SAW to introduce a 'Forum on Failure (FOF)' that celebrates setbacks as a way of normalizing conversations regarding difficulties. The first FOF was in-person in 2019, then 2020 was a virtual event and 2021 was a hybrid experience. The goal is to emphasize that setbacks do not define the person but are part of the common experience in medical training. Medical student attendees have described this as a very humanistic dialogue and have appreciated the frank, vulnerable discussions by practising physicians. This event aims to humanize the medical student experience and challenge the macho and glory culture of medicine.

Pairing students with mentors can enhance the feeling of community. SAW, in collaboration with the MD Alumni Office, connects incoming first-year students with alumni who have expressed a keen interest in mentorship. The objectives of the programme are twofold. First, SAW provides our medical students with a safe, welcoming relationship with someone who can provide support and guidance. This also offers our mentors the opportunity to play a meaningful role in the life of a medical student, offering the feeling of being part of a larger whole.

Conclusion

The findings of our pre-COVID-19 survey and COVID-19 survey on medical student wellness, psychiatric morbidity, and burnout are similar. The level of exhaustion in our medical students is significant (74%) and similar to the pre-COVID-19 survey. A majority (81%) of the surveyed group recognized academic pressures as a source of stress, and relationship (62%) and money worries (35%) and housing (10%) were also notable which may reflect the challenges inherent in residency applications. Financially, our students at the University of Calgary have higher than average debt and this was a significant stressor for students in the last phase of the programme in the first survey (60% of respondents in clerkship versus 26% in pre-clerkship).

In Canada, the COVID-19 pandemic has had a profound impact on the social fabric of society, including the universities highlighting the inequities across the country. The burden of increased isolation imposed by COVID-19 can only worsen the prevalence of anxiety and depression our survey reveals and speaks to the issue of the importance of timely access to mental health counselling and support from the Student Wellness Office and the wider community. Our results also suggest a need for advice for financial planning. This finding of increasing numbers of university students in general, not just medical students struggling with anxiety and depression has been well documented by Haidt in 2018 and Twenge in 2017. Both our surveys reported a pre-university prevalence of around 26% for diagnosed mental health disorders (28% in the first survey and 27% in the second).

Similar numbers in each survey reported currently taking medication for their mental health, suggesting significant need for timely access to medical services. It is worrisome to see high CAGE positive rates at 13.9%, however, this is lower than the first survey results of 22%. This may be because during the COVID-19 pandemic lockdown there was less chance to socialize or participate in sports events. Nevertheless, this highlights the importance of informed counselling about the risks and benefits of alcohol use as well as for a variety of other substances. The latter now includes legalized cannabis which is widely available, but also more serious, illegal drugs such as ecstasy, psilocybin, amphetamines, ketamine, cocaine, and opiates.

In Alberta, some of the mitigating organizational factors include active partnerships with the Alberta Medical Association (AMA) and the University Calgary Cummings Medical School to look at burnout through both educational activities and social activities including lunch and learn activities addressing issues of racism in medicine and the decolonization of the medical curriculum. The AMA also promotes access to timely mental health services through the 'Physician Wellness Programme' and the Student Wellness Office. This represents a subtle shift from the medical paradigm of pathogenesis to salutogenesis as a theory to guide health promotion. Antonovsky in his 1996 publication emphasized that health is a state of optimal physical, mental, and social wellbeing, not merely the absence of disease and infirmity. This can be facilitated with a strong sense of coherence when confronted with stressors by developing comprehensibility, coping strategies, and meaningfulness.

Hopefully, this destigmatizes mental illness and the need to seek help or explore underlying risk factors, such as culture, family, and personal choices that may undermine resilience and competence. Corey Keyes in 2007 has argued for the conception and diagnosis of a two continua model of mental health and illness. This calls for the second adoption of the promotion of genuine mental health as flourishing. Arguing that people can be free of mental illness but not mentally healthy and not flourishing and may even be languishing, burnt out, and with no motivation. Keyes defined flourishing as living an authentic life with joy and passion, a condition that all medical students feel when they get into medical school. However, Keyes found that in the States that the prevalence of flourishing is barely 20%. Perhaps at this point, it is a timely reminder that other disciplines, such as social work, have published work on the role of the family of origin in vocational choice.

Let us give the last word regarding cultural factors impacting medical student wellness to a great thought leader, Jonathan Rauch. In his book, the Constitution of knowledge, he argues that all people, and students in particular, need to check their facts and not just their privilege, return to the neutral objectivity of liberal science, and retreat from the moral clarity of social justice, identity politics, and intersectionalism, and defend our liberal science tradition. Jonathan Rauch (2021) argues that we need a reality-based network which consists of the big four pillars of academia and science, law, government, and journalism to help us correct our confirmational and conformity biases. This larger community promotes a critical persuasion with viewpoint diversity in the reality-based community in the spirit of collaboration and replaces the personal and tribal networks by the liberal network. The reality-based community is a counterpoint to the silos and fragmentation of student bodies in the educational sections with its confirmation and conformity biases. This can be addressed by viewpoint diversity and having retreats that share an interlocking mission statement and that work within identified organizational structures, thus addressing the antecedents of burnout and stress through the promotion of a positive culture of personal agency and resilience. Consideration should be given to Balint groups, which may be able to reduce burnout and help students and faculty to feel a part of a community where stresses can be shared.

Acknowledgements

Thanks to the Canadian Organization of Undergraduate Psychiatric Educators, COUPE, for sharing of information on medical student wellness across Canada. Especially Dr Kathryn Fung at UBC, Vancouver and Dr Sandra Northcott, Associate Dean at Western University.

References

Antonovsky, A. The Salutogenic model as a theory to guide health. Health promotion international. *Oxford University press.* 1996. Vol 11. No. 1. 11–18.

Ashton, C. & Kamali, F. (1995). Personality, lifestyles, alcohol and drug consumption in a sample of British medical students. *Medical Education*, 29(3), pp.187–192.

Cherak, S., Brown, A., Kachra, R., Makuk., Sudeshan, S., Paget, M., and Kassam,A. (2021) Exploring the impact of the COVID-19 pandemic on medical learner wellness: a needs assessment for the development of learner wellness interventions. *Canadian Medical Education Journal*. https://pub med.ncbi.nlm.nih.gov/34249191/ https://doi.org/10.36834/cmej.70995

Dyrbye, L., Thomas, M. and Shanafelt, T. (2006). Systematic Review of Depression, Anxiety, and Other Indicators of Psychological Distress Among U.S. and Canadian Medical Students. *Academic Medicine*, 81(4), pp.354–373.

Dyrbye, L., Thomas, M., Massie, F., Power, D., Eacker, A., Harper, W., Durning, S., Moutier, C., Szydlo, D., Novotny, P., Sloan, J. and Shanafelt, T. (2008). Burnout and Suicidal Ideation among U.S. Medical Students. *Annals of Internal Medicine*, 149(5), p.334.

Edward H. The relationship between false self-compliance and the motivation to become a professional helper. Part 1. *Smith College Studies*, 60. 1990-Issue 2: 169–184. Published online 2009. https://doi.org/10.1080/00377319009516672.

El Hawary H, Salimi A, Barone N, Alam P, Thibaudeau S. (2021) The effect of COVID-19 on medical students education and wellbeing; a cross-sectional survey. *Canadian Medical Education Journal*, (CMEJ) https://doi.org/10.36834/cmej.71261

Glauser, W. (2017). Medical schools addressing student anxiety, burnout and depression. *Canadian Medical Association Journal*, 189(50), E1569–E1570. doi:10.1503/cmaj.109-5516 [Cross ref], [Web of Science ®], [Google Scholar]

Goldberg, D., Gater, R., Sartorius, N., Ustun, T., Piccinelli, M., Gureje, O. and Rutter, C. (1997). The validity of two versions of the GHQ in the WHO study of mental illness in general health care. *Psychological Medicine*, 27(1), pp.191–197.

Gould, E. 2003 The University in a Corporate Culture. *Yale University Press*. April

Haidt Jonathan. Universities must choose between the Telos of Truth and Social Justice. https://www.theatlantic.com/ideas/archive/2018/11/academics-truth-justice/574165/

Twinge, J. The i Gen Population. Chapter 4, The New Mental Health Crisis. 2017 *Atria Books*.

Kachra R., Brown Allison, Paget Mike. Sharma Nishan, Low Joshua, Brockman Kathryne, Urquhart Zachary. Using Design Thinking To Re-Invent The Delivery of Undergraduate Medical Education 2020 Abstracts *Canadian Medical Education Journal* 11(2) 2020 doi.org/10.36834/cmej.v11i20.

Keyes, C. (2007). Promoting and protecting mental health as flourishing. *American Psychologist*. February–March. 62(2): 95–108.

Lackie, B. (1983). The families of origin of social workers. *Clin Soc Work J* 11, 309–322. https://doi.org/10.1007/BF00755898

Lukiannoff Greg and Haidt, Jonathan. 2018. *Penguin Books*. The Coddling of the American Mind.

Macleans, 2016. 'Medical school in Canada: What does it take to get in?' Oct. Medical school in Canada: What does it take to get in? (macleans.ca)

Moir, F., Yielder, J., Sanson, J., and Chen, Y. (2018). Depression in medical students: current insights. *Advances in Medical Education and Practice*, Volume 9, pp.323–333.

The National College Health Assessment group, NCHA. The Canadian Reference group 2019. Executive summary. https://www.cacuss.ca/files/Research/NCHA-II%20SPRING%202019%20CANADIAN%20REFERENCE%20GROUP%20EXECUTIVE%20SUMMARY.pdf

Newbury-Birch, D., Walshaw, D. and Kamali, F. (2001). Drink and drugs: from medical students to doctors. *Drug and Alcohol Dependence*, 64(3), pp.265–270.

Okoniewsa Basia, Ladha Malika A., Ma Irene W.Y. Journey of candidates who were unmatched in the Canadian Residency Matching Service (CaRMS): A phenomenological study. *CMEJ* 2020, 11(3) e82–e91 Special Issue.

Pattni, Vijay, Phillips, Jeff, Saha, Rajnish. Balint groups could be one way to prevent burnout during COVID-19. *The BMJ opinion*. May 2020.

Peterson, U., Demerouti, E., Bergström, G., Samuelsson, M., Åsberg, M. and Nygren, Å. (2008). Burnout and physical and mental health among Swedish healthcare workers. *Journal of Advanced Nursing*, 62(1): pp.84–95.

Rate of Doctor Burnout in Canada has doubled since before pandemic. https://www.cma.ca/news-releases-and-statements/physician-burnout-nearly-doubles-during-pandemic

Rauch, J. In defense of truth. 2021. *The Brooking Institute*. *The Constitution of knowledge*. June.

Rennie, S. (2003). Differences in medical students' attitudes to academic misconduct and reported behaviour across the years--a questionnaire study. *Journal of Medical Ethics*, 29(2), pp.97–102

Saipanish, R. (2003). Stress among medical students in a Thai medical school. *Medical Teacher*, 25(5): 502–506.

Sherina, M., Rampal, L. and Kaneson, N. (2004). Psychological stress among undergraduate medical students. *Med J Malaysia*, 59(2), pp.207–11.

Smith S., Kassam A, Griggs L., Rizzuti F, Horton J, Brown A. Teaching Mindfulness-based stress management techniques to medical leaners through simulation. *Can Med Educ.* J. 2021 Feb 26;12(1): e95–e97.

Szeto ACH, Henderson L, Lindsay B L, Knaak S, Dobson KS. Increasing resiliency and reducing mental illness stigma in post-secondary students: A meta-analytic evaluation of the inquiring mind program. *J Am Coll Health. 2021 Dec 7*;1–11 doi: 10.1080/07448481.2021.2007112

The Munk Debates, podcast. https://podcasts.apple.com/ca/podcast/be-it-resolved-modern-universit ies-are-a-threat-to/id1486184902?i=1000551144503

Vogel, L. (2018). Even resilient doctors report high levels of burnout, finds CMA survey. *Canadian Medical Association Journal*, 190(43), pp.E1293–E1293.

Wilkes, C. Lewis, T. Brager, N. Bulloch, A. MacMaster, Paget, M. Holm, J. Farrell, S. (2022). Ventriglio M. Wellbeing and mental health amongst medical students in Canada. October 2019. *International Review of Psychiatry* 31(2):1–4. OI:10.1080/09540261.2019.1675927

Woloschuk, W., Harasym, P. and Temple, W. (2004). Attitude change during medical school: a cohort study. *Medical Education*, 38(5), pp.522–534.

Woods, Allan. 2017 The tragic case of Dr Robert Chu, Toronto Star. June https://www.thestar.com/ news/canada/2017/06/17/tragic-case-of-robert-chu-shows-plight-of-canadian-medical-school-grads.html?rf

8

Denmark

Medical Student Wellbeing in Denmark

Jesper Nørgaard Kjær

Background

Denmark is a small country in Northern Europe. It has a welfare state and a very large public sector that includes healthcare, education, state pension, and other public services. Denmark is a high-income group country. The population is ethnically quite homogenous with 85 % Danes. Around 17,000 Inuits from Greenland and 22,000 Faroese live in Denmark. The majority of other ethnic groups are migrants or refugees from Europe or the Middle East (see Box 8.1 for information on demographics).

The life expectancy for men is close to 80 years and for women 83 years. In 2018, the most common causes of death were chronic obstructive pulmonary disease, lung cancer, and ischaemic heart disease (World Health Organization, 2021). Nine out of ten of the most common causes are non-communicable diseases. The only communicable disease is pneumonia. In 2020 2.5% of mortality were caused by COVID-19, which was the eighth leading cause of death. Not all healthcare services are free-of-charge. In 2017 around 14% of all healthcare costs were paid for by the user. Most of the costs were for prescription drugs or dental care that are only partly covered by public health insurance.

In the World Happiness Report from 2022, Denmark was ranked second (Helliwell et al., 2022). Asked to rank their current lives as a whole using the mental image of a ladder, Danes on average answered 7.6 on the scale going from zero (worst possible life) to ten (best possible life). Since the annual data were first collected in 2005, the average answer has been stable in the range of 7.5 to 8.0. Regression analysis finds that 71% of the average answer can be explained by six factors: high GDP per capita, strong social support, healthy life expectancy at birth, freedom to make life choices, low perceptions of corruption, and generosity (mentioned in the order of the most to the least important factor).

The Mental Health of Medical Students in Denmark

General information about medical schools in Denmark can be found in Box 8.2. Results from two large studies of medical students are presented in this chapter. The British Medical Association (BMA) and Oxford Health NHS Foundation Trust led an international collaboration that surveyed medical students internationally, including in Denmark (Kjær et al., 2022). A total of 647 medical students from Denmark participated in the BMA survey. The

Jesper Nørgaard Kjær, *Denmark* In: *The Mental Health of Medical Students.* Edited by: Andrew Molodynski, Sarah Marie Farrell, and Dinesh Bhugra, Oxford University Press. © Oxford University Press 2024. DOI: 10.1093/oso/9780192864871.003.0008

Box 8.1 Demographics

- Population: 5.8 million
- Languages: Danish, Faroese, Inuit, German (small minority). English is the predominant second language
- Ethnic groups: Danish (85.6%) includes Faroese and Inuit minorities, non-Danish (14.4%) includes Turkish, Polish, Syrian, Romanian, German, and Iraqi minorities
- Religion: Christianity (75.8%), No religion (19.1%), Islam (4.4%), other (0.7%)
- GDP per capita: 68,094 USD
- Government: Constitutional monarchy
- Life expectancy: Women 83.4 years, men 79.6 years
- Employed medical doctors: 23,290 (65% specialists)

Box 8.2 Medical school in Denmark

- No. of medical schools: 4
- 6 years of education
- Enrolled medical students: 9,438 (as of October 1, 2021)
- Sex: 68% females (2017)
- Mean age at enrolment: 21 years (2017)
- Average years to graduation: 7.7 years (2017)

---

survey was conducted from February to August 2020. The other survey was conducted by the organization for medical students in Denmark (FADL). The FADL survey included 2,928 medical students in 2021 and 1,716 in 2019 (Holm-Nielsen et al., 2021).

Psychological Distress and Burnout

High levels of psychological distress and burnout among medical students were found in Denmark. In the BMA survey, six to seven out of ten scored as 'cases' of psychological distress measured by the General Health Questionnaire-12. More females (69%) than males (64%) reached caseness. Burnout, as rated with the Oldenburg Burnout Inventory (OLBI), was for disengagement similar for males and females (71% and 70%), while exhaustion was markedly higher for females (72%) compared with males (62%). Figure 8.1 shows the rates across the years of medical school, indicating a decreasing prevalence of psychological distress as the students get more experience, a better social network, and do clinical rotations in the later years. Another reason for the decline could be survivorship bias, as students with more distress progressively drop out. OLBI disengagement increased from year one to three, then declined by 23% from year three to four, before increasing again in years five and six. The rising disengagement in the first three years could be due to heavy reading

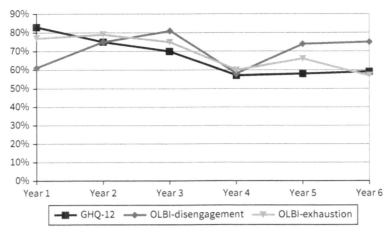

Figure 8.1 Rates of caseness for GHQ-12, OLBI-disengagement, and OLBI-exhaustion.

Source: data from Kjær JN, Molodynski A, Bhugra D, Lewis T. Wellbeing, psychiatric morbidity and psychological distress amongst medical students in Denmark. *International Journal of Social Psychiatry.* 2022;68(6):1289–1294.

of theoretical subjects such as physiology and biochemistry. At most Danish universities, clinical rotations start during year four and that could be a reason for the improved engagement. While OLBI-exhaustion decreased in the last three years, it is concerning that disengagement increased again in the last two years of medical school. Reasons for this could be exposure to excruciating clinical work without yet having any responsibility, thus not experiencing the same rate of exhaustion. Instead, the students could be worrying about their future work as a doctor.

The FADL survey used the WHO-5 Wellbeing Index. In 2019, 70% of students who responded scored above 50, which indicates wellbeing and that they were not at risk of depression or psychological distress. Sixteen per cent (16%) scored 36–50, which indicates a risk of depression or psychological distress, and 10% scored below 36, which indicates high risk. Four per cent (4%) did not answer. In 2021, wellbeing decreased to 59%, and the prevalence of at risk and high risk increased to 22% and 14%, respectively. Five per cent (5%) did not answer. FADL considers that the decreased wellbeing could be due to the COVID-19 pandemic that took place in-between their two surveys. However, the BMA survey was conducted during the pandemic and did not find a major increase of psychological distress for those answering the survey after the lockdown. On the contrary, after the lockdown, a reduction in exhaustion rates were observed (75% before and 67% after). The FADL survey also asked the participants if they had experienced mental health issues (defined as exam anxiety, social isolation, impaired, exhaustion, anxiety, depression, etc.) during medical school. In 2019, 60% answered yes and 2 years later, a minor increase to 62% was found, which did not indicate a major influence of the pandemic. Those results are more in line with the proportions of psychological distress and burnout from the BMA survey. In the FADL survey, the students were able to elaborate their answer and in 2021, the most prevalent answers were psychological distress (67%), sadness (52%), lack of motivation (49%), and concentration difficulties (48%).

Mental Disorders

Around one-third of the students had visited a professional regarding their mental health before medical school, according to the BMA survey. Diagnosed mental disorders were less common. Eleven per cent (11%) reported one or more mental disorders prior to starting medical school. Depressive disorders (5%), anxiety disorders, and OCD (4%), and eating disorders (3%) were most frequent. One per cent (1%) reported attention deficit hyperactivity disorder (ADHD), autism spectrum disorder, and stress-related disorder. Personality disorder, complex post-traumatic stress disorder (PTSD), bipolar disorder, and psychotic disorder were all reported by less than 1% of the participants. Nine per cent (9%) had been prescribed medication for their mental health prior to starting medical school. Antidepressants were by far most prevalent (6%). One per cent (1%) or less had been prescribed either ADHD medication, anxiolytic medication (non-antidepressant class), antipsychotic medication, benzodiazepine, z-drug, or mood stabilizer.

Whilst at medical school, more students reported being diagnosed with a mental disorder (16%). Depressive disorder (7%), anxiety disorder (8%), and stress-related disorder (3%) were most prevalent. Eating disorders (1%) were less reported. Personality disorder, complex PTSD, bipolar disorder, and psychotic disorder were stable at less than 1% of the participants. Six per cent (6%) of the medical students reported using prescription drugs for their mental health at the time of inquiry. Antidepressants were again most prevalent (4%) while other psychopharmacological drugs were prescribed to 1% or less of the participants.

Substance Use

Alcohol use is a known public health issue in Denmark. Therefore, it was not surprising that 13% of participants in the BMA survey screened positive for an alcohol use problem using the CAGE questionnaire. Almost one in five males (18%) screened positive, while 11% females screened positive. Alcohol use problem is not that prevalent in the general population. A survey of 16- to 24-year-olds from 2021 found that around 12% of males and 7% of females had an alcohol use problem according to the modified CAGE-C (Christensen et al., 2021). CAGE-C only screens for alcohol-related problems within the last year, making the proportions of CAGE (lifetime) and CAGE-C less comparable. Of other substances, previous use of cannabis was most prevalent (18%). Cocaine (3%), ecstasy (2%), amphetamine (1%), ketamine (1%), and opiates (1%) were much less prevalent. Four per cent (4%) reported that they had worried about their substance use, and 4% reported that someone else had worried about their substance use.

Causes of Psychological Distress

Causes of significant stress as reported by the BMA survey are shown in Figure 8.2. By far the most prevalent cause of stress was studying. More than eight out of ten indicated that studying was a significant cause of stress. This could partly be explained by one in five medical students experiencing inadequate language proficiency while reading textbooks or

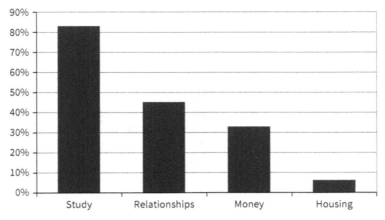

Figure 8.2 Causes of significant stress.

Source: data from Kjær JN, Molodynski A, Bhugra D, Lewis T. Wellbeing, psychiatric morbidity and psychological distress amongst medical students in Denmark. *International Journal of Social Psychiatry.* 2022;68(6):1289–1294.

Reported causes of significant stress by medical students in Denmark participating in the BMA survey.

academic literature, according to a report from 2017 (Kristensen & Brændgaard, 2017). Half of respondents did not feel able to explain medical language to laymen. The experience of inadequate language proficiency was attenuated in students that did not grow up speaking Danish as their primary language. They experienced a lack of proficiency in written and oral communication, and experienced not being understood because of their accent or limited vocabulary.

Significant stress from studying could also explain why six per cent (6%) of respondents had paused a whole semester and 19% had prolonged their time at medical school by taking fewer classes than required in at least one semester, according to the FADL survey. The reasons for prolonging study were to do research, work full-time, ease the study burden, or take time off.

Clinical rotations can also be a cause of stress. In 2021, one in five students were dissatisfied with clinical rotations as reported in the FADL survey. They report fear of having too many days off due to illness as they then would not get the rotation approved and would have to postpone exams. Some reported feeling discouraged when the doctors did not have time to supervise or when it was only possible to watch by the side without trying any clinical work independently. Furthermore, it is a cause of stress that the clinical rotations interfere with major holidays and preparations for exams.

Study Drugs

The use of study drugs to enhance academic performance was not common. In the BMA study, 4% reported having taken a non-prescription substance to enhance performance. Only 1% reported daily usage. Two per cent (2%) reported using ADHD medication, and less than 1% used beta-blockers. The FADL survey reports a minor decline, as 7% used performance enhancers in 2019 and 6% in 2021. Around seven out of ten only used the enhancers doing exams or in preparation for exams. The low prevalence of study drugs was also found among Danish students in general by a register-based study (Butt et al., 2017). Only 0.14% of healthy students claimed a prescription for a beta-blocker during the exam period from 1996 to 2012. However, the validity of the surveys in this regard are questionable and Danish media has reported an increase of the illegal import of study drugs, mostly ADHD medication, from 2016 to 2020 (Krog, 2021).

Initiatives and Policies

An Interprofessional Training Unit

In 2004, the first interprofessional training unit was established in Denmark (Jakobsen et al., 2010). In the first two years, nursing, occupational therapy, and physiotherapy students were in the unit and in 2006 medical students were added. A unit of eight beds managed by the students under the supervision of trained staff. The unit develops both clinical skills and experience with interpersonal collaboration of the attending medical students. The unit was evaluated as a safe learning environment. This initiative meets the demand for independent clinical work that the medical students requested in the FADL survey. Nationwide, the number of training units has not been determined. They are not present at every teaching hospital even though the training unit was found cost-effective and had no differences in complications or patient-reported quality of life compared to a conventional unit (Hansen et al., 2009).

Medical Students Mentoring Medical Students

FADL organizes a nationwide mentor programme (FADL, 2022). Mentees can apply for any reason, and it is free-of-charge for members of FADL The mentor programme is advertised to help with any problems and mentions loneliness, social issues, and learning difficulties as examples, but is also advertised for those without any major problems that want to improve as a student. The mentors are other students that have taken an introductory course on how to be a mentor. There is no salary given to the mentors, instead they are given a diploma at the end of the semester. FADL matches mentors and mentees according to their priorities and experiences. The mentor and mentee meet three to four times each semester and can also attend social events with other mentors and mentees. Mentees express gratitude for the shared experience of the mentor, for example, because they can avoid some of the mistakes that the mentor made. The mentor programme is part of creating a pleasant study environment at the universities.

Abolishment of the Four-year Rule

In 2008, the Danish government regulated specialization so that medical doctors had to begin specialization no more than four years after graduation. The regulation was named the four-year rule and its purpose was to force doctors to choose specialties that might not have been their first priority (Hansen, 2014). In Denmark, after graduation, all doctors have a one-year internship to gain authorization. Afterwards, you apply for one-year introduction positions in different specialties. You need to finish a one-year position in the specialty before you can apply for the main specialization position that lasts four to five years. Depending on the popularity of the specialty you might need a lot of experience to qualify for a main specialization position. Therefore, junior doctors often take a lot of time to do research or clinical work to improve their CVs. The four-year rule instead forced medical students to improve their CVs while studying if they wanted to be sure to get into a certain specialty. The organizations for medical students and junior doctors opposed the rule. They argued that the rule caused unnecessary pressure on medical students to not only pass their exams but also to do other relevant activities to improve their CV. The government abandoned the rule in 2019 and it was seen as an achievement for the wellbeing of medical students (Gundersen, 2019).

Conclusion

High levels of psychological distress and burnout among medical students are threats to the future workforce of doctors in Denmark. Initiatives to improve education have been implemented. However, as the main cause of distress is studying, more is needed. For example, students request better time for supervision during clinical rotations and improved planning of clinical rotations and exams.

References

Butt, J.H., Dalsgaard, S., Torp-Pedersen, C., Køber, L., Gislason, G.H., Kruuse, C., & Fosbøl, E.L. (2017). 'Beta-blockers for exams identify students at high risk of psychiatric morbidity'. *J Child Adolesc Psychopharmacol* 27: 266–273.

Christensen, A., Ekholm, O., & Thrige, D. (2021). 'Danskernes Sundhed—Tal fra den nationale sundhedsprofil'. Syddansk Universitet. https://www.danskernessundhed.dk/Kontakt.html (Accessed 11 April 2022).

FADL (2022). 'FADLs Mentorordning'. https://fadl.dk/fadl-aarhus/lokale-fordele-aarhus/mediciner skabets-og-fadls-mentorordning/ (Accessed 11 April 2022).

Gundersen, R. (2019). 'Nu bliver seksårsfristen afskaffet'. Dagens Medicin. https://dagensmedicin.dk/ nu-bliver-seksaarsfristen-afskaffet/ (Accessed 11 April 2022).

Hansen, S. (2014). 'Forhadt fireårsregel til forhandling'. Uniavisen. https://uniavisen.dk/forhadt-fireaa rsregel-til-forhandling/ (Accessed 11 April 2022).

Hansen, T.B., Jacobsen, F., & Larsen, K. (2009). 'Cost effective interprofessional training: an evaluation of a training unit in Denmark'. *J Interprof Care* 23: 234–241.

Helliwell, J., Layard, R., Sachs, J., De Neve, J., Aknin, L., Wang, S., & Paculor, S. (2022). 'The World Happiness Report 2022'. https://worldhappiness.report/ (Accessed 11 April 2022).

Holm-Nielsen, L., Bengtsson, E., Lassen, L., Mellergaard, C., Andersen, S., Christiansen, S., Schaldemose, P., Jacobsen, A., Møller, E., Sørensen, H., & Hansen, S. (2021). 'FADLs Studieundersøgelse 2021'. https://fadl.dk/fadl/politisk-arbejde/studieundersoegelse/ (Accessed 11 April 2022).

Jakobsen, F., Larsen, K., & Hansen, T. (2010). 'This is the closest I have come to being compared to a doctor: Views of medical students on clinical clerkship in an Interprofessional Training Unit'. *Med Teach* 32: e399–e406.

Kjær, J.N., Molodynski, A., Bhugra, D., & Lewis, T. (2022). 'Wellbeing, psychiatric morbidity and psychological distress amongst medical students in Denmark'. *Int J Soc Psychiatry* 68: 1289–1294.

Kristensen, A. & Brændgaard, N. (2017). 'Sprogbehov på medicinuddannelsen'. Københavns Universitet. https://cip.ku.dk/projekter-og-samarbejdsaftaler/sprogstrategisk-satsning/formidling/rapporter/medicinstudiet/ (Accessed 11 March 2022).

Krog, S. (2021). 'Mathias købte study drugs for bitcoins, men hans krop betalte prisen'. https://www.dr.dk/nyheder/indland/mathias-koebte-study-drugs-bitcoins-men-hans-krop-betalte-prisen (Accessed 11.4.22).

World Health Organization (2021). 'Denmark: Country Health Profile 2021'. https://eurohealthobservatory.who.int/publications/m/denmark-country-health-profile-2021 (Accessed 11 April 2022).

9

Wales

Initiatives to Support Medical Students' Mental Health in Wales

Umakant Dave, Andrew Grant, Liz Forty, Chris Horn, and Sara Hunt

Wales

Wales is one of the four nations that make up the United Kingdom. In 2020 Wales had an estimated population of 3,170,000. Since 1999 the government in Wales has been devolved to the Welsh parliament or 'Senedd'. Between 20% and 30% of people speak Welsh and all government and official business is carried out bilingually.

The population of Wales is concentrated in the Southeast near the cities of Newport, Cardiff, and Swansea and along the North Wales coast where the largest city is Wrexham.

Wales played a key role in the industrial revolution, during which time its population grew exponentially. Wales was a major producer of, first, iron, then coal. Large areas of Wales were and still are under agricultural use.

The landscape and the economy of Wales are changed greatly following the closure of the coal mines and steelworks. The economy, history, and landscape of Wales place specific needs on the providers of undergraduate medical education. Some of the available clinical placements need to be provided in rural settings that necessitate students travelling long distances and/or being resident on site. Cardiff and Swansea medical schools offer a track within their respective programmes where students spend a whole academic year situated with a primary care team. The purpose of these 'Extended clerkships' is to give students a prolonged period of working in the front line with community-based healthcare professionals. It is hoped that some students who follow these tracks will develop a sense of the challenges and rewards of working in a rural and/or remote setting.

A 2019 survey commissioned by the British Medical Association (described elsewhere in this book) was completed by 266 students in Wales (12% of the Welsh medical student population) (Farrell et al., 2019). It is very likely that some of the students who completed this survey were motivated by personal experience of mental health problems and the results, therefore, cannot be assumed to be representative. The results showed that (% in brackets, of the 266 respondents); 44 students (15%) received a mental health diagnosis whilst at medical school; 31 had experienced depression (one specified a bipolar illness), 9 anxiety, 2 obsessive compulsive disorder, and 2 attention deficit hyperactivity disorder (ADHD). Of the 266 respondents 56 (21%) reported that they were currently seeing a GP regarding their mental health.

Sixty-five students (24%) exhibited concerning drinking habits. Sixty-one (23%) reported cannabis use, but there was no difference in use of cannabis among students who had a mental health diagnosis and those who did not.

Umakant Dave, Andrew Grant, Liz Forty, Chris Horn, and Sara Hunt, *Wales* In: *The Mental Health of Medical Students*. Edited by: Andrew Molodynski, Sarah Marie Farrell, and Dinesh Bhugra, Oxford University Press. © Oxford University Press 2024. DOI: 10.1093/oso/9780192864871.003.0009

Table 9.1 Use of drugs by medical students in Wales, numbers, and percentages

Substance	#	%
Cannabis	61	23%
Ecstasy	21	8%
Cocaine	15	6%
Ketamine	12	5%
Amphetamines	7	3%
Other—KAT, LSD, etc.	6	2%
Opiates	3	1%
Total (Any substance)	76	28.6%

Reproduced with permission from Farrell, S., Molodynski, A., Cohen, D., Grant, A., Rees, S., Wullshleger, A., Lewis, T. & Kadhum, M. 2019. Wellbeing and burnout among medical students in Wales. *International Review of Psychiatry* 33:1–2, pages 37–42.

Twenty-five students (10%) had taken non-prescription substances or prescribed medication outside of its intended use to feel better or to raise their mood (see Table 9.1). When focussing on drugs and non- prescription medication to increase concentration and improve study, five students (2%) reported to have used Modafinil and another 2% similar substances.

In this chapter we describe initiatives that have been introduced at two Welsh medical schools in Cardiff and Swansea to enhance wellbeing and raise medical students' awareness of available sources of support.

Cardiff University School of Medicine offers three undergraduate medicine programmes: Medicine MBBCh, with an annual intake of over 300; Medicine Graduate Entry MBBCh, with an annual intake between 10-20; and Medicine North Wales (in collaboration with Bangor University) with an annual intake of approximately 20. Swansea University Medical School (SUMS) offers a Graduate Entry Medical Programme with an annual intake of approximately 154. For the remainder of this chapter, 'Cardiff' refers to Cardiff University School of Medicine and 'Swansea' refers to SUMS. From 2024 students will be able to study medicine at Bangor University

Student Support at Welsh Medical Schools

Students are supported, both academically and pastorally, throughout their studies at both medical schools. At Cardiff, this is carried out by a wide range of individuals including personal tutors, case-based learning (CBL) facilitators, year directors, and coordinators, module leads, and clinical placement educational supervisors and coordinators across Wales. Support mechanisms at Swansea are delivered by a similar network of individuals, which includes personal academic mentors, year leads, and cohort leads. Students at both medical schools have access to a wide range of generic support services through campus-based university health and wellbeing services.

In this chapter we describe activities which contribute to student wellbeing at Cardiff and Swansea. A randomized controlled study evaluating Enhanced Stress Resilience Training (ESRT) in graduate-entry medical students is being carried out at Swansea. We give the reasons why we believe this mindfulness intervention meets medical students' needs. We describe the creation of completely new programmes which provide help and support for student wellbeing at both medical schools. We describe the use of reflective learning, and activities that encourage the delivery of peer support initiatives by medical students.

A Specialized Support Service for Medical Students

The MyMedic—Learning Development Unit (LDU) at Cardiff Medical School provides a holistic service, working to ensure that students' journeys through medical school are designed around each unique student. The multidisciplinary team includes doctors, psychologists, communication experts, and experienced professional services support (PSS) staff. Students who are referred are allocated a MyMedic Advisor (MMA) who ensures that the student is able to access all relevant support within and external to the university. MyMedic Advisors offer advice and signposting, supporting students to manage their studies alongside other issues and challenges they may be dealing with. The service provides continuity of support for students throughout their time at medical school. MyMedic-LDU also provides access to Occupational Psychologists who provide support in relation to study skills/work-life balance/time management-planning. Students may also be referred to MyMedic's expert in language. MyMedic-LDU does not provide treatment or counselling but will direct students to appropriate university and healthcare services. MyMedic-LDU liaise with relevant individuals and teams within the medical school, as well as with wider university health and wellbeing services (Occupational Health (OH) and Disability and Dyslexia Support (DDS) in particular), and external services/organizations, to ensure a coordinated approach to student support and wellbeing.

Student Engagement with MyMedic-LDU

Self-referrals to MyMedic-LDU have increased significantly over time. In 2011–2012, 19% of all referrals were self-referrals, with this figure increasing to 89% in 2020–2021. The reasons for self-referral since 2012 have also shifted from primarily educational reasons to the need for health and personal support. Table 9.2 presents the reasons for students accessing the MyMedic-LDU Service between 2013/14–2020/21. The increase in the number of Cardiff medical students declaring mental health issues over this time period is consistent with the increase seen in the general student population over this time period (UCAS, 2021).

The number of students accessing MyMedic-LDU have also increased, from 165 students in 2015/16 to 194 students in 2020/21 (with cohort numbers remaining relatively stable over this period). Approximately one-quarter of medical students at Cardiff are, at the time of

Table 9.2 Most frequent reasons for students presenting to the MyMedic service (2013/14–2020/21). (NB: Students often present with more than one issue)

	2013/14	2014/15	2015/16	2016/17	2017/18	2018/19	2019/20	2020/21
Examination issues (%)	33	24	13	9	12	14	9	10
Work/Life balance (%)	10	11	14	15	14	17	14	10
Physical health (%)	9	16	12	12	8	8	9	8
Mental health (%)	10	13	12	17	17	17	20	20
Psychological wellbeing (%)	15	25	35	36	38	33	40	41

NB: Other issues that students present with have included time management/personal organization, language skills, communication skills, assertiveness/confidence, and probity.

Source: data from MYMEDIC, Cardiff Medical School.

writing, registered with MyMedic-LDU (N = 383), although only a proportion of these (227) (15% of all medical students at Cardiff) are actively receiving support.

Box 9.1 includes representative quotes from students who have accessed MyMedic-LDU illustrating how they value a specialized service for medical students, that breaks down barriers and normalizes support-seeking for medical students, who are often reluctant to seek help, particularly in relation to mental health concerns.

Box 9.1 Medical student feedback about the value of MyMedic—LDU—highlighting some of the reasons why a bespoke service for medical students can be beneficial

---

- *Medical students have different needs and stressors to other university students, and I think a specialized service that understands these needs means it is more accessible and people are more likely to use it.*
  - *The service specifically addresses needs related to placement, difficult course content, more professional/intense university experience than peers and the potential for trauma & difficult experiences whilst on the course.*
  - *Having support from people that understand the nuances and challenges of medicine is invaluable.*
  - *MyMedic reassures medical students that there is support for them too, that it's okay to need a little extra help and that seeking advice doesn't mean you are not resilient enough to do it.*

Mindfulness and ESRT

Evidence has demonstrated the significant benefits of mindfulness/meditation practice to wellbeing, resilience, and adaptation to stressful situations. The findings of lower depression and mood disturbance among medical students participating in Mindfulness-Based Stress Reduction (MBSR) show that it can reduce stress, depression, anxiety, and distress (Rosenzweig et al., 2003). Although the overall magnitude of the effect of MBSR on psychological distress when compared to the usual-treatment arm noted by Van Dijk et al. in medical students was small to moderate (small reduction of psychological distress and dysfunctional cognitions and a moderate increase of positive mental health, life satisfaction, and mindfulness skills) what was striking was that these changes were still detectable at 20-month follow-up indicating that mindfulness training provides lasting rather than temporary benefits (van Dijk et al., 2017).

Lebares and colleagues argued that the time-compressed, high-stakes environment of surgical training required culturally appropriate, time-sensitive mindfulness training. ESRT is a modified form of MBSR training which has been streamlined, tailored, and contextualized for surgeons. The first iteration of ESRT was found feasible and acceptable in surgery interns (Lebares et al., 2018). There is significantly reduced time commitment compared to MBSR (five, 1-hour sessions at weekly intervals and home practice starting from three minutes daily compared with eight, 2.5 hours weekly sessions and 40 minutes daily practice in MBSR). ESRT is also skills-based rather than enquiry-based training. This makes ESRT much more accessible to busy medical students. Results of a pilot randomized clinical trial demonstrated potential benefits to wellbeing and executive function in surgery residents (Lebares et al., 2019). ESRT focuses on the complex skills of interoception, emotional regulation, and perspective taking. These skills typically taught through formal training in ESRT, appear to yield *Neurological* and cognitive changes that can enhance compassion, self-regulation, executive function, and performance. ESRT was chosen as time constraints are real in a graduate-entry medicine course, and skills-based training may suit medical students better.

The randomized controlled trial of (ESRT) currently being carried out at Swansea includes an evaluation of whether the effects of mindfulness are sustained after 6 months. This is measured by a pack of validated psychological questionnaires as well as monitoring of heart rate variability (HRV). Full results will be available in late-2023. Promotion of and recruitment to the trial has increased normalization of the discussion about stress and wellbeing in medical students. See Box 9.2.

Box 9.2 Individual feedback from participants on the ESRT trial

- *'The way that I react to things, and the way that I speak to people, in the way that I engage in placements has really changed more than I expected.'*
- *'I'd say I'm definitely a lot calmer in general, I am more positive, I do feel happier in general, I do feel like I've got a bit more purpose.'*
- *'I accept stressful events more easily now. Especially with exams this week, I found, it's probably the easiest exam season I've been through.'*

> **Box 9.3 Short mindfulness training offered to year 1 students at Swansea**
>
> - Short practice: **Attend to what is.** The first step invites attending broadly to one's experience, (physical sensation, thoughts, feelings) noting it, but without the need to change what is being observed.
> - **Focus on the breath.** The second step narrows the field of attention to a single, pointed focus on the breath in the body.
> - **Attend to the body.** The third step widens attention again to include the body as a whole and any sensations that are present.

Stress, Burnout, and Wellbeing in the Curriculum

Since 2017, year 1 medical students at SUMS are offered an hour-long session which includes stress, burnout, and mental health issues in medical students and the potential role of mindfulness. A short practice-based mindfulness training is also included (see Box 9.3). In these sessions a number of activities that improve wellbeing and resilience and ways to incorporate them in daily lives are discussed (Dave & Taylor-Robinson, 2022).

Reflective Practice

Self-reflection encourages positive outcomes on medical student wellbeing and clinical skills as well as improvements in levels of empathy and respect for patients, ability to self-reflect, cultural competency, and communication skills (Chen & Forbes, 2014). Higher levels of emotional intelligence have been associated with positive psychological wellbeing (Ruiz-Aranda et al., 2012; Sanchez-Alvarez et al., 2015).

Reflective practice is a core component in the undergraduate/graduate-entry medical programmes in Cardiff and Swansea.

Introduction to Reflective Writing

Students are introduced to the process of reflection early in both the Cardiff and Swansea programmes. They go onto develop these skills in clinical practice. All Cardiff students attend the workshop 'Becoming a doctor, staying a person', which builds further on supporting students to develop their emotional intelligence, self-awareness, and skills in self-reflection and regulation. This session was developed based on the work of Schön—The Reflective Practitioner (Schön, 1983). Students learn about reflecting 'in action' (in the moment), and 'on' action. Students write their own 'change stories' which they can choose to submit to the tutor.

Reflective writing with detailed personal feedback is a key component of professionalism in teaching in the graduate-entry medical programme at SUMS. This helps students to express the fear, concerns, frustrations, uncertainty, and joy of clinical practice without fear of being judged. A senior clinician/academic provides detailed personal feedback to help students make sense of the complex clinical world and support their personal development. A recent modification (2021) means that the same faculty provides the feedback over the entire course leading to the development of longer-term connections and Socratic dialogue between students and faculty.

Balint Groups

Students in years 3 and 4, at Cardiff, have the opportunity to engage with Balint groups (Monk et al., 2018) where a group of students meet, with a facilitator, to discuss cases/patients. Groups usually focus on the doctor–patient relationship, and the group are asked to reflect on the emotional impact an interaction had for both the patient and for them. Balint groups have been shown to reduce burnout and improve the management of stress and anxiety (Bar-Sela et al., 2012).

Analysis of Student Reflective Writing

Since 2009 Swansea students' written reflections have provided an opportunity to appreciate the difficulties, subtleties, uncertainties, and paradoxes of medical practice, and to challenge pre-conceived ideas. Since this requirement was introduced, around 3,000 pieces of reflective writing have been collected (Charlton et al., 2017).

Analysis of these reflections was used to formalize a resilience programme based around shared experience of common challenges.

Preparing for Clinical Practice: Resilience Training in the Curriculum

Common themes were identified through analysis of students' reflective writings. These highlighted a need to prepare the students more specifically for some of the challenges they would face in their future medical careers (see Box 9.4).

These themes formed the core of the 'Preparation for Clinical Practice' (PCP) programme.

Box 9.4 Themes arising from the reflective writings of Swansea medical students

---

a) Self-care
b) Personal/professional difficulties (relationships, financial, etc.)
c) Dealing with uncertainty, risk management
d) 'Mistakes'
e) Need for peer/mentor support
f) Illness (physical/mental)
g) Professional development and competence
h) Failure to progress
i) Bullying

The Preparation for Clinical Practice Programme

Initially introduced as a pilot, for first-year Medicine (GEM) students, eight sessions were offered across the year which were voluntary and not assessed. The module was sensitively designed to ensure that comprehensive tutor support was available, should the topic areas evoke uncomfortable or difficult feelings. There was an average of 51 students at each session (65% of the cohort).

Each session followed a similar format:

- Introduction and video clips (e.g. TED Talk) appropriate to the subject matter
- Tutor role play depicting a challenging, yet not atypical situation
- External speaker (often a near-peer student or postgraduate) describing lived experience and narrative with opportunity for student questioning and thought sharing
- Group discussion between students and speaker and facilitated by tutors. In small groups or across the whole group or both.

The programme built on ideas in the literature of reflecting and sharing experiences whilst combining this with personal stories of tutors and past students. The programme aimed to enable students to develop resilience in the face of future challenges.

After each session, participants rated to what extent each component of the session had affected their confidence to cope, awareness of available support, and understanding of attending to self-care.

Evaluation of the PCP Programme Pilot

Students suggested that the programme had raised awareness of mental health problems amongst medical students, and had encouraged them to ask for help when needed:

The difficulty with self-care, is that we know we should all do that, but often, by the time we are in difficulty, it is difficult to know which way is up and which way is down, so learning about how to ask for help, who to ask for help and that you can ask for help is important whilst you are feeling good. PCP achieved that.

Lived Experience Describe by Near Peers

The lived experience aspect of the course evoked the greatest number of comments from students:

The lived experience part of the sessions was by far the most valuable. You know, the issues people came across, how they felt about them, what impact it had on them and how they sought help to climb out of that situation.

All the comments relating to the lived experience were positive, with students noting the value of these experiences for their learning. Students found the talks inspiring and gained practical tips from the speakers.

Videos/TED Talks

In relation to the videoed talks students' feelings were mixed. Some students felt they were helpful and their position at the start of the session put students at ease, others found them less helpful.

Role Play

The role plays also received a mixed reaction with the students:

Sometimes, I felt the role plays were too simplistic, where there was an obvious right and wrong way to go about things, there could have been more nuance to some of them.

Facilitated Discussion

Some students were very positive about the group discussion, whilst others felt that there should have been more opportunity to explore this. Some felt that the effectiveness of group discussion was dependent on the mix of students in the different groups:

Sometimes, it was difficult to get a discussion going in the facilitated group sessions as some people, felt uncomfortable about speaking up and other times, you had a dominant character who took over.

Conclusions from Evaluation of PCP Pilot

The evaluation suggested that the most compelling component of this programme involved the lived experience by peers/near peers based on actual events where experience, hope, and strength are shared.

Integrating Health and Wellbeing Throughout the Curriculum

SUMS has recognized the importance of the PCP programme, which has, now, been integrated into the [compulsory] curriculum. PCP provides some insights for the development of programmes designed to build resilience in medical students. The value and enthusiasm for the programme was seen in the numbers who attended voluntarily. The need for programmes to be practical and relevant to the students is paramount, for the PCP programme.

This was achieved by using student reflections and including past experiences from former students. Hearing and sharing experiences face-to-face was seen as particularly valuable and had an additional benefit of being an opportunistic time for students to raise any problems within a safe environment. The sessions now revolve largely around the shared experience of visiting clinicians with ample opportunity for discussion and questions—facilitated by clinical tutors. Videos, such as topic-specific TED talks, are used solely as an introduction to the session, if at all. The role plays enacted by the tutors have been removed.

At Cardiff, the Embedding Mental Wellbeing in the Curriculum project recommends keeping the curriculum in focus, with mental wellbeing being core to the curriculum in the way it is taught (Houghton & Anderson, 2017). The aim is to promote health and wellbeing throughout the curriculum, to support all students whether they decide to disclose a disability or seek support. Near-peer sessions are delivered in year 1, including 'Talking about mental health and seeking support' and also in year 3 'Preparing for Placements/Dealing with Death'.

'I think in the moment, you're just focused on what's going on around you, and the situation you're in. You almost forget all the potential support/suggestions on how to deal with these things available to you. The Dealing with Death talk was helpful later on when you're still thinking about what you have experienced and how to move forward.'
'My very first day on placement, I was put in a difficult situation seeing two deaths in ITU. Had I not had this talk, I would have felt completely lost.'

In year 2, the MyMedic Team deliver a session focused on 'Maintaining your Wellbeing throughout medical school', providing practical techniques that students can use to manage stress, worries, and anxiety. Wellbeing is a core focus within professionalism workshops, where students are guided through scenarios and consider dilemmas related to professionalism. Equality, diversity, and inclusivity (EDI) training runs through each year of the MBBCh, where scenarios are focused on encountering prejudice and discrimination as a medical student. They encourage reflection and discussion and include a significant focus on student health and wellbeing. A key focus is encouraging students to seek support appropriately and to feel safe to raise their concerns (School of Medicine 'Raising Concerns' Policy https://sway.office.com/H6WFoxMCrkcZur1r).

Peer Support and Near-peer Mentoring

Peer support is one of the most valuable resources in maintaining student wellbeing. Peers are likely to be the first to notice and respond to distressed peers. Initiating and providing peer support does not come easily to many medical students unless there are pre-existing social relationships (Graves et al., 2022).

Transition to learning in a clinical environment is well-recognized as a challenging period for medical students (Malau-Aduli et al., 2020; Prince et al., 2005). A near-peer mentoring scheme was introduced at Cardiff with the aim of easing this transition. All year 3 and year 5 students are invited to participate. Each year 3 student mentee is paired with a year 5 volunteer mentor. Where possible, student pairs are matched based on placement location to facilitate face-to-face meetings. In 2021/22, there were 36 mentee/mentor pairs. Mentors are given an introductory presentation and handbook containing information, learning resources, and further support contacts.

Demographics of Students Who Choose to Access Near-peer Mentoring

Demographic data were collected to determine which students were more likely to access the mentoring programme. The percentage of students in years 3 and 5 respectively who identify as female are 68% and 66%. Of the volunteer mentees, 95% identified as female with 70% of the mentors identifying as female. In terms of sexual orientation, 26% of the mentees identified as homosexual, bisexual, or pansexual This rate appears significantly higher than the rate in the UK general population of 16–24-year-olds identifying as lesbian, gay, or bisexual of 8% (ONS, 2020). All mentors identified as heterosexual. Of the mentees, 43% identified as being from an ethnic minority background, compared to 33% of the full year 3 cohort. Despite 32% of the year 5 cohort being from ethnic minority backgrounds, only 13% of the year 5 mentors were from an ethnic minority background. These data suggest that students from minority groups may be more likely to voluntarily access near-peer mentorship, but less likely to volunteer as mentors. The major reasons that students sought near-peer mentorship were related to increasing confidence/reassurance, academic advice—particularly around placements and assessments, and developing social networks. 82% of mentees agreed that the near-peer mentoring reduced their anxiety or stress levels.

An Award for Peer Support

At Swansea, since 2017, an annual award has been established to raise the profile of peer support and to reward good practice. Any student or faculty can nominate a student who has provided or facilitated peer support to GEM students. Shortlisted candidates make a presentation to a panel and a winner/joint winners are identified. Many outstanding peer support initiatives have been brought to light through this process. Examples include: tea and empathy groups, examination training, revision classes, one-to-one support, peer-assisted learning in Swansea (PALS), sharing personal stories of struggles, sharing resources, running mock exams, and acting as year representative.

Case-based Professionalism Teaching

A Mental Health Case and Student Wellbeing

A case focused on students'/practitioners' mental health is a core part of the CBL curriculum in years 1 and 2 at Cardiff (Hassoulas et al., 2017). Students consider the case scenario within facilitated small group sessions. The mental health case is based around the scenario of a fictional university student, who during his time at university, develops depressive symptoms and later on psychotic features. Four video diaries are used to portray the student's journey covering the range, progression, and impact of his symptoms, which were created to help students identify with the experiences of the patient case. Due to the sensitive nature of the videos and case content, students are provided with the contact details of relevant support services and encouraged to seek support should they feel that they need to.

'The videos before each of the case sessions really helped put the case in context as you could put into perspective that the mental health problems where those of a real person and not just a scenario.

The mental health case also includes a seminar where people with personal experience of mental illness, including former students, share their experiences around mental health. Students complete an online module 'Medics and Mental Health' and consider content around disclosing mental health issues, seeking appropriate support and GMC guidance around this area. This module is focused on challenging some of the myths around medics and mental health, particularly student concerns around fitness to practice (Winter et al., 2017) encouraging the disclosure of mental illness and enabling students to seek support appropriately.

'Thank you for this case, I understand that some students may have found this case difficult, but the university and the case leads made sure that the students were aware of where they need to go to get support.'
'Case 10 was an interesting one. I felt the topic may be difficult to discuss with peers and patients, but actually found the opposite. Initially people were unsure about what to say but the sessions did well in highlighting the importance of talking about mental health.'

Professionalism Dilemmas Through Case Discussion

Professionalism teaching is given importance in SUMS from the outset. Some aspects of professionalism teaching relate to wellbeing improvement (e.g. self-care, teamwork, admitting mistakes and learning from them). Case-based professionalism teaching is a way of helping students learn from professionalism dilemmas witnessed by themselves and their peers (Monrouxe et al., 2017). This is facilitated in small group-based sessions, where students are encouraged to bring their own professionalism dilemmas. This hybrid plan starts with a facilitator discussing a case with professionalism issues and then students share their own professionalism related dilemmas from the clinical world in a safe space. This open discussion helps students to make meaning of the complex clinical world.

Supervision of Medical Students' Health and Wellbeing

MBBCh Health and Wellbeing Curricular Developments

At Cardiff MyMedic-LDU work closely with curriculum teams and students within the medical school to ensure that student health and wellbeing is considered in relation to both curriculum design and delivery.

Both Cardiff and Swansea medical schools have Health and Conduct (H&C) committees who work primarily to identify students who need additional support (health, academic, personal issues). All students who have failed significant exams, have health concerns, low-level professionalism concerns, or significant personal issues are monitored by the committee. Referral to H&C comes from numerous sources with no restriction and its primarily role is seen as supportive. Membership includes year leads, cohort leads, wellbeing lead, chair of H&C committee, head of the programme.

Support Structure Within the School

The Student Experience and Information Team within the Faculty of Medicine, Health, and Life Science, Swansea University, work in partnership with academic staff and other professional services and departments to deliver the highest level of professional support in the following functions:

- Student information and student enquiries—this will cover a wide range of topics across all programmes in the faculty
- Student Welfare and Wellbeing Signposting and Triage
- Student communications
- Extenuating circumstances
- Processing transfers/suspensions/withdrawals
- Enabling services—supporting students with differing needs including alternative assessment
- Student attendance and study engagement
- Student experience to include but not limited to student representative, student feedback, student events, subject/academic student societies, peer mentoring

Within the team there are student information and support officers who act as first port of call for students with non-academic and wellbeing issues. The support officers can provide advice, support, and guidance on a wide range of welfare issues to students throughout their time at university, e.g. bereavement, mental health concerns, and relationship issues. They signpost students to a variety of support and resources available within the university and externally.

Acknowledgements

The authors would like to thank Steve Daniels for preparing the section on student support within the medical school.

References

Bar-Sela, G., Lulav-Grinwald, D., & Mitnik, I. (2012). Balint group' meetings for oncology residents as a tool to improve therapeutic communication skills and reduce burnout level. *J Cancer Educ* **27**: 786–789.

Charlton, R., Hayward, C., Rees, J., & Weston, C. (2017). *A Human Touch Anthology of prose and Poetry. The undergraduates of Swansea University Medical School*, Hampton-in Arden: Hampton-in Arden Publishing.

Chen, I. & Forbes, C. (2014). 'Reflective writing and its impact on empathy in medical education: systematic review'. *J Educ Eval Health Prof* 11: 20.

Dave, U. & Taylor-Robinson, S. (2022). 'Maintaining resilience in today's medical environment: personal perspectives on self-care'. *Int J Gen Med* 15: 2475–2478.

Farrell, S., Molodynski, A., Cohen, D., Grant, A., Rees, S., Wullshleger, A., Lewis, T., & Kadhum, M. (2019). 'Wellbeing and burnout among medical students in Wales'. *Internl Rev Psychiatry* 31(7–8): 613–618.

Graves, J., Flynn, E., & Woodward-Kron, R. (2022). 'Supporting medical students to support peers: a qualitative interview study'. *BMC Med Educ* 22: 300.

Hassoulas, A., Forty, L., Hoskins, M., Walters, J., & Riley, S. (2017). 'A case-based medical curriculum for the 21st century: the use of innovative approaches in designing and developing a case on mental health'. *Med Teach* 39: 505–511.

Houghton, A. & Anderson, J. (2017). Embedding mental wellbeing in the curriculum:maximising success in higher education [Online]. Higher Education Academy. https://www.advance-he.ac.uk/knowledge-hub/embedding-mental-wellbeing-curriculum-maximising-success-higher-education [Accessed 17 August 2023].

Lebares, C., Guvva, E., Olaru, M., Sugrue, L., Staffaroni, A., Delucchi, K., Kramer, J., Ascher, N., & Harris, H. (2019). 'Efficacy of mindfulness-based cognitive training in surgery additional analysis of the mindful surgeon pilot randomized clinical trial'. *JAMA Netw Open* 2: e1 194108.

Lebares, C., Hershberger, A., & Guvva, E. (2018). 'Feasibility of formal mindfulness-based stress-resilience training among surgery intern: a randomized clinical trial'. *JAMA Surg* 153: e182734.

Malau-Aduli, B., Roche, P., Adu, M., Jones, K., Alele, F., & Drovandi, A. (2020). 'Perceptions and processes influencing the transition of medical students from pre-clinical to clinical training'. *BMC Med Educ* 20(1): 279.

Monk, A., Hind, D. & Crimlisk, H. (2018). 'Balint groups in undergraduate medical education: a systematic review'. *Psychoanalytic Psychotherapy* 32: 61–86.

Monrouxe, L., Shaw, M., & Rees, C. (2017). Antecedents and consequences of medical students' moral decision making during professionalism dilemmas. *AMA J Ethics* 19: 568–577.

Prince, K., Boshuizen, H., Van Der Vleuten, C., Van Der Vleuten, F., & Scherpbier, A. (2005). 'Students' opinions about their preparation for clinical practice'. *Med Educ* 39: 704–712.

Rosenzweig, S., Reibel, D., Greeson, J., Brainard, G., & Hojat, M. (2003). 'Mindfulness based stress reduction lowers psychological distress in medical students'. *Teach Learn Med* 15: 88–92.

Ruiz-Aranda, D., Castillo, R., Salguero, J. M., Cabello, R., Fernandez=Berrocal, P., & Balluerka, N. (2012). 'Short-and midterm effects of emotional intelligence training on adolescent mental health'. *J Adolesc Health* 51: 462–467.

Sanchez-Alvarez, N., Extremera, N., & Fernandez-Berrocal, P. (2015). 'Maintaining life satisfaction in adolescence: affective mediators of the influence of perceived emotional intelligence on overall life satisfaction judgments in a two-year longitudinal study'. *Front Psychol* 6: 1892.

Schön, D. (1983). *The Reflective Practitioner: How Professionals Think in Action*. New York: Basic Books.

UCAS 2021. (2021). End of Cycle data showing the number of disability declarations from all UK applicants between 2011 and 2020. Data table: UK applicants disability declarations 2011–2020. UCAS.

Van Dijk, I., Ucassen, P., Akkermans, R., Van Engelen, B., Van Weel, C., & Speckens, A. (2017). 'Effects of mindfulness-based stress reduction on the mental health of clinical clerkship students: a cluster-randomized controlled trial'. *Acad Med* 92(7): 1012–1021.

Winter, P., Rix, A., & Grant, A. (2017). Medical student beliefs about disclosure of mental health issues: a qualitative study. *J Vet Med Educ* 44(1): 147–156.

10

Egypt

Burnout, Mental Health, and Wellbeing Among Egyptian Students

Tarek Okasha, Nermin Shaker, and Dina Aly El-Gabry

Introduction

Mental health has recently come into increasing focus, attracting the interest of both the public sector and the scientific community. In Egypt, mental health research among university students dates back to the 1970s. The early work of Okasha et al. (1977) provided insightful perspectives on the subject, carrying out research on 1,050 students, 139 of which attended the faculty of medicine. Students visiting the student health centre were referred from a multitude of sources: family recommendations, personal motivation, general health practitioners, or their faculties. The study found anxiety to be the most frequent diagnosis, encountered in 36% of the cases. Anxiety was found to act as a reactive function to either maturational or environmental stressors, the most common participating factors being relationship problems with either fellow students or tutors, as well as difficulty in mastering the subject studied. Common symptoms included the inability to learn effectively and adequately, lack of concentration, and social discomfort paired with insomnia or excessive complaints. Although the study diagnosed students only clinically, excluding the use of rating scales and referred to the general student population at Ain Shams University rather than the faculty of medicine per se, the results provide us with a dependable point of reference about common problems faced by students at that time.

Undergraduate Programmes for Medical Students in Egypt

In the last two decades, international medical education has been experiencing a range of challenges and changes that have called for significant reforms; globalization, and advances in information technology, best evidence, evidence-based practice, quality practices and quality assurance, and accreditation. In Egypt there are 28 medical schools offering medical undergraduate education, including two of the largest educational medical institutions in Africa and the Middle East: Cairo University (first founded in 1827) and Ain Shams University (first founded in 1928) (Okasha & Shaker, 2020).

The first two private medical schools were established in 1996. Due to concerns about the quality of clinical teaching and training of interns, it took an additional 20 years to establish

Tarek Okasha, Nermin Shaker, and Dina Aly El-Gabry, *Egypt* In: *The Mental Health of Medical Students*.
Edited by: Andrew Molodynski, Sarah Marie Farrell, and Dinesh Bhugra, Oxford University Press. © Oxford University Press 2024.
DOI: 10.1093/oso/9780192864871.003.0010

the third private medical school, which opened in 2016. Almost all medical schools in Egypt have well-established teaching hospitals, and most confine the clinical training of students to these hospitals. However, a small number of schools use Ministry of Health hospitals or other health provision outlets affiliated with governmental or non-governmental agencies (Abdelaziz et al., 2018).

Until 2018, Egyptian medical schools comprised a six-year programme of undergraduate medical education. This system featured a clear preclinical—clinical dichotomy. A Bachelor of Medicine and Surgery (MBBCh) was awarded upon graduation, but graduates were required to attend a full-year internship programme before obtaining their licence to practice as general practitioners. This system adopted a discipline-based curriculum, in which didactic large-group lectures and apprenticeship approaches to clinical teaching were the main methods of instruction (Abdelaziz et al., 2018). The new system, developed in 2018–2019, requires 7 years to get a medical degree: 5 years of integrated medical education and 2 years of internship. Teaching methods include lectures, case scenarios, case presentations, role play, self-learning, and clinical training. Methods of assessment include Objective Structured Clinical Exam (OSCE), Multiple Choice Questions (MCQ), Modified Short Assay Questions, projects, and assignments. This integrated curriculum features innovative instructional methods, including simulation, early clinical exposure, and project-based learning, in addition to problem-based learning, shifting towards integration, and student-centredness (Okasha & Shaker, 2020).

The Egyptian Medical System and its Impact on Medical Students

Egyptian medical students face an abundance of psychosocial stressors, both academic and non-academic, which significantly contribute to the development of chronic stress symptoms. To begin with, the competitive nature of pre-med admission due to a lack of a premedical university preparatory programme (UPP) presents students with adjustment difficulties. Understanding and learning a dense and complex syllabus can be a further barrier for students to overcome, aggravated by the fact that not all of those enrolled are proficient in English, the language of instruction in all medical schools in Egypt. To date, Egyptian medical schools have followed the French model, comprising a 6-year programme of undergraduate medical education. Most undergraduate programmes use didactic large-group lectures and apprenticeship approaches to clinical teaching as the main methods of instruction. Students hence face major difficulties on several levels: long teaching hours, lack of leisure or recreation time, learning difficulty or language-based obstacles with absorbing the curriculum, irregular schedules, high frequency of tests, peer competition, and anxiety related to academic performance, achievement, and fear of failure. The grading system of Egyptian medical education is rigorous and stress-inducing, calculating the final grade at graduation based on the cumulative scores of the exams over each of the 6 years of education (El-Gabry et al., 2022). As such, the competitive selection process, challenging learning environment, and rigorous grading system place huge demands on each student's mental and physical health. Psychosocial stressors are also significant due to high parental expectations, home sickness, adjustment to new accommodation, new social circles, financial strain, and fear of future failure in students' medical career.

Stress, Anxiety, and Depression Among Egyptian Medical Students

Unfortunately, comprehensive epidemiological data on the psychological health of undergraduate medical students in Egyptian universities remains scarce. Only recently has research regarding mental wellbeing among medical students been conducted at different universities in different cities across Egypt (Mansoura, Tanta, Assuit, Menoufyia, Al Fayoum, Cairo). However, a national survey regarding mental wellbeing among medical students does not exist as of now (El-Gabry et al., 2022; Fawzy & Hamed, 2017).

El-Gabry et al.'s (2022) study on 547 medical students from two universities in Cairo investigated one governmental and one private university: Ain Shams University and Misr University for Science and Technology, respectively. The study's results showcased that 16% of medical students were diagnosed with mental illness while in medical school, in comparison to 7% that had been diagnosed prior to starting medical school. More than half of these students reported that their studies were the leading source of stress.

A cross-sectional study of 700 medical students carried out at Assuit University similarly found high frequencies of depression (60%), anxiety (73%), and psychological stress (59.9%) as common occurrences using the Depression Anxiety Stress Scale (DASS 21). Using the same scale at Menoufyia University in first-year medical students, the prevalence of depression, anxiety, and stress among students was 63.6%, 78.4%, and 57.8%, respectively (Abdallah & Gabr, 2014) and 60.8%, 64.3%, and 62.4% at a study performed on 442 medical students at Al Fayoum University (Abdel Wahed & Hassan, 2017). Stressors were reported by 94.5% of the total sample of medical students at Mansoura University (Amr et al., 2008), using administrating questionnaires covering different stressors, perceived stress scale, physical wellbeing factors, the Hospital Anxiety and Depression scale, as well as neuroticism and extraversion subscales of the Eysenck Personality Questionnaire. Based on these results, psychosocial stressors clearly play a significant role in the mental health landscape of Egyptian medical students.

Burnout Symptoms in Medical Students

El-Gabry et al.'s (2022) study highlighted very high levels of distress among medical students, finding 88% screening positive for burnout using the Oldenburg Burnout Inventory (OLBI), 64% of those interviewed reached the same threshold as those cases studied in the short version of the general health questionnaire (GHQ-12). The high prevalence of burnout in this study is consistent with a previous study conducted in Egypt, which reported a burnout prevalence of 79.9% (Atlam, 2018) and other African countries such as Uganda (Kajjimu et al., 2021). However, these results are unfortunately higher compared to the results for medical students' burnout in other parts of the Arab world, such as Morocco, Jordan, Bahrain, Oman, Saudi Arabia (Aboalshamat et al., 2017; Al Ubaidi et al., 2018; Al-Alawi et al., 2019; Albalawi et al., 2015; Almalki et al., 2017; Altannir et al., 2019; Lemtiri Chelieh et al., 2019; Mahfouz et al., 2020; Masri et al., 2019).

These differing results could be attributed to methodological differences, such as the use of different scales to identify burnout symptoms. Alternatively, the effect of different cultural and educational systems across the Middle East could contribute to a differently nuanced interpretation of outcomes. Given the high chronic stress that medical students in Egypt face, the diagnosis of mental and psychological exhaustion are not surprising. These ailments can ultimately lead to feelings of incapacity, symptoms of mental illness, and manifestations of depression and burnout. Unfortunately, this already high percentage may in fact mask a much more pervasive problem: students commonly approach their professors informally in their private clinics (away from the university), as there is a fear of mental illness stigma which is deeply rooted in Egyptian culture and social expectations.

Case Report

A 20-year-old previously medically free single Egyptian female second-year medical student presented to the outpatient clinic, complaining of recurrent intrusive distressing thoughts of sexual content. These thoughts would occur most of the day nearly every day and have been occurring over the past 9 months. She knew that these thoughts were silly and she did not want to think about them, however, could not stop them. She would react by reciting prayers for redemption all the time to try and compensate for these thoughts and relieve the distress she experienced. This impaired her ability to study, and she started becoming isolated and avoided going out. She had failed to study for an upcoming exam so she presented to the clinic to try and seek help for her condition.

This was her second time seeking psychiatric advice, whereas a year ago, she had sought advice for feeling extremely drained and unable to study. She was overwhelmed with the course load and the recurring exams and could not study for all of them. She had found herself spending long hours studying a small amount of material and she would repeat individual sentences in her books repeatedly. She stopped pursuing her interests such as reading and drawing and stopped enjoying studying medicine. She felt like she was not herself anymore as she started failing her module exams for the first time in her life, which made her feel like a failure. She started feeling sad most of the day, spontaneously crying whenever alone. She started avoiding going to university and stayed in bed most of the day, with normal sleep and appetite. There were no other mood, anxiety, or obsessive-compulsive-related symptoms at the time. She had sought psychiatric advice, was prescribed an antidepressant and referred to cognitive behavioural therapy (CBT) for which she never showed up and ended up failing two subjects in her finals.

Substance Misuse and Abuse Among Medical Students

The British Medical Association has identified drug use as a worldwide problem, finding it to be at least equal to the population level in each country and in many cases, much higher (Bhugra et al., 2019). Only scarce data concerning substance misuse among Egyptian medical students exists. In a recent study by El-Gabry et al. (2022), 9% of students were CAGE-positive, indicating a problematic level of alcohol consumption. This is higher than the prevalence of alcohol use disorders in other studies carried out in the Arab world, such as 8% in Jordan (Masri et al., 2019) and 5% in a Moroccan study (Lemtiri Chelieh et al., 2019). Forty-two students (7.7%) reported taking a non-prescription substance or prescription medication outside its intended use (to improve wellbeing or uplift their mood), whereas 76 students (13.9%) described using medication to enhance concentration, study, or academic performance. This indicates that most of these students probably use medication as a form of self-medication, due to addiction to the drug, or a mixture of both. This occurs despite students being in the best possible place to understand the consequences of drug and substance abuse and face the consequences of its physical, mental, and societal damage (Molodynski et al., 2019).

Future Horizons

Research data clearly indicates a high tendency towards psychosocial stress, mental health difficulties, and burnout symptoms in Egyptian medical students. A few initiatives aimed at improvement have been launched recently, introducing the application of integrated modular-based programmes in medical schools and particularly at the faculties of medicine, such as at Ain Shams University, Cairo University (Kasr El Ainy) and Mansoura University (Abdelaziz et al., 2018). These initiatives also aim to integrate international standards on medical education, which place increasing importance on psychological support for students. Student psychiatric and mental health support service started in February 2019 to provide Ain Shams University students with appropriate counselling and psychological support aiming at early detection and management of students' psychiatric disorders, assisting students who were experiencing stressful events to promote better adaptation to their college life (Okasha & Shaker, 2020).

However, a profound gap between the service provided and students' needs being met remains. This is an alarming sign of a high risk of mental illness in a population who unfortunately represents the future backbone of our healthcare system. Decision-makers and the scientific community in Egypt would be well advised to prioritize and approach this problem in the near future. The health of our society depends on competent doctors are able to fulfil their duties and tackle challenges efficiently and effectively whilst being in good health themselves.

References

Abdallah, A.R. & Gabr, H.M. (2014). 'Depression, anxiety and stress among first year medical students in an Egyptian public university'. *Int Res J Med Med Sci* **2**(1): 11–19.

Abdel Wahed, W.Y. & Hassan, S.K. (2017). 'Prevalence and associated factors of stress, anxiety and depression among medical Fayoum University students'. *Alex J Med* **53**(1): 77–84.

Abdelaziz, A. et al. (2018). 'Medical education in Egypt: Historical background, current status, and challenges'. *Health Prof Educ* **4**(4): 236–244.

Aboalshamat, K. et al. (2017). 'The relationship between burnout and perfectionism in medical and dental students in Saudi Arabia'. *J Dent Special* **5**(2): 122–127.

Al-Alawi, M., Al-Sinawi, H., Al-Qubtan, A., Al-Lawati, J., Al-Habsi, A., Al-Shuraiqi, M., Al-Adawi, S., & Panchatcharam, S.M. (2019). 'Prevalence and determinants of burnout Syndrome and Depression among medical students at Sultan Qaboos University: a cross-sectional analytical study from Oman'. *Arch Environ Occup Health* **74**(3): 130–139.

Albalawi, A.E. et al. (2015). 'The assessment of the burnout syndrome among medical students in Tabuk University, a cross-sectional analytic study'. *BRJMCS* **6**(1): 14–19.

Almalki, S.A., Almojali, A.I., Alothman, A.S., Masuadi, E.M., & Alaqeel, M.K. (2017). 'Burnout and its association with extracurricular activities among medical students in Saudi Arabia'. *Int J Med Educ* **8**: 144–150.

Altannir, Y., Alnajjar, W., Ahmad, S.O., Altannir, M., Yousuf, F., Obeidat, A., & Al-Tannir, M. (2019). 'Assessment of burnout in medical undergraduate students in Riyadh, Saudi Arabia'. *BMC Med Educ* **19**(1): 34.

Al Ubaidi, B.A., Jassim, G., & Salem, A. (2018). 'Burnout syndrome in medical students in the kingdom of Bahrain'. *Glob J Health Sci* **10**(11): 86–94.

Amr, M., El Gilany, A.H., & El-Hawary, A. (2008) 'Does gender predict medical students' stress in Mansoura, Egypt?' *Med Educ Online* **13**(1): 4481.

Atlam, S.A. (2018). 'Burnout syndrome: determinants and predictors among medical students of tanta university, Egypt'. *EJCM* **36**(01): 61–73.

Bhugra, D., Sauerteig, S.O., Bland, D., Lloyd-Kendall, A., Wijesuriya, J., Singh, G., Kochhar, A., Molodynski, A., & Ventriglio, A. (2019). 'A descriptive study of mental health and wellbeing of doctors and medical students in the UK'. *Int Rev Psychiatry* **31**(7–8): 563–568.

El-Gabry, D.A., Okasha, T., Shaker, N., Elserafy, D., Yehia, M., Aziz, K.A., Bhugra, D., Molodynski, A., & Elkhatib, H. (2022). 'Mental health and wellbeing among Egyptian medical students: a cross-sectional study'. *Middle East Curr Psychiatry* **29**(1). doi: 10.1186/s43045-022-00193-1

Fawzy, M. & Hamed, S.A. (2017). 'Prevalence of psychological stress, depression and anxiety among medical students in Egypt'. *Psychiatry Res* **255**: 186–194.

Kajjimu, J., Kaggwa, M.M., & Bongomin, F. (2021). 'Burnout and associated factors among medical students in a public university in Uganda: a cross-sectional study'. *Adv Med Educ Pract* **12**: 63–75.

Lemtiri Chelieh, M., Kadhum, M., Lewis, T., Molodynski, A., Abouqal, R., Belayachi, J., & Bhugra, D. (2019). 'Mental health and wellbeing among Moroccan medical students: a descriptive study'. *Int Rev Psychiatry* **31**(7–8): 608–612.

Mahfouz, M.S., Ali, S.A., Alqahtani, H.A., Kubaisi, A.A., Ashiri, N.M., Daghriri, E.H., Alzahrani, S.A., Sowaidi, A.A., Maashi, A.M., & Alhazmi, D.A. (2020). 'Burnout and its associated factors among medical students of Jazan University, Jazan, Saudi Arabia'. *Ment Ill* **12**(2): 35–42.

Masri, R., Kadhum, M., Farrell, S.M., Khamees, A., Al-Taiar, H., & Molodynski, A. (2019). 'Wellbeing and mental health amongst medical students in Jordan: a descriptive study'. *Int Rev Psychiatry* **31**(7–8): 619–625.

Molodynski, A., Ventriglio, A., & Bhugra, D. (2019). 'A crisis brewing for the healthcare system and a crisis already happening for our students'. *Int Rev Psychiatry* **31**(7–8): 545–547.

Okasha, A., Kamel, M., Sadek, A., & Lotaif, Z.B. (1977). 'Psychiatric morbidity among university students in Egypt'. *Br J Psychiatry* **131**(2): 149–154.

Okasha, T. & Shaker, N. (2020). 'Psychiatric education and training in Arab countries'. *Int Rev Psychiatry* **32**(2): 151–156.

11
Georgia

Mental Health and Wellbeing of Medical Students in Georgia

Ekaterine Berdzenishvili, Eteri Machavariani, and Eka Chkonia

Introduction

Medical education is a rigorous and prolonged process that involves certain levels of stress and personal sacrifice. It is well established that the rates of burnout and psychiatric morbidity are higher among medical students than those of peers of the same age (Moir et al., 2018), and medical students from Georgia are no different. A number of potentially stressful factors have been reported among medical undergraduates. These include a highly stressful environment, competitiveness, excessive workload, sleep deprivation, peer pressure, and many other personal, curricular, institutional, and affective factors (Tempski et al., 2012). Factors known to be associated with mental health problems in medical students include maladaptive personality traits (Yates et al., 2008), financial difficulties, pre-existing mental health problems (Guthrie et al., 1998), and exposure to an older, fragmented, and more theoretical curricular structure (Kaufman et al., 1998). These findings suggest that certain aspects of medical education have harmful consequences on students' mental health and wellbeing, thereby hindering the aim of medical education to produce medical doctors with the desired personal qualities and professional competency.

Local Context

Georgia is an upper-middle-income country in the Eastern European Region. There are three registered medical universities and 25 medical programmes in the country (Universities and Programs Catalog, 2022). According to the National Statistics Office of Georgia, 22,501 students and residents are attending medical or veterinarian degree programmes or undergoing residency training as of 2022, out of which 6,505 are international students (Higher Education—National Statistics Office of Georgia, 2022). Most of them are citizens of India, Iraq, Nigeria, Turkey, Azerbaijan, and Russia, mostly living in Tbilisi (95%), Kutaisi (2.2%), and Batumi (1.8%). The most expensive and popular course is medical education (Kinkladze & Chitaladze, 2019).

Medical Students living and studying in Georgia have to overcome the general challenges of medical school life like burnout, stress of achieving, and attaining high academic standards, as well as problems relevant to the country, such as economic instability and political turmoil. For international students, stress is further exacerbated by an unfamiliar environment and the

Ekaterine Berdzenishvili, Eteri Machavariani, and Eka Chkonia, *Georgia* In: *The Mental Health of Medical Students*. Edited by: Andrew Molodynski, Sarah Marie Farrell, and Dinesh Bhugra, Oxford University Press. © Oxford University Press 2024. DOI: 10.1093/oso/9780192864871.003.0011 need to adjust to the new country, culture, and language. Finally, the COVID-19 pandemic, which devastated the world, affected Georgia as well, taking a toll on the healthcare system and leading to a high rate of infections and deaths and many lockdowns, movement restrictions, and uncertainty. In this situation of the usual stressors combined with the COVID-19 pandemic, it is especially important to understand the mental health of medical students in the country, determine modifiable factors that exacerbate stress, and introduce strategies that will increase resilience and provide essential mental healthcare for the medical student population.

There are few studies about medical student mental health in Georgia. The most prevalent data that we have on this group come from studies looking at international students. It appears that mental health problems are highly prevalent among international medical students. One study, looking at stress and sleep disturbances determined a high prevalence of both among international medical students (Soyakin et al., 2019), while another one showed that 38% and 43% of surveyed participants scored positively on the anxiety and depression questionnaires respectively (Rekhviashvili et al., 2021). The same study found that almost half of the study population had pre-hypertension. The cause-and-effect relationship between stress and raised blood pressure is to be determined in this high-stress environment. Poor lifestyle choices and non-healthy eating habits are also prevalent among medical students, suggesting that not only mental health service access is lacking for this group, but primary care access as well.

The situation among Georgian nationals does not differ significantly from their international peers. High stress levels, especially in the first (predominantly basic science based and pre-clinical) 4 years of medical education, was a noticeable finding of a study of Georgian medical students (Abashishvili et al., 2022). Students in different stages of education tended to have different stressors, ranging from coursework and exams in the early years to financial struggles later. Stress seemed to decrease after the completion of the pre-clinical part and the beginning of the clinical courses, which generally are regarded as less stressful in Georgian medical schools teaching in a traditional way (programmes that do not have a US MD teaching style).

COVID-19

It is important to note the exacerbated stress caused by the COVID-19 pandemic. The situation was especially tough for students as the educational system was first paralysed and then transitioned to online teaching. Many international students were stranded without further notice. Pandemic affected the mental health of the student population all over the world, with increasing prevalence of depression, anxiety, and stress (Holm-Hadulla et al., 2021; Hamaideh et al., 2022). According to a cross-sectional survey conducted during the pandemic, anxiety and depression levels were skyrocketing, with factors like fear of infection, inadequate supplies, boredom, stigmatization, financial concerns, and expectation-related worries, academic-related concerns were added to the long list of usual suspects of medical students' stressors (Nadareishvili et al., 2022).

Methods

In 2021, in collaboration with colleagues from Oxford University and King's College, we conducted a study looking at stress, wellbeing, and burnout in Georgian medical students

(Berdzenishvili et al., 2021). This was a part of the second wave of a large international initiative to measure stress, burnout, psychological problems, and substance misuse among thousands of students across many countries. The instrument to measure stress and burnout was a survey, which was an exact replica of the online survey used in other countries, translated into Georgian. The survey contained questions to collect demographic details and information about sources of stress. It also contained the General Health Questionnaire 12 (GHQ12) (Goldberg & Blackwell, 1970), the Oldenburg Burnout Inventory (OLBI) (Demerouti & Bakker, 2008), and the CAGE questionnaire (Ewing, 1984) to measure levels of psychiatric symptoms, burnout (disengagement and exhaustion), and problematic alcohol use, respectively. A score of 2 or greater on the GHQ12 was chosen as a cutoff to indicate caseness in line with other similar studies (Almeida et al., 2019) and scores of 2.10 and 2.25 were used as the cutoffs for disengagement and exhaustion respectively on the OLBI. A score of 2 or more on the CAGE questionnaire was chosen as a cutoff to indicate the presence of problematic alcohol use. All replies were anonymous.

Results

41 students responded to the survey and all students responded to all questions in the survey. All were from the Tbilisi State Medical University. Basic demographic details and parental educational level are shown in Table 11.1.

We asked students about four major domains of life and whether they were causes of stress to them. The highest rates of stress were reported for housing and study, at 92% and 82%, respectively, but money and relationships were also stress to many (Figure 11.1).

About 8% of students reached caseness using the GHQ12 and 80% and 83% scored as being disengaged and exhausted, respectively, using the OLBI. Rates of reported substance misuse were low with only 12% of students being positive for alcohol problems using the

Table 11.1 Demographic characteristics of study participants

Total number of participants	41
Gender	
Female	20 (51%)
Male	21 (49%)
Parental education level	
High school	1 (2%)
Undergraduate	9 (22%)
Postgraduate	31 (76%)
Currently working alongside studies	
Yes	4 (10%)
No	37 (90%)

Adapted with permission from Berdzenishvili, E., et al. (2021) 'Stress, Well-being, and Burnout in Georgian Medical Students: A Brief Report'. *World Social Psychiatry* 3(2): 114.

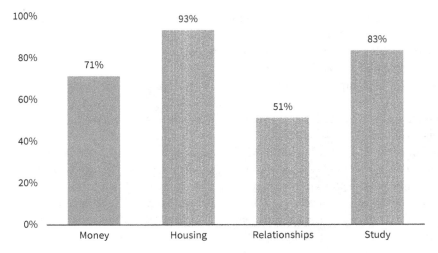

Figure 11.1 Reported sources of stress (percentages).
Adapted with permission from Berdzenishvili, E. et al. (2021) 'Stress, Well-being, and Burnout in Georgian Medical Students: A Brief Report', *World Social Psychiatry* 3(2), p. 114.

CAGE questionnaire and only 10% admitting the current illicit drug use. These results are shown in Table 11.2.

Discussion

Our study had limitations, principally the small sample size. It was also a convenience sample, so caution is needed when interpreting the results. Our results are, however, in line with those from the other countries involved in this programme (Chelieh et al., 2019; Farrell

Table 11.2 Results of the CAGE,[1] GHQ-12[2], and OLBI[3] scales

Total number of participants	41
Alcohol problems (CAGE positive)	5 (12%)
Current drug use	4 (10%)
GHQ-12 caseness	28 (68%)
Disengaged (OLBI)	33 (80%)
Exhausted (OLBI)	34 (83%)

1. CAGE questionnaire for substance abuse

2. General health questionnaire 12

3. Oldenburg burnout inventory

Adapted with permission from Berdzenishvili, E. et al. (2021) 'Stress, Well-being, and Burnout in Georgian Medical Students: A Brief Report'. *World Social Psychiatry* 3(2): 114.

et al., 2019; Masri et al., 2019) as well as other studies from Georgia (Abashishvili et al., 2022; Nadareishvili et al., 2022; Rekhviashvili et al., 2021; Soyakin et al., 2019). The small number of students taking part in the research could be explained with stigma related to mental illness, which is highly prevalent not only in the general population, but also among medical professionals in Georgia. Anti-stigma interventions during the first educational years at the university could reduce prejudice, improve knowledge, and attitudes towards the mental illness, helping medical students to identify and communicate their mental health problems (Waqas et al., 2020).

The majority of medical students who responded had parents who had achieved postgraduate education (76%) compared to 37% of the overall population aged over 25. We found similar disparities in all countries, suggesting that social mobility is an issue that affects the medical workforce and those in training. At the same time educated parents may support their children better than less educated parents, perhaps because they went through a similar experience (Yusoff, 2013). Improving the awareness and knowledge of parents about the challenges of being a medical student could help to increase emotional and social support from family members and have positive effects on students' mental health and wellbeing (SAMHSA, 2021).

Students reported high levels of stress and many reported multiple stressors. The highest rates were reported for housing and study, which could have several explanations.

There are some factors contributing to increased stress among medical students in Georgia. During the last decade the private and state institutions providing higher educational programmes in Georgia, started to conduct medical high educational programmes in the English language, trying to adjust their curricula to the United States Medical Licensing Examination (USMLE) (Tbilisi State Medical University USMD Program, no date) in order to cater to the increased demand from the national and international student populations. Within the framework of a 6-year curriculum there are three cycles (a basic (preclinical) cycle, a clinical-theoretical cycle, and the more practical internship cycle). Most students studying on English programmes are involved in a learning process which is conducted in their non-native language, creating even more pressure in the high demanding, intense environment of medical education. Besides, students studying medicine on Georgian programmes in their native language need sufficient English language skills to update medical knowledge, as English remains the international language for science and medicine. Moreover, due to multicultural environment in medical high educational institutions, having sufficient English language skills became essential for social communication.

Although proficiency in English is part of admission requirements in Georgian Universities, the language skills of students often are not enough to overcome the difficulties related to learning process and communication in medical education. For example, Yasin et al. found that the Arab students, who studied medicine in English but were nor proficient enough in the language, were experiencing significantly more difficulties in studying, compared to those considered proficient (Tayem et al., 2020). Studies on medical students' English language needs in Taiwanese higher education institutions showed that English was perceived as important for students' academic studies and their future work (Chia et al., 1999). Here the students studying medicine in Georgia are not an exception.

Educational institutions providing medical programmes either in English or Georgian languages should conduct an analysis on the needs of the English language among students, accordingly embed diverse strategies and offer medical or general English courses to support further development of language skills. This could reduce the stress associated with language barriers in the educational process and communication in multicultural environments, thus paving the way for professional development and improvement in social connections, essential for wellbeing.

At the same time, providing medical education in English has made Georgian universities an attractive place for international students. In 2022 of overall bachelor's degree medical students represent 4%, of 159,842 students in Georgia, with half of those being foreign students (Higher Education—National Statistics Office of Georgia, 2022) with different ethnical, cultural backgrounds, and almost 70 different geographical origins. It can be assumed that the migration process accompanied by the environmental and cultural changes also has an impact on mental health and wellbeing of international medical students leading to unfavourable results at personal or professional level (Oyeniyi et al., 2021). Housing problems created by high rental prices and lack of contacts in new social circumstances could be attributed to the high number of international students' migration. At the same time universities in Georgia lack the necessary accommodation and policies to solve this problem. Nowadays it is only Tbilisi State University that has shared accommodation for 320 students (Tbilisi State University, 2017). Providing strategies to support students more in these domains would be beneficial. High educational institutions should have housing possibilities in campus areas or mediate to find accommodations in affordable rent prices to reduce housing insecurities of students (Sackett et al., 2016).

High levels of stress were associated with very high levels of reported psychiatric symptoms and burnout. These results are in line with those from many countries. They suggest that Georgian medical students are not immune in any way from the global crisis in medical student wellbeing. Medical schools should therefore observe their students at the end of the first year, to determine whether they need psychological support. A brief intervention such as a psychological consulting might be beneficial. This could at the same time serve as a preventive measure to recognize more severe mental health problems at the early stages, where universities could suggest a referral to mental health professionals. Besides, group therapies like Mindfulness Based Stress Reduction could reduce the level of stress and improve academic performance (Worsley et al., 2020). Creating extracurricular activities to enhance social networking between students could help them develop personal and professional skills to better deal with the intense, demanding medical-education environment.

Substance Use

Despite high levels of stress and burnout, substance misuse among medical students was low. This may be an artefact of the small sample size of the study or may be a sign that respondents had found more positive ways to cope with difficult emotions. Another explanation could be the absence of stimulants on the Georgian pharmaceutical market. The prescribed and illicit stimulants, as cognitive enhancers and mood improvers, are one of the most widely misused substances among medical students (Sabbe et al., 2022), though access to them is highly restricted due to law regulations in Georgia.

Conclusion

Despite the limited number of studies conducted among medical students in Georgia, the results show high levels of stress, sleep disorders, psychiatric symptoms, and burnout. This can significantly impair quality of life and empathy of students, have serious impact on capacity to organize highly demanding study hours, socialize, and perform academically. Among students of the health professions, this could affect patient care, since empathy and professionalism might be impaired (Dyrbye et al., 2012; Neumann et al., 2011).

We hope that the results at hand will encourage a stronger focus on student wellbeing and more work to ascertain the level of the problem so that strategies and interventions can be developed to help reduce the stress factors and improve wellbeing of medical students in Georgia.

References

Abashishvili, L., et al. (2022). 'Stress level among medical students in Georgia and its causative factors'. *Exp Clin Med Georgia* (2).

Almeida, T., et al. (2019). 'A descriptive study of mental health and wellbeing among medical students in Portugal'. *Int Rev Psychiatry* **31**(7–8): 574–578.

Berdzenishvili, E., et al. (2021) 'Stress, well-being, and burnout in Georgian medical students: a brief report'. *World Social Psychiatry* **3**(2): 114.

Chelieh, M.L., *et al.* (2019). 'Mental health and wellbeing among Moroccan medical students: a descriptive study'. *Int Rev Psychiatry* **31**(7–8): 608–612.

Chia, H.-U., Johnson, R., Chia, H.-L., & Olive, F. (1999). 'English for college students in Taiwan: a study of perceptions of english needs in a medical context'. *English for Specific Purposes* **18**(2): 107–119.

Demerouti, E. & Bakker, A.B. (2008). *The Oldenburg Burnout Inventory A Good Alternative to Measure Burnout and Engagement, Handbook of Stress and Burnout in Health Care.* https://www.scirp.org/ (S(czeh2tfqw2orz553k1w0r45))/reference/referencespapers.aspx?referenceid=2865496 (Accessed 25 August 2022).

Dyrbye, L.N., et al. (2012). 'A Multi-institutional study exploring the impact of positive mental health on medical students' professionalism in an era of high burnout'. *Acad Med* **87**(8): 1024–1031.

Ewing, J.A. (1984). 'Detecting alcoholism. The CAGE questionnaire'. *JAMA* **252**(14): 1905–1907.

Farrell, S.M., et al. (2019) 'Wellbeing and burnout in medical students in India; a large scale survey'. *Int Rev Psychiatry* **31**(7–8): 555–562.

Goldberg, D.P. & Blackwell, B. (1970). 'Psychiatric illness in general practice: a detailed study using a new method of case identification'. *Br Med J* **2**(5707): 439.

Guthrie, E., et al. (1998). 'Psychological stress and burnout in medical students: a five-year prospective longitudinal study'. *J R Soc Med* **91**: 237–243.

Hamaideh, S.H., et al. (2022). 'Depression, anxiety and stress among undergraduate students during COVID-19 outbreak and "home-quarantine"'. *Nursing Open* **9**(2): 1423–1431.

Higher Education - National Statistics Office of Georgia (2022). https://www.geostat.ge/en/modules/cat egories/61/higher-education (Accessed 24 August 2022).

Holm-Hadulla, R.M., et al. (2021). 'Well-being and mental health of students during the COVID-19 pandemic'. *Psychopathology* **54**(6): 291–297.

Kaufman, D. M., Mensink, D., & Day, V. (1998). 'Stressors in medical school: relation to curriculum format and year of study'. *Teach Learn Med* **10**(3): 138–144.

Kinkladze, R. & Chitaladze K. (2019). 'Foreign students in Georgia and their impact of the country's economics'. https://dspace.tsu.ge/bitstream/handle/123456789/556/Foreign%20students%20in%20

Georgia%20and%20their%20impact%20of%20the%20country%27s%20economics.pdf?sequence=1&isAllowed=y (Accessed 10 September 2022).

Masri, R., et al. (2019). 'Wellbeing and mental health amongst medical students in Jordan: a descriptive study'. *Int Rev Psychiatry* 31(7–8): 619–625.

Moir, F., et al. (2018). 'Depression in medical students: current insights'. *Adv Med Educ Pract* 9: 323–333.

Nadareishvili, I., et al. (2022). 'University students' mental health amidst the COVID-19 pandemic in Georgia'. *Int J Soc Psychiatry* 2022(5): 1036–1046.

Neumann, M., et al. (2011). 'Empathy decline and its reasons: a systematic review of studies with medical students and residents'. *Acad Med* 86(8): 996–1009.

Oyeniyi, O.F., Bain, S.F., & Furgerson, K.L. (2021). 'Stress factors experienced by international students while attending a South Texas university'.

Rekhviashvili, A., et al. (2021). 'Anxiety and depression among international students studying in Georgia'. *Int J Adv Res* 9(04): 886–893.

Sabbe, M., et al. (2022). 'Use and misuse of prescription stimulants by university students: a cross-sectional survey in the French-speaking community of Belgium, 2018'. *Arch Public Health* 80(1): 1–10.

Sackett, C., Goldrick-Rab, S., & Broton, K. (2016). *Strategies for Colleges and Universities to Help Students with Housing Instability*. https://housingmatters.urban.org. https://housingmatters.urban.org/research-summary/strategies-colleges-and-universities-help-students-housing-instability (Accessed 10 September 2022].

SAMHSA (2021). Evidence-based resource guide series: Prevention and Treatment of Anxiety, Depression, and Suicidal Thoughts and Behaviors Among College Students I Prevention and Treatment of Anxiety, Depression, and Suicidal Thoughts and Behaviors Among College Students Prevention and Treatment of Anxiety, Depression, and Suicidal Thoughts and Behaviors Among College Students Acknowledgments. https://store.samhsa.gov/sites/default/files/SAMHSA_Digital_Download/PEP21-06-05-002.pdf (Accessed 10 September 2021).

Soyakin, B. et al. (2019). 'Sleep disturbances and stress among the foreign medical students of European university, Georgia'. *Sleep Medicine* 64: S331–S332.

Tayem, Y. *et al.* (2020). Language barriers to studying medicine in English: perceptions of final-year medical students at the Arabian Gulf University. World Health Organization—Regional Office for the Eastern Mediterranean. http://www.emro.who.int/emhj-volume-26-2020/volume-26-issue-2/language-barriers-to-studying-medicine-in-english-perceptions-of-final-year-medical-students-at-the-arabian-gulf-university.html [Accessed 10 September 2022].

Tbilisi State Medical University USMD Program (n.d.). https://tsmu.edu/ts/images/dxp/diplomirebuli-medikosis-amerikuli-programa-5b06b54aca5c7.pdf (Accessed 24 August 2022).

Tempski, P., et al. (2012) 'What do medical students think about their quality of life? A qualitative study'. *BMC Med Educ* 12(1): 1–8.

Universities and Programs Catalog (2022). https://unicatalog.ge/ (Accessed 24 August 2022).

Tbilisi State University (2017). https://tsu.ge/ka/domitory/page (Accessed 10 September 2022).

Waqas, A., et al. (2020). 'Interventions to reduce stigma related to mental illnesses in educational institutes: a systematic review'. *Psychiatric Quarterly* 91(3): 887.

Worsley, J., Pennington, A., & Corcoran, R. (2020). What interventions improve college and university students' mental health and wellbeing? A review of review-level evidence For the What Works Centre for Wellbeing About the What Works Centre for Wellbeing. University of Liverpool. https://whatworkswellbeing.org/wp-content/uploads/2020/03/Student-mental-health-full-review.pdf (Accessed 10 September 2022).

Yates, J., James, D., & Aston, I. (2008) 'Pre-existing mental health problems in medical students: a retrospective survey'. *Med Teach* 30(3): 319–321.

Yusoff, M.S.B. (2013). 'Associations of pass-fail outcomes with psychological health of first-year medical students in a Malaysian medical school'. *Sultan Qaboos University Medical Journal* 13(1): 107.

12

Hong Kong

Medical Student Wellbeing in Hong Kong

Julie Chen, Linda Chan, and Weng Chin

Introduction

From medical school through postgraduate training and into medical practice, doctors at every stage of professional development experience stress and distress that can affect personal wellbeing, academic outcomes, and patient care. At the undergraduate level, wellbeing has received significant attention in recent years with documentation of the significant prevalence of psychological distress such as mood disorders and burnout among students, the factors contributing to this problem, its impact on student mental health, as well as approaches to address this pressing problem in medical schools worldwide. These issues have also been explored in Hong Kong (HK) with sobering but also encouraging results.

Hong Kong is a Special Administrative Region of China, with 15,200 medical doctors serving a population of 7.3 million residents, as of 2022. Most practising doctors are graduates of The University of Hong Kong (HKU) or the Chinese University of Hong Kong (CUHK), public tertiary education institutions that house the only two medical schools in the city. There is a long history of formal Western medical education in Hong Kong that was introduced with the founding of the Hong Kong College of Medicine for Chinese in 1887. It was later named the Hong Kong College of Medicine, the forerunner to the Li Ka Shing Faculty of Medicine at HKU. Among its first graduating class was Dr Sun Yat-sen who would become known as the father of modern China.

Both Hong Kong medical schools offer a 6-year bachelor's degree with each now admitting a cohort of 300 new medical students each year. Most are admitted directly from local secondary schools and are often the top performers in Hong Kong's university entrance exam, the Diploma of Secondary Education (DSE), and the highest achieving graduates of local international schools. Medical students undertake a modern and progressive curriculum taught in English except for communication skills and clinical teaching which is conducted in Cantonese, the local dialect. Undergraduate medical studies in Hong Kong are strenuous and academic stress is a major problem alongside cultural factors and societal changes that exert unique pressures on medical student wellbeing in Hong Kong.

Julie Chen, Linda Chan, and Weng Chin, *Hong Kong* In: *The Mental Health of Medical Students*. Edited by: Andrew Molodynski, Sarah Marie Farrell, and Dinesh Bhugra, Oxford University Press. © Oxford University Press 2024. DOI: 10.1093/oso/9780192864871.003.0012

The Landscape of Medical Student Wellness in Hong Kong

Based on studies already conducted and those ongoing in our setting, a concerning proportion of medical students in Hong Kong (HK) experience stress and burnout and describe psychological symptoms suggestive of depression and anxiety. Protective qualities like grit and resilience are seen at comparatively lower levels than international counterparts.

Stress and Burnout

Excessive stress in students can lead to psychological distress and have negative consequences such as poorer academic outcomes (Henning et al., 2018). The Perceived Stress Scale (PSS-10) has been validated in HK medical students (Chen et al., 2021a) to assess how unpredictable, uncontrollable, and overloaded they find their lives. A study in HKU highlighted that even in their first year, medical students had higher perceived stress compared to the HK general population, other HK university students, as well as medical students in the USA (Chen et al., 2021d; Chua et al., 2004; Kwok & Ng, 2016; Worly et al., 2019). Longitudinally, their stress level gradually increased and peaked at Year 2, before decreasing thereafter. By Year 6, medical student stress level was still higher than the stress level reported for healthcare workers during the 2003 Severe Acute Respiratory Syndrome (SARS) outbreak (Chen et al., 2021c; Lee et al., 2007) (Figure 12.1).

Potential reasons for peaking of perceived stress in Year 2 may be related to the advanced depth coupled with the amount of knowledge to be learned, in addition to adjustment challenges. Most students reported study-related workload and examinations as the two

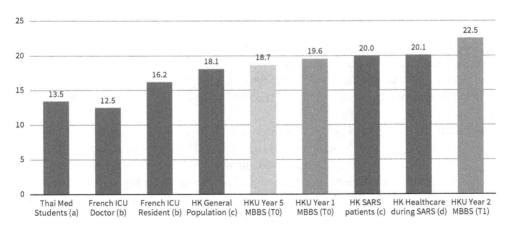

References:
(a) Wongpakaran N & Wongpakaran T. Biopsychosoc Med. 2010;e4(6).
(b) Jones G, et al. Int J Nurs Stud. 2015;52(1):250–259.
(c) Chua SE, et al. Can J Psychiat. 2004;49(6):391–393.
(d) Lee AM, et al. Can J Psychiat. 2007;52(4):233–240.

Figure 12.1 Perceived stress (PSS-10) of HK medical students compared with different populations.

commonest sources of stress. Additional academic reasons included students perceiving the teaching and learning to be less practical than expected, insufficient feedback given on performance, plus challenges with administrative arrangements (Chen, 2018; Chen et al., 2018). Other factors frequently reported included challenging interpersonal relationships such as family conflicts and negative interactions with faculty members, a lack of rest, their own and relatives' health issues, and financial difficulties (Chen, 2018; Chau et al., 2019).

Research into burnout among a broader range of HK medical students revealed significantly different rates depending on the instrument employed. For example, the proportion of medical students with burnout ranged from 27.9% using the Maslach Burnout Inventory, to 95% utilizing the Oldenburg Burnout Inventory (Chau et al., 2019; Lee et al., 2020). This is consistent with Erschens and colleagues' report that the global prevalence of burnout among medical students ranged from 7.0% to 75.2% depending on the instrument used (Ercshens et al., 2019) and another estimation of 44.2% among this population worldwide (Frajerman et al., 2019). Among HK medical students, lifestyle characteristics such as sleep quality and exercise level were significantly associated with the presence of burnout, whereas sociodemographic factors were not (Lee et al., 2020).

Depressive and Anxiety Symptoms

A longitudinal evaluation of medical student wellbeing at HKU began in 2020–2021 and is still ongoing. Students completed sequential surveys on their mood and resilience at three time points (on entry, midway, and end of year) over the academic year. During their first year of study, the proportion of this cohort who screened positive for depression (Patient Health Questionnaire (PHQ-9) score ≥10) increased from 31.5% to 49.2% over the course of the year. At a cut-point of ≥10, the sensitivity and specificity for major depression are both 88% respectively (Kroenke et al., 2001). This was notably higher than the proportion meeting this cut-off among HK university students (27.0%) (Lun et al., 2018) and medical students in China (11.0%) (Sobowale et al., 2014). It was also higher than global estimates for the pooled prevalence of depression or depressive symptoms (27.2%) (Rotenstein et al., 2016). Of greater concern, the proportion of medical students who thought they were better off dead or had suicidal thoughts increased from 19.3% at the beginning of their first academic year to 29.1% by year-end. This was higher than the estimated pooled prevalence of suicidal ideation among medical students globally (11.1%) (Rotenstein et al., 2016) and that reported in the UK (16.6%) (Knipe et al., 2018).

Similarly, for generalized anxiety disorder (GAD), a seven-item anxiety scale (GAD-7) score of ≥10 has good sensitivity (89%) and specificity (82%) for identifying GAD (Spitzer et al., 2006). The proportion of medical students who scored GAD-7 ≥10 rose from 25.5% to 45.4% during their first academic year. These figures were both higher than that among HK university students (20.0%) (Lun et al., 2018), UK medical students (24.9%) (Knipe et al., 2018), and the pooled prevalence of anxiety among medical students worldwide (33.8%) (Quek et al., 2019). Furthermore, Chau et al. found that 87% of HK medical students screened positive for minor psychiatric disorders based on the 12-item General Health Questionnaire (GHQ-12) with a few students also reporting to have developed other psychiatric conditions, for example, post-traumatic stress disorder and bulimia (Chau et al., 2019) (Figure 12.2).

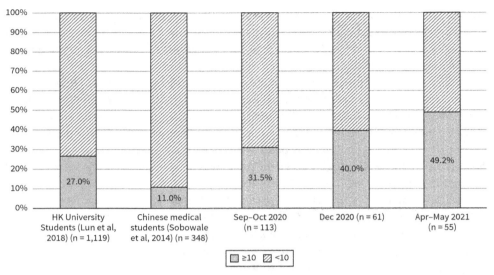

Figure 12.2 The proportion of first-year HK medical students who screened positive for depression (PHQ-9) at different time points vs. comparable student populations.

Grit and Resilience

Grit reflects the passion and perseverance one has in the pursuit of long-term goals despite challenges (Duckworth et al., 2007). HK medical students reported lower levels of protective qualities such as grit and resilience compared to their counterparts in the USA. HK medical students' scores ranged from 3.32 to 3.41 on the 12-item Grit scale, and while there is no cut-off score for this scale, the higher, the better. The range was lower than that in US graduating medical students (4.01) (Miller-Matero et al., 2018), but it is possible this is a function of maturity and life experience because grit increases with age.

Resilience can be defined as, 'the process of effectively negotiating, adapting to, or managing significant sources of stress or trauma' (Windle, 2011, p.163). It was measured by the 2-item Connor-Davidson Resilience Scale (Vaishnavi et al., 2007) with HK medical students' resilience levels over the academic year (5.16–5.22) being in the same range as age-matched peers in the HK general population (5.2) (Ni et al., 2016). Again, these levels were lower than those of first-year US medical students whose resilience levels ranged from 6.6 to 6.7 (Dyrbye et al., 2017).

Sociocultural Considerations

The high levels of stress, distress and suicidal ideation for this cohort may be exacerbated by the double-whammy of socio-political events in HK and the global pandemic. There may have been residual effects from the 2019–2020 social unrest in HK that was a significant stressor for many and could lead to mental health sequelae at baseline and beyond (Ni et al., 2020). The unrest was truncated by the 2020 COVID-19 pandemic that was full-blown by the time they started medical school and disrupted learning to a large extent. A HKU medical student-led study reflected the view that medical school became a 'lonely battle' in which the loss of face-to-face contact, online-learning fatigue, insufficient institutional support and communication, and uncertainty about their future combined to have a negative impact on mental health (Poon et al., 2021).

The first year of study can be a challenge for medical students as they need to adapt to the rigours of medical study, including the volume of material and the new terminology and concepts being introduced. It also requires transitioning to a more independent learning style that promotes small group discussion and critical thinking and is less didactic than what many of those educated in local secondary schools are accustomed to. This may result in a form of moral distress in which the student knows that they should speak up but is held back by engrained beliefs that the teacher is always right.

Cultures comprise unique sets of characteristics, beliefs, and social norms that exert a strong influence on those socialized within it. A recent study used Hofstede's cultural framework to characterize the cultural dimensions among medical students and trainees from different countries (Monrouxe et al., 2021). This may help understand why medical students in this context are suffering. HK medical students scored high for *power distance*, indicating an acceptance of hierarchical order. Teachers and authority figures are respected and even feared; therefore, asking questions can be perceived as challenging authority and considered disrespectful. They also had a high score in the *masculinity* dimension suggesting that the culture is assertive and prioritizes competitiveness and success. Failure is frowned upon and seen as a weakness. The fear of failure is pervasive and even relatively small academic shortcomings may lead to extreme reactions.

Molodynski and colleagues found that the most common stressor troubling HK medical students are their academic studies (Molodynski et al., 2021) and is the highest rated stressor among twelve countries. This is consistent with the observations of the medical school student wellness team who also cite exam and academic stress as the most common cause of psychological distress. Some of the pressure is self-inflicted as many students are high-achieving and used to success but some struggle because they are not motivated to study medicine. The student may feel pressured to defer to parents' wishes and enter a highly regarded and financially rewarding profession such as medicine though it may not be the career path the student envisions for themselves. Within Hofstede's cultural dimensions (Monrouxe et al., 2021), HK medical students skew towards *collectivism* which values the group's interests over the individual suggesting attitudes and behaviours that support a tight-knit community are favoured. This will go a long way in maintaining family harmony and meeting society's expectations. This is also in line with the Confucian conception of filial piety prevalent in HK society (King & Bond, 1985) which at the most basic level is to not bring disgrace to one's family and at the highest level is to demonstrate virtue by performing one's expected social roles well.

Help-seeking Among HK Medical Students

Help-seeking Behaviours

Medical students are a high-risk group with unmet needs due to a high prevalence of poor psychological wellbeing coupled with inadequate or inappropriate health-seeking behaviours

(Givens & Tjia, 2002). Previous studies show that even when help and support resources are available, many students who could benefit from professional mental health interventions either delay seeking help or do not seek it at all (Dyrbye et al., 2015; Gulliver et al., 2010; Ruud et al., 2020; Thistlethwaite et al., 2010). Amongst those who do seek help, many prefer to approach alternative sources such as untrained family and friends or try to cope by themselves using self-help techniques (Chang et al., 2012; Chew-Graham et al., 2003; Dyrbye et al., 2010). Within a cultural context, these behaviours appear to be more prominent amongst Asian students than among American students (Chang, 2008; Li et al., 2013).

At HKU, we examined help-seeking attitudes and behaviours as part of a survey which was administered annually for six years to a cohort of students who entered medical school in 2014 (Chen et al., 2021b). Data on self-perceived help-seeking needs and behaviours were collected using two questions:

1. Have you felt the need to seek support for non-academic reasons (e.g. social issues, stress, other psychological reasons)?
2. Have you ever actually sought any support for non-academic reasons outside the classroom?

From the 895 cumulative responses returned, there were 309 positive reports of a self-perceived need for help, out of which only 151 (48%) reported having sought support for non-academic reasons outside the classroom. These findings were comparable to help-seeking rates reported in other settings (Dyrbye et al., 2015; Ruud et al., 2020). There were gender differences observed with more female students reporting a need for help (35% of female responses vs. 29% of males), and reporting having sought help (23% females vs. 15% males); however, these differences were not statistically significant. Amongst those reporting a need for help, a similar proportion (16% of males and 17% of females) did not seek help.

Students were also asked, 'If you actually sought help, who did you turn to for support?'. Responses revealed that very few students sought professional help with 58% seeking help from friends outside of medical school, 48% from family, 46% from classmates and 14% from a counsellor or social worker. Only 5% sought help from a teacher.

We observed that significantly more medical students reported needing help and sought help during their clinical years (vs. pre-clinical). Students who reported needing help had higher levels of stress on the PSS-10 and lower quality of life as measured by the WHOQOL-BREF across all domains. This profile was also observed amongst students who had sought help. We also found that students who reported needing help but did not seek help had the highest levels of perceived stress and lowest quality of life across all domains.

Barriers to Help-seeking

From the international literature, students needing support but not seeking help may be unable to distinguish the difference between medical school stress and psychological symptoms (Rosenthal & Okie, 2005). Students with higher levels of psychological symptoms may be more reluctant to seek help due to poorer motivation levels to seek help (Chang, 2008). From an Asian context, studies have found that cultural values and behaviours may be a significant reason why students avoid seeking help. The Chinese have been described as a family-orientated culture (King & Bond, 1985) valuing the family over the individual. Consequently, revealing personal distress to outsiders may be perceived as shaming one's entire family (Kung, 2003). Such perceived pressure may influence our students to conceal embarrassing life events from their families. Therefore, students may believe that they should try to resolve their psychological problems within their family-friend system or by themselves to avoid inflicting stress on the family (Volet & Karabenick, 2006). A qualitative study by Li et al. found that Chinese students may hold misperceptions that make them reluctant to seek help, such as beliefs that counselling mainly involves sharing personal information with a stranger, that counselling is primarily for solving problems, and that counselling is primarily for those who have no one else to help them (Li et al., 2013). Many Asian cultures also consider emotional self-control and resiliency to be virtuous, especially during complex lifetime events (King & Bond, 1985). This may be another reason why our Chinese medical students avoid seeking help when experiencing high levels of stress.

Despite our growing awareness of students' unmet needs and the increased availability of mental health services, there are still many barriers impeding the support of student wellbeing. Through interactions with students, our student wellness counsellors have identified four key reasons for why they may be hesitant to use the school's support services (Chen et al., 2021b). Firstly, medical students do not want to be recognized as having a mental illness or being unable to cope. Students worry about the stigma of a mental health diagnosis and are concerned regarding the confidentiality of counselling. Some fear that it may compromise their future career prospects. Second, many students lack awareness or may be in denial that they are experiencing psychological distress and do not realize they need help or delay seeking help until symptoms become very severe. Third, students often do not understand what is involved in the counselling process. As a result, they may not believe that it will be useful or relevant. Fourth, students may perceive that counselling is very time and work-intensive and that it will not be feasible to balance counselling with their already overburdened study timetable. Most of these barriers have also been observed in the literature from other settings (Gulliver et al., 2010; Roberts et al., 2000; Thistlethwaite et al., 2010).

Facilitating Help-seeking

To help overcome these barriers, our student wellness team uses a range of strategies to promote a culture that enables those who recognize they need help to feel safe in doing so (Chen et al., 2021b). As many Chinese students prefer a less active role in the help-seeking process, our wellbeing team primarily utilizes outreach and wellbeing promotion activities to establish initial interactions and familiarize students with mental health services. To help normalize mental wellbeing help-seeking, our team delivers psychoeducational information using social and informal group formats. This requires our team to be familiar with the common perceptions and stigmas held by our students and carefully select the location and content focus of outreach activities. Delivering psychoeducation is also essential for addressing student misperceptions and promoting a better understanding of what is involved in counselling. It also allows students to ask questions for clarification. To encourage students to feel more open to talking about their emotions, the wellness team will try to create an engaging and culturally appropriate atmosphere, such as giving students the choice of communicating in Cantonese, Mandarin, or English. As confidentiality is a key concern for students, our wellness services are kept separate from teaching and learning spaces. Students can opt to meet with counsellors wherever it is mutually convenient such as in their school hall of residence, by Zoom, or by phone. Flexibility in the time and location for interacting with wellness counsellors helps make their services more accessible for students who typically have packed timetables.

A Multilevel Approach to Nurturing Learner Wellbeing in Medical School: A Case Example

Published and internal data have helped capture the problem's scope among HK medical students. Both medical schools in HK have set up a dedicated student wellness team to serve medical and healthcare sciences students within the faculty to support students in need (Chinese University of Hong Kong Student Support, 2022; LKS Faculty of Medicine Student Wellness, 2022). A multipronged approach that provides support for the students but also recognizes the important role of the context in which the students are learning and living, will help to provide a framework for promoting wellness. Swenson et al. propose an organizational approach to address the challenge of healthcare professional burnout drawing on the principles of quality improvement and systems engineering (Swenson & Shanafelt, 2020). The blueprint for this process comprises three main areas: mitigating the drivers of burnout, cultivating a culture of wellness, and bolstering individual and organizational resilience. Taking reference from this, we present a framework for student wellness that guides the approach at the medical school in HKU as a case example of a work in progress.

The framework situates the student at the centre, with the primary contact being individual interventions such as counselling support that is focused on mental health and coping skills. The personalized individual level support is buoyed by outreach to the broader learning community, of which the student is a part, through health promotion and education. The community is, in turn, embedded within a learning culture that seeks to engage all members to do their part to promote a positive and respectful wellness culture in which learners can thrive (Figure 12.3).

Individual Support

Recognizing the prevalence of medical student psychological distress and the unique needs of this population, a core student wellness team (SWT) was first established at the Faculty of Medicine as an adjunct to the services of the university medical and psychological support services. It began with a single counsellor in 2017 and has since evolved to the current complement of five mental health professionals with backgrounds in clinical psychology, social work, family therapy, and counselling. They use a diverse range of clinical approaches such as cognitive behavioural therapy, transformational systemic therapy, mindfulness, or narrative-based techniques to cater to the needs and characteristics of the individual student they serve. They also have the support of designated student wellness psychiatrists who provide additional support for students with more complex issues. A strong focus is on

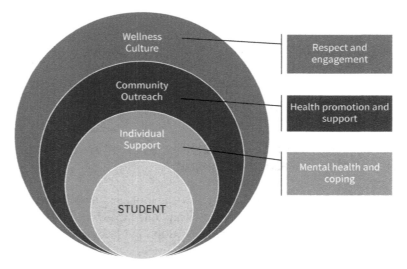

Figure 12.3 A framework for student wellness in a medical school.

resilience-building and recognizing and augmenting strengths. A proportion of students do not have 'problems' but proactively seek advice to better themselves. Logistical arrangements to overcome barriers and to encourage help-seeking are described in the previous section but include offering a range of communication platforms and a friendly accessible centre on the medical campus within student housing, extended hours, choice of language, and strict confidentiality.

Community Outreach

The SWT aims to be visible and approachable. It targets locations where students usually gather such as the student learning common (a communal study space) and residential halls to converse and offer informal advice. This helps to put a friendly face on the counsellor and draws from the 'Let's Talk' initiative pioneered at Cornell University that effectively increased student access to mental health services (Boone et al., 2011). Mental health awareness and education are framed in casual and non-threatening ways, such as fun wellness events that include meeting the university therapy dog Jasper (Figure 12.4), snack and stress-ball giveaways during exam time, wellness tips taped to study carrels in the medical library, drop-in craft sessions like making postcards with inspirational messages to send to peers, and art-jamming. Special events centred around dates like World Mental Health Day and collaborating with events led by colleagues from university health services help tie in mental health awareness activities initiated on the medical campus to the broader mental health context. The SWT regularly liaises with student societies as well as the departments/ schools of the faculty to offer tailored mental health seminars or workshops on request. This has the dual impact of providing education on recognizing and helping students in distress and developing personal relationships with front-line teachers and administrators who will also serve as the eyes and ears in the classrooms to detect students who may need help.

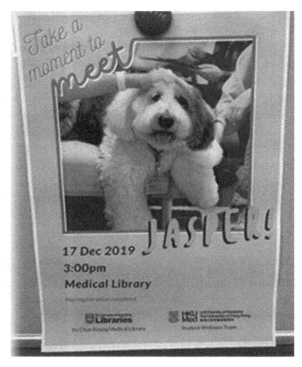

Figure 12.4 Jasper, HKU Libraries resident therapy dog.

Wellness Culture

The culture in which learning takes place, such as the engrained hierarchy of medical school, the perception that failure is not an option, and the subconscious biases and stereotypes that exist can all have a negative impact on wellness, as discussed earlier. Making these elements of the 'hidden curriculum' (Hafferty, 1998) visible and calling them out as detrimental is an important step towards nurturing a wellness culture. Particularly impactful are sharing sessions and workshops to learn from local examples (e.g. abusive behaviour on the ward) or the lived experience (e.g. a transgender doctor who underwent physical transition while in medical school) and how to address it. The power of role models can be harnessed, for example, by enlisting senior professors to share stories of their fallibility and 'failure CV'. Integrating these sharing sessions as well as workshops on self-care such as mindful practice and resilience building, into the medical curriculum as part of a wellness thread, as we do in the medical humanities programme, can further underscore the importance of these topics as part and parcel of medical education. Engaging students as partners in wellness is crucial as peers have an impact and unique access to the student body. Every year interested students are invited to train as peer supporters to reach out to potentially struggling peers in classrooms and online. They undertake the formal Mental Health First Aid training course together with basic communication and counselling skills workshops by the SWT and meet periodically throughout the year to debrief and share experiences.

To further shape wellness culture, openly discussing mental health from the first day of medical school sets the tone that wellness is a priority. As part of a broader conversation about learner wellbeing, the Assistant Dean presents the results of the voluntary, anonymous wellness survey completed by this class when they first enrolled. These data show there are a proportion of students who have already been screened positive for depression or anxiety and who already have had suicidal thoughts even before starting medical school. They are encouraged to do a wellness check-in via periodic completion of wellness screening tools, recognize that it is ok to not be ok, know that they are not alone in feeling distressed over the course of their studies, and most importantly, identify that it is a strength to seek and accept help that is readily available.

These efforts can feel disjointed without a set of unifying principles to underpin them. Towards this end, we specifically sought the input of student societies, student focus groups, faculty and staff interested in wellness, and other members of the learning community to discuss and describe the wellness culture that we are striving for. This resulted in a teaching and learning charter that articulated the communal guiding principles, grounded in mutual respect, that the faculty has formally adopted. It is posted prominently across campus and is the home screen for all the computers in the teaching venues. All members of the learning community need to take personal ownership and responsibility for a positive learning culture conducive to wellness and to make it a place where we wish to study and work and where we can all flourish.

Conclusion

Hong Kong medical students are not unlike their peers around the world in suffering significant rates of psychological distress but the reasons for their mental unwellness and help-seeking behaviour may be found deeply embedded in culture. Like their peers though, they are also resilient. This, combined with the efforts to support, promote, and engrain wellness attitudes and thinking in the medical school culture as well as concrete initiatives in medical education, gives reason to hope.

References

Boone, M.S., Edwards, G.R., Haltom, M., Hill, J.S., Liang, Y.-S., Mier, S.R., Shropshire, S. Y., Belizaire, L.S., Kamp, L.C., Murthi, M., Wong, W.-K., & Yau, T.Y. (2011). 'Let's talk: getting out of the counseling center to serve hard-to-reach students'. *Journal of Multicultural Counseling and Development* 39: 194–205.

Chang, E., Eddins-Folensbee, F., & Coverdale, J. (2012). 'Survey of the prevalence of burnout, stress, depression, and the use of supports by medical students at one school'. *Acad Psychiatry* 36: 177–182.

Chang, H. (2008). 'Help-seeking for stressful events among Chinese college students in Taiwan: roles of gender, prior history of counseling, and help-seeking attitudes'. *Journal of College Student Development* 49: 41–51.

Chau, S.W., Lewis, T., NG, R., Chen, J.Y., Farrell, S.M., Molodynski, A., & Bhugra, D.J.I. R.O.P. (2019). 'Wellbeing and mental health amongst medical students from Hong Kong'. *Int Rev Psychiatry* 31: 626–629.

Chen, J.Y. (2018). Medical student stress at The University of Hong Kong: What does it look like? In: Chen, J.Y. & Chin, W.Y. (eds) *Learner Wellbeing Across the Continuum* (pp. 28–33). Hong Kong: The University of Hong Kong.

Chen, J.Y., Chin, W.-Y., Tiwari, A., Wong, J., Wong, I.C., Worsley, A., Feng, Y., Sham, M.H., Tsang, J.P.Y., & Lau, C.S. (2021a). 'Validation of the perceived stress scale (Pss-10) in medical and health sciences students in Hong Kong'. *The Asia Pacific Scholar* 6: 31–37.

Chen, J.Y., Chin, W.-Y., Tsang, J.P.Y. & Lau, C.S. (2021b). 'Wellbeing and support-seeking in undergraduate medical students'. *AMEE 2021 Virtual Conference*

Chen, J.Y., Chin, W.Y., Chan, L.K., Tiwari, A., Wong, J., Worsley, A.J., Feng, Y., Sham, M.H., Tsang, J.P.Y., & Lau, C.S. (2018). Stress and quality of life of students in the Lks Faculty of Medicine. *Bau Institute of Medical and Health Sciences Education Research Meeting*. Hong Kong, SAR.

Chen, J.Y., Chin, W.Y., Tiwari, A., Wong, J., Tsang, J.P.Y., & Lau, C.S. (2021c). 'Stress, motivation and academic achievement in undergraduate medical and nursing students: a longitudinal cohort study'. *International Conference for Medical Education*. Virtual Conference Yogyakarta, Indonesia: Li Ka Shing Faculty of Medicine, The Universoty of Hong Kong.

Chen, J.Y., Chin, W.Y., Tiwari, A., Wong, J., Tsang, J.P.Y., & Lau, C.S. (2021d). 'Stress, motivation and academic achievement in undergraduate medical and nursing students: a longitudinal cohort study'. *International Conference on Medical Education*. Virtual conference Yogyakarta, Indonesia.

Chew-Graham, C.A., Rogers, A., & Yassin, N. (2003). '"I wouldn't want it on my CV or their records": medical students' experiences of help-seeking for mental health problems'. *Med Educ* 37: 873–80.

Chinese University of Hong Kong Student Support. Chinese University of Hong Kong. https://www.med.cuhk.edu.hk/study/current-students/student-wellness/student-support [Accessed 2022].

Chua, S.E., Cheung, V., Cheung, C., Mcalonan, G.M., Wong, J.W.S., Cheung, E.P.T., Chan, M.T.Y., Wong, M.M.C., Tang, S.W., & Choy, K.M. (2004). 'Psychological effects of the Sars outbreak in Hong Kong on high-risk health care workers'. *Can J Psychiatry* 49: 391–393.

Duckworth, A.L., Peterson, C., Matthews, M.D., & Kelly, D.R. (2007). 'Grit: perseverance and passion for long-term goals'. *J Pers Soc Psychol* 92: 1087.

Dyrbye, L.N., Eacker, A., Durning, S.J., Brazeau, C., Moutier, C., Massie, F.S., Satele, D., Sloan, J.A., & Shanafelt, T.D. (2015). 'The impact of stigma and personal experiences on the help-seeking behaviors of medical students with burnout'. *Acad Med* 90: 961–969.

Dyrbye, L.N., Power, D.V., Massie, F.S., Eacker, A., Harper, W., Thomas, M.R., Szydlo, D.W., Sloan, J.A., & Shanafelt, T.D. (2010). 'Factors associated with resilience to and recovery from burnout: a prospective, multi-institutional study of US medical students'. *Med Educ* 44: 1016–1026.

Dyrbye, L.N., Shanafelt, T.D., Werner, L., Sood, A., Satele, D., & Wolanskyj, A.P. (2017). 'The impact of a required longitudinal stress management and resilience training course for first-year medical students'. *J Gen Int Med* 32: 1309–1314.

Erschens, R., Keifenheim, K.E., Herrmann-Werner, A., Loda, T., Schwille-Kiuntke, J., Bugaj, T.J., Nikendei, C., Huhn, D., Zipfel, S., & Junne, F. (2019). 'Professional burnout among medical students: systematic literature review and meta-analysis'. *Med Teach* 41: 172–183.

Frajerman, A., Morvan, Y., Krebs, M.-O., Gorwood, P., & Chaumette, B. (2019). 'Burnout in medical students before residency: a systematic review and meta-analysis'. *Eur Psychiatry* 55: 36–42.

Givens, J.L. & Tjia, J. (2002). 'Depressed medical students' use of mental health services and barriers to use'. *Acad Med* 77: 918–921.

Gulliver, A., Griffiths, K.M., & Christensen, H. (2010). Perceived barriers and facilitators to mental health help-seeking in young people: a systematic review. *BMC Psychiatry* 10: 113.

Hafferty, F.W. (1998). 'Beyond curriculum reform: confronting medicine's hidden curriculum'. *Acad Med* 73: 403–407.

Henning, M., Krägeloh, C., Booth, R., Hill, E.M., Chen, J., & Webster, C. (2018). 'An exploratory study of the relationships among physical health, competitiveness, stress, motivation, and grade attainment: pre-medical and health science students'. TAPS 3(3): 5–16.

King, A.Y.C. & Bond, M.H. (1985). The Confucian paradigm of man: a sociological view. In: Tseng, W.-S. & Wu, D.Y.H. (eds) *Chinese Culture and Mental Health* (pp. 29–45). Orlando, FL: Academic Press.

Knipe, D., Maughan, C., Gilbert, J., Dymock, D., Moran, P., & Gunnell, D. (2018). 'Mental health in medical, dentistry and veterinary students: cross-sectional online survey'. *Bjpsych Open* 4: 441–446.

Kroenke, K., Spitzer, R.L., & Williams, J.B.W. (2001). 'The Phq-9: validity of a brief depression severity measure'. *J Gen Int Med* 16: 606–613.

Kung, Winnie W. (2003). 'Chinese Americans' help seeking for emotional distress'. *Soc Serv Rev* 77: 110–134.

Kwok, J.M.Y. & Ng, D.K.S. (2016). 'A study of the perceived stress level of university students in Hong Kong'. *Int J Psychol Stud* 8: 91–106.

Lee, A.M., Wong, J.G.W.S., Mcalonan, G.M., Cheung, V., Cheung, C., Sham, P.C., Chu, C.-M., Wong, P.-C., Tsang, K.W.T., & Chua, S.E. (2007). 'Stress and psychological distress among SARS survivors 1 year after the outbreak'. *Can J Psychiatry* 52: 233–240.

Lee, K.P., Yeung, N., Wong, C., Yip, B., Luk, L.H.F., & Wong, S. (2020). 'Prevalence of medical students' burnout and its associated demographics and lifestyle factors in Hong Kong'. *PLoS One* 15: e0235154.

Li, P., Wong, Y.J., & Toth, P. (2013). 'Asian international students' willingness to seek counseling: a mixed-methods study'. *International Journal for the Advancement of Counselling* 35: 1–15.

LKS Faculty of Medicine Student Wellness. The University of Hong Kong. https://www.med.hku.hk/en/teaching-and-learning/student-wellness [Accessed 2022].

Lun, K.W.C., Chan, C.K., Ip, P.K.Y., Ma, S.Y.K., Tsai, W.W., Wong, C.S., Wong, C.H.T., Wong, T.W., & Yan, D. (2018). 'Depression and anxiety among university students in Hong Kong'. *Hong Kong Med J* 24: 466–472.

Miller-Matero, L.R., Martinez, S., Maclean, L., Yaremchuk, K., & Ko, A.B. (2018). 'Grit: A predictor of medical student performance'. *Educ Health* 31: 109.

Molodynski, A., Lewis, T., Kadhum, M., Farrell, S.M., Lemtiri Chelieh, M., Falcão De Almeida, T., Masri, R., Kar, A., Volpe, U., Moir, F., Torales, J., Castaldelli-Maia, J.M., Chau, S.W.H., Wilkes, C., & Bhugra, D. (2021). 'Cultural variations in wellbeing, burnout and substance use amongst medical students in twelve countries'. *Int Rev Psychiatry* 33: 37–42.

Monrouxe, L.V., Chandratilake, M., Chen, J., Chhabra, S., Zheng, L., Costa, P.S., Lee, Y.M., Karnieli-Miller, O., Nishigori, H., Ogden, K., Pawlikowska, T., Riquelme, A., Sethi, A., Soemantri, D., Wearn, A., Wolvaardt, L., Yusoff, M.S.B., & Yau, S.Y. (2021). 'Medical students' and trainees' country-by-gender profiles: Hofstede's cultural dimensions across sixteen diverse countries'. *Front Med (Lausanne)* 8: 746288.

Ni, M.Y., Li, T.K., Yu, N.X., Pang, H., Chan, B.H., Leung, G.M., & Stewart, S.M. (2016). 'Normative data and psychometric properties of the Connor–Davidson Resilience Scale (CD-RISC) and the abbreviated version (CD-RISC2) among the general population in Hong Kong'. *Qual Life Res* 25: 111–116.

Ni, M.Y., Yao, X.I., Leung, K.S.M., Yau, C., Leung, C.M.C., Lun, P., Flores, F.P., Wing Chung, C., Cowling, B.J., & Leung, G.M. (2020). 'Depression and post-traumatic stress during major social unrest in Hong Kong: a 10-year prospective cohort study'. *Lancet* 395: 273–284.

Poon, S.H.L., Chow, M.S., & Lam, W.W. (2021). 'Medical education and mental wellbeing during COVID-19: a student's perspective'. *Med Sci Educ* 31: 1183–1185.

Quek, T.T.-C., Tam, W.-S., Tran, B.X., Zhang, M., Zhang, Z., Ho, C.S.-H., & Ho, R.C.-M. (2019). 'The global prevalence of anxiety among medical students: a meta-analysis'. *Int J Environ Res Public Health* 16: 2735.

Roberts, L.W., Warner, T.D., Carter, D., Frank, E., Ganzini, L., & Lyketsos, C. (2000). 'Caring for medical students as patients: access to services and care-seeking practices of 1,027 students at nine medical schools. Collaborative Research Group on Medical Student Healthcare'. *Acad Med* 75: 272–277.

Rosenthal, J.M. & Okie, S. (2005). 'White coat, mood indigo—depression in medical school'. *N Engl J Med* 353: 1085–1088.

Rotenstein, L.S., Ramos, M.A., Torre, M., Segal, J.B., Peluso, M.J., Guille, C., Sen, S., & Mata, D.A. (2016). 'Prevalence of depression, depressive symptoms, and suicidal ideation among medical students: a systematic review and meta-analysis'. *JAMA* 316: 2214–2236.

Ruud, N., Løvseth, L.T., Isaksson Ro, K., & Tyssen, R. (2020). 'Comparing mental distress and help-seeking among first-year medical students in Norway: results of two cross-sectional surveys 20 years apart'. *BMJ Open* 10: e036968.

Sobowale, K., Zhou, A.N., Fan, J., Liu, N., & Sherer, R. (2014). 'Depression and suicidal ideation in medical students in China: a call for wellness curricula'. *Int J Med Educ* 5: 31.

Spitzer, R.L., Kroenke, K., Williams, J.B., & Löwe, B. (2006). 'A brief measure for assessing generalized anxiety disorder: the Gad-7'. *Arch Int Med* 166: 1092–1097.

Swenson, S.J. & Shanafelt, T.D. (2020). *Mayo Clinic Strategies to Reduce Burnout: 12 Actions To Create The Ideal Workplace*. USA: Oxford University Press.

Thistlethwaite, J., Quirk, F., & Evans, R. (2010). 'Medical students seeking medical help: a qualitative study'. *Med Teach* **32**: 164–166.

Vaishnavi, S., Connor, K., & Davidson, J.R. (2007). 'An abbreviated version of the Connor-Davidson Resilience Scale (CD-RISC), the CD-RISC2: psychometric properties and applications in psycho-pharmacological trials'. *Psych Res* **152**: 293–297.

Volet, S. & Karabenick, S.A. (2006). *Help Seeking in Cultural Context. Help Seeking in Academic Setting: Goals, Groups, and Contexts*. Lawrence Erlbaum Associates Publishers.

Windle, G. (2011). 'What is resilience? A review and concept analysis'. *Rev Clin Gerontol* **21**: 152–169.

Worly, B., Verbeck, N., Walker, C., & Clinchot, D.M. (2019). 'Burnout, perceived stress, and empathic concern: differences in female and male Millennial medical students'. *Psychol Health Med* **24**: 429–438.

13
India

Stress and Burnout Amongst Medical Students in India

*Avinash Shekhar, Sharad Philip, Santosh Kumar Chaturvedi,
and Dinesh Bhugra*

Introduction

With a population of 1.4 billion people, India has one of the largest pools of aspiring and trained doctors. Coveted by many, medical training brings with it social prestige and financial stability—it is fiercely competitive. However, little is known and even less is understood about the impact of medical training on the wellbeing of doctors in India. It is not uncommon to hear of doctors and medical students suffering from mental health conditions—sometimes even leading to death by suicide.

Across the country, 604 institutions (306 government, 288 private, and 10 semi- private) provide undergraduate medical training for 90,675 medical students (NMC, 2022). Typically, students in standards 11th and 12th at school (equivalent to A levels in the UK) begin training for the national level competitive exam known as National Eligibility-cum-Entrance Test Under Graduation (NEET UG). The following numbers provide an idea of the scale. In 2019, 1.41 million students attempted the NEET; 797,000 qualified and only 75,000 got selected for the MBBS course (Philip et al., 2021). A further 50,000 students were selected for undergraduate courses in Ayurveda, Unani, Siddha, and Homeopathy (alternative systems of medicine).

Stress and Indian Medical Education

Seeking admission into affordable government funded institutions, aspiring doctors compete for better rankings and scores on this test. The cost of medical training in privately run institutions ranges from USD 40,000 to 130,000 (Grover, 2018). These figures are three to four times higher than fees charged in many other countries. Understandably, 20,000–25,000 Indian students go abroad to study medicine every year (Nagarajan, 2022). Tuition amounts thereafter become sources of financial stress for both the students and their families as few scholarships are available. Other stressors for medical students include moving away from home and changing support systems with consequent loneliness and 'culture shock'. Ragging, bullying, hazing rituals, etc. also contribute as stressful experiences. In spite of prohibitive laws, infractions continue to occur (NDTV, 2019). This adds to new students' stress and making new friendships and new relationships can cause difficulties in adjustments and settling down.

Avinash Shekhar, Sharad Philip, Santosh Kumar Chaturvedi, and Dinesh Bhugra, *India* In: *The Mental Health of Medical Students*.
Edited by: Andrew Molodynski, Sarah Marie Farrell, and Dinesh Bhugra, Oxford University Press. © Oxford University Press 2024.
DOI: 10.1093/oso/9780192864871.003.0013

During the MBBS (Bachelor of Medicine, Bachelor of Surgery) course, the whole year is usually packed with lectures, assignments, presentations, assessments, examinations, and clinic-based practicals. In many colleges, students continue to report unsatisfactory hostel facilities, inadequate library facilities, frequent excess examinations, excessively competitive attitudes among students, political conflicts, jealousy and peer rivalry as contributing to their stress (Nandi et al., 2012) which can then lead to high levels of burnout. MBBS education involves 19 subjects with university examinations crammed into around four and half years with another year of internship at the end. Internship is the 1-year period after the final professional MBBS examinations where students participate actively and provide clinical services with limited or no supervision in different specialties. They are usually the frontline doctors who see the patients first and have on-call and emergency duties. Internship can be especially hectic in government hospitals, with large patient loads and limited human and financial resources. Frequently, junior doctors and interns become the victims of violence perpetrated by irate relatives of patients. Overwhelming numbers and poor support systems often lead to compassion fatigue (Mishra, 2021). Most states mandate obligatory periods of rural or remote area service—freshly minted doctors grapple with administrative, academic, and clinical challenges with minimal guidance at these locations, further exacerbating the stress and distress. In addition, often the focus in these placements is on infection control exposing interns to further stress and worry.

Undergraduate medical trainees, towards the end of their course begin preparations for their postgraduate (PG) medical training and beyond. Performance in the MBBS course may affect their selection in their chosen specialty, thus further adding to stress. Trainees must again focus on their performance relative to peers and seniors across the country. 'Selection pressures' imply that only 1 in 5 trainees will get an opportunity to pursue postgraduate (PG) medical training (more than 150,000 students compete for about 30,000 seats yearly). Many non-clinical and basic sciences PG training programmes continue to have vacancies as most trainees tend to aspire for clinical disciplines due to better financial returns, personal interest, etc. Many coaching institutions groom medical students and post-internship trainees through additional classes and examinations. Some of these institutes are known to run parallel medical training/teaching programmes from the first year onwards (DBMCI, 2022). Thus, medical students often sacrifice leisure, recreation, and vacation periods to attend these classes. Hence, from the time of entry to MBBS till the exit at internship, medical students face a variety of stressors.

Table 13.1 provides a brief description of important studies assessing wellbeing of medical students in India over the last decade.

Stress and Burnout and Coping in Indian Medical Students

Burnout has been defined elsewhere in this volume at length. Just to remind ourselves it is characterized as a state of increasing psychological distress, mental and physical exhaustion, increased mental distress, cynicism and pessimism intermixed with apathy and indifference and reduced proficiency in various aspects of life (World Health Organization, 2019). As noted above in Table 13.1, Burnout remains an occupational hazard for those in the healthcare professions. Stress often leads to decreased sleep quality, which along with the already difficult schedule of medical students, contributes to the aforementioned exhaustion. Persistent stress

Table 13.1 Indian medical students and their mental health: research at a glance

Study details	Important Findings
(Agrawal et al., 2021) Cross-sectional, single centre government medical college, 323 undergraduate students	Moderate to high stress was reported in medical students. Academic pressure and the health of the family were major concerns
(Saraswathi et al., 2020) Longitudinal, single centre, private medical college, 252 undergraduate students on follow up	Significant increase in prevalence of levels of anxiety and stress. COVID 19 in family/ friends and interactions with patients with COVID 19 predicted high stress
(Vidhukumar & Hamza, 2020) Cross-sectional, single centre, government medical college, 375 undergraduate medical students	Having hobbies helped in reducing stress/ mitigating burnout
(Pharasi & Patra, 2020) Cross-sectional, single centre, government medical college, 196 undergraduate medical students	Higher resilience scores were significantly associated with low emotional exhaustion in burnout score
(Farrell et al., 2019) Cross-sectional, multicentre, government, and private medical colleges. 597 undergraduate students	62% of the respondents reported a GHQ score >2. 88% and 81% of the respondents reported disengagement and exhaustion respectively as per the OLBI scale. 8% CAGE positive for problematic alcoholic usage
(Patil et al., 2018) Cross-sectional, single centre, private medical college, 200 year one, two, and three students	Prevalence of depression was found to be higher in 1st year students
(Garg et al., 2017) Cross-sectional study, single centre, government medical college, 251 undergraduate students	Worry about future, endurance, and capacity was rated the highest among the final year students
(Chowdhury et al., 2017) Cross-sectional, single centre, government medical college, 460 undergraduate students	Mean score was highest in 1st year and lowest in 3rd year
(Singh et al., 2016) Cross-sectional, single centre, government medical college, 100 final year students	Coping strategies include positive and negative strategies like substance use were noted. Positive strategies correlated with lower stress level
(Yuvraj et al., 2016) Cross-sectional, single centre, government medical college, 210 year one and two medical students	47% of the participants were found to have some mental health problem and required counselling. Of these, 28% required detailed evaluation
(Bute et al., 2016) Cross-sectional, single centre, private medical college, 737 undergraduate students	66% of the students had significant anxiety, depression, somatic symptoms, and social dysfunction. Interns were worst affected
(Goel et al, 2016) Longitudinal, single centre, government medical college, 160 students—all year one students	Depression and stress increased after one year. Disengagement dimension of burnout increased
(Iqbal et al., 2015) Cross-sectional study, single centre, government medical college, 353 undergraduate students	Morbidity was found to be more in 5th semester students rather than students of 2nd semester. Perception of self-assessment in academics was strongly associated with the higher score

Table 13.1 Continued

Study details	Important Findings
(Jena & Tiwari, 2015) Cross-sectional and comparative, multicentre—government and private medical college, 182 year one students	Prevalence of stress was higher in the government college than the private college
(Shad et al., 2015) Online survey, cross-sectional, 112 medical and 102 non-medical students	Medical students had higher levels of burnout and sleep impairment
(Manjunath & Kulkarni, 2013) Cross-sectional, single centre, private medical college, 211 year one and two students	Stress increased with the number of years in training
(Nandi et al., 2012) Cross-sectional, single centre, government medical college, 215 students in 3rd, 6th, and 9th semester	Social interactions of highly stressed respondents suffered in comparison to their non-stressed peers

is also associated with repetitive negative thinking and worry (Rosenkranz et al., 2020) and can predispose to cynicism and indifference (Viljoen & Claassen, 2017). Often substance misuse and other maladaptive coping mechanisms exacerbate burnout, resulting in dysfunction and even dropouts. Suicidal ideation and mental health morbidity are strongly associated with burnout (Vidhukumar & Hamza, 2020). Poor mental health literacy and apprehensions of stigma and discrimination delay help seeking. Medical students most often approach peers or immediate seniors for advice and help (Mishra, 2021) seldom seeking out mental health professionals. Rigid schedules and time pressures also reduce the opportunities for help seeking. Students in medical schools show significantly poorer levels of sleep quality and wellbeing when compared to schools of alternate medicine. Students mostly blamed academic load for their poor sleep and wellbeing (Kukade et al., 2022). With regard to their training, modern medicine schools differ from traditional disciplines in the extent of preparedness imparted regarding medical emergencies (Patwardhan et al., 2011). A study from rural medical college surveyed 177 medical students through their education careers for precipitating and protective factors against depression and anxiety (Sharma et al., 2018). These authors found that academic studies, friends, and financial problems were the common precipitating factors while sports, hobbies, yoga, and meditation were used as coping strategies (Sharma et al., 2018).

Medical students in the first year of studies at an urban medical college were noted to have reduced activity levels and increased screen use and this was associated with negative emotional health (Yadav et al., 2022). Another study from eastern India examined the effect of mindfulness traits in mitigating against depression and anxiety states. Trait mindfulness was found to be associated with lower depressive and anxiety states (Sampath et al., 2019).

Impact of the Pandemic

COVID19 brought a wide range of occupational stressors to doctors and medical students along with other healthcare professional in India. Medical students in their final years and those in internship were recruited during the COVID-19 crisis to work on the inpatient wards. Furthermore, their final year and other examinations were postponed including the NEET-PG entrance exam in 2021. Most medical students and doctors were co-opted to assist in COVID-19 care. Unsurprisingly, they reported feeling underprepared to manage patients with COVID-19 and their families. The urgency and rapidity with which these measures were implemented meant training was inadequate with substandard supervision and poor support systems (Sharma & Narayan, 2021). Some interns reported that even during this period of unprecedented demand on service, their monthly stipends were not being paid on time and no incentives were being given to the students who were part of the frontline healthcare teams thereby further adding to financial stress. Interns also faced a reduction of the routine cases in their posting and were seeing only COVID-19 patients. This may impact their acquisition of other relevant clinical skills. There was a concern that they would not develop their skills in handling the usual illnesses and were just used as cheap labour to handle the shortage in these special wards.

For the students in their early MBBS, all classes became online activities. This meant that students missed out on any hands-on practical postings. Owing to academic pressures, resumption of offline teaching also saw truncation of the usual study durations and reduced vacations and breaks (The Times of India, 2022), making their hectic schedules worse (Agrawal et al., 2021; Menon et al., 2021; Saraswathi et al., 2020). There were no nationwide studies done in India that compared burnout in students from different parts of the country.

National Survey Findings

NIMHANS conducted a national survey amongst medical students in India as part of a larger international effort to evaluate wellbeing of medical students. The survey link was disseminated through medical student groups across the country, predominantly by reaching out to student leadership and through WhatsApp chat groups. A message accompanied the link to introduce the survey and its aims, assuring confidentiality and anonymity. Consenting respondents provided information about basic demographic details such as year of study, level of parental education, hours of work outside of student activities, current and past mental health difficulties, prescribed and ongoing medications, and basic details of substance use.

The survey relied on innovative methods for dissemination such as signposting on social media. The survey was open from 09/02/20 until 31/08/20. Fortnightly reminders were sent. The short version of the 'General Health Questionnaire' (GHQ-12) (Goldberg & Blackwell, 1970; Goldberg et al., 1997), the Oldenburg Burnout Inventory (OLBI) (Demerouti & Bakker, 2008) and the CAGE questionnaire (Ewing, 1984) were used.

Survey Results

A total 341 medical students reported across all years of medical training 12% reported that they were currently having a mental health condition with diagnoses ranging from mood disorders, anxiety disorders. This was a steep increase as only 2% of the respondents reported having a mental health condition prior to medical training. Furthermore 7% of the respondents reported being on prescription psychotropics. Alarmingly, the frequency of new mental health diagnoses increased as the medical training progressed with the largest increase noted in and after year 3. Students were more likely to be stressed due to academic pressures (70%)—with 6% even reporting use of cognitive performance enhancing substances without prescriptions. This was followed by relationships (50%) and financial issues (25%)—most reported a combination of stressors. The most concerning survey result showed that 70% of all respondents reported high scores on GHQ-12, indicating a need for clinical evaluation for depression. This was worse during transition periods like the first and last years of medical training. High levels of burnout were noted amongst 80% and 86% of all respondents fulfilling criteria for exhaustion and disengagement, respectfully. Further details regarding the survey and the results for India can be obtained from the published article (Philip et al., 2021).

This survey found that medical students were indeed at great risk of developing mental ill health. Stress of medical training was noted to be associated with an increase in mental health morbidity for students. Increase in the number of respondents being diagnosed after entering medical training warrants further exploration and research. Risk of mental health morbidity seemed to increase with medical training. Transitional periods, especially the first year and internship are noted to have additional stressors. Such transitional periods must be an added focus for mental and occupational healthcare services. The timing of the survey fell between the period of onset of the COVID-19 pandemic but we were not in a position to compare pre- and post-data.

Mental Health Promotion and Wellbeing

As is well recognized 75% of psychiatric disorders in adulthood start below the age of 24—exactly the age group most medical students belong to. Hence it is vital that their mental health and wellbeing are looked after. Many strategies have been proposed. Stress management training which includes relaxation techniques, assertive training, self-awareness of one's stress and maintaining work–life balance has been shown to be effective in improving stress and exhaustion levels in Indian medical students (Nebhinani et al., 2021).

The National Medical Commission (NMC) functions as the premier medical education regulator in India. Alongside the curriculum it stipulates extracurricular activities during various stages of medical training. These are purposed towards demonstrating the importance of a work–life balance early on and they provide mandated opportunities for physical activities too. Commencing in the first year, the foundation course for one month stipulates a compulsory four hours per week for sports and two hours per week for extracurricular activities, adding up to a total of 22 hours of time protected from academics. For the first two years of training, the NMC mandates 4% of the teaching hours be dedicated to sports and extracurricular activities including yoga. Sessions on time and stress management alongside stress relief techniques are included as part of the foundation course (Medical Council of India, 2019). Many medical colleges/universities have annual intercollegiate events emphasizing sports and recreation. In some instances, a group of colleges in a state will have sporting or cultural festivals (The Times of India, 2019; Manipal, 2022).

Some colleges appoint mentors for incoming students to ease them into their medical training. These are often members of the teaching faculty with whom some students may not feel comfortable sharing mental health problems and may thus avoid honest disclosures. In some medical colleges, student counsellors (trained psychologists) are appointed to address students' mental health concerns. Still other colleges have set up student wellness centres. Meant to be accessible by all students, these centres provide professional health and counselling services. India's premier government funded medical education institution, All India Institute of Medical Sciences (AIIMS), New Delhi runs a Student Wellness Centre (AIIMS, 2022). Services provided include individual counselling, group counselling sessions, 24/7 helpline, self-help programmes, community support, and virtual sessions. Similar services are seen in other AIIMS and some other private medical colleges. Medical Students Association of India undertakes various projects for student wellbeing. Many of them were during the COVID-19 pandemic to counter the rising stress and burnout in medical students who were recruited for managing the crisis. Beat the Burnout 2.0 was an interactive online activity which was aimed to improve the quality of life of medical students by gauging the stress levels amongst them during the COVID-19 pandemic and by demonstrating effective stress relieving strategies. Tools like reflective narratives was utilized by psychologists to engage medical students during the pandemic at a leading medical college. Multiple styles allowed for narrations and expressions of prevailing concerns of medical students. Students wrote essays, poems, and playscripts highlighting their introspections on empathy, loss, and related tragedies and lockdown measures. These provided students improved peer connectedness—something on short supply during the pandemic and related restrictions.

Distressed students benefit from such divergent techniques of expressing themselves. Hence such workshops need to be conducted periodically for other stressful situations considering the very positive feedback reported (Vaz, 2021). Beyond stress management, another activity, 'PANDAmic' informed on pandemic preparedness and various e-learning platforms (Medical Students Association, 2021). Other medical training institutes brought out do-it-yourself simple easy manuals on stress relief (Chandran & Sreedaran, 2020; Janardhana et al., 2020). As of August 2022, data regarding the results and evaluation of these programmes remain unavailable.

The Way Forward

It is clear that medical students in modern medical schools in India demonstrate high rates of burnout. Currently some strategies address these concerns with the largest focus being on health promotion. This focus can become a driver for further positive change.

At an Individual Level

We recommend incorporation of extracurricular activities to promote cohesion and development of secondary and tertiary support systems in the colleges. A study amongst dental students examining the role of extracurricular activities reported that active participation in such activities protected against burnout (Kumar, 2021). Extracurricular activities included participation in various clubs, arts, performances, music, sports, volunteer, and community activities. Participation in after-college volunteer activities may be beneficial in the reduction of stress and burnout prevention. However, these can add on to demands on daily time. Various hobbies and recreational activities can be encouraged even during college. Regular yoga and meditation activities conducted in group formats can also be beneficial (Ganpat & Nagendra, 2011). Students requesting periods of absence from academics ought not to be denied. In all medical colleges, students are expected to attend 75% of classes and the Indian medical education curriculum does not allow gap periods or extended breaks. Breaks from academic work can be useful in reducing stress and giving a breather for medical students. An option for yearlong sabbaticals would be useful for medical students without the need for explanation of the gaps in training as is done in many Western countries where students are actively encouraged to spend periods in different healthcare systems. Exchange and elective programmes too can be incorporated. Students will benefit from a choice of extended duration of medical education in blocks of six months.

Resilience building strategies like problem solving, stress management, active coping, connection making, and building self-efficacy would help in reduction of burnout in medical students. Emphasis on physical activity and sleep hygiene should be retained. Technology can play a role in reducing stress and burnout with online peer networks complementing the traditional networks. Robust peer mentoring systems and training of faculty members may aid in surveillance and early detection of mental health issues. This may subsequently reduce morbidity for those affected and reduce dropout rates. Mental health promotion should also be focused on student welfare activities.

Group Level

Academic stress is the most common stressor identified by students. Competitiveness amongst medical students may hamper social interactions and limit avenues for peer support Cooperative learning is a suggestion that has been put forward to build peer support and improve social interaction among students (Mishra, 2021).

Institutional Level

Every medical college would do best to have student wellness centres established according to local needs. Programmes for improving awareness and destigmatizing mental health problems are needed to reduce the barriers to help seeking from mental health professionals. 24/7 helplines are another feature that could be initiated, with counsellors available at all times to help in periods of crisis. Support for minority and marginalized groups, i.e. gender, sexuality, religion, caste, lingual, race, and diversity initiatives, would be a welcome step that would help medical students.

Students could be encouraged to take up parallel courses or dual degree programmes in psychology, social work, data sciences, public health, health administration, etc. that would add value to young doctors. Range of such choices can provide increased exposure, life skills, and resilience. However, it must be balanced with existing workload, deadlines, and related stresses. Peer support networks and facilitators can be trained in low intensity psychological interventions with aims of improving self-awareness, self-practice, and even peer delivery. Examples of low intensity psychological interventions include healthcare activity programmes, problem-solving therapy, and stress management. Zero bullying and anti-hazing policies should be strictly enforced in all medical colleges. In addition, training of all faculty, hostel wardens and other stakeholders in awareness of mental health issues is needed in medical colleges to eliminate the stigma, making them more approachable for students. Initiatives that can facilitate early identification of students at risk or those with mental health/substance use disorders would be useful. Education modules like life skills and education about substance use could be provided in the foundation course and periodically for all students on a regular basis. However, this must be respectful and rights based in its approach. Medical students can be provided a platform to share lived experience, this would be especially useful for priming incoming trainees. Sharing of coping strategies and challenges may help in identifying best practices that could be shared to improve coping. Development of peer support groups for the students through voluntary participation should be encouraged. They should be trained in identifying early signs, knowing when to contact mental health professionals and gatekeeper training for preventing suicide These services need to be made easily accessible to all students. Students and faculty mentors can be involved in making these services and supports most accessible.

Policy Level

Another move that would help students would be an increase in accessible and affordable medical education to limit the financial stress on students. Establishment of such centres would also decrease the number of Indian students studying outside India and prevent events like the Indian student evacuation crisis that happened due to the conflict in Ukraine. Ensuring that medical institutes have adequate infrastructure and trained staff to educate medical students is also a must. Better hostel facilities and nutritious food services would contribute in decreasing the small daily stresses that can occur in medical students. Facilitated exchange and gap programmes may further benefit their psychological wellbeing. Rightful accommodations to vulnerable students such as those with disabilities and support would help them navigate the medical education on similar footing as other students. To achieve a good work–life balance, support may be provided for those students with families, for example, day-care for children. This would help students to be able to continue their medical education without worry of neglecting the family or cost of childcare. Adequate maternity and paternity leave should be included for undergraduate medical students.

Conclusion

As illustrated, burnout rates are high among medical students, the future medical work force. It is crucial to support them in this vulnerable period. Actions are needed at individual, group, policy, and institutional levels. Inclusion of strategies of early identification and redressal of burnout can help medical professionals throughout their career. Professional development alongside health, especially mental health promotion are urgent needs. Medical educators and policy makers ought to focus on increasing the degree of targeted support around mental health. Mental health promotion activities ought to incorporate stigma reduction in order to enhance access and uptake.

References

Agrawal, N., Sharma, H. Dabas, A. and Mishra, A. (2021) 'Perceived Stress Among Medical Students and Doctors in India During COVID-19 Pandemic', *MAMC Journal of Medical Sciences*, 7(1), p. 14.

AIIMS (2022) 'About Us – Student Wellness Centre', *Student Wellness Centre*. Available at: https://swc.aiims.edu/about-us/ (Accessed: 20 April 2022).

Bute, J., Bachhotiya, A., Arora, V.K. and Kori, S. (2016) 'A cross-sectional study of mental well-being among undergraduate students in a Medical College, in Central India', *International Journal of Medical Science and Public Health*, 5(9), p. 1775.

Chandran, S. and Sreedaran, P. (2020) *Breathe-A handbook for the wellbeing of healthcare workers during the pandemic and beyond*.

Chowdhury, R., Mukherjee, A., Mitra, K., Naskar, S., Karmakar, P.R. and Lahiri S.K. (2017) 'Perceived psychological stress among undergraduate medical students: Role of academic factors', *Indian Journal of Public Health*, 61(1), p. 55.

Demerouti, E. and Bakker, A.B. (2008) 'The Oldenburg Burnout Inventory: A good alternative to measure burnout and engagement', *Handbook of Stress and Burnout in Health Care* [Preprint].

Ewing, J.A. (1984) 'Detecting Alcoholism: The CAGE Questionnaire', *JAMA*, 252(14), pp. 1905–1907.

Farrell, S.M., Kar, A., Valsraj, K. Mukherjee, S. Kunheri, B., Molodynski, A. and George, S. (2019) 'Wellbeing and burnout in medical students in India; a large scale survey', *International Review of Psychiatry (Abingdon, England)*, 31(7–8), pp. 555–562.

DBMCI 2022 *Fundamental Batch – For 1st Prof Students* (2022) *DBMCI*. Available at: https://www.dbmci.com/fundamental-combo-batch (Accessed: 20 April 2022).

Ganpat, T.S. and Nagendra, H.R. (2011) 'Integrated yoga therapy for improving mental health in managers', *Industrial Psychiatry Journal*, 20(1), pp. 45–48.

Garg, K., Agarwal, M. and Dalal, P.K. (2017) 'Stress among medical students: A cross-sectional study from a North Indian Medical University', *Indian Journal of Psychiatry*, 59(4), pp. 502–504.

Goel, A.D., Akarte, S.V, Agrawal, S.P. and Yadav, V. (2016) 'Longitudinal assessment of depression, stress, and burnout in medical students', *Journal of Neurosciences in Rural Practice*, 7(4), pp. 493–498.

Goldberg, D.P., Gater, R., Sartorius, N., Ustun, T.B., Piccinelli, M., Gureje, O. and Rutter, C. (1997) 'The validity of two versions of the GHQ in the WHO study of mental illness in general health care', *Psychological Medicine*, 27(1), pp. 191–197.

Goldberg, D.P. and Blackwell, B. (1970) 'Psychiatric Illness in General Practice: A Detailed Study Using a New Method of Case Identification', *BMJ*, 2(5707), pp. 439–443.

Grover, S (2018) *Physician burnout: Are we taking care of ourselves enough!* Available at: https://www.jmhhb.org/article.asp?issn=0971-8990;year=2018;volume=23;issue=2;spage=76;epage=77;aulast=Grover (Accessed: 20 April 2022).

Iqbal, S., Gupta, S. and Venkatarao, E. (2015) 'Stress, anxiety and depression among medical undergraduate students and their socio-demographic correlates', *The Indian Journal of Medical Research*, 141(3), pp. 354–357.

Janardhana, N., Joseph, S.J., R, T.K., Mehrotra, S., Kumar, A., Chand, P.K., Desai, G. and Cherian, A.V. (2020) 'Psychosocial care for frontline health care workers during covid-19' (2020), p. 56.

Jena, S. and Tiwari, H. (2015) 'Stress and mental health problems in 1st year medical students: A survey of two medical colleges in Kanpur, India', *International Journal of Research in Medical Sciences*, p. 1.

Kukade, A.S., Mathad, M.D. and K, R.S. (2022) 'Sleep Quality, Wellbeing and Happiness in Medical Undergraduates in Western India', *National Journal of Community Medicine*, 13(05), pp. 298–303.

Kumar, Y.S., Ramanarayan, V., Rajesh, R., Francis, S.T.V., Ganesan, S., Kumar, S.V. (2021) *Association of extracurricular activities and burnout among students in a dental teaching institution in India*. Available at: https://www.jiaphd.org/article.asp?issn=2319-5932;year=2021;volume=19;issue=4;spage=294;epage=298;aulast=Kumar (Accessed: 20 April 2022).

Cultural-Activities, Manipal. Available at: https://manipal.edu/kmc-manipal/about-kmc/Cultural-Activities.html (Accessed: 20 April 2022).

Manjunath, R. and Kulkarni, P. (2013) 'Mental Health Status and Depression Among Medical Students in Mysore, Karnataka – An Untouched Public Health Issue', *National Journal of Community Medicine*, 4(01), pp. 50–53.

Medical Council of India (2019). Foundation Course for the Undergraduate Medical Education Program, 2019: pp 1-46. 'FOUNDATION-COURSE-MBBS-17.07.2019.pdf' (no date). Available at: https://www.nmc.org.in/wp-content/uploads/2020/08/FOUNDATION-COURSE-MBBS-17.07.2019.pdf (Accessed: 20 April 2022).

Medical students association (2022). Available at: https://www.msaindia.org/Activities/currentprojects (Accessed: 20 April 2022).

Menon, B., Sannapareddy, S. and Menon, M. (2021) 'Assessment of Severity of Stress Among Medical and Dental Students During the COVID-19 Pandemic', *Annals of Indian Academy of Neurology*, 24(5), pp. 703–707.

Mishra, S., Padhy. S.K. and Sinha, A.K. (2021) *Stress, distress, and burnout among medical trainees: An institutional approach*. Available at: https://www.indjsp.org/article.asp?issn=0971-9962;year=2021;volume=37;issue=2;spage=162;epage=167;aulast=Mishra (Accessed: 20 April 2022).

Nagarajan (2022) *Why students from India go abroad to study medicine | India News – Times of India*. Available at: https://timesofindia.indiatimes.com/india/why-students-from-india-go-abroad-to-study-medicine/articleshow/89910988.cms (Accessed: 20 April 2022).

Nandi, M., Hazra, A., Sarkar, S., Mondal, R., & Ghosal, M.K. (2012) 'Stress and its risk factors in medical students: an observational study from a medical college in India', *Indian Journal of Medical Sciences*, 66(1–2), pp. 1–12.

NDTV (2019) *MCI Received Six Complaints Of Ragging In Medical Colleges In 2019-20, NDTV.com*. Available at: https://www.ndtv.com/education/mci-received-six-complaints-of-ragging-in-medical-colleges-in-2019-20-2155970 (Accessed: 20 April 2022).

Nebhinani, N., Kuppili, P.P., and Mamta (2021) 'Stress, Burnout, and Coping among First-Year Medical Undergraduates', *Journal of Neurosciences in Rural Practice*, 12(03), pp. 483–489.

NMC (2022) 'List of College Teaching MBBS. Available at: https://www.nmc.org.in/information-desk/for-students-to-study-in-india/list-of-college-teaching-mbbs/ (Accessed: 20 April 2022)

Patil, K., Chande, D., Pratinidhi, S.A., & Bhat, A. (2018) 'A Study to assess Depression levels in MBBS Students', *Indian Journal of Mental Health*, 5, p. 296.

Patwardhan, K., Gehlot, S., Singh, G., & Rathore, H.S.C. (2011) 'The Ayurveda Education in India: How Well Are the Graduates Exposed to Basic Clinical Skills?', *Evidence-based Complementary and Alternative Medicine: eCAM*, 2011, p. 197391.

Pharasi, S. & Patra, S. (2020) 'Burnout in medical students of a tertiary care Indian medical center: How much protection does resilience confer?'. *Indian Journal of Psychiatry*, 62(4), pp. 407–412.

Philip, S., Molodynski, A., Barklie, L., Bhugra, D., & Chaturvedi, S.K. (2021) 'Psychological well-being and burnout amongst medical students in India: a report from a nationally accessible survey', *Middle East Current Psychiatry*, 28(1), p. 54.

Rosenkranz, T., Takano, K., Watkins, E.R., & Ehring, T. (2020) 'Assessing repetitive negative thinking in daily life: Development of an ecological momentary assessment paradigm', *PLOS ONE*, 15(4), p. e0231783.

Sampath, H., Biswas, G.B., Soohinda, G., & Dutta, S. (2019) 'Mindfulness and its role in psychological well-being among medical college students', *Open Journal of Psychiatry & Allied Sciences*, 10(1), p. 52.

Saraswathi, I., Saikarthik, J., Kumar, K.S, Srinivasan, K.M., Ardhanaari, M., & Gunapriya, R. (2020) 'Impact of COVID-19 outbreak on the mental health status of undergraduate medical students in a COVID-19 treating medical college: a prospective longitudinal study', *PeerJ*, 8, p. e10164.

Shad, R.S., Thawani, R., & Goel, A. (2015) 'Burnout and Sleep Quality: A Cross-Sectional Questionnaire-Based Study of Medical and Non-Medical Students in India', *Cureus* [Preprint].

Sharma, S., Bokariya, P., Kothari, R., & Kothari, V. (2018) 'Study of Psychological Wellbeing of Medical Students at Mahatma Gandhi Institute of Medical Sciences', p. 8.

Sharma, Y. & Narayan, K. (2021) *Medical students suspend studies to help in COVID crisis, University World News*. Available at: https://www.universityworldnews.com/post.php?story=20210506152611911 (Accessed: 13 June 2022).

Singh, S., Prakash, J., Das, R.C., & Srivastava, K. (2016) 'A cross-sectional assessment of stress, coping, and burnout in the final-year medical undergraduate students', *Industrial Psychiatry Journal* **25**(2), p. 179.

The Times of India (2019) '"Burnout 3.0" kicks off at MSU's pavilion ground', 28 November. Available at: https://timesofindia.indiatimes.com/city/vadodara/burnout-3-0-kicks-off-at-msus-pavilion-gro und/articleshow/72267400.cms (Accessed: 20 April 2022).

The Times of India (2022) 'To make up for Covid delay, more classes for MBBS 1st-year students', 4 February. Available at: https://timesofindia.indiatimes.com/india/to-make-up-for-covid-delay- more-classes-for-mbbs-1st-year-students/articleshow/89332527.cms (Accessed: 20 April 2022).

Vaz, M. (2021) 'Reflective narratives during the Covid-19 pandemic: an outlet for medical students in uncertain times', *Indian Journal of Medical Ethics*, pp. 1–3.

Vidhukumar, K. & Hamza, M. (2020) 'Prevalence and Correlates of Burnout among Undergraduate Medical Students – A Cross-sectional Survey', *Indian Journal of Psychological Medicine* **42**(2): 122–127.

Viljoen, M. & Claassen, N. (2017) 'Cynicism as subscale of burnout', *Work (Reading, Mass.)* **56**(4): 499–503.

World Health Organization (2019) *Burn-out an 'occupational phenomenon': International Classification of Diseases* (2019). Available at: https://www.who.int/news/item/28-05-2019-burn-out-an-occup ational-phenomenon-international-classification-of-diseases (Accessed: 20 April 2022).

Yuvaraj B. Y., Poornima S., & Rashmi S. (2016) 'Screening for overall mental health status using mental health inventory amongst medical students of a government medical college in North Karnataka, India', *International Journal of Community Medicine and Public Health*, pp. 3308–3312.

Yadav, A., Yadav, K., Punjabi, P., Sankhla, M., & Shukla, J. (2022) 'Analysing the Effect of Lockdown on Physical Activity, Screen Time, and Emotional Wellbeing Among Young Medical Students of India During the COVID-19 Pandemic', *Journal of Medical Education*, 21(1).

14

Indonesia

Supporting Indonesian Medical Student Wellbeing in Medical Education: A Call to Action to Address Burnout

Theresia Citraningtyas, Rossalina Lili, Darien Alfa Cipta, and Nabila Ananda Kloping

Burnout Among Medical Students in Indonesia

In early 2020, our team conducted a descriptive study to understand more about wellbeing, burnout, anxiety, and depression among medical students in Indonesia (Lili et al., 2021). Data from 1,729 medical students from 29 universities showed 93% of respondents to be disengaged with their studies and 95% to be exhausted; 87% expressed that they felt tired even before arriving at their university/hospital. As many as 82% reported that they now required significantly more time to de-stress, relax, and recover compared to the time prior to medical school. About 79% reported an inability to tolerate pressures from their study; 68% were emotionally drained. Also, 69% described feeling disconnected from their studies and 77% felt sickened by the tasks they needed to complete. Despite that, 80% of the respondents felt they could still overcome their problems and 86% reported they could come across something new and exciting in their respective work conditions.

In this study, 77 (4.4%) medical students reported being diagnosed with mental disorders at the time of the survey. Depressive disorder, anxiety disorder, and mixed anxiety and depression disorder made up 59% of the diagnoses. Other diagnoses included bipolar disorder, borderline personality disorder, schizophrenia, and unspecified diagnoses. Note that 12% of respondents reported having visited a general practitioner or psychiatrist regarding their mental health problems prior to medical school, even though not all received a formal diagnosis.

Respondents reported the primary stressor to be academic work (68%). Almost half also reported their family to be a source of stress (45%), and/or financial issues (29%). We will now provide an overview of the medical education system in order to look into some factors which may contribute to these high rates, with the aim of identifying potential areas for further research and action.

The Process of Becoming a Doctor in Indonesia

The process of becoming a doctor is known to be lengthy, arduous, and costly, with minimal breaks compared to other academic majors. In order to obtain a medical doctor degree

Theresia Citraningtyas, Rossalina Lili, Darien Alfa Cipta, and Nabila Ananda Kloping, *Indonesia* In: *The Mental Health of Medical Students*. Edited by: Andrew Molodynski, Sarah Marie Farrell, and Dinesh Bhugra, Oxford University Press. © Oxford University Press 2024. DOI: 10.1093/oso/9780192864871.003.0014 (*dokter* 'dr.' pre-nominal title), senior high school graduates have to complete a four-year Bachelor of Medicine (*Sarjana Kedokteran—S.Ked*) programme followed by two years of apprenticeship/clerkship/professional clinical training. These medical graduates are then required to go through internship to be able to practice as general practitioners. Those who then want to pursue a particular medical specialization would need to apply to and complete four to five years at a university-based residency programme (Program Pendidikan Dokter Spesialis—PPDS), mainly in public-owned universities. Another two to three years of subspecialization would give them the additional title of consultant.

The undergraduate programme consists of blocks focusing on a system (such as musculoskeletal) or field (such as emergency medicine) with interdisciplinary components (e.g. anatomy, physiology, pathology, orthopaedics, internal medicine). The national medical education competency standards (*Standar Nasional Pendidikan Profesi Dokter Indonesia—SNPPDI*, 2019, previously *Standar Kompetensi Dokter Indonesia—SKDI*, 2012) outlines expected clinical skill sets based on capacity levels (1: knowing to 4: executing/treating) for different health problems, diagnoses, and medical procedures (Konsil Kedokteran Indonesia, 2019b). The standards are translated into national clinical practice guidelines and becomes the reference for medical schools to develop their competency-based curriculum, first outlined by the Indonesian Medical Council in 2006 (Bustamam et al., 2012).

Students learn this in blocks and include several weeks of combined lectures, problem-based learning (PBL), and skills labs. For every block, students are expected to produce presentations, write a report for their PBLs, attend skill labs and skill lab examinations, and take standardized (multiple-choice question) tests. Attendance requirements are strict. In many medical schools, missing a single PBL or skill lab session or introductory lecture could mean having to repeat an entire block. This also possibly impedes the student from being able to participate in subsequent blocks for which the previous one is a prerequisite. There are additional financial repercussions, as students are required to pay tuition per block as well as per semester.

Students are assessed at the end of each block using computer-based (or written) and skills lab examinations. This situation creates a potential discrepancy between what the students are interested in learning as presented during PBLs and what they would need to study for the test. There are also different integrated examinations across blocks, such as the Objective Structured Clinical Examinations (OSCE) and Structured Objective Case Analysis (SOCA). Students also need to complete a research project ('*skripsi*'), which includes proposal presentation examination, ethical clearance, data collection, and analysis towards a final thesis examination (Bustamam et al., 2012).

After obtaining their bachelor's degree, students enter their clerkship starting with a few weeks of introductory training, followed by rotations through different medical departments (which generally include stations in different clinical settings organized by the university at designated teaching hospitals and/or community health centres). Students are supervised to examine actual patients and are assessed accordingly (Bustamam et al., 2012).

At the end of medical training, students are assessed using the medical student competency test (*Ujian Kompetensi Mahasiswa Program Pendidikan Dokter—UKMPPD*) administered by the Directorate General of Higher Education in collaboration with the Ministry of Health, the Indonesian Medical Council, the Indonesian Doctors Association, and the Association of Indonesian Medical Education Institutions (Kementerian Pendidikan, 2023).

The computer-based test and OSCE is run four times a year. This final medical competency exam is arguably the most crucial test for medical students.

The Bigger Picture: Medical Education in an Archipelago of Disparity

Indonesia is the world's fourth most populous and third-largest country in Asia, with a population of over 276 million (World Bank, 2022) spread across approximately 1,690 populated islands (Ministry of Marine Affairs and Fisheries, 2012) in an archipelago of 17,508 islands (Government of Republic of Indonesia, 1996). Over 56% of the population reside on the island of Java, and 22% in Sumatra (Badan Pusat Statistik, 2021). Social and educational discrepancies across the archipelago are profound. While urban medical centres compete at an international level, some of the smaller outer islands struggle to access basic medical care and even proper nutrition, with nutritional stunting still being a major public health concern (World Bank, 2015). Catering for the needs of doctors against this backdrop is not an easy feat.

There are currently 92 medical schools in Indonesia (LAM-PTKes, 2022), each accepting approximately 150 new medical students per year (Indonesian Consortium of Health Science, 2013). Approximately 60% are in private universities and follow a market-based system and decentralized policy (Harimurti et al., 2017). According to the 2020 Statistic report from the Directorate General of Higher Education (Directorate General of Higher Education, 2020), there are 63 public universities and over 3,000 private universities throughout the country. Medical schools are mainly located on the islands of Sumatra and Java, where it is most populated, with 12 being in Jakarta alone.

One way to address the problem of geographic distribution of medical personnel has been through regional internship placement (Ministry of Health Republic of Indonesia, 2017). This replaced the previous scheme of mandatory placement of doctors as temporary workers (*Pegawai Tidak Tetap—PTT*) in public community health centres and regional hospitals. The internship programme changes the concept to an extended period of learning in a paid position. This provides a temporary solution but does not solve the more crucial problem of the lack of permanent doctors, especially for rural and regional Indonesia.

Policies related to medical education are linked to concerns around the quantity and quality of the healthcare workforce. The Minister of Health, Mr. Budi Gunadi, has stated that in order to meet the WHO (Kumar & Pal, 2018) recommendation of at least 1:1,000 physicians/population ratio, Indonesia needs at least 130,000 more doctors. The minister is thus collaborating with the Minister of Education to push for more medical schools in the country (Ministry of Health Republic of Indonesia, 2022).

This move to increase quantity is a total reversal of previous policy. In a press conference in 2019, the head of the Health Workforce Directorate of the Ministry of Health (*BPPSDMK Kemenkes RI*) had stated that Indonesia had a surplus of medical doctors with 12,000 annual graduates (JPNN, 2017). Together with the ministry of higher education, the body had imposed a quota on medical graduates and a moratorium on the founding of new medical schools. The leadership of the Indonesian Medical Council appeared to support this view at that time (Fitri, 2016).

The rationale for the past moratorium was related to concerns of quality, measured from the high number of retakers of the national competency exam (UKMPPD), as illustrated in Figure 14.1. Over 10% of students fail their first attempt. Students can retake the test multiple times until they pass.

This competency exam had been changed from what used to be the Indonesian Doctors Competency Exam (*Ujian Kompetensi Dokter Indonesia—UKDI*) which was considered a prerequisite for medical graduates to obtain their licence to practice. Instead, the new exam determines their graduation, putting more pressure on students and the onus on medical schools for quality control. Failure rates are an issue of serious concern since test retakers cannot graduate with a medical degree and must continue paying tuition until they pass/ drop out. Romadhoni et al. (2021) emphasized the need for academic and psychological support for test retakers. We argue that the need for such support is necessary for everyone who has to take the test.

Most multiple retakers come from medical schools with the lowest, or 'C' accreditation status (LAM-PTKes, 2022). Medical schools are accredited according to criteria from the Directorate of Higher Education, previously categorized to levels 'A', 'B', and 'C', recently revised to 'superior', 'very good', 'good', and 'not accredited' (BAN-PT, 2020). The problem of quality among graduates from low accredited universities has been a subject of public debate (Prasetya & Suharlim, 2016). The Indonesian Medical Association (*Ikatan Dokter Indonesia/ IDI*) had once suggested for medical schools with C accreditation to be closed down—a move that was not approved by policymakers (Harimurti et al., 2017).

According to the Indonesian Medical Council, only 28% of students were enlisted in 'A' accredited medical schools (Konsil Kedokteran Indonesia, 2019a). This number has increased slightly in 2022, with 35 medical schools having achieved 'A' accreditation standard (LAM-PTKes, 2022). The more recent push toward more medical students may potentially create new issues related to the quality of intake with less stringent admission and the limited availability of teaching hospital facilities (Mustika et al., 2019).

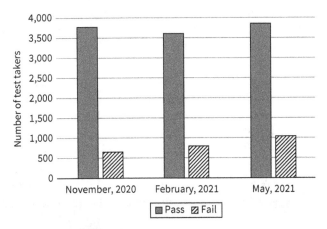

Figure 14.1 The UKMPPD Passing Statistics.

Source: data from Ministry of Education and Culture (2022) Registrars Online Uji Kompetensi Mahasiswa Program Profesi Dokter, Ministry of Education and Culture Republic of Indonesia. Available at: https://pnukm ppd.kemdikbud.go.id/index.php/statistik (Accessed: 4 June 2022).

Interestingly, our study, which compared rates of burnout across different medical schools and regions, found that students from Sumatera Island had lower rates of burnout than those on other islands (Kloping et al., 2021). The pattern also unfortunately corresponds with lower passing rates in the national competency exam. Thus, there need to be solutions that tackle burnout by increasing learning effectiveness, rather than reducing the study load in a way that negatively impacts quality.

Historical Perspective

This discrepancy in the quality and distribution of the medical workforce is related to the nature of Indonesian geography and political history. The first medical schools in Indonesia were established during the Dutch colonial era (Citraningtyas, 2019; Sysling, 2019) as a training ground for local medics in response to a pandemic at the turn of the last century (Pols, 2018). These first institutions have become the Ivy league public universities that determine the standard today. With time, more and more private universities with medical schools were founded. Some target wealthy more academic urban students, while others cater for their less privileged regional counterparts. Competition is highest to enter public universities, which generally provide a high standard of training at a lesser cost.

Several nationwide reforms have taken place in medical education in Indonesia in the last few decades to improve the quality of medical education. One of the biggest reforms in medical education was arguably the switch from traditional discipline-based lectures to integrated PBL. The move was initially trialled at the Faculty of Medicine, Universitas Indonesia in 1995, based on the first author's firsthand experience. After three semesters of divided staff support, student results using old-fashioned tests were deemed unsatisfactory. The system reverted to traditional lectures, with six semesters of preclinical studies packed into three. The batch considered themselves medical education guinea pigs/lab rats—the Indonesian term being experimental rabbits; hence, they proudly call themselves 'The Rabbits'. Interestingly, more 'Rabbits' have become researchers and academics than other batches. It remains a question whether having been a part of real-world experimentation might have propelled the development of a research mindset and an orientation towards teaching-learning. It took another decade for medical education across the country to finally adopt PBL.

Meant to make learning self-directed and relevant, PBL places the responsibility of knowing what to learn more on the students. While intended to increase student involvement in learning, the change from passive to active learning also requires more from students. The quality of learning is also contingent on the students' capacity and active participation. Socioeconomic disparities across the archipelago translates to discrepancies in the quality of potential student intake. Affirmative action is needed to meet the need for doctors in Indonesia's peripheries, yet this can create problems when rural and regional students are expected to perform to the same level as more academically privileged urban peers.

Some other reforms were ignited through the Worldbank Health Taskforce and Services project in 2002, which brought together medical schools across the country. One major reform was the development of a national standardized competency exam as previously described. Previously, students from public universities automatically graduated after passing their required courses, while students from private universities had to sit a comprehensive final exam at a public university in order to graduate. The reform required all students to sit a standardized national competency exam led by a team of assessors from different universities.

In many medical schools, the curriculum is now transitioning towards implementing a newly developed curriculum based on the latest standard (Konsil Kedokteran Indonesia, 2019b) from the previous 2012 version (Konsil Kedokteran Indonesia, 2012). The preamble of this new standard explicitly states that it has a higher target for undergraduate medical students. For example, while the previous standard only focuses on clinical competencies, the new standard also emphasizes skills to become educators and researchers. There is also an increase in the expectation of competence for each diagnosis. To illustrate, in mental health/psychiatry, the SKDI requires a medical doctor to have level 4 competence for mild-moderate depression from a previous level 2 competence (to diagnose and refer only) in 2012 (Konsil Kedokteran Indonesia, 2019a). To add to the complexity, higher education across the country are now expected to roll out Independent Learning Curriculum (Kurikulum Merdeka Belajar) which technically should allow students to spend up to one semester (20 credits) studying at a different study programme and two semesters (40 credits) in various activities of their choice at other universities, or even in different type of non-academic contexts in lieu of the traditional teaching-learning processes.

The new standards depict a move towards quality improvement, to enhance the role of university graduates in general and primary care doctors in particular in alignment with international standards and real-world needs. At the same time, it requires considerate and innovative implementation for this competence to be achieved without imposing further academic stress that possibly increases burnout among already stretched medical students.

The parliament is currently drafting a new Medical Education Bill to address some of these issues. One important point in the proposed draft is to allow medical students to graduate without passing the current competency exam (UKMPPD). The bill reemphasizes the autonomy of each university to determine whether or not their students are able to graduate (Baleg DPR RI, 2019). However, the draft has not concretely instated a mechanism to maintain the quality of graduates, who theoretically could thus get the title of medical doctor despite failing the competency exam.

At the Level of the Individual: Psychosocial Issues

Aside from systemic issues imposed by the medical education requirements, personal issues may also contribute to burnout among individual students. Personal issues include adverse life events as well as psychological aspects that increase the risk of burnout. Students have reported family issues such as abuse, parental divorce, major illnesses in the family, and the death of close family members. There is a significant relationship between negative personal life events and professional burnout (Dyrbye *et al.*, 2006).

Medicine is one of the most competitive fields to enter, generally luring bright and compassionate young persons who are not deterred by strenuous education and who have the resources to support them. There is a tendency for this group to feel the need to constantly prove themselves, placing academic achievement as a token of self-worth, often related to family expectations. In accordance with a Brazilian study (Pacheco et al., 2017), we often found in counselling sessions with medical students that they complained about the pressure from parents as a source of stress. Some students stated that their initial wish and passion is not in medicine, a profession imposed by their parents.

In our study of medical students, 45% of the respondents' parents have a postgraduate degree. This high standard may carry high expectations of academic success for the students. A study found that perceptions of parental affection is not a protective factor for anxiety among medical students (Zainal, 2019), potentially because of a sense of pressure to make their parents proud. Stress related to academic competition has been known to be a contributor to burnout (Frajerman et al., 2019).

Students from rural and regional areas also have to deal with significant adjustments, as described in Kloping et al. (2021). These students are physically disconnected from their usual psychological support, family members, or friends. They might also struggle to adapt to the urban culture, where people are perceived as more individualistic and competitive.

Socioeconomic Disadvantage

Aside from academic pressures and personal issues, the high cost of medical education could also contribute to the stress and burnout level among medical students (Frajerman et al., 2019). It is well known that entrance examinations and fees create a disadvantage for poorer applicants and high school graduates outside of major cities (Harimurti et al., 2017). Aside from the cost of tuition, they also need to have additional financial resources for living costs and travel to the urban centres where the medical schools are located.

Some students have obtained financial support from charities and religious organizations. More recently, various tuition scholarship schemes are available (Kompas, 2022; LPDP, 2021). Despite support for tuition, students still need to have independent resources to cover living cost during years of training. Some scholarship schemes also require students to meet minimum academic performance, which means that students who are struggling academically would be compounded by financial pressures. Students may even be obliged to return the money in case of failure.

Students have been known to have to take various jobs to supplement family support or scholarships. These students are at high risk of burnout and poor academic performance due to lack of time to study and rest. Some students have had to discontinue or defer their studies when their family suffer from financial setbacks.

Following medical school, residency entry and training is even more challenging. Residents are regarded primarily as students and have no position in the medical profession at teaching hospitals, described by Harimurti et al. (2017) as 'operating outside the standards of workforce employment'. Residents are expected to pay tuition while providing medical services at the hospital. It has only been since 2016 that residents at some teaching hospitals receive a meagre compensation despite long hours and heavy responsibilities, at an amount far less than minimum wage. This becomes a potential deterrent for some medical graduates from continuing their studies.

Changes During the Pandemic

The beginning of the pandemic cost the lives of hundreds of doctors. Late-stage medical students were deployed to the frontlines to deal with the disease at its deadliest. Early year students had to master the skills online by watching and making videos. They were less able to get together with peers. Students with limited internet access became seriously disadvantaged. Clinical-stage medical students were subject to greater exposure to sick patients, imposing a threat to themselves, their families, and contacts. Health workers faced discrimination; some were evicted from rental places for fear of bringing infections. Surveys conducted amid the pandemic showed that 83% of Indonesian health workers experienced moderate to severe burnout, contributing to emotional exhaustion, reduced empathy, and lower confidence in themselves (Fahrial Syam, 2021; Winurini, 2021).

During the COVID-19 pandemic, from April to May 2021, our team conducted a similar online survey to measure burnout among medical students across the country. We found that among 1947 active medical students registered as a member of the Asian Medical Students Association (AMSA), 35.5% reported experiencing burnout, which we defined as having a high level of emotional exhaustion and/or high-level depersonalization (Cipta et al., 2022, in submission). Other studies found burnout among interns and residents ranging from 25.6% to 56.67% (Daryanto et al., 2022; Nurikhwan et al., 2022).

The results appear to differ significantly from our pre-pandemic study (Lili et al., 2021). Much of this difference may be related to the use of different measurement tools and the exclusion of students who had previously been diagnosed with other mental conditions. The tool used in this study was the Maslach Burnout Inventory—Student Survey (MBI-SS), which has been validated in the Indonesian student population (Arlinkasari & Akmal, 2017; Daryanto et al., 2022), in contrast to our previous study that used the OLBI in the English language as a part of an international study (Lili et al., 2021). It also needs to be ascertained whether more students have become diagnosed with psychiatric conditions that made them excluded from the study. It also needs to be ascertained whether our second study recruited students with lesser rates of burnout because participants in the first study with high burnout rates might not have participated in the second study.

Taking this into account, it would be interesting to study whether changes during the pandemic might actually have reduced burnout in some cases. Among early year students, the switch to online learning allowed students to learn from the comfort of their homes and provided extra time which would have otherwise been spent commuting. Skill lab exams, which usually must be completed in one try of 8-10 minutes, were replaced with video submissions of examining family members, which allowed students multiple retakes. At the same time, the social isolation and disconnection have greatly impeded cooperative learning processes, at a stage in life where peer groups are most important. Many students have expressed difficulty focusing on their academic studies and a deterioration of wellbeing from a lack of friends.

Financially, the COVID-19 pandemic also propelled the Ministry of Health to provide a significant amount of financial support to health workers, including residents (Ministry of Health Republic of Indonesia, 2020). Long hours were reduced to shorter shifts to limit potential exposure to coronavirus. At the same time, based on the experience of the third author, the clinical workload for some departments increased significantly due to patient load increment or covering up the responsibility of peers who got infected by COVID-19.

A Call to Action

The systemic, social, and individual factors that contribute to burnout provide points for potential improvement. We propose a call to action along three levels as proposed by Rochais, a humanistic educationist focused on the growth of persons (PRH International, 2015) as illustrated in Figure 14.2.

The issue of burnout is a concern for the medical field as a whole, students being part of the larger context. The implicit message that burnout is 'normal' for medical professionals needs to be reverted. Self-care and wellbeing are often forgotten as part of a physician's professionalism. This topic has gained momentum following the pandemic. Initiatives include a workshop on self-care and wellbeing for medical professionals during the annual scientific psychiatric meeting (PDSKJI Jaya, 2022). Beyond emphasizing this through continuing medical education, efforts need to be taken to integrate wellbeing into the medical education and healthcare system rather than place the sole responsibility on individuals.

From the medical education system point of view, stakeholders need to consider the element of wellbeing in the discussion of curriculum development, directly alongside discourse on competency improvement (quality) and service provision (quantity and distribution). The national competency exam, currently considered a single-point quality assurance tool, may need to be adjusted to a more longitudinal quality assessment. Regarding this type of assessment, the recent implementation of the student stage exams (known as '*Ujian Tahap Bersama*'), in year 2 and year 4, starting from year 2021, reflects that the Association of Indonesian Medical Education Institutions (AIPKI Wilayah IV, 2019) has considered and accepted input from various academic circles and lawmakers (Baleg DPR RI, 2019). In addition, medical students could be more actively involved as stakeholders in designing the curriculum and examination objectives. Pre-medical academic support programmes might be needed for rural and regional students.

It is important to identify and assess students' psychological status and wellbeing at earlier points, probably at admission, and ensure that they receive adequate support. Counselling and psychotherapy need to be accessible for medical students who need it, and its utilization

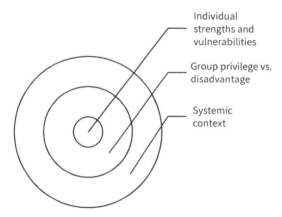

Individual strengths and vulnerabilities

Group privilege vs. disadvantage

Systemic context

Figure 14.2 Three target levels for resilience-building.
Adapted with permission from PRH International (2015) *PRH Helping Relationship And The Growth of Persons.*

should be endorsed rather than stigmatized. Currently, counselling is generally for students who are considered 'problematic' and referred by academic staff. Students may thus fear repercussions of having a diagnoses or mental health problems on their assessments for further study. Students need to be able to access independent services that ensure full confidentiality.

Alongside better design and university support, student support likely plays an essential part in students' mental health. To overcome the problem of the limited number of counsellors and mental health professionals, several medical schools have included student peer support in the counselling pathway.

At the university where the third author works, the Universitas Pelita Harapan (UPH) the peer support was originally developed for sexual and reproductive health. A survey of this group of students showed they wanted to extend their service to support mental health and wellbeing, as a response to the need they see among themselves. These students thus require training and supervision to provide adequate peer support (e.g. in active listening, psychological first aid).

Another model of intervention on the individual level was conducted in Universitas Kristen Krida Wacana (UKRIDA), in collaboration with Personality and Human Relations (*Personnalité et Relations Humaines—PRH*), to provide workshops that focus on personal development. Participants reported rediscovering meaning in their professional calling, developing positive ways to cope with their situation, and feeling more solid in their identity, thus reducing burnout (Citraningtyas, 2017; Citraningtyas and Lili, 2019; Lili & Citraningtyas, 2019). Further research and scale up of this type of interventions are an important step to address burnout.

At the Faculty of Medicine, Universitas Indonesia, a 4 x 90 minute module 'Transition and Adaptation Towards Resilience: Recognizing Stress and Strengthening Mental Health in the Adaptation Process of New Students at the Faculty of Medicine' was developed based on in-depth interviews of 20 students and a delphi method with 12 experts (Kaligis, 2022). The module covered: 1) How to develop independence and adapt to a new environment, study skills, time management, and friendships; 2) Stress and stress management, 3) Recognizing mental disorders, and 4) Obtaining mental health support. Twenty randomly selected first-year students participated in a quasi-experimental model to be assessed at weeks 0, 4, 8, and 12. Cortisol measurement decreased significantly in the treatment group (Wilcoxon test, $p < 0.001$), while salivary alpha-amylase enzyme levels were not significantly different. Resilience measured using CD-RISC increased significantly in the treatment group compared to the control group at weeks 4, 8, 12 (ANOVA two-way test, $p < 0.001$). There was a significant decrease (ANOVA two-way, $p < 0.001$) in perceived stress scores (PSS) as well as depression, anxiety, and stress scores (DASS) at week 12 showed significant differences (Wilcoxon test, $p < 0.001$). There were significant improvement in knowledge, attitudes and behaviour toward mental health (ANOVA two-way, $p < 0.001$) as measured using a targeted instrument (CVI range 0.7–1.0, S-CVI value for each questionnaire 0.87; 0.90 and 0.99; reliability using Cronbach's alpha 0.521; 0.780; and 0.852.). Student's satisfaction with the module (CSQ-I) was 37.4 (SB 3.81) out of a maximum score of 40.

Focusing on individuals, however, must not diminish the importance of systemic improvements. Aside from that, the issue of medical school financing also needs attention. Student grants and loan schemes need to be further developed as well as a social security to buffer financial shocks. The potential of crowdfunding to invest in future generations of healthcare professionals may need to be considered.

Beyond that, an interesting research question is also how much burnout in medical students is related to burnout among their lecturers. Expectations for each faculty member to maintain higher education's three pillars (teaching, research, and community 'service—'the *Tridharma*') and respective bureaucratic procedures have diverted faculty members' attention from their students in relational terms. Academics are required to participate in rigorous certification processes and provide detailed reporting. Clinicians are also expected to meet the requirements posed by the professional bodies to retain their medical registration and licence as well as tend to their clinical practice. While meant to ensure the quality of higher education and clinical practice, some argue that the time spent to handle the bureaucracy could be better allocated to teaching and mentoring students and developing ways to prevent burnout and enhance wellbeing.

References

Arlinkasari, F. and Akmal, S. Z. (2017) 'Hubungan antara School Engagement, Academic Self-Efficacy dan Academic Burnout pada Mahasiswa', *Humanitas (Jurnal Psikologi)*, 1(2), pp. 81–102. doi: 10.28932/HUMANITAS.V1I2.418.

Badan Pusat Statistik (2021) *Hasil Sensus Penduduk 2020, 2020*.

Baleg DPR RI (2019). Jakarta.

BAN-PT (2020) *Peraturan Badan Akreditasi Nasional Perguruan Tinggi No 1 Tahun 2020*. Jakarta: LLDIKTI WILAYAH VI.

Bustamam, N. *et al.* (2012) 'Hubungan Kurikulum Pendidikan Tahap Sarjana terhadap Kompetensi Mahasiswa pada Tahap Profesi di Rumah Sakit Pendidikan', *Jurnal Pendidikan Kedokteran Indonesia: The Indonesian Journal of Medical Education*, 1(3), pp. 175–182. doi: 10.22146/JPKI.25103.

Cipta, D. A. *et al.* (2022) 'Burnout Prevalence and Degree among Medical Students in Indonesia During COVID-19 Pandemic: A Cross-Sectional Descriptive Survey', *International Journal of Social Psychiatry*, 68(6), pp. 1232–1237.

Citraningtyas, T. (2017) 'Pilot Workshop to Facilitate Personal Development for the Medical Profession', in *Asian Medical Education Association Symposium*. Hong Kong.

Citraningtyas, T. (2019) 'Nurturing Indonesia: medicine and decolonisation in the Dutch East Indies, by Hans Pols', 43(3), pp. 575–576. doi: 10.1080/10357823.2019.1632778.

Citraningtyas, T. and Lili, R. (2019) 'Experiencing "Who Am I" as an Intercultural, Interfaith Group Dynamic in Indonesia', in *World Association of Social Psychiatry Congress*.

Daryanto, B. *et al.* (2022) 'Burnout syndrome among residents of different surgical specialties in a tertiary referral teaching hospital in Indonesia during COVID-19 pandemic', *Clinical Epidemiology and Global Health*, 14, p. 100994. doi: 10.1016/J.CEGH.2022.100994.

Directorate General for Higher Education, Ministry of Education and Culture, Republic of Indonesia (2020) *Higher Education Statistics*.

Directorate General for Higher Education, Ministry of Education and Culture, Republic of Indonesia (2020) *Guide Book: Independent Learning, Independent Campus (Buku Panduan Merdeka Belajar, Kampus Merdeka)*. Jakarta : Direktorat Jenderal Pendidikan Tinggi Kemdikbud RI.

Dyrbye, L. N., Thomas, M. R., Huntington, J. L., et al. (2006) 'Personal life events and medical student burnout: A multicenter study', *Academic Medicine*, 81(4), pp. 374–384. doi:10.1097/00001888-200604000-00010

Fahrial Syam, A. (2021) 'Indonesian Health Workers during COVID-19 Pandemic', *The Indonesian Journal of Community and Occupational Medicine*, 1(2), pp. 41–3. doi: 10.53773/ijcom.v1i2.25.41-3.

Fitri (2016) *Kendalikan Jumlah Fakultas Kedokteran, LLDIKTI WILAYAH XII*. Available at: https://kopertis12.or.id/2016/04/28/kendalikan-jumlah-fakultas-kedokteran.html (Accessed: 4 June 2022).

Frajerman, A. *et al.* (2019) 'Burnout in medical students before residency: A systematic review and meta-analysis', *European Psyc*, 55, pp. 36–42.

Government of Republic of Indonesia (1996) *Undang-Undang no 6 Tahun 1996 tentang 'Perairan Indonesia'*. Jakarta: Badan Pembinaan Hukum Nasional.

Harimurti, P., Prawira, J. and Hort, K. (2017) 'The Republic of Indonesia Health System Review Asia Pacific Observatory on Health Systems and Policies', *Health Systems in Transition*, 7(1), pp. 65–170.

Indonesian Consortium of Health Science (2013) *Perkembangan pendidikan kedokteran di Indonesia - Sistem pendidikan kedokteran di Indonesia menuju 2045 (Development of medical education in Indonesia:medical education system in Indonesia toward 2045)*.

JPNN (2017) *2018 Diprediksi Ada 12.000 Sarjana Kedokteran di Indonesia - Pendidikan JPNN.com*, *Jawa Post National Network*. Available at: https://www.jpnn.com/news/2018-diprediksi-ada-12000-sarjana-kedokteran-di-indonesia (Accessed: 4 June 2022).

Kaligis, F. M. (2022) Development and Effectiveness of the Module for Strengthening Mental Health on Resilience to Stress in Transitional-Age-Adolescent Medical Students. Dissertation. Doctoral Program in Medical Science. Universitas Indonesia Faculty of Medicine.

Kementerian Pendidikan, K. R. dan T. (2023) *Layanan Uji Kompetensi*. Jakarta: Direktorat Jenderal Pendidikan Tinggi, Riset, Dan Teknologi.

Kloping, N. A. *et al.* (2021) 'Mental health and wellbeing of Indonesian medical students: A regional comparison study', *The International journal of social psychiatry*, 68(6), pp. 1295–1299. doi: 10.1177/00207640211057732.

Kompas (2022) *Beasiswa Kedokteran di 6 PTN dan PTS, Simak Persyaratannya Halaman all - Kompas.com*, *Kompas*. Available at: https://www.kompas.com/edu/read/2022/03/04/170742671/beasiswa-kedokteran-di-6-ptn-dan-pts-simak-persyaratannya?page=all (Accessed: 4 June 2022).

Konsil Kedokteran Indonesia (2012) *Standar Kompetensi Dokter Indonesia*. Jakarta: Konsil Kedokteran Indonesia (Indonesian Medical Council). Available at: http://www.kki.go.id/assets/data/arsip/SKD I_Perkonsil,_11_maret_13.pdf.

Konsil Kedokteran Indonesia (2019a) *Profil Konsil Kedokteran Indonesia*, Indonesian Medical Council. Available at: http:/kki.go.id/index.php/subMenu/983.

Konsil Kedokteran Indonesia (2019b) *Standar Pendidikan Profesi Dokter Indonesia*, Indonesian Medical Council.

Kumar, R. and Pal, R. (2018) 'India achieves WHO recommended doctor population ratio: A call for paradigm shift in public health discourse!', *Journal of Family Medicine and Primary Care* 7(5): 841.

LAM-PTKes (2022) *Database Hasil Akreditasi*. Available at: https://lamptkes.org/Database-Hasil-Akreditasi (Accessed: 28 May 2022).

Lili, R. *et al.* (2021) 'Wellbeing and mental health among medical students in Indonesia: A descriptive study':, *https://doi-org.ezproxy.is.ed.ac.uk/10.1177/00207640211057709*. doi: 10.1177/00207640211057709.

Lili, R. and Citraningtyas, T. (2019) 'Strength-based Group Meeting Approach for Patients with Anxiety and Depression: a Pilot Study in Indonesia'. *World Association of Social Psychiatry Congress*.

LPDP (2021) *Komponen yang didanai oleh Lembaga Pengelola Dana Pendidikan (LPDP) pada program beasiswa Magister/Doktoral/Spesialis Kedokteran—Knowledgebase / Program Beasiswa (Umum)—Layanan Informasi dan Bantuan LPDP*, LPDP Indonesian Endowment Fund for Education, Ministry of Finance Republic of Indonesia. Available at: https://bantuan.lpdp.kemenkeu.go.id/kb/articles/komponen-yang-didanai-oleh-lembaga-pengelola-dana-pendidikan-lpdp-pada-program-beasiswa-magist (Accessed: 4 June 2022).

Ministry of Health Republic of Indonesia (2017) *Effectuation of Internship Program for Doctor and Dentist in Indonesia - Ministry of Health Regulation (Permenkes) Number 39 Year 2017*. Indonesia.

Ministry of Health Republic of Indonesia (2020) *Provision of Incentives and Death Compensation for Health Personnel that Handles COVID-19 Diseases - Ministry of Finance Regulation Number HK 01.07 Year 2020*. Jakarta: Kementerian Kesehatan Republik Indonesia.

Ministry of Health Republic of Indonesia (2022) *Percepat Pemenuhan Tenaga Kesehatan, Kemenkes Buka Program Bantuan Pendidikan Untuk Dokter Spesialis dan Dokter Gigi Spesialis*, Ministry of Health Republic of Indonesia. Available at: https://www.kemkes.go.id/article/view/22060200008/percepat-pemenuhan-tenaga-kesehatan-kemenkes-buka-program-bantuan-pendidikan-untuk-dokter-spesialis-.html (Accessed: 3 June 2022).

Ministry of Marine Affairs and Fisheries (2012) *Direktori Pulau-pulau Kecil Indonesia, Direktorat Pemberdayagunaan Pulau-pulau Kecil*. Available at: http://www.ppk-kp3k.kkp.go.id/direktori-pulau/index.php/public_c/pulau_data (Accessed: 14 June 2022).

Mustika, R. *et al.* (2019) 'The odyssey of medical education in Indonesia', *The Asia Pacific Scholar*, 4(1), pp. 4–8. doi: 10.29060/TAPS.2019-4-1/GP1077.

Nurikhwan, P. W., Felaza, E. and Soemantri, D. (2022) 'Burnout and quality of life of medical residents: A mixedmethod study', *Korean Journal of Medical Education*, 34(1), pp. 27–39. doi: 10.3946/KJME.2022.217.

Pacheco, J. P. G. *et al.* (2017) 'Mental health problems among medical students in Brazil: a systematic review and meta-analysis', *Brazilian Journal of Psychiatry*, 39(4), pp. 369–378. doi: 10.1590/1516-4446-2017-2223.

PDSKJI Jaya (2022) 'Pertemuan Ilmiah Tahunan (PIT) 1 PDSKJI Jaya', in *Pertemuan Ilmiah Tahunan (PIT) PDSKJI Jaya*. Medan: Perhimpunan Dokter Spesialis Kedokteran Jiwa Indonesia.

Pols, H. (2018) *Nurturing Indonesia: Medicine and Decolonisation in the Dutch East Indies*. Cambridge.

Prasetya, N. L. and Suharlim, C. (2016) *National competency: Poor quality of medical graduates - Mon, November 7 2016 - The Jakarta Post, The Jakarta Post*. Available at: https://www.thejakartapost.com/news/2016/11/07/national-competency-poor-quality-medical-graduates.html (Accessed: 4 June 2022).

PRH International (2015) *PRH Helping Relationship And The Growth of Persons*. Poitiers France: Personality and Human Relations.

Romadhoni, R., Retno Rahayu, G. and Khoiriyah, U. (2021) 'Identifikasi Motivasi Dan Dukungan Yang Diperlukan Mahasiswa Retaker Uji Kompetensi Mahasiswa Program Profesi Dokter', *Jurnal Pendidikan Kedokteran Indonesia: The Indonesian Journal of Medical Education*, 10(1), p. 75. doi: 10.22146/jpki.48329.

Sysling, F. (2019) 'Nurturing Indonesia: Medicine and Decolonisation in the Dutch East Indies', *Isis*, 110(4), pp. 849–850.

Winurini, S. (2021) *Burn Out Among Indonesian Medical Workers During Pandemic*. Jakarta.

World Bank (2015) *The World Bank Health, Nutrition and Population Global Practice Indonesia Country Management Unit East Asia and Pacific Region*. USA: The World Bank.

World Bank (2022) *Population, total - Indonesia | Data, World Bank*. Available at: https://data.worldbank.org/indicator/SP.POP.TOTL?locations=ID (Accessed: 5 June 2022).

Zainal, S. N. B. (2019) *Hubungan Persepsi Mahasiswa Kedokteran FKIK UKRIDA Angkatan 2016, 2017, dan 2018 terhadap Kasih Sayang Orangtua dengan Taraf Kecemasan*. Universitas Kristen Krida Wacana.

15
Italy

Mental Health and Wellbeing Among Italian Medical Students

Antonio Ventriglio, Gaia Sampogna, and Andrea Fiorillo

Introduction

University students are a vulnerable group as they are exposed to a large amount of stress, competition, and expectation. It has been argued that up to 35% of students may report psychological distress and/or mental health-related disorders (Auerbach et al., 2018). In particular, medical students (MSs) are tomorrow's healthcare professionals and their role becomes relevant in the course of training with an increasing awareness, a new identity, and an increase in autonomy and responsibility (Cuijpers et al., 2019). They report higher rates of mental health problems, including depressive symptoms, anxiety, and substance abuse, with a significant impact on academic performance and subjective quality of life (Mousa et al., 2016; Moutinho et al., 2019; Rotenstein et al., 2016). A set of risk factors for mental disorders among MSs includes: female sex, stressful life events, excessive use of technology (including smart phones and social networks), and/or poor sleep (Lemola et al., 2015). It has also been argued that the long and challenging educational training may lead to burnout with overwhelming exhaustion, depersonalization, and reduced personal efficiency (Frajerman et al., 2019; Kiekens et al., 2019).

In the last decade, an increasing consumption of tobacco and illicit drugs has been noted among MSs, with increases during the years of medical school (Mas et al., 2004). Also, it is of interest that these misuses or dependences are associated with a higher risk of depressive or behavioural symptoms (Fluharty et al., 2017). A specific use/abuse of psychostimulants, energy drinks in order to improve cognitive performance and learning and to reduce the subjective need for sleep has been reported (Azagba et al., 2014). Despite the prevalence of mental distress, mental disorders, and substance abuse among MSs, the rate of help-seeking is low, mostly because of fear of stigma or exposure to peers' and professors' judgement. Barriers to help-seeking may be even higher after graduation due to the fear of stigma and discrimination in the work environment (Mehta et al., 2018).

Italian MSs

According to a recent review of literature by Sampogna et al. (2020), sixteen studies have described mental health issues among Italian MSs in the last two decades (2000–2020). Sample sizes ranged from 44 to 794 students assessed in a cross-sectional and multicentre design. The

Antonio Ventriglio, Gaia Sampogna, and Andrea Fiorillo, *Italy* In: *The Mental Health of Medical Students*.
Edited by: Andrew Molodynski, Sarah Marie Farrell, and Dinesh Bhugra, Oxford University Press. © Oxford University Press 2024.
DOI: 10.1093/oso/9780192864871.003.0015

mean prevalence of depressive symptoms ranged between 2.5 and 21.4% and suicidal idea-tion, as disclosed by respondents, has been screened in 17% of the samples. Other disorders rated: adjustment disorders (36%)>psychotic disorders (14.3%)> dysthymia and panic dis-orders (7.1%). Additionally, rates for substance misuse were 15.3–31.4% for cigarettes, 22–75% for energy drinks, and 13–86% for alcohol.

A survey conducted among MSs at the University of Siena (Italy) between 2005 and 2015 concluded that their perceived quality of life was lower than in the same-age general popu-lation, with both a worse perception of their own health status and higher discomfort due to the emotional burden during the course of the medical training (Messina et al., 2016).

A more recent survey from the University of Modena (Italy) has reported that an un-precedented 74.7% of MSs have been using substances or cognitive enhancers to improve their cognitive functions and study performances during the course of their training (Pighi et al., 2018). Also, Italian MSs seem to show lower levels of multidimensional wellbeing when compared to a sample of MSs in Serbia (Lietz et al., 2018). It is well known that stigma against mental illness and mentally ill patients remains high among medical practitioners and MSs as confirmed in a sample of MSs from the University of Modena and Reggio Emilia tested with the Attribution Questionnaire 27—Italian Version (AQ-27-I) (Pingani et al., 2016).

Volpe et al. (2019) surveyed 360 MSs from Ancona and Foggia, 58.33% females and 41.67% males, in a cross-sectional study. An online survey was launched through the insti-tutions' email servers to all MSs. There was a response rate of 88.6% in Ancona and 11.4% in Foggia. Students were assessed for their general health and burnout with the following in-struments: Oldenburgh Burnout Inventory (OLBI); General Health Questionnaire (GHQ); CAGE (Cutdown/Annoyed/Guilty/Eye Opener). The authors reported that 8.6% of respond-ents reported mental disorders with the following prevalence: 5% anxiety disorder; 2.5% de-pression; 0.28%: burnout syndrome; 8.9% alcohol related problems; 33% cognitive enhancers users. These findings show that a certain percentage of Italian MSs present psychological conditions with alcohol misuse and use of drugs to cope with their condition.

Solano et al. (2019) reported on 552 MSs in Genoa, 59% females and 41% males, collecting data during classrooms with a response rate of 82.3%. Authors screened respondents in order to evaluate the presence of suicidal thoughts/behaviours, coping strategies, temperament, and attitude towards suicidality. Tools employed were the Suicide Opinion Questionnaire (SOQ), the Coping Orientation to Problems Experienced (COPE), and the Temperament Evaluation of the Memphis (TEMPS-A). 17% of the sample reported severe suicidal thoughts and behaviours. Respondents with poor coping strategies were more likely to be males, have poor academic achievement, and were less likely to have a parent working in the medical or mental health fields.

Rapinesi et al. (2018) published a case-control study on 98 students from University La Sapienza in Rome comparing 49 helpseekers vs. 49 controls. In order to evaluate tempera-ment, attention deficit/hyperactivity disorder traits and depressive symptomatology, they used the Beck Depression Inventory-II, the Temperament and Character Inventory-Revised, and the Adult ADHD Self-Report Scale. 17.1% of helpseekers reported depressive symptoms vs. 10.1% in control group (p < 0.001).The ADHD total score was 3.7 in the help-seeking group vs. 2.5 in control group (p < 0.001).

Lamberti et al. (2017) in Naples reported on 641 MSs (mean age of 26.2 years old; 59.1% females and 40.9% males) interviewed during medical examinations in their medical course with a response rate of 100%. They employed the Alcohol Use Disorders Identification Test (AUDIT-C) to assess the prevalence of alcohol drinking: 85.5% were regular alcohol users; 16.6% regular smokers; 91%: habitual coffee consumers. The findings show a need to assess alcohol use in healthcare professionals and to recognize risky behaviours in order to develop effective preventive interventions.

Armstrong et al. (2017) published findings from a multicentre cross-sectional study based in Bologna that involved 527 students from Italy and America (43% males) in order to evaluate the prevalence of tobacco use, attitudes, clinical skills, and tobacco related experiences. 29.5% of respondents reported smoking habits with Italian students less likely to receive smoking cessation training compared to American students.

Casuccio et al. (2015) involved 794 students in Palermo (mean age 21.9 years old) in order to assess the levels of knowledge and attitudes related to energy drink consumption and the prevalence of related side effects. 22% of their sample reported energy drink use. Female students presented high levels of somatization, obsessive-compulsive symptoms, depressive, and anxiety symptoms, with a higher prevalence among students who used energy drinks regularly.

Luca et al. (2015) reported on 200 MSs from Catania assessed for levels of alcohol consumption in relation with sociodemographic and psychopathological variables. Tools employed were: Alcohol Use Disorders Identification Test (AUDIT-C); Self-Report Symptom Inventory-Revised (SCL-90-R); General Symptomatic Index (GSI). 27% of their sample reported mental health issues with 13% demonstrating alcohol use disorder.

In a small sample from Rome (44 MSs), Lia and Cavaggioni (2013) reported the following rates of mental health disorders: 35.7%, adjustment disorders> 21.4%, depressive syndromes > 14.3%, psychotic disorders> 7.1%, dysthymia> 7.1%, anxiety> 7.1%, panic attacks > 7.1%: bipolar disorders> 7.1%, single episode of mania.

Saulle et al. (2013) reported on 730 MSs from different cities in Italy (Turin, Padua, Florence, Brescia, Ferrara, Varese Udine, Palermo, Salerno). They employed the Global Health Professions Student Survey (GHPSS) in order to evaluate smoking prevalence, knowledge, and attitudes among Italian MSs. 20.4% were current smokers with 87.7% believing that health professionals need to receive specific training on smoking cessation; 65% believed that health professionals had a role in giving advice or information about smoking cessation.

Grassi et al. (2012), published findings from a cross-sectional study involving 439 MSs from Rome, Udine, and Verona, aimed to evaluate smoking behaviour and levels of knowledge about smoking related mortality, the harmful effects of cigarette smoking and the efficacy of counselling techniques. 15.3% were current smokers and 9.6% previous smokers; the level of knowledge on tobacco use was low as well as a great proportion of students did not know how to provide proper counselling to smokers.

Gualano et al. (2012) reported on a multicentre cross-sectional study involving 744 students from Rome, Chieti, Turin, and Palermo, aimed to evaluate the prevalence of tobacco use, the levels of knowledge and attitudes about tobacco smoking cessation training with The GHPSS questionnaire: Findings demonstrated that 31.4% were current smokers while the majority (90%) considered health professionals as role models for patients as well as they have a role in giving information about smoking cessation.

La Torre et al. (2012) reported on 655 MSs from Palermo, Rome, and Turin. They used the Global Tobacco Surveillance System form to assess smoking prevalence, the levels of knowledge, and attitudes toward smoking and the availability of tobacco cessation training. 29.3%

reported smoking habits, with 57.2% of participants believing that health professionals are role models for patients, 89.8% reported to be aware of smoking cessation interventions.

In 2010 in Florence, Lucenteforte et al. reported on 194 university students interviewed with the Modified Instrument of the World Health Organization about tobacco smoking for healthcare givers. The aim was to assess the impact of university choice on smoking habits. 20.1% reported smoking habits with 32.5% of MSs reporting at least one parent who smoked. Respondents were more conscious regarding the negative effects of smoking and tobacco related diseases than other students.

Oteri et al. (2007) published findings from the University of Messina regarding 450 MSs anonymously interviewed with an ad-hoc questionnaire regarding energy drink consumption in order to evaluate the levels of knowledge related to the use of energy drinks (alone or in association with alcohol). 56.9% were energy drink users; 48.4% reported using energy drinks associated with alcohol; the use of energy drinks and alcohol is frequent and brings a higher risk of developing alcohol dependence (Oteri et al., 2007).

Factors Associated with poor Mental Health Among Italian MSs

Giusti et al. (2021) explored sociodemographic, psychological, and psychosocial differences between 130 medical and 86 health professional students and their empathic abilities using the Patient Health Questionnaire-9, Interpersonal Reactivity Index, Integrative Hope Scale, and the UCLA Loneliness Scale. In both groups, 15% of students reported previous contact for psychological problems. 23.3% of health professional students reported depressive symptoms *vs.* 10% of MSs with female non-MSs reporting more intense feelings of loneliness than other subgroups of students. In both groups, women were particularly prone to personal distress. Associated factors for poor self-assessed affective emphatic skills were: previous contact for psychological problems, feelings of loneliness, emphasizing the need to test psychosocial models to better understand empathic skills among students.

Ardenghi et al. (2022) reported findings from a multicentre cross-sectional study examining emotional intelligence as a mediator between attachment security and empathy in preclinical MSs. 253 MSs (56.13% female), aged 19- to 29, were involved. Findings have shown that attachment security positively correlated to empathic and perspective taking as well as negatively to personal distress. Participants with the same level of attachment security and higher scores for the emotional quotient reported higher scores on empathy and a lower score on personal distress.

The same group (Ardenghi et al., 2021) also explored whether the extent of emotional dysregulation predicted empathy and patient centredness in MSs in northern Italy. They used the Difficulties in Emotion Regulation Scale (DERS), the Interpersonal Reactivity Index (IRI) and the Patient-Practitioner Orientation Scale—8 Items—Italian version (PPOS-8-IT). They demonstrated that DERS scores were associated to a significant variance in both IRI and PPOS-8-IT components beyond gender. Emotional dysregulation was positively associated with Personal Distress, whereas Empathic Concern, Perspective Taking, and the patient centredness were negatively correlated with emotional regulation difficulties.

The role of gender on emotional distress and psychiatric drug use among students has been assessed in 694 Italian MSs from Turin (Carletto et al., 2021). This study reported that depression, anxiety, and stress symptoms rated 52.6%, 61.7% and 78.5%, respectively among MSs. Female students reported higher rates of depression than males. Also, rates of stress were consistently higher in females than in males whereas no gender differences were described in substances use rates.

It has been argued that mindfulness facets may play a protective role from perceived stress, psychosomatic burden, and sleep-wake quality in MSs. 349 respondents from Bologna completed self-report questionnaires examining personality traits as well as physical and psychological wellbeing (Fino et al., 2021) Findings showed that mindfulness facets mitigate the negative consequences of trait anxiety on medical student wellbeing especially in high-pressure periods and when self-regulation is needed the most.

Recently, Limone and Toto (2022) reviewed the literature regarding predisposing factors among undergraduates to develop mental health difficulties. They concluded that social, psychological, biological, and/or lifestyle-based factors as well as academic factors are involved. The pressure to achieve academic excellence was found to particularly affect those with disadvantaged family background, chronic illness, injuries, or substances abuse.

Parental bonding and its role in depression and suicidal ideation has been explored by Tugnoli et al. (2022) in an Italian sample of MSs. In a sample of 671 students (182 males and 489 females), females experienced more distress and self-injurious behaviours, while males reported higher rate of drugs or alcohol abuse. The Beck Hopelessness Scale scores as well as Beck Depression Inventory II (BDI-II) scores correlated positively with the Parental Bonding Instrument (PBI) score for 'protection' and negatively with the 'care' score.

Donisi et al. (2022) reported on a training programme in communication and emotion handling skills, delivered for MSs, and its impact on empathy, emotional intelligence, and attachment style. A 16-hour Emoty-Com training was delivered to MSs in Verona and Milan. An assessment of empathy, attachment style, and emotional intelligence was performed with three questions on attitudes towards doctors' emotions, before and after the training: 264 students reported a reduction in worry about managing emotions during doctor-patient relationships.

Finally, being a second victim in a patient safety incident may have an impact on health of MSs and residents. A cross-sectional study based on an online questionnaire among MSs and residents has been conducted in Novara (Rinaldi et al., 2022). 62.6% of the sample experienced symptoms related to being a second victim: the feeling of working badly (51.52%), hypervigilance (51.52%). Authors concluded that this experience may have a significant impact on their future professional and personal lives.

COVID-19 and Mental Health among MSs in Italy

Some studies have now explored the impact of COVID-19 pandemic on MSs' mental health in Italy. Carletto et al. (2022) reported findings from a sample of 1,359 MSs from Turin. The prevalence rates of anxiety, depressive symptoms, moderate perceived stress, and severe perceived stress during the COVID-19 pandemic were 47.8%, 52.1%, 56.2%, 28.4%, respectively. Associate factors were female gender, family history of psychiatric disorders, living off-site, competitive/hostile climates and unsatisfying friendships among classmates, poor relationships with cohabitants, negative judgement of medical school choice, fear of COVID-19 infection, feelings of loneliness, distressing existential reflections.

De Micheli et al. (2021) enrolled 509 MSs during the second outbreak of COVID-19 in Italy. The assessment of psychological symptoms was based on the 12-item General Health Questionnaire (GHQ-12) as well as 'readiness to fight the pandemic' and their emotional reactions to the pandemic using visual analogue scales. Perceived control reduced psychological symptoms and had a positive effect on the willingness to fight the pandemic. Age and concern for patients had a significant positive impact on respondents' readiness to fight the pandemic, while years of attendance had a significant but negative impact.

Quarta et al. (2022) collected data during the COVID-19 outbreak (April–May 2021) among 939 students and 238 employees through an online survey. Findings have shown that MSs exhibited higher levels of anxiety, depression, and stress, and lower levels of subjective wellbeing (< 0.001 for all domains) compared to staff members. Also, mediation analyses indicated that the time spent in nature, social relationships, and levels of energy were mediating factors between sport practice and wellbeing.

Patrono et al. (2022) reported findings on a sample of 3,533 students from a university in Northern Italy that explored the mental health emergency among students during the COVID-19 pandemic. Participants reported headaches, depression, and sadness, digestive disorders, a fear of COVID-19, and anxiety/panic crises. The time spent in isolation was associated with an increased risk of digestive disorders, headaches, and COVID-19 fear. Factors such as female gender, medium-intense telephone usage, sleep quality, memory difficulties, and performance reduction were associated with an increased risk of health issues.

Finally, Lo Moro et al. (2022) reported on the consequences of the pandemic on MSs' depressive symptoms and their perceived stress in a repeated cross-sectional survey. The first study aimed to explore whether MSs had higher levels of depressive symptoms and stress during the pandemic compared with a pre-pandemic period (data from 2018). The second step was designed to identify whether MSs had higher levels of these conditions during the pandemic compared with their same-year peers during a pre-pandemic period. The first study reported higher levels of depressive symptoms and stress during the pandemic than in 2018; these rates were confirmed in the second study with a confirmatory analysis of poor mental health, worsened psychological state, and economic repercussions due to the pandemic.

Conclusions

This review of studies regarding the mental health of Italian MSs confirms that many report psychopathological conditions with misuse of tobacco, alcohol, and drugs to cope with their own condition. The COVID-19 pandemic has led to an additional mental health burden and perceived stress. Gender and emotional dysregulation may play a role, among other factors, in the vulnerability for mental illness of MSs. Since the health of the next generation of doctors is relevant, faculties of medicine in Italy (as in the rest of the world) should promote an effective and accurate surveillance strategy on MSs and trainees' mental health. The early detection of risk factors and early intervention in cases of mental distress or drug abuse are crucial. Further research is needed to describe associated factors and variables related to risk for mental disorders among MSs, and more specific systematic preventive and therapeutic interventions should be promoted in the university settings.

References

Ardenghi, S., Rampoldi, G., Montelisciani, L., Antolini, L., Donisi, V., Perlini, C., Rimondini, M., Garbin, D., Piccolo, L.D., & Strepparava, M.G. (2022). 'Emotional intelligence as a mediator between attachment security and empathy in pre-clinical medical students: A multi-center cross-sectional study'. *Patient Educ Counsel* **105**(9): 2880–2887.

Ardenghi, S., Russo, S., Bani, M., Rampoldi, G., & Strepparava, M.G. (2021). 'The role of difficulties in emotion regulation in predicting empathy and patient-centeredness in pre-clinical medical students: a cross-sectional study'. *Psychol Health Med* 1–15. Advance online publication. https://doi.org/10.1080/13548506.2021.2001549

Armstrong, G.W., Veronese, G., George, P.F., Montroni, I., & Ugolini, G. (2017). 'Assessment of tobacco habits, attitudes, and education among medical students in the United States and Italy: a cross-sectional survey. *J Prev Med Public Health = Yebang Uihakhoe chi* **50**(3): 177–187.

Auerbach, R.P., Mortier, P., Bruffaerts, R., Alonso, J., Benjet, C., Cuijpers, P., Demyttenaere, K., Ebert, D.D., Green, J.G., & Hasking, P. (2018). 'WHO World Mental Health Surveys International College Student Project: prevalence and distribution of mental disorders'. *J. Abnorm Psychol* **127**: 623–638.

Azagba, S., Langille, D., & Asbridge, M. (2014). 'An emerging adolescent health risk: caffeinated energy drink consumption patterns among high school students'. *Prev Med* **62**: 54–59.

Carletto, S., Lo Moro, G., Zuccaroli Lavista, V., Soro, G., Siliquini, R., Bert, F., & Leombruni, P. (2022). 'The impact of COVID-19 on mental health in medical students: a cross-sectional survey study in Italy'. *Psychol Rep* 332941221127632. Advance online publication. https://doi.org/10.1177/00332941221127632

Carletto, S., Miniotti, M., Persico, A., & Leombruni, P. (2021). 'Emotional distress and psychiatric drug use among students in an Italian medical school: assessing the role of gender and year of study'. *J Educ Health Promo* **10**: 451.

Casuccio, A., Bonanno, V., Catalano, R., Cracchiolo, M., Giugno, S., Sciuto, V., & Immordino, P. (2015). 'Knowledge, attitudes, and practices on energy drink consumption and side effects in a cohort of medical students'. *J Addict Dis* **34**(4): 274–283.

Cuijpers, P., Auerbach, R.P., Benjet, C., Bruffaerts, R., Ebert, D., Karyotaki, E., & Kessler, R.C. (2019, January 9). 'Introduction to the special issue: the WHO World Mental Health International College Student (WMH-ICS) initiative'. *Int J Methods Psychiatric Res* **28**(2): e1762.

De Micheli, G., Vergani, L., Mazzoni, D., & Marton, G. (2021). 'After the pandemic: the future of italian medicine. the psychological impact of COVID-19 on medical and other healthcare-related degrees students'. *Front Psychol* **12**: 648419.

Donisi, V., Perlini, C., Mazzi, M.A., Rimondini, M., Garbin, D., Ardenghi, S., Rampoldi, G., Montelisciani, L., Antolini, L., Strepparava, M.G., & Del Piccolo, L. (2022). 'Training in communication and emotion handling skills for students attending medical school: Relationship with empathy, emotional intelligence, and attachment style'. *Patient Educ Couns* **105**(9): 2871–2879.

Fino, E., Martoni, M., & Russo, P.M. (2021). 'Specific mindfulness traits protect against negative effects of trait anxiety on medical student wellbeing during high-pressure periods'. *Adv Health Sci Educ* **26**(3): 1095–1111.

Fluharty, M., Taylor, A.E., Grabski, M., & Munafò, M. (2017). 'The association of cigarette smoking with depression and anxiety: a systematic review'. *Nicotine Tob Res* **19**: 3–13.

Frajerman, A., Morvan, Y., Krebs, M.O., Gorwood, P., & Chaumette, B. (2019). 'Burnout in medical students before residency: a systematic review and meta-analysis'. *Eur Psychiatry* **55**: 36–42.

Giusti, L., Mammarella, S., Salza, A., Ussorio, D., Bianco, D., Casacchia, M., & Roncone, R. (2021). 'Heart and head: profiles and predictors of self-assessed cognitive and affective empathy in a sample of medical and health professional students'. *Front Psychol* **12**: 632996. https://doi.org/10.3389/fpsyg.2021.632996

Grassi, M.C., Chiamulera, C., Baraldo, M., Culasso, F., Ferketich, A.K., Raupach, T., Patrono, C., & Nencini, P. (2012). 'Cigarette smoking knowledge and perceptions among students in four Italian medical schools'. *Nicotine Tob Res* **14**(9): 1065–1072.

Gualano, M.R., Siliquini, R., Manzoli, L., Firenze, A., Cattaruzza, M.S., Bert, F., Renzi, D., Romano, N., Ricciardi, W., & Boccia, A. (2012). 'Tobacco use prevalence, knowledge and attitudes, and tobacco cessation training among medical students: results of a pilot study of Global Health Professions Students Survey (GHPSS) in Italy'. *J Public Health* 20: 89–94.

Kiekens, G., Hasking, P., Claes, L., Boyes, M., Mortier, P., Auerbach, R.P., Cuijpers, P., Demyttenaere, K., Green, J.G., Kessler, R.C., Myin-Germeys, I., Nock, M.K., & Bruffaerts, R. (2019). 'Predicting the incidence of non-suicidal self-injury in college students'. *Eur Psychiatry* 59: 44–51.

La Torre, G., Kirch, W., Bes-Rastrollo, M., Ramos, R.M., Czaplicki, M., Gualano, M.R., Thümmler, K., Ricciardi, W., Boccia, A., & GHPSS Collaborative Group (2012). 'Tobacco use among medical students in Europe: results of a multicentre study using the Global Health Professions Student Survey'. *Public Health* 126(2): 159–164.

Lamberti, M., Napolitano, F., Napolitano, P., Arnese, A., Crispino, V., Panariello, G., & Di Giuseppe, G. (2017). 'Prevalence of alcohol use disorders among under- and post-graduate healthcare students in Italy'. *PloS One* 12(4): e0175719. https://doi.org/10.1371/journal.pone.0175719

Lemola, S., Perkinson-Gloor, N., Brand, S., Dewald-Kaufmann, J., & Grob, A. (2015). 'Adolescents' electronic media use at night, sleep disturbance, and depressive symptoms in the smartphone age'. *J Youth Adolesc* 44: 405–418.

Lia, C., & Cavaggioni, G. (2013). 'L'iter di selezione nella Facoltà di Medicina: l'utilità di una valutazione psicoattitudinale' [The selection process in the Faculty of Medicine: the usefulness of a psychological and aptitude assessment]. *La Clinica Terapeutica* 164(1): 39–42.

Lietz, F., Piumatti, G., Mosso, C., Marinkovic, J., & Bjegovic-Mikanovic, A.V. (2018). 'Testing multidimensional well-being among university community samples in Italy and Serbia'. *Health Promot Int* 33(2): 288–298.

Limone, P., & Toto, G.A. (2022). 'Factors that predispose undergraduates to mental issues: a cumulative literature review for future research perspectives'. *Front Public Health* 10: 831349.

Lo Moro, G., Carletto, S., Zuccaroli Lavista, V., Soro, G., Bert, F., Siliquini, R., & Leombruni, P. (2022). 'The consequences of the pandemic on medical students' depressive symptoms and perceived stress: a repeated cross-sectional survey with a nested longitudinal subsample'. *J Clin Med* 11(19): 5896.

Luca, M., Ruta, S., Signorelli, M., Petralia, A., & Aguglia, E. (2015). 'Variabili psicologiche e consumo di alcol in un campione di studenti di medicina: differenze di genere' [Psychological variables and alcohol consumption in a sample of students of medicine: gender differences]. *Rivista di psichiatria* 50(1): 38–42.

Lucenteforte, E., Vannacci, A., Cipollini, F., Gori, A., Santini, L., Franchi, G., Terrone, R., Ravaldi, C., Mugelli, A., Gensini, G.F., & Lapi, F. (2010). 'Smoking habits among university students in Florence: is a medical degree course the right choice?'. *Prev Med* 51(5): 429–430.

Mas, A., Nerín, I., Barrueco, M., Cordero, J., Guillén, D., Jiménez-Ruiz, C., & Sobradillo, V. (2004). 'Smoking habits among sixth-year medical students in Spain'. *Arch Bronconeumol Engl Ed* 40: 403–408.

Mehta, S.S. & Edwards, M.L. (2018). 'Suffering in silence: mental health stigma and physicians' licensing fears'. *Am J Psychiatry Resid J* 1: 1–4.

Messina, G., Quercioli, C., Troiano, G., Russo, C., Barbini3, E., Nisticò, F., & Nante, N. (2016). 'Italian medical students quality of life: years 2005–2015'. *Ann Ig* 28(4): 245–251.

Mousa, O.Y., Dhamoon, M.S., Lander, S., & Dhamoon, A.S. (2016). 'The MD blues: under-recognized depression and anxiety in medical trainees'. *PLoS ONE* 11: e0156554.

Moutinho, I.L.D., Lucchetti, A.L.G., da Ezequiel, O.S., & Lucchetti, G. (2019). 'Mental health and quality of life of Brazilian medical students: Incidence, prevalence, and associated factors within two years of follow-up'. *Psychiatry Res* 74: 306–312.

Oteri, A., Salvo, F., Caputi, A.P., & Calapai, G. (2007). 'Intake of energy drinks in association with alcoholic beverages in a cohort of students of the School of Medicine of the University of Messina'. *Alcohol Clin Exp Res* 31(10): 1677–1680.

Patrono, A., Renzetti, S., Manco, A., Brunelli, P., Moncada, S.M., Macgowan, M.J., Placidi, D., Calza, S., Cagna, G., Rota, M., Memo, M., Tira, M., & Lucchini, R.G. (2022). 'COVID-19 aftermath: exploring the mental health emergency among students at a Northern Italian university'. *Int J Environ Res Public Health* 19(14): 8587.

Pighi, M., Pontoni, G., Sinisi, A., Ferrari, S., Mattei, G., Pingani, L., Simoni, E., & Galeazzi, G.M. (2018). 'Use and propensity to use substances as cognitive enhancers in Italian medical students'. *Brain Sci* **8**(11). pii: E197.

Pingani, L., Catellani, S., Del Vecchio, V., Sampogna, G., Ellefson, S.E., Rigatelli, M., Fiorillo, A., Evans-Lacko, S., & Corrigan, P.W. (2016). 'Stigma in the context of schools: analysis of the phenomenon of stigma in a population of university students'. *BMC Psychiatry* **16**: 29.

Quarta, S., Levante, A., García-Conesa, M.T., Lecciso, F., Scoditti, E., Carluccio, M.A., Calabriso, N., Damiano, F., Santarpino, G., Verri, T., Pinto, P., Siculella, L., & Massaro, M. (2022). 'Assessment of subjective well-being in a cohort of university students and staff members: association with physical activity and outdoor leisure time during the COVID-19 pandemic'. *Int J Environ Res Public Health* **19**(8): 4787.

Rapinesi, C., Kotzalidis, G.D., Del Casale, A., Ferrone, M., Vento, A., Callovini, G., Curto, M., Ferracuti, S., Sani, G., Pompili, M., Familiari, G., Girardi, P., & Angeletti, G. (2018). 'Depressive symptoms, temperament/character, and attention deficit/hyperactivity disorder traits in medical students seeking counseling'. *Psychiatria Danubina* **30**(3): 305–309.

Rinaldi, C., Ratti, M., Russotto, S., Seys, D., Vanhaecht, K., & Panella, M. (2022). 'Healthcare students and medical residents as second victims: a cross-sectional study'. *Int J Environ Res Public Health* **19**(19): 12218.

Rotenstein, L.S., Ramos, M.A., Torre, M., Bradley Segal, J., Peluso, M.J., Guille, C., Sen, S., Mata, D.A. (2016). 'Prevalence of depression, depressive symptoms, and suicidal ideation among medical students a systematic review and meta-analysis'. *JAMA J Am Med Assoc* **316**: 2214–2236.

Sampogna, G., Lovisi, G.M., Zinno, F., Del Vecchio, V., Luciano, M., Gonçalves Loureiro Sol, É., Unger, R.J.G., Ventriglio, A., & Fiorillo, A. (2021). 'Mental health disturbances and related problems in italian university medical students from 2000 to 2020: an integrative review of qualitative and quantitative studies'. *Medicina* **57**: 11.

Saulle, R., Bontempi, C., Baldo, V., Boccia, G., Bonaccorsi, G., Brusaferro, S., Donato, F., Firenze, A., Gregorio, P., Pelissero, G., Sella, A., Siliquini, R., Boccia, A., & La Torre, G. (2013). 'GHPSS multicenter Italian survey: smoking prevalence, knowledge and attitudes, and tobacco cessation training among third-year medical students'. *Tumori* **99**(1): 17–22.

Solano, P., Aguglia, A., Caprino, M., Conigliaro, C., Giacomini, G., Serafini, G., & Amore, M. (2019). 'The personal experience of severe suicidal behaviour leads to negative attitudes towards self- and other's suicidal thoughts and behaviours: a study of temperaments, coping strategies, and attitudes towards suicide among medical students'. *Psychiatry Res* **272**: 669–675.

Tugnoli, S., Casetta, I., Caracciolo, S., & Salviato, J. (2022). 'Parental bonding, depression, and suicidal ideation in medical students'. *Front Psychol* **13**: 877306.

Volpe, U., Ventriglio, A., Bellomo, A., Kadhum, M., Lewis, T., Molodynski, A., Sampogna, G., & Fiorillo, A. (2019). 'Mental health and wellbeing among Italian medical students: a descriptive study'. *Int Rev Psychiatry* **31**(7–8): 569–573.

16
Jordan

Medical Student Wellbeing in Jordan

Rawan Masri and Almu'atasim Khamees

Overview about Jordan

Jordan is an Arab country located in southwest Asia. It covers an area of 89,000 square kilometres (Central Intelligence Agency Government Publications Office, 2015) and as of the year 2021 its population size measured 11,057,000 (Jordanian Department of Statistics, 2021). According to the Jordanian Department of statics in 2021, 52.9% of Jordanians are males. It's mainly a country of the young with about 44.3% of the population under the age of 20, 44.0% between the age of 20 and 50 years old, and only 5.5% above the age of 65 years old (Jordanian Department of Statistics, 2021).

Jordan consists of 12 governorates including Amman, the capital of Jordan, which is divided into central, north, and south administrative parts. About 90.3% of the Jordanian population live in urban areas with 42.0% living in Amman and only 8.0% living in the southern Jordanian governorates (Jordanian Department of Statistics, 2021).

Using the economic classification of the World Bank, Jordan is considered an upper middle-income country (The World Bank, 2020). However, Jordan has many challenges in its economy such as inflation and insufficient natural resources like oil (Idris, 2016). Also, Jordan has a limited water resource and a water crisis considered the second most severe in the world (UNICEF Jordan). 22.8% of Jordanians were unemployed in the first quarter of 2022 (Jordanian Department of Statistics, 2021).

Jordanian Education and Medical Education

Jordan has a 98% literacy rate (MacroTrends, 2022), which indicates the importance of education among the Jordanian population. Jordanian school education consists of 2 years of pre-primary education followed by 10 years of basic education, then 2 years of secondary and higher education (World Education Network). Moreover, about 97% of Jordanian children have primary education at schools (UNICEF). Regarding higher education, Jordan has 10 public universities, 19 private universities, and 45 community colleges distributed through all governorates (Jordanian Ministry of Higher Education and Scientific Research, 2022). Likewise, six medical schools were appointed in public universities with no private medical schools until this time. The medical education system in Jordan consists of six years, three preclinical and three clinical years. Medical students are

Rawan Masri and Almu'atasim Khamees, *Jordan* In: *The Mental Health of Medical Students*. Edited by: Andrew Molodynski, Sarah Marie Farrell, and Dinesh Bhugra, Oxford University Press. © Oxford University Press 2024. DOI: 10.1093/oso/9780192864871.003.0016 introduced to the basic medical sciences in the first three years and the majority of medical specialties in the last three years (Khamees et al., 2022a, Tamimi and Tamimi, 2010). Medical students have their clinical years in mandatory rotations in the different departments of Jordanian hospitals. The total number of hospitals in Jordan is 121, distributed into 33 government hospitals, 15 military hospitals for royal medical services, 71 private and two university hospitals (Jordanian Private Hospitals Association, 2022). Medical students and general physicians face many stressors like the high cost of studying medicine, the medical education system, the rapid growth in numbers of undergraduate and postgraduate doctors, and a lack of opportunities to take jobs or subspecialties. Medical faculties in Jordan are overloaded with medical students and are deficient in trained teaching staff due to the low salaries in the country. These stressors can have a negative psychological impact on medical students.

The Mental Health of Medical Students Before the COVID-19 Pandemic

In 2008, the Jordanian ministry of health in collaboration with the World Health Organization (WHO) developed their first national policies and action plans regarding mental health services (WHO, 2019). The WHO determined that Jordan needed intense support for reinforcing the mental health system and selected Jordan to be the first country to enforce the 'WHO's mental health action programme (mhGAP)' (WHO, 2019).

Jordanian undergraduate students showed moderate to high levels of stress, depression, and anxiety. Despite that, about half of them were not aware of what psychological services were available (Dalky and Gharaibeh, 2019). One major factor for not seeking mental health support was the stigma of mental illness. Jordanian students from non-medical specialties showed significantly more shame and stigma toward mentally ill patients in comparison to medical students (Al-Natour et al., 2021). This highlighted the importance of curricular modification and the addition of specific tailored courses and programmes to raise awareness of mental health and to fight the shame against mental health patients.

Medical students showed high-stress levels, especially among female students. Students with stressful social circumstances, low socioeconomic status, and those who were obliged to enter the faculty of medicine were at higher risk (Munir et al., 2015).

In 2019, A descriptive study was conducted on 479 Jordanian medical students to assess for psychiatric disorders and burnout using the GHQ-12 and OLBI questionnaires respectively (Masri et al., 2019). The study discovered that 2% of students were diagnosed with mental disorders prior to entering medical school while 11% were diagnosed during their medical studies. 92% of medical students were considered positive with the GHQ-12 questionnaire. This is significantly higher than the results found in a study conducted on Jordanian women which showed that 39% of Jordanian women were psychologically distressed (Daradkeh et al., 2006). The level of burnout among Jordanian medical students showed high disengagement and exhaustion at 87% and 91% of students respectively. Only 8% of medical students showed problematic alcohol drinking behaviours (Masri et al., 2019). Additionally, another Jordanian study in which 838 healthcare students completed a questionnaire about symptoms of mental health problems and their associated factors reported that 65.3% of students showed anxiety symptoms, and 62.2% had mild to severe depression. Moreover, 54.2% had stress symptoms and these were significantly higher among female students (P-value < 0.01) (Almhdawi et al., 2018). Furthermore, the students' mental stress was associated with a low level of quality of life (Almhdawi et al., 2021b).

When asking Jordanian medical students about the factors that increase stress, 68% reported that financial factors associated with studying medicine were the main stressor. About 52% stated that their stress was due to problematic intimate relationships during medical school. However, only 15% of students reported that study difficulties were the main factor for their stress and 10% cited housing factors (Masri et al., 2019).

In order to study suicidal ideation and attempts among university students, an international cross-sectional comparative study enrolled 8,417 university students from Jordan and another eleven Muslim countries. The total number of Jordanian students was 700. The rate of suicidal ideation among Jordanian students was 12.4%, and the attempted suicide rate was 5.6%. These percentages were similar to that recorded in Lebanon (12.3% and 5.1% respectively). However, other countries that bordered or are located near Jordan, like Saudi Arabia, Palestine, and Egypt, recorded higher percentages compared to Jordan. Students from Saudi Arabia, Palestine, and Egypt showed suicidal ideation among 38.7%, 23.6%, and 17.5% of their students respectively, while suicidal attempts were reported among 13.4%, 17.6%, and 7.1% of students respectively. Although suicidal behaviours were more commonly reported by female students, male students required more medical attention (Eskin et al., 2019). Again, these alarming results among a young, educated population highlight the importance of mental health awareness for different society members, especially university students.

The Mental Health of Medical Students AFTER the COVID-19 Pandemic

Coronavirus disease 2019 (COVID-19) is caused by the severe acute respiratory syndrome coronavirus 2 (SARS-CoV-2), which is considered one of the most highly pathogenic infections. At the end of 2019, the WHO recognized this pandemic in Wuhan, China. After that, it spread rapidly reaching all world countries and causing an international lockdown. As a result, millions of deaths were confirmed with a mortality rate of 11% (Khamees et al., 2022c).

Jordan was one of the countries affected early by the COVID-19 pandemic. On March 2, 2020, Jordan reported its first confirmed case of COVID-19. Following this case, a slowly progressive increment in COVID-19 cases was recorded until the WHO classified Jordan as having a 'cluster of cases'. This led Jordanian authorities to announce an emergency national lockdown and insisted on the isolation of all governorates to control the spread of this highly contagious virus. Also, the Jordanian ministry of health declared obligatory quarantine for confirmed cases in governmental-funded institutions continued by quarantine for at least one week at the patient's home (Al-Balas et al., 2021). Other protocols such as closing borders and introducing online education resulted in widespread employment problems and difficulties. This lockdown and its consequences were associated with a negative impact on the lifestyle of Jordanians with nutritional habits, exercising, smoking, and sleeping behaviours being affected (Khamees et al., 2022b). Only Jordanian armed forces, medical staff, and medical students in their clinical years could move freely during the lockdown (Seetan et al.,

2021). Consequently, these specific COVID-19 protocols caused extra pressure on medical students that could affect their mental health. In addition, medical students showed low satisfaction levels with the online teaching system during the COVID-19 pandemic, complained more of neck pain, stress, and depression symptoms, resulting in a low level of health-related quality of life (Almhdawi et al., 2021a).

A Jordanian study was conducted during the COVID-19 pandemic among 553 medical students from six medical schools. More than half of the students reported that COVID-19 had a negative impact on their studying, stress level, physical activity, financial situation, eating habits, sleeping habits, social relationships, and relationships with friends ((68%), (56%), (73%), (51%), (54%), (51%), (66%), and (54%), respectively) (Seetan et al., 2021). Moreover, about two-thirds of medical students worried about their family members contracting COVID-19 while 32.5% had anxiety about being infected themselves. Furthermore, 41.8% had worries about long-time isolation and 30.7% had worries about travel restriction preventing them from doing exams or elective courses outside Jordan. Regarding the effect of COVID-19 on medical education, 58.4% of students showed concerns about not gaining enough clinical skills or attending labs, 20.8% showed difficulties in using new technologies or attending online classes, 23.1% had anxiety about the inability to graduate from medical school, and 17.9% had fear of dropping out (Seetan et al., 2021). When asking students about activities that can improve their mental health during the COVID-19 pandemic, 68.9% had chosen activities such as cooking, baking, and music. Likewise, 60.0% had chosen praying and mediation, 54.1% did physical activities, 45.0% chose social media, and 15.6% tried to learn a new language to decrease stress. However, only 14.3% stated that visiting a psychiatrist would improve their mental health in this pandemic (Seetan et al., 2021).

As a result of the COVID-19 pandemic, 50.3% of Jordanian medical students had severe psychological distress whilst 20.1% had moderate symptoms. This psychological distress was significantly associated with age (21 to 23 years), male gender, and with students in their clinical years (Seetan et al., 2021). Accordingly, it is a priority to improve students' mental health in parallel with facing any pandemic and its negative impact on health, mental health, and other lifestyle habits.

In another Jordanian study, medical students from all medical schools in the country participated. 47.3% of students said that the COVID-19 pandemic had a negative impact on their academic grades. When asking students about the reasons for this decline in their grades, 71.0% stated that online teaching and the associated fluctuation and variation in the time of classes was the main factor. More than half of students reported that online teaching had restricted feedback and made motivation hard. Technical problems contributed to stress. Also, 34.0% of students had financial problems due to the pandemic that prevented them from paying their university fees. Consequently, 70.4% of students stated that their mental health was negatively affected by this pandemic, 65.1% were more anxious and depressed, and 49.5% had an obsession with having the disease (Al-Husban et al., 2021). Obsessions related to COVID-19 preventive methods were significantly higher in female students and in students who participated in the presentation of COVID-19-related lectures. Despite that, students with these obsessions had significantly more knowledge about COVID-19 disease and how to prevent the infection (Al-Shatanawi et al., 2021).

Policies

Owing to its stability in a region that is struggling both financially and politically, the Hashemite Kingdom of Jordan is acknowledged as the second uppermost refugee host country worldwide (Elkahlout and Hadid, 2021) hosting 1.26 million Syrians of which 670,000 are enrolled as refugees with UNHCR (UNHCR, 2022), 66,000 Iraqi refugees with UNHCR and over 2 million Palestinian refugees registered with UNRWA (UNRWA, OCHA, 2022).

International policies about mental health in Jordan are still evolving. Mental health services in Jordan are struggling due to the heavy load coming from the unceasing flow of refugees in view of the current situation in Syria and surrounding countries in the middle east (WHO, 2020).

It was not until 2011 that the national mental health policy was developed. It was revised in 2016 and a new action plan is expected soon. The national mental health and substance use action plan (2018–2021) was developed through this policy. This policy addresses the importance of integrating mental health services into the primary healthcare setting through WHO mhGAP being the main action plan used to train general practitioners, family doctors, and nurses. The policy also relies on mhGap for the prevention, diagnosis and treatment of mental health patients (WHO, 2020).

There is a definite shortage of mental health staff in Jordan, Jordan has about 200 doctors offering their service per 100,000 populations, but as few as one psychiatrist per 100,000 (WHO, 2020). There are approximately 6.2 mental health practitioners per 100,000 Jordanian population (WHO, 2011). Even though mental healthcare is considered free for all Jordanian citizens through the Ministry of Health clinics under article 24 of Jordanian law, there is still a limited mental health budget and limited psychotropic medication availability in primary healthcare (WHO, 2020).

As a result, there has been an increasing focus on tertiary care services in place of primary care in Jordan, as described by the World Health Organization (WHO) Annex 1 pyramid on the optimal mix of mental health services (Jordanian MOH, 2011).

This had drawn international non-government organizations (NGOs) to Jordan, offering different services including mental health and psychological support. International medical corps (IMC), an NGO established in 1984, located in many regions all over the world including Jordan (International Medical Corps, 2022a, International Medical Corps, 2022b), is well known for its vast healthcare, emergency, women and children's health, and mental health services. IMC has integrated its mental health clinics with community health centres in order to serve refugees as well as Jordanian citizens (International Medical Corps, 2022c, International Medical Corps, 2022d).

In 2022, the IMC in collaboration with the Ministry of Social Development (MoSD) and the Ministry of Health (MoH) launched a platform through an application named Relax app to overcome stigma, enhance awareness about mental health and facilitate the delivery of mental health services to those in need by providing a hotline support service and a map for different mental health clinics in Jordan. This app is supported by MOH staff that are trained about MHGAP Intervention Guide Action Programme (mhGAP) (Jordan Health Information Systems and MHPSS teams, 2022).

As for local policies regarding students' wellbeing, the medical school of Yarmouk University has started a mental health initiative and named it 'Yarmouk Soul'. In cooperation with the psychology department at Yarmouk University, the medical school there started open day lectures, student meetings, and mental health discussions for medical and non-medical students. Looking at wellbeing and what obstacles they might encounter during their school years that might affect their mental health. It aims to increase awareness and education about preventive measures regarding mental health. Also, this initiative offers psychological counselling, support groups, and psychiatric clinical referrals to those in need. One of the aims of 'Yarmouk Soul' is to train medical staff and medical students to offer counselling to the students and advise them to see a psychiatrist if needed (Yarmouk University Faculty of Medicine, 2022a).

Yarmouk university plans to develop a psychiatric clinic inside the medical school that offers its services for medical students, which will accelerate the management and treatment of students who suffer from mental health problems rather than delay this process through referrals to other clinics. Also, they are in the process of starting counselling for students by a professional psychologist from the psychology department at the university to try to facilitate a more rapid intervention as opposed to being referred to a state/private psychologist.

Medical schools all over Jordan are currently revising the medical curriculum in order to decrease the redundancy in the basic sciences in the first three years of medical studies (Aborajooh et al., 2020, Tamimi & Tamimi, 2010). This will hopefully aid in decreasing dropouts from medical schools and decreasing part of the time, energy and stress imposed on medical students by integrating problem-based learning (PBL) with basic sciences.

There is currently cooperation with Yarmouk FM broadcasting radio station which is situated on the university campus. There are recorded and live programmes discussing the most common mental health disorders that students are facing. These programmes aim to spread awareness about physical and mental health problems and how to overcome academic and social stressors that affect students. They are mainly covered by doctors working in the Yarmouk school of medicine (Yarmouk University Faculty of Medicine, 2022b).

There is a current emphasis on involving medical students in different committees at the administrative level, such as the student support psychological committee and the academic committee, that take into account the students' feedback on different issues concerning problems that face the students and also take their feedback on curricular issues.

Yarmouk university had signed a contract agreement with the International Medical Corps (IMC) organization. This agreement allows the students to train in psychiatric clinics that are part of the IMC. They are also allowed to observe counselling sessions by psychologists so that they are exposed to different types of mental health disorders and their management (Yarmouk University Faculty of Medicine, 2021). One of the suggestions is that these students would be able to be treated in these clinics and there is a plan for opening a special clinic for medical students and their needs.

Drama students are now merging drama with medical education. A partnership with the school of arts and the school of medicine at The University of Jordan was initiated in 2017 as part of evolving medical education. Competent drama students were trained to simulate the role of a grieving patient, and the medical student was given the chance to play the role of the doctor breaking the bad news after having learnt it theoretically in the family medicine rotation during their fifth year of their studying (Jaber et al., 2019).

As a recommendation, acting out different scenarios regarding mental health disorders in collaboration with the medical school would be beneficial. The scenarios should be revised by the psychiatrists in the faculty before they are publicized.

Improving academic teaching under extraordinary circumstances and pandemics should be highlighted by national and international institutions. Future plans for improving tele-medicine and tele-education platforms for new emerging situations should be considered to accommodate the students' needs for remote medical learning in order not to impair the usual teaching system. One suggestion is allowing access to Electronic Medical Records (EMR) in order to follow up with patients, view their charts, and be able to discuss the case and its management with the attending physician. Virtual rounds alongside E-learning should be considered and students should be trained thoroughly in how to conduct tele-education and telemedicine (Franklin et al., 2021).

Medical students' mental health should be the core of our focus for the present time and for the future. Early detection programmes and prevenattive measures should be highlighted. Furthermore, establishing a solid social support system starting in medical school and fighting stigma as an approach method for easy and rapid access to mental health support.

References

Aborajooh, E., AL-Taher, R., Tarboush, N. A., AL-Ani, A., Qasem, N., Ababneh, S., Ababneh, G., AL-Ahrash, A., AL-Saeedi, B., AL-Husaini, S., & Bucheeri, A. (2020). 'A cross-sectional study of basic education influence on the clinical training: Attitudes and perception among Jordanian medical students'. *Ann Med Surg (Lond)* **60**: 456–461.

Al-Balas, M., AL-Balas, H. I., Alqassieh, R., AL-Balas, H., Khamees, A., AL-Balas, R., & AL-Balas, S. 2021. Clinical Features of Covid-19 Patients in Jordan: A Study of 508 Patients. *Open Respir Med J*, 15, 28–34.

AL-Husban, N., Alkhayat, A., Aljweesri, M., Alharbi, R., Aljazzaf, Z., AL-Husban, N., Elmuhtaseb, M. S., AL Oweidat, K., & Obeidat, N. 2021. Effects of Covid-19 pandemic on medical students in Jordanian universities: A multi-center cross-sectional study. *Ann Med Surg (Lond)*, 67, 102466.

AL-Natour, A., Abuhammad, S., & AL-Modallal, H. 2021. Religiosity and stigma toward patients with mental illness among undergraduate university students. *Heliyon*, 7, e06565.

AL-Shatanawi, T. N., Sakka, S. A., Kheirallah, K. A., AL-Mistarehi, A. H., AL-Tamimi, S., Alrabadi, N., Alsulaiman, J., AL Khader, A., Abdallah, F., Tawalbeh, L. I., Saleh, T., Hijazi, W., Alnsour, A. R., & Younes, N. A. 2021. Self-Reported Obsession Toward Covid-19 Preventive Measures Among Undergraduate Medical Students During the Early Phase of Pandemic in Jordan. *Front Public Health*, 9, 719668.

Almhdawi, K. A., Alazrai, A., Obeidat, D., Altarifi, A. A., Oteir, A. O., Aljammal, A. H., Arabiat, A. A., Alrabbaie, H., Jaber, H., & Almousa, K. M. 2021a. Healthcare students' mental and physical well-being during the Covid-19 lockdown and distance learning. *Work*, 70, 3–10.

Almhdawi, K. A., Kanaan, S. F., Khader, Y., AL-Hourani, Z., AL-Jarrah, M. D., Almomani, F., & Alqhazo, M. T. 2021b. Mental and physical health-related quality of life and their associated factors among students of a comprehensive allied health institution. *Work*, 70, 63-73.

Almhdawi, K. A., Kanaan, S. F., Khader, Y., AL-Hourani, Z., Almomani, F., & Nazzal, M. 2018. Study-related mental health symptoms and their correlates among allied health professions students. *Work*, 61, 391–401.

Central Intelligence Agency Government Publications Office. 2015. The World Factbook 2014-15, Government Printing Office. Isbn: 0160925533.

Dalky, H. F. & Gharaibeh, A. 2019. Depression, anxiety, and stress among college students in Jordan and their need for mental health services. *Nurs Forum*, 54, 205–212.

Daradkeh, T. K., Alawan, A., AL MA'Aitah, R., & Otoom, S. A. 2006. Psychiatric morbidity and its sociodemographic correlates among women in Irbid, Jordan. *East Mediterr Health J*, 12 Suppl 2, S107–S117.

Elkahlout, G. & Hadid, A. 2021. Stable Jordan: How A Monarchy Survived Disorder. *Asian Affairs*, 52, 852–871.

Eskin, M., Albuhairan, F., Rezaeian, M., Abdel-Khalek, A. M., Harlak, H., EL-Nayal, M., Asad, N., Khan, A., Mechri, A., Noor, I. M., Hamdan, M., Isayeva, U., Khader, Y., AL Sayyari, A., Khader, A., Behzadi, B., Ozturk, C. S., Hendarmin, L. A., Khan, M. M., & Khatib, S. 2019. Suicidal Thoughts, Attempts and Motives Among University Students in 12 Muslim-Majority Countries. *Psychiatr Q*, 90, 229–248.

Franklin, G., Martin, C., Ruszaj, M., Matin, M., Kataria, A., HU, J., Brickman, A., & Elkin, P. L. 2021. How the Covid-19 Pandemic Impacted Medical Education during the Last Year of Medical School: A Class Survey. *Life (Basel)*, 11.

Idris, I. 2016. Economic Situation in Jordan. Available: https://assets.publishing.service.gov.uk/media/5b97f50ae5274a1391b13967/K4D_Hdr_Economic_Situation_in_Jordan.pdf

International Medical Corps. 2022a. Mental Health and Psychosocial Support (Mhpss) in Humanitarian Settings [Online]. Available: https://internationalmedicalcorps.org/where-we-work/.

International Medical Corps. 2022b. Who we are. Available: https://internationalmedicalcorps.org/who-we-are/.

International Medical Corps. 2022c. Integrating mental health into primary healthcare [Online]. Available: https://internationalmedicalcorps.org/program/mental-health-psychosocial%20support/integrating-mental-health-into-primary-healthcare/.

International Medical Corps. 2022d. Our work [Online]. Available: https://internationalmedicalcorps.org/what-we-do/our-work/.

Jaber, R. M., Abu-Hassan, H. H., AL Raie, J., Tayseer, A., Alghzawi, A. O., Salameh, H. H., & Massad, I. 2019. Merging drama with medical education: simulation in learning breaking bad news pre-and post-study. *Open Journal of Nursing*, 9, 620.

Jordanian Department Of Statistics. 2021. Statistical YearBook Of Jordan 2021 [Online]. Available: http://dosweb.dos.gov.jo/DataBank/Population_Estimares/PopulationEstimates.pdf.

Jordanian Ministry of Higher Educationand Scientific Research. Higher Education in Jordan [Online]. Available: https://mohe.gov.jo/EN/Pages/Higher_Education_in_Jordan

Jordanian Moh. 2011. National Mental Health Policy. Available: https://www.mhinnovation.net/sites/default/files/downloads/innovation/reports/National-Mental-Health-Policy-Jordan.pdf

Jordanian Private Hospitals Association. Healthcare System Overview [Online]. Available: https://phajordan.org/EN-article-3809-#:~:text=Currently%

Jordan Health Information Systems and Mhpss teams. 2022. Supporting the Mental Health System in Jordan with a New Smart Phone App [Online]. Available: https://internationalmedicalcorps.org/story/supporting-the-mental-health-system-in-jordan-with-a-new-smart-phone-app/.

Khamees, A., Awadi, S., AL Sharie, S., Faiyoumi, B. A., Alzu'BI, E., Hailat, L., & AL-Keder, B. 2022a. Factors affecting medical student's decision in choosing a future career specialty: A cross-sectional study. *Ann Med Surg (Lond)*, 74, 103305.

Khamees, A., Awadi, S., Rawashdeh, S., Talafha, M., Bani-Issa, J., Alkadiri, M. A. S., AL Zoubi, M. S., Hussein, E., Fattah, F. A., Bashayreh, I. H., & AL-Saghir, M. 2022b. Impact of Covid-19 pandemic on the Jordanian eating and nutritional habits. *Heliyon*, 8, e09585.

Khamees, A., Bani-Issa, J., Zoubi, M. S. A., Qasem, T., Abualarjah, M. I., Alawadin, S. A., AL-Shami, K., Hussein, F. E., Hussein, E., Bashayreh, I. H., Tambuwala, M. M., AL-Saghir, M., & Cornelison, C. T. 2022c. Sars-CoV-2 and Coronavirus Disease Mitigation: Treatment Options, Vaccinations and Variants. *Pathogens*, 11.

Macrotrends 2022. Jordan Literacy Rate 1979-2022. Available: https://www.macrotrends.net/countries/Jor/jordan/literacy-rate

Masri, R., Kadhum, M., Farrell, S. M., Khamees, A., AL-Taiar, H., & Molodynski, A. 2019. Wellbeing and mental health amongst medical students in Jordan: a descriptive study. *Int Rev Psychiatry*, 31, 619-625.

Munir, A., Husam, A., Muhammad, A., Mohammad, H., Fadi, A., & Zouhair, A. 2015. Sources and predictors of stress among medical students in Jordan. *Bull Environ Pharmacol Life Sci*, 4, 113-21.

Ocha. 2022. *Registered People of Concern Refugees and Asylum Seekers in Jordan - Iraqi Refugees (as of 31 March 2022)* [Online]. Available: https://reliefweb.int/report/jordan/registered-people-concern-refugees-and-asylum-seekers-jordan-iraqi-refugees-31-march.

Seetan, K., AL-Zubi, M., Rubbai, Y., Athamneh, M., Khamees, A., & Radaideh, T. 2021. Impact of Covid-19 on medical students' mental wellbeing in Jordan. *PLoS One*, 16, e0253295.

Tamimi, A. F. & Tamimi, F. 2010. Medical education in Jordan. *Med Teach*, 32, 36-40.

The World Bank. 2020. The world by income [Online]. Available: https://datatopics.worldbank.org/world-development-indicators/the-world-by-income-and-region.html#:~:text=The%20World%20Bank%20classifies%20economies,%2Dmiddle%2C%20and%20high%20income.

Unhcr 2022. Jordan issues record number of work permits to Syrian refugees. Available: https://www.unhcr.org/news/press/2022/1/61effaa54/jordan-issues-record-number-work-permits-syrian

Unicef Education in Jordan. Available: https://www.unicef.org/jordan/education

Unicef Jordan. Water, sanitation and hygiene [Online]. Available: https://www.unicef.org/jordan/water-sanitation-and-hygiene#

Unrwa. *Where WE Work* [Online]. Available: https://www.unrwa.org/where-we-work/jordan.

Who 2011. Who-Aims Report ON Mental Health System IN Jordan. Available: https://www.ecoi.net/en/file/local/1130531/1788_1308390842_mh-aims-report-jordan-jan-2011-en.pdf

Who. 2019. *Mental health in Jordan* [Online]. Available: http://www.emro.who.int/jor/jordan-news/mental-health-in-jordan.html

Who 2020. Jordan Who Special Initiative for Mental Health Situational Assessment. Available: https://cdn.who.int/media/docs/default-source/mental-health/special-initiative/who-special-initiative-country-report---jordan---2020_414542ae-ce5d-4f1d-bf40-fe1b1cbf8003.pdf?sfvrsn=e813985_4

World Education Network. Snapshot of Jordan Education System [Online]. Available: https://www.jordaneducation.info/education-system/jordan-education-overview.html

Yarmouk University Faculty of Medicine. 2021. Agreement of collaboration with Imc in fields of training in mental health [Online]. Available: https://medicine.yu.edu.jo/index.php/about-faculty-en/faculty-news-archive-en/604-agreement-imc-en.

Yarmouk University Faculty of Medicine. 2022a. Launching (Yarmouk Soul) initiative with a lecture by Dr. Sqour [Online]. Available: https://medicine.yu.edu.jo/index.php/about-faculty-en/faculty-news-archive-en/864-yu-soul-en.

Yarmouk University Faculty of Medicine. 2022b. Your Health @ Yarmouk FM [Online]. Available: https://medicine.yu.edu.jo/index.php/it-faculty/faculty-news-center/619-your-health-yarmoukfm-en.

17

Morocco

Mental Health Among Moroccan Medical Students

Maha Lemtiri Chelieh, Redouane Abouqal, and Jihane Belayachi

Medical Studies and Health Systems Challenges

Health System Challenges

The Moroccan Kingdom is located in the northwest of Africa and has 36 million inhabitants. Morocco is ranked among lower-middle income countries, with 24% of its population being considered poor or at risk of poverty (World Bank, 2019).

The Moroccan health system provides medical care through a public and a private sector. It faces a number of issues.

One of the issues is a shortage of human ressources.

In the past 50 years Morocco has had substantial population growth, which has led to an increase in our elderly population and an increase of chronic diseases. This phenomenon has led to an increase in the population demand for healthcare services. A study carried out in 2007 showed that Morocco was still among countries suffering from an acute deficit in human health resources, both quantitatively and qualitatively. The medical and paramedical density barely exceeded 1.64 per 1,000 inhabitants, whereas the critical threshold set by the World Health Organization (WHO) at the time was 2.5 health workers per 1,000 inhabitants (Evans & Weltgesundheitsorganisation, 2006). In order to face this shortage in human resources, especially in terms of medical personnel, the Moroccan Government has adopted a national initiative to train 3,300 doctors per year by 2020 (Ministère de la santé du Maroc, 2009). The initiative, which has created new faculties of medicine and increased the number of admissions, should make up for the lack of medical staff and ensure care for the population in the best conditions. Additionally to the faculties of Rabat, Casablanca, Fes, and Marrakech, the faculties of Oujda (2009), Tanger (2015), Agadir (2015) and private faculties in Rabat, Casablanca and Marrakech were created with their university's hospitals (Fourtassi et al., 2020; Ministère de la Santé du Maroc, 2009; L'économiste, 2013)).

In the WHO report of 2017, the shortage of human resources continued, with a density of 1.52 per 1,000 inhabitants (0.62 of physicians per 1,000 inhabitants and 0.97 of nursing and midwifery per 1,000 inhabitants in the public sector) which is way below the minimum threshold of health workers (4.45 per 1,000 inhabitants) recommended by the WHO. Based on the SDG (Sustainable Development Goals) critical threshold, the Ministry of health

Maha Lemtiri Chelieh, Redouane Abouqal, and Jihane Belayachi, *Morocco* In: *The Mental Health of Medical Students*. Edited by: Andrew Molodynski, Sarah Marie Farrell, and Dinesh Bhugra, Oxford University Press. © Oxford University Press 2024. DOI: 10.1093/oso/9780192864871.003.0017 estimates a deficit of medical and paramedical staff at 129,548, and of medical doctors alone at 32,387 (WHO, 2016).

The low total health expenditure to GDP (5.8%) can explain much of this shortage as it is below the average in WHO member countries (6.8%) and also below the average in OECD countries (8.9%) (Fourtassi et al., 2020; World Bank, 2017).

The emigration of skilled health workforce also exacerbates this shortage. The National Human Rights Council (CNDH) drew up an alarming observation in its report: between 600 and 700 Moroccan doctors leave the country every year to European, American, and Asian countries. 23,000 doctors are practising in Morocco and between 10,000 and 14,000 Moroccan doctors work abroad, particularly in Europe. Thus, 1 out of 3 Moroccan doctors practice abroad, despite the 'pressing need' of the Kingdom in terms of health professionals. The migration is explained by the pursuit of better salaries and more comfortable working environment (National Human Rights Council and Amina Bouayach, 2022).

A cross-sectional study carried out in 2021 in the Faculty of Medicine of Casablanca found that 70.1% of final year students had intentions to leave the country. Foreign countries were attractive because of better training (97.6%), better working conditions (99%) and quality of life (97.2%). The dissatisfaction about quality of medical education (95.2%) and salary (97%), alongside the denigration of doctors in media (83.6%) were reason for leaving the country. Germany was the favourite destination (34%) (Sylla et al., 2021).

Despite the increase of medical infrastructures, the geographical inequality of healthcare services is still an issue: 20% of the population travel a distance of over 10 kilometres to find the nearest health facility, especially in rural areas. There is also an under-use of curative services because of the shortage of human resources (WHO, 2016).

Morocco is currently in the process of reforming his healthcare system.

The first part of the reform is on a governmental level with the creation of three entities:

The creation of the 'High Authority of Health' to watch over the quality of health services
The creation of a 'Medicines Agency' who will implement the national pharmaceutical policy and will developed the production of medicines
The creation of a 'Blood Agency' that will be responsible for the management of the blood stock and blood transfusion.

The second part of the reform is on a human resources level. Currently the rate of of qualifying doctors who then work in the public sector does not go beyond 12%. Morocco wants to exceed in 2025 the objectives of the WHO to reach the goal of 24 doctors for 10,000 inhabitants.

Strategies adopted to increase this rate include remuneration by providing in addition to the fixed salary a supplement calculated on the basis of medical acts performed by the doctor each month and the right to conclude work contracts with doctors in the private sector.

The third component of the reform concerns the upgrading of the healthcare system by the restoration of 1,400 health centres in cities and rural communities.

The fourth axis is related to the digitalization of the health system, through the implementation of an integrated computer system for the entire health sector, including the various health institutions and the managers of the health insurance (Alaoui & Moussaaid, 2022).

Only 62% of the Moroccan population is granted health insurance. Reforms aim to introduce universal health coverage with the challenge of the extension of coverage of uncovered populations (WHO, 2016).

Medical Studies

Morocco has 10 faculties of medicine, 7 of which are part of the public system, located in 7 different regions of Morocco (Table 17.1) (Fourtassi et al., 2020). (la liste des établissements d'enseignements supérieur au Maroc, 2018) (Liste des universités privées autorisées par le ministère de l'éducation nationale, de la formation professionnelle, de l'enseignement supérieur et de la recherche scientifique, 2018).

As in many countries, medical studies in Morocco are a long path.

The admission process involves two important steps: a preselection process, based on students' grades in the baccalaureate (national high school graduation exam) and an entrance exam.

The general curriculum consists of three cycles. The first cycle (first and second year) is only theoretical and basic sciences are studied. The second cycle (third, fourth, and fifth year) is theoretical and practical and pathology is studied. The third cycle (sixth and seventh year) is purely clinical. The reorientation to another field between the cycles is not possible. Clinical rotations occur in university hospitals. There are two different exam sessions and the clinical rotation periods are validated after a clinical assessment. The basic medical degree is obtained after passing a licensing exam and defending a thesis.

At the end of the general curriculum, medical students can graduate as General Practitioners and start medical practice or aim for specialization. In order to pursue specialization, 'Residency' is mandatory. Residency take 3 to 5 years depending on the specialization. During the residency, residents must take an exam at the end of the first year of residency and a final exam at the end of the specialty to become specialist.

There are two ways to be accepted into a specialty/residency programme.

The first way is after completing the general curriculum. Doctors of medicine take a 2-steps written exams called 'residency competition'. The doctors who pass this residency

Table 17.1 Morocco's 10 Faculties of Medicine with their University's affiliation

City	University
Public institutions	
Rabat	University Mohammed V
Casablanca	University Hassan II
Marrakech	University Cadi Ayyad
Fes	University Sidi Mohammed Ben Abdellah
Oujda	University Mohammed Ier
Tanger	University Abdelmalek Saadi
Agadir	University Ibn Zohr
Private institutions	
Rabat	International University Abulcasis of health of science
Casablanca	International University Mohammed VI of health of science
Marrakech	Private University of Marrakech

Source: data from Fourtassi, M. et al. (2020) 'Medical education in Morocco: Current situation and future challenges', Medical Teacher, *42*(9), pp. 973–979.

competition are named 'residents by competition'. The choice of specialty is depending of the rank at the competition.

The second way is before completing the general curriculum but after completing the first 5 years of medical studies. Medical students can take a 2-steps written exams called 'internship competition'. The doctors who pass this competition are named 'residents on title' and access immediately the residency programme after completing the general curriculum, with priority in the choice of specialty (Figure 17.1) (Faculté de Médecine de Marrakech, 2015).

The existence of these two distinct paths aimed to distinguished between residents who will pursue a university career and residents who will not: only those who take the 'internship competition' were allowed to pursue a university career in order to be medical professors. The existence of the internship path was intended to provide excellence and the access to the university teaching curriculum. By this means, this pathway put the interns in a physical and psychological pressure. Today, these two paths still exist despite the fact that the university career is no longer exclusive to the internship path. The only remaining advantage of the internship path is the priority in the choice of specialty. The advantage of exclusivity to access to a university career is no longer in effect (El Khamlichi, 2014).

A reform of medical studies was undertaken in 2015 with the adoption of a newly organized manual of pedagogical standards.

Unfortunately, only some changes were implemented: new modules were introduced to the curriculum and the curriculum content in each semester among all the faculties of medicine were harmonized. However, teaching methods remain mainly lecture-based and teacher-centred.

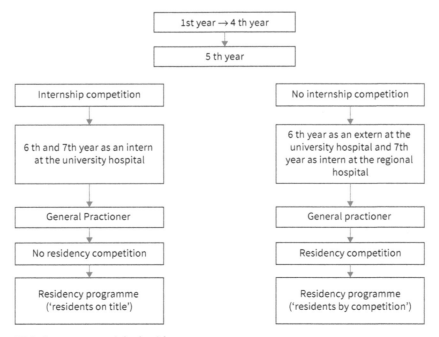

Figure 17.1 Access to specialty/residency programme.
Source: data from Faculté de Médecine de Marrakech, (2015) 'Les études médicales'.

Other important changes were the establishment of an LMD system (licence, master, PhD) allowing the reorientation of medical students (the reorientation was previously not possible), the transition from general medicine to family medicine as a specialty and the shortening of medical studies from 7 years to 6 years (Faculté de Médecine et de Pharmacie de Marrakech, 2015).

The university path is accessible after a validated residency and attending to the competition of assistant professor.

Mental Health Among Medical Students

Table 17.2 summarizes the main results of studies on different aspects of the mental health of Moroccan medical students such as psychological distress, psychiatric disorders, and suicide.

Table 17.3 table summarizes the main results of studies on substance use among Moroccan medical students.

Table 17.4 summarizes the main results of studies on educational environment of Moroccan medical students.

Weaving Bibliometric Analysis of Medical Study In Morocco

We conducted a bibliometric analysis of related to medical study in Morocco literature based on the Web Of Science (WOS) database. A weaving bibliometric analysis aimed to discover trending topics and scholars focus in the field.

In this study we followed the general bibliometric analysis workflow that consists of five stages (Börner et al., 2005; Zupic & Čater, 2015). In the study design stage, our main research question was: What was the bibliometric of medical study field research, which were published by scholars with Moroccan affiliations, and indexed in the WOS until October 2022.

The data collection stage is divided into three sub-stages: Data collection, data filtering, and data cleaning. The author team performed a search from the WOS database; searching keywords for the field included: Medical Students OR Student, Medical OR Medical Student. Searching keywords for the field excluded: Students Health Occupations; Students Dental; Students Nursing; Students Premedical; Students Public Health. Search is limited to author's keywords, and document types are limited to: articles written in English. After filtering the data, the number of remaining records was 24. Measurements were conducted on this data.

Various analytical techniques have been applied to extract the information about the collection of publications. General statistics provide quantitative information such as the number of annual publications and publication trends, journals with the top number of publications, and authors or organizations with the highest productivity. Tools used in data visualization stage were, VOS viewer version 1.6.12. and Bibliometrix package in R (Aria & Cuccurullo, 2017; van Eck & Waltman, 2010).

After data filtering according to inclusion criteria, we proceeded to analytics and plots for four different level metrics including: sources; authors; documents; and clustering by coupling. Firstly, descriptive analyses were conducted to evaluate the characteristics and types of articles retrieved. We present a performance analysis of matrix normalization, mapping

Table 17.2 Mental health among medical students: psychological distress, psychiatric disorders, and suicide

Name of first author, year of publication	Design of study: type of study, period, sample	Scale	Prevalence or mean +/- SD of mental health parameters	Other results
(Essangri et al., 2021)	Cross-sectional study; 2020; 439 medical students of the Faculty of Medicine of Rabat from 1st to 7th year.	Nine item Patient Health Questionnaire (PHQ-9); seven-item Generalized Anxiety Disorder Scale (GAD 7); seven-item Insomnia Severity Index; six-item Kessler psychological distress scale.	- Depression (74.6%); - Anxiety (62.3%); - Insomnia (62.6%); - Psychological distress (69%).	- Female gender is a risk factor for severe symptoms of anxiety, depression, and insomnia. - Preclinical level of enrolment is a risk factor for depression, insomnia, and distress. - Living in high COVID-19 prevalence locations was a risk factor for severe anxiety and depression.
(Barrimi et al., 2020)	Cross-sectional and multicentre study among medical students from 1st to 7th year in Morocco; 2017.	Open questions	- 5% had made at least one suicide attempt; - 31% had suicidal thoughts. - Students rate their mental health as poor in 13% cases, fair in 40% cases and good in 47% cases.	- Association of suicidal thoughts with substance use, poor mental health, and suicide attempts. - Association of suicide attempts with poor mental health and the presence of a long-term illness.
(Lemtiri Chelieh, 2020)	Cross-sectional study; 2019; 637 medical students of the Faculty of Medicine of Rabat from 1st to 7th year.	- Perceived Stress Scale (PSS) - Perceived Health— Patient Health Questionnaire 4 (PHQ-4) - Short Form 12 (SF12) from the medical outcome study - Open questions regarding suicide	- Stress: low stress (1.4%), moderate stress (82.1 %), high stress (16, 5%); - Depression (35.60%), - Anxiety (36.10%); - Quality of life: mean mental quality of life (34.72 ± 11.19); mean physical quality of life 51.32 ± 8.72. - Suicide: Suicidal ideation (25.4%); Planning a suicide attempt (6.9%); Unsuccessful suicide attempt (2.5%).	No analysis

(Abdeslam et al., 2019)	Cross-sectional study; 2017–2018; 358 medical students of the Cadi Ayyad University from 3d to 8th year.	- Open questions	- Psychological distress (66.76%); - Need of psychological help (53%); - Use of stress management methods (70.1%).	Strong association between the use of stress management methods and the need for psychological help.
(Azzouzi et al., 2019)	Cross-sectional study; 2013–2014; 710 medical students of the Faculty of Medicine of Fes from 1st to 6th year.	- SCOFF (Sick, Control, One Stone, Fat, Food) questionnaire - The Eating Disorder Inventory 2 (EDI2)	- According to BMI: 11.1% of cases being underweight, 13.4% overweight, and 1.8% obese. - The prevalence of EDs in students was 32.8%; - Weight-control behaviour (18.5%): diet (6.5%), fasting (7%), appetite suppressants (3%), induced vomiting (1.7%), laxatives (0.7%) and diuretics (0.6%).	Increased body-mass index values were significantly associated with dieting, fasting, and the use of appetite suppressants.
(Chichou, 2018)	Cross-sectional descriptive and analytical study with 380 students (3rd, 4th, 5th, 6th, 7th and 8th year) from the Faculty of Medicine and Pharmacy of Marrakech.	GHQ-12	The average GHQ score was 6.37 ± 3.484, with a psychological distress rate of 66.76%.	Psychological distress is strongly associated to a poor perception of the educational environment, the use of stress management methods and the need for psychological help.
(El Mibrak, 2018)	Cross-sectional and multicentre study of 1,731 medical, law, agronomic students of University Mohammed V of Rabat; 2017.	Spielberger inventory	Severe anxiety: medical students (40%), law students (23.1%) and agronomic institute students (16.1%)	- Association of high anxiety with female sex and the presence of a personal psychiatric history among all students. - Association of anxiety with educational level and substance among medical students.

(continued)

Table 17.2 Continued

Name of first author, year of publication	Design of study: type of study, period, sample	Scale	Prevalence or mean +/− SD of mental health parameters	Other results
(Idrissi Kaitouni, 2018)	Cross-sectional study among 500 students of the Faculty of Medicine of Marrakech in 2017.	Open questions	- Stress (77.1%), depressed mood (22.6%), loss of personal accomplishment (63%), emotional exhaustion (60.3%), depersonalization (16.9%), poor quality of life (8.7%). - Suicidal thoughts (19.4%), at least one suicide attempt (3.3%). - Regular consumption: tobacco (9.9%); alcohol (9.6%), cannabis (7.1%), 2.6% smoking shisha 2.6%), 'hard' drugs (1.6%) - A climate of violence in the performance of their duties (39.8%); a rather negative view of the future (30.4%); physically feeling unhealthy (25.8%)	No analysis
(Ouchtain, 2016)	Cross-sectional study among 350 students of the Faculty of Medicine of Marrakech.	- Beck–Depression–Inventory (BDI) - Mini-Interview-Neuropsychiatric-Review (MINI) - Open questions for consumption of substances	- Depression (35.1%) - Characterized anxiety disorders: social phobia - General anxiety disorder - Obsessive compulsive disorder - Agoraphobia - Post-traumatic stress disorder (54%) - Smoking (15.4%) - Hashish (6.2%) - Alcohol (15.4%)	- Association with a high rate of depression and characterized anxiety disorders: female sex, socioeconomic level, and the presence of a personal or family psychiatric history. - Association of anxiety and depression with the level of study and the consumption of toxic substances.

Study	Design/Population	Instrument	Results	Findings
(Lahlou et al., 2015)	Cross-sectional study; 2014; 178 medical students of 5th year of Faculty of Medicine of Rabat.	- MBI (Maslash Burnout Inventory) - PSS (Perceived Stress Scale)	- Burnout (44%); - Mean stress score: 24±7.18 - Average daily working hours: 8.33 ± 2.74 hours; - Average daily number of sleeping hours: 7 ± 1.1 hours	- Positive correlation between the number of hours worked burnout score; - Negative correlation between the number of hours of sleep and burnout.
(Azzaoui et al., 2013)	Cross-sectional and multicentre study; 2012–2013; 198 medical students from 3d to 7th year of Faculty of Medicine of Rabat, Casablanca and Fes.	MBI	Burnout (64.4%)	- Association of burnout with exams, course overload, long study duration, problems with teachers, and perfectionism - Statistically significant consequences of burnout: feelings of irritability and guilt, alcohol, and cannabis use, relational impact, and the idea of dropping out of studies
(Bounsir, 2008)	Cross-sectional study among 240 students of the Faculty of Medicine of Marrakech in 2006.	MBI	High emotional exhaustion (39.5%), high dehumanization (29%), low personal accomplishment (18.5%)	- The female sex helps to protect from the depersonalization. - Spare time activities contribute to the diminution of the emotional exhaustion and to the increase of the personal accomplishment. - The auto medication fosters dehumanization. - The students who choose to study medicine out of conviction are not exposed to the burnout syndrome.

(continued)

Table 17.3 Consumption of substances and use of psychoactive substances among medical students

Name of first author, year of publication	Design of study: type of study, period, sample	Scale	Prevalence or mean +/− SD	Results
(Barrimi et al., 2020)	Cross-sectional and multicentre study among medical students from 1st to 7th year in Morocco; 2017.	Open questions	- Consumption of psychoactive substances (12%): only tobacco (3 %), only alcohol (1.8%), consumption of many substances at the same time (tobacco, alcohol, cannabis, and others) (20%).	- Association of suicidal thoughts with substance use.
(El Yaakoubi, 2016)	Cross-sectional and descriptive study among 371 students of the Faculty of Medicine of Rabat in 2014-2015	- Open questions for substance consumption - The Fagerström Test for Nicotine Dependence	- Tobacco (17%); Cannabis (13%); Alcohol (12%); psychotropic drugs (3.8%); other drugs (3.8%) - Nicotine dependence (57.6%): Low (30.3%) Moderate (21.2%) High (6.1%)	No analysis
(Kouara, 2013)	Cross-sectional and descriptive study among 445 students from 1st to 6th year of the Faculty of Medicine of Fes in 2012–2013	- Open question for Nicotine Consumption - The Fagerström Test for Nicotine Dependence	- Smokers (10.6 %) - Dependence: Low (77%) Moderate (22%) High (0%)	The proportion of smokers increases significantly according to the year of study going from 0% in the 1st year to 20.5% in the 6th year and also according to the age going from 0% for the students between 17 and 19 years old up to 15.4 % for students between 23 and 27 years old.
(Zaghba et al., 2013)	Cross-sectional and descriptive study among 712 students from 1st to 6th year of the Faculty of Medicine of Casablanca in 2009-2010	Questionnaire of the International Union against Tuberculosis and Lung Disease, intended for health personnel, and adapted to medical students	- Permanent smokers (4.4%) - Occasional smokers (3.5 %)	No analysis

Table 17.4 Educational environment among medical students

Name of first author, year of publication	Design of study: type of study, period, sample	Scale	Prevalence or mean +/− SD	Other results
(Lemtiri Chelieh, 2020)	Cross-sectional study; 2019; 637 medical students of the Faculty of Medicine of Rabat from 1st to 7th year	Open questions: assessment by a visual scale from 1 to 10	-Failure:	Frequency of occasional failure at (63.30%) and absence of failure (36.70%) during their academic studies; Typ of failure: rates of 49.80%, 8.80%, 2.20%, 1.40%, 1.40% of retaking exams, failure in the internship competition, failure in clinical examinations, bad marks, failure at the training exam(s) respectively; level of fear of academic failure: mean of 6.75, a median of 7 with an interquartile range of [5; 9] (10 =maximum fear)
				- Help from faculty to understand failure: mean of 2.15, a median of 1 with an interquartile range of [1; 3] (10= the best help)
				- Course accessibility: mean of 3.83, a median of 3 with an interquartile range of [1; 6] (10= the best accessibility)
				- Workload: mean of 7.84, a median of 8 with an interquartile range of [7; 10] (10 =maximum workload)
				- Teaching is centred on student: mean of 3.31, a median of 3 with an interquartile range of [1; 5] (10= the best focus on students)
				- Student participation in decision-making: mean of 2.16, a median of 1 with an interquartile range of [1; 3] (10=the best participation)
				- Contribution of the faculty to the preparation for a medical career: mean of 2.99, a median of 3 with an interquartile range of [1; 4] (10=the best preparation)
				- Contribution of the faculty to the preparation for a medical career: mean of 2.99, a median of 3 with an interquartile range of [1; 4] (10=the best preparation)
				- Certain future in terms of specialization: mean of 3.09, a median of 2 with an interquartile range of [1; 5] (10 = certain future)
				- Quality of the majority of teacher-student relationships: non-existent (74.41%), negative (5.02%), positive (20.57%).

(continued)

Table 17.4 Continued

Name of first author, year of publication	Design of study: type of study, period, sample	Scale	Prevalence or mean +/− SD	Other results
(Rahmouni, 2018)	Cross-sectional study among 216 students from 1st to 7th from the Faculty of Medicine of Fes in 2016	Conditional Associative Learning Morocco test (CALM): to assess learning abilities	-	The performance of undergraduate students is higher than those of the second cycle; the amplitude of performance increases again during the third cycle; the performance of students with the same level of education increases with the socioeconomic level and sport.
(Chichou, 2018)	Cross-sectional descriptive and analytical study among 380 students (3rd, 4th, 5th, 6th, 7th, and 8th year) from the Faculty of Medicine of Marrakech	Dundee Ready Education Environment Measure (DREEM)	Mean total score: 86.5 ± 29.194/200 (200 represent a perfect educational environment, a score of 51–100 indicates a considerable number of problems)	- Item 3 "There is a good support system for students when they experience stress" had the lowest score - The factors associated with a poor perception of the educational environment are the female gender, the age >21 years, the existence of a psychological distress, the use of stress management methods.
(Chaouche, 2014)	Cross-sectional study among 632 students (3rd, 4th, 5th and 6th year) from the Faculty of Medicine of Fes	DREEM	Mean total score: 99.20 ± 27,521/200	Association of DREEM with psychological distress.
(Moufawaq, 2005)	Cross-sectional study among 274 students (5th and 6th year) from the Faculty of Medicine of Fes	Open questions	-	- The relationship between core disciplines and clinical practice is not evident to many students (40.2%); the lack of parallelism between theoretical teaching and clinical teaching (98.4%); 50.6% attended the lecture; dissatisfaction with their lectures (66.1%); little satisfaction or dissatisfaction with the practical training (86.1%); little satisfaction or dissatisfaction with their evaluation method (79.7%); suggestions from students to improve their medical education (58%).

and clustering set-theoretic normalization methods have been used to measure the similarities of the items (author's keywords.) After the normalization of the raw co-occurrence matrix, mapping, and clustering was conducted. The multidimensional scaling (MDS) is used to transform the matrix into a two-dimension space, and the Euclidean distance-based map was used to show the similarities between each knowledge unit. Knowledge units are still mapped into a two-dimension space, with the link strength being used to show the similarities of each unit. After locating the units into the two-dimensional space, cluster methods are applied to divide the units into different groups. We utilized bibliographic coupling to describe the intellectual structure of the field. We explored the thematic structure of the field through an analysis of the co-occurrence of the authors' keyword. Finally, we conduct a content analysis to identify the literature's theoretical lenses and trends, and suggest avenues for future research (Bretas & Alon, 2021).

Thematic Mapping

Figure 17.2 shows the thematic map of the field of medical study in Morocco mental health, which is essentially split into four quadrants (Q1 to Q4). The upper right quadrant (Q1) represents driving themes, the upper left quadrant (Q2) is the very specialized themes, the lower left quadrant (Q3) is emerging or disappearing themes and the lower right quadrant (Q4) is underlying themes.

From the thematic map, the main topics that medical students in Morocco were concerned about mental health as basic themes, niche theme are sleep privation and knowledge. However, neither motor themes nor emerging themes were individualized in a thematic map (Figure 17.2).

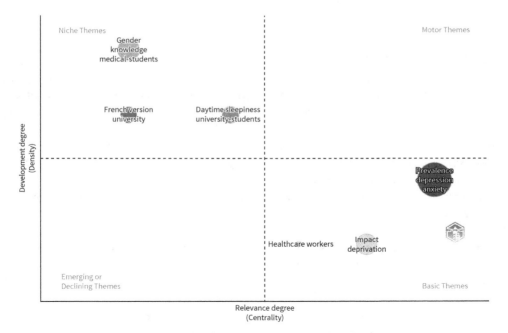

Figure 17.2 Thematic map.

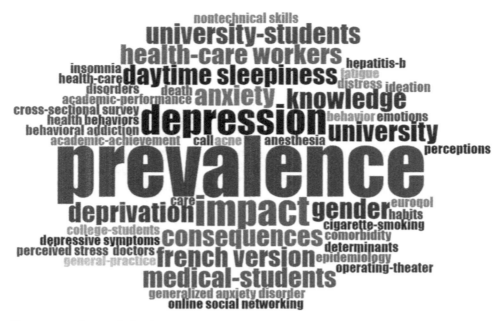

Figure 17.3 The word-cloud.

Keywords Analysis

The word-cloud shows frequently used keywords in medical study publications in Morocco. These are some of the highest numbers of recurring keywords within the field, as shown in (Figure 17.3).

Factorial Analysis

The conceptual structure of the keywords compresses extensive data with multiple variables into a low-dimensional space to form an intuitive two-dimensional graph that utilizes plane distance to reflect the relation between the keywords. The results are interpreted based on the relative positions of the points and their arrangement along the dimensions; as words are more similar in distribution, the closer they are represented in the map.

Co-occurrence network and factorial analysis concluded that the most frequent terms which represents the main topics that which can be divided in two main research areas, including (Figure 17.4):

- The first cluster (on the left side) contains 17 key words and focuses on research on mental health in medical student in Morocco. Some of the concerning subjects in this cluster were: psychological distress, psychiatric disorders, suicide attempts, use of psychoactive substances, medical education, and occupational diseases.
- The second cluster (on the right side) contains seven key words and focuses on research on information technology in medical study in Morocco.

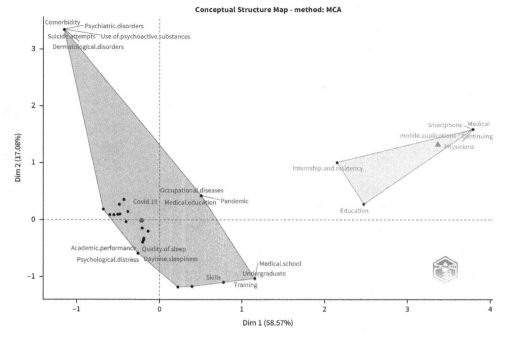

Figure 17.4   Conceptual structure map of keywords.

Factorial Analysis of Most Cited Documents

From the factorial map of most cited documents, we observe that the top cited articles were divided into the two clusters (Figure 17.5).

For cluster one, five papers are detected:

Ben Loubir D, 2014: Prevalence of Stress in Casablanca Medical Students: A Cross-Sectional Study

This cross-sectional study sought to determine the prevalence of stress among Casablanca Medical students and to investigate if there is an association between stress and academic skills. Among the participants, 52.7% were stressed by examinations. The study showed a negative association between stress and academic competence, test competence, time management and strategic study (Ben Loubir et al., 2014).

Chelieh ML, 2019: Mental Health and Wellbeing Among Moroccan Medical Students: A Descriptive Study

Some of the main results of this cross-sectional study among medical students of the Faculty of Medicine and Pharmacy of Rabat (FMPR) were: 47% of medical students had a minor psychiatric disorder; regarding the dimensions of burnout, 68% had disengagement and 93% suffer from exhaustion. The consumption of alcohol and substances in the last 12 months was 20.1% and 8.3% respectively. Concerning the diagnosis of a mental health condition prior and during medical school was 3.9% and 15.5% respectively (Lemtiri Chelieh et al., 2019).

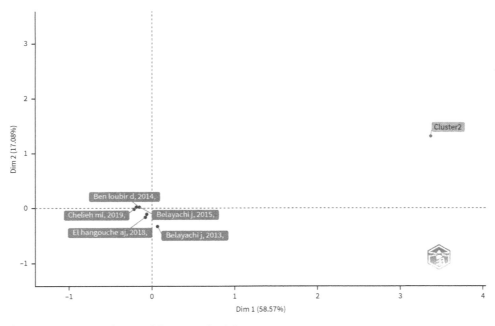

Figure 17.5 Factorial map of the most cited documents.

Belayachi J, 2015: Moroccan Medical Students' Perceptions of Their Educational Environment

This cross-sectional study among medical students from the FMPR shows that the total mean DREEM score was 90.8 out of 200, which means that students perceived the educational environment as having many problems (Belayachi et al., 2015).

El Hangouche AJ, 2018: Relationship Between Poor Quality Sleep, Excessive Daytime Sleepiness, and Low Academic Performance In Medical Students

This purpose of this study was to determine the prevalence of excessive daytime sleepiness, sleep quality, and psychological distress and their association with low academic performance among medical students from the FMPR.

Regarding the quality of sleep the results showed a prevalence of 58.2% and 36.6% of poor sleepers and excessive daytime sleepiness, respectively. Psychological distress was among 86.4% of medical students. The study found an association of being a poor sleeper with poor academic performance (El Hangouche et al., 2018).

Belayachi J, 2013: Self-Perceived Sleepiness in Emergency Training Physicians: Prevalence and Relationship With Quality Of Life

This study was a prospective survey conducted among emergency training physicians in University Hospital Center Ibn Sina. The results found 24.7% of sleepiness, 39.5% of excessive sleepiness and 35.8% of severe sleepiness.

Concerning the different dimensions of quality of life: 33.4% of physicians have mobility problems, 9.9% self-care problems, 59.2% usual activities problems, 59.2% suffer from pain or discomfort, and 59.3% have anxiety or depression.

Poor quality life index was associated with 4 independent variables: unmarried, no physic exercise, shift-off sleep hour less than 6 hours, and severe sleep deprivation (Belayachi et al., 2013).

There were no impacting papers in cluster 2.

Descriptive Results of The Bibliometric Research

Table 17.5 resumes different parameters of the scientific production concerning the mental health of medical students in Morocco.

Table 17.5 Descriptive results of the bibliometric research

Description	Results
MAIN INFORMATION ABOUT DATA	
Timespan	2008:2022
Sources (journals, books, etc)	21
Documents	24
Annual growth rate %	8.16
Document average age	3.38
Average citations per doc	5.542
References	594
DOCUMENT CONTENTS	
Keywords Plus (ID)	73
Author's keywords (DE)	69
AUTHORS	
Authors	101
Authors of single-authored docs	1
AUTHORS COLLABORATION	
Single-authored docs	1
Co-Authors per doc	5.46
International co-authorships %	12.5
DOCUMENT TYPES	
article	22
editorial material	1
meeting abstract	1

Conclusions

The Moroccan healthcare system faces many issues. To overcome those issues, the Moroccan healthcare and education systems are undergoing reform. This reform includes both the healthcare system and medical studies.

The literature review shows that medical students face many psychological issues. These different forms of psychological stress will of course affect each other.

We aimed to determine the relationship between stress, anxiety, depression, burnout, and quality of life among medical students at the Faculty of Medicine of Rabat in 2019.

We assessed the model fit by using a SEM (Structural Equation Modelling).

Our results show that:

Stress has a direct impact on anxiety and exhaustion and an indirect impact on depression, disengagement, and quality of life.

Anxiety has a direct impact on depression and quality of life and an indirect impact on burnout and quality of life.

Depression has a direct impact on exhaustion and mental health related quality of life and an indirect impact on disengagement and quality of life.

Exhaustion has a direct impact on disengagement and quality of life.

Disengagement has no impact on quality of life.

These impacts are positive correlations except for the relationships between different mental health parameters and the quality of life, which are negative correlations (Figure 17.6) (Lemtiri Chelieh, 2020).

In the same study, medical students expressed several needs such as: training in work methodology (69.9%), training in managing emotions (71.3%), training in communication with patients (78%), the need for a guidance structure (79.1%) and the need for a support structure (68.8%). No students expressed a need for individualized educational coaching (Lemtiri Chelieh, 2020).

The results of the literature review concerning medical education show that medical students perceived the educational environment as having many problems.

These results show the need for interventions.

Several types of interventions for medical students could be established: institutional interventions and student interventions (group or individual).

There could be alterations to the academic curriculum, so they can intervene on the type of learning, the mode of evaluation, and/or on behaviour towards the students.

Interventions on an individual level are those that directly concern the student's wellbeing, such as stress management/psycho-educational groups facilitated by psychiatrists, discussion and skill training sessions, annual speech about mental health, and screening systems of mental health issues for medical students (Frajerman, 2020).

Some faculties offers a support structure like the faculties of Marrakech and Fes and a structure of mentoring like the faculty of Marrakech ('Cellule d'écoute—Faculté de Médecine et de Pharmacie de Marrakech', 2020) ('Vie éstudiantine—Faculté de Médecine et de Pharmacie de Marrakech', 2020). The activity and the contribution of these entities are not studied.

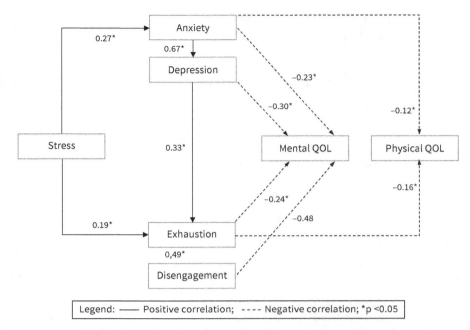

Figure 17.6 Model of path analysis the relationships between stress, anxiety, depression, burnout, and quality of life among medical students of Rabat with standardized coefficients.

Reproduced from Lemtiri Chelieh, M. (2020) 'La Sante Mentale Des Etudiants En Medecine De Rabat De La 1ere A La 7eme Annee: Revue De Litterature Et Etude Transversale A Visee Descriptive Et Analytique'. © Maha Lemtiri Chelieh

The interventions regarding mental health of Moroccan medical students are still poor and more interventions both institutional and personal should be established.

References

Abdeslam, B., et al. (2019) 'Mental Health Status Among Moroccan Medical Students at the Cadi Ayyad University', *International Journal of Psychiatry Research*, 2(1).

Alaoui, M.C. and Moussaaid, B. (2022) 'Réforme de la santé: tout ce qu'il faut savoir sur le projet de loi-cadre adopté en conseil des ministres', Le 360, 24 July. Available at: https://fr.le360.ma/politique/reforme-de-la-sante-tout-ce-quil-faut-savoir-sur-le-projet-de-loi-cadre-adopte-en-conseil-des-264 149?fbclid=IwAR0iS5EwvIIBVwPNCQnjmf5o8V57x6n9J1skCqfS0Daz6vaFFfahPmjzunM.

Aria, M. and Cuccurullo, C. (2017). 'bibliometrix: An R-tool for comprehensive science mapping analysis', *Journal of Informetrics*, 11(4), pp. 959–975.

Azzaoui, L. et al. (2013) '*Le burnout chez l'étudiant en Médecine Marocain: quels constats?* quelles solutions?' Hôpital Arrazi-CHU IBN SINA.

Azzouzi, N. et al. (2019) 'Eating disorders among Moroccan medical students: cognition and behavior', *Psychology Research and Behavior Management*, 12, pp. 129–135.

Barrimi, M. et al. (2020) 'Les idées et les tentatives de suicide chez les étudiants en médecine au Maroc: résultats d'une étude multicentrique', *Annales Médico-psychologiques, revue psychiatrique*, 178(5), pp. 481–486.

Belayachi, J. et al. (2013) 'Self-perceived sleepiness in emergency training physicians: prevalence and relationship with quality of life', *Journal of Occupational Medicine and Toxicology*, 8(1), p. 24.

Belayachi, J. et al. (2015) 'Moroccan medical students' perceptions of their educational environment', *Journal of Educational Evaluation for Health Professions*, 12, p. 47.

Ben Loubir, D. et al. (2014) 'Prevalence of stress in Casablanca medical students: a cross-sectional study', *The Pan African Medical Journal*, 19, p. 149.

Börner, K., Chen, C. and Boyack, K.W. (2005) 'Visualizing knowledge domains', Annual Review of Information Science and Technology, *37*(1), pp. 179–255.

Bounsir, A. (2008) Burnout chez les étudiants de la faculté de médecine et de pharmacie de Marrakech. Université Cadi Ayad.

Bretas, V.P.G. and Alon, I. (2021) 'Franchising research on emerging markets: Bibliometric and content analyses', Journal of Business Research, *133*, pp. 51–65.

'Cellule d'écoute – Faculté de Médecine et de Pharmacie de Marrakech' (2020). Available at: http://www.fmpm.uca.ma/?page_id=303 (Accessed: 30 October 2020).

Chaouche, M. (2014) La santé mentale et l'environnement éducatif des étudiants en médecine de Fès. Université Hassan II.

Chichou, H. (2018) L'environnement éducatif et la santé mentale des étudiants en médecine de Marrakech. Université Cadi Ayad.

van Eck, N.J. and Waltman, L. (2010) 'Software survey: VOSviewer, a computer program for bibliometric mapping', *Scientometrics*, 84(2), pp. 523–538.

El Hangouche, A.J. et al. (2018) 'Relationship between poor quality sleep, excessive daytime sleepiness and low academic performance in medical students', *Advances in Medical Education and Practice*, Volume 9, pp. 631–638.

El Khamlichi, A. (2014) CHU en détresse. Formation médicale en danger. *Editions la croisée des chemins.*

El Mibrak, L. (2018) Anxiété en milieu estudiantin: étude transversale sur une population d'étudiants en médecine, en droit et en agronomie. Université Mohammed V de Rabat.

El Yaakoubi, A. (2016) Toxiphilie, enquête auprès des étudiants de la faculté de médecine et de pharmacie de Rabat. Université Mohammed V de Rabat.

Essangri, H. et al. (2021) 'Predictive Factors for Impaired Mental Health among Medical Students during the Early Stage of the COVID-19 Pandemic in Morocco', *The American Journal of Tropical Medicine and Hygiene*, 104(1), pp. 95–102.

Evans, T. and Weltgesundheitsorganisation (eds) (2006) Travailler ensemble pour la santé. Genève: Organisation Mondiale de la Santé (Rapport sur la santé dans la monde, 2006).

Faculté de Médecine de Marrakech (2015) 'Les études médicales'. Available at: http://wd.fmpm.uca.ma/fmpm/formation/init/etud_th/etud_med.pdf.

Faculté de Médecine et de Pharmacie de Marrakech (2015) *RÉFORME MÉDICALE*. Available at: http://www.fmpm.uca.ma/?page_id=249 (Accessed: 5 June 2022).

Fourtassi, M. et al. (2020) 'Medical education in Morocco: Current situation and future challenges', *Medical Teacher*, 42(9), pp. 973–979.

Frajerman, A. (2020) 'Quelles interventions pour améliorer le bien-être des étudiants en médecine? Une revue de la littérature', *L'Encéphale*, 46(1), pp. 55–64.

Idrissi Kaitouni, Z. (2018) La santé de l'étudiant en médecine à la FMPM de la première à la sixième année d'étude. Université Cadi Ayad.

Kouara, S. (2013) Tabagisme chez les étudiants en médecine de Fes. Université Sidi Mohammed Ben Abdellah.

Lahlou, L. et al. (2015) '« Burn out » et stress chez les étudiants en médecine de Rabat, Maroc', *Revue d'Épidémiologie et de Santé Publique*, 63, p. S83.

Lemtiri Chelieh, M. et al. (2019) 'Mental health and well-being among Moroccan medical students: a descriptive study', *International Review of Psychiatry*, 31(7–8), pp. 608–612.

Lemtiri Chelieh, M. (2020) 'La sante mentale des etudiants en medecine de rabat de la 1ere a la 7eme annee: revue de litterature et etude transversale a visee descriptive et analytique'. http://ao.um5.ac.ma/xmlui/handle/123456789/18268 (Accessed: 18 July 2022).

Ministère de la santé du Maroc (2009) *Ministère de la santé. La démographie médicale et paramédicale à l'horizon 2025.* https://www.sante.gov.ma/Documents/Demographie-Medicale.pdf.

Moufawaq, S. (2005) Appréciation du programme des études médicales: point de vue des étudiants. Université Hassan II.

National Human Rights Council and Amina Bouayach (2022) *L'effectivité du droit à la santé: Défis, enjeux et voies de renforcement.*

Ouchtain, A. (2016) La prévalence et les caractéristiques des troubles anxieux et dépressifs chez les étudiants de la faculté de médecine et de pharmacie de Marrakech. Université Cadi Ayad.

Rahmouni, J. (2018) Evaluation de l'évolution des capacités d'apprentissage chez les étudiants en médecine (étude la FMPF). Université Hassan II.

Sylla, A. et al. (2021) 'Migration intention of final year medical students', *European Journal of Public Health*, 31(Supplement_3), p. ckab165.448.

'Vie éstudiantine – Faculté de Médecine et de Pharmacie de Marrakech' (2020). Available at: http://www.fmpm.uca.ma/?page_id=299 (Accessed: 30 October 2020).

WHO (2016) *Stratégie de coopération OMS-Maroc 2017-2021.* https://extranet.who.int/iris/restricted/bitstream/handle/10665/254588/CCS_Maroc_2016_fr_19364.pdf;jsessionid=B5BBF797B8B67 07269E22995B7732E8E?sequence=5.

World Bank (2017) *Current health expenditure (% of GDP) | Data.* https://data.worldbank.org/indicator/SH.XPD.CHEX.GD.ZS?view=map (Accessed: 6 April 2022).

World Bank (2019) Poverty & equity and macroeconomics, trade & investment global practices. Available at: http://pubdocs. worldbank.org/en/919381570664049212/EN-MPO-OCT19-Morocco. pdf.

Zaghba, N. et al. (2013) 'Comportement des étudiants en médecine de Casablanca vis-à-vis du tabac en 2010', *Revue des Maladies Respiratoires*, 30(5), pp. 367–373.

Zupic, I. and Čater, T. (2015) 'Bibliometric Methods in Management and Organization', *Organizational Research Methods*, 18(3), pp. 429–472.

18
Nepal

Medical Student Wellbeing in Nepal

Bikram Kafle

Introduction

Nepal is a landlocked country situated in South Asia between India and China. It became a federal republic with the promulgation of the constitution in 2015. It is ethnically diverse, with 125 ethnic groups and approximately 123 languages spoken. Nepal has diverse geography that includes the Terai or flat river plain in the south, central hill regions, and mountainous Himalayas in the north. The country has a federal parliamentary republic and is made up of seven provinces (Pradesh) with the nation's capital located in Kathmandu. The total population is 29,675,000(United Nations, Department of Economic and Social Affairs, Population Division, 2019).

The current healthcare delivery system is organized as a tiered referral system. At the basic level are community health units, health posts, urban health clinics and primary hospitals (including primary health centres). More complex and serious cases are referred to secondary-level hospitals, tertiary-level hospitals (provincial and above) and eight specialized hospitals. The Ministry of Health and Population (MoHP) formulates overall health policies/plans and regulates, monitors, and evaluates health activities and outcomes. In 2018, the Epidemiology and Disease Control Division (EDCD) of the Department of Health Services (DoHS) was designated as the focal unit to oversee mental health in Nepal. The mental health programmes in the country are operationalized by the Non-Communicable Disease and Mental Health Section

Mental Healthcare System in Nepal

Mental health services in Nepal started out in general hospital settings. The first psychiatric outpatient services started in 1962 and in-patient treatment in 1964 (Upadhyaya, 2015:60). A mental hospital was established in 1984 and it moved to its current location in Lagankhel, Lalitpur, in 1985. It is the only mental hospital in Nepal and has a capacity of 50 beds. Nepal never had a 'mental asylum'. Mental health services are provided by the psychiatric units of medical colleges, provincial government hospitals, and a few private hospitals. The total number of in-patient psychiatric facilities is 25 and the overall number of beds is 500. Clinics have been initiated in different subspecialties, such as child, memory, headache, and addiction. The Child and Adolescent Psychiatry Unit at Kanti Children's Hospital is the only

Bikram Kafle, *Nepal* In: *The Mental Health of Medical Students*. Edited by: Andrew Molodynski, Sarah Marie Farrell, and Dinesh Bhugra, Oxford University Press. © Oxford University Press 2024. DOI: 10.1093/oso/9780192864871.003.0018 full-time outpatient clinic for children in Nepal. There is no dedicated in-patient unit for children. Non-governmental organizations (NGOs) have played a vital role in the delivery of mental health services (Upadhaya et al., 2014:113). Community mental health services were initiated in the 1980s by the United Mission to Nepal (Jha et al., 2018). In the 1990s and early 2000s, NGOs such as the Centre for Victims of Torture, Nepal (CVICT), the Centre for Mental Health and Counselling—Nepal (CMC-Nepal) and the Transcultural Psychosocial Organization Nepal (TPO Nepal) provided mental health and psychosocial care to the victims of civil conflict and the Bhutanese refugee crisis. NGOs have also contributed to the scaling up of community mental health programmes, in collaboration with the MoHP. See Table 18.1.

There are currently no programmes in Nepalese medical school curricula to screen for poor mental health or to help people cope with the stress of being a medical student. Improved understanding of mental health among medical students will encourage the development and integration of student wellness programmes to prevent negative outcomes of poor mental health.

There are eighteen medical schools and all except four are in the private sector. Among government-run schools, the National Academy of Medical Sciences (NAMS) is a postgraduate training institution attached to Bir Hospital, the oldest hospital in Nepal. The Institute of Medicine (IOM) was the first medical school to be started in the late 1970s. IOM admits students from other countries who are paying privately to the undergraduate medical (MBBS) course. The other two schools, BP Koirala Institute of Health Sciences (BPKIHS)

Table 18.1 Mental health services and resources in Nepal

	2020	2008 (Shyangwa and Jha 2008:36)
Health budget as a proportion of national budget	6.15%	6.5%
Mental health budget as a proportion of the total health budget	1%	0.8%
Number of registered doctors in Nepal	26 346	6719
Number of psychiatrists	200	39
Number of in-patient psychiatric facilities	25	–
Number of psychiatric beds	500	385
Child psychiatrists	3	0
Old age psychiatrists	0	0
Clinical psychologists	30 (MPhil) 200 (MA)	>9
Psychiatric nurses	50	48
Psychosocial counsellors (trained using the 780 h curriculum of NGOs)	700	–
Community-based psychosocial workers (trained in basic emotional support)	>300	–

and Patan Academy of Health Sciences (PAHS) admit students paying partial and full tuition to the MBBS course. The duration of the MBBS course is four and half years followed by a year of rotating internship which foreign students can do in their home countries. At PAHS, the MBBS course is of six years duration (with internship). The medical schools are affiliated with and follow the curriculum of two Nepalese universities, Tribhuvan University, a government university, and Kathmandu University, a private university. BPKIHS and PAHS are autonomous institutions. (Shankar, 2011:8) The postgraduate course is of 3 years duration.

Data regarding the status of mental health among Nepalese medical students and residents is limited, and few studies have been conducted here. A few studies on the prevalence of anxiety and depressive disorders among medical students have been done in Nepal which revealed a high prevalence of anxiety and depressive disorders (Adhikari et al., 2017:7; Dhami et al., 2018:32; Kunwar et al., 2016:22).

Medical education is long and both physically and emotionally demanding. Before entering medical school, the mental health of medical students is similar to that of the general populationor even better (Carson et al., 2000:115). Inside the medical school, they are exposed to various academic and psychosocial stressors thought to be typical of the medical school environment. Medical students are exposed to multiple stressors that may detrimentally affect their mental health, such as study, difficult academic environments, heavy workload, sleeplessness, and exposure to serious illness. They are also exposed to substantial tuition fees leading to financial difficulties, constant travel raising housing concerns, and/or a lack of recreational activities (Dyrbye et al., 2005:1613; Levey, 2001:142) In addition to these, they also face personal life events, beyond the control of the medical school authorities like illness, marriage, the birth of a child, and/or death of family members. These issues may result in significant anxiety or mood disorders, compromise academic attainment, and heighten the risk of medical errors, dropout, alcohol and substance abuse, and tragically in some cases suicide (Combes et al., 2000:1178; Mandal et al., 2012:126; Tyssen et al., 2001: 69). The poor health-related quality of life among medical students is contributed mainly by the mental component (Lins et al., 2015:149).

Findings from Our Survey

Prior to joining medical school, 4% of students had been diagnosed with a mental health condition. This increased to 8% within medical school. Two-thirds of students cited their academic studies as their leading source of stress. The CAGE test showed that 14% screened positive for problem drinking and potential alcohol problems. Twenty-three students (14%) described taking medication to enhance concentration or to feel better, while 11% of students reported the use of recreational drugs. The prevalence of mental health problems using the GHQ-12 was around 50%. Studies from Nepal have previously reported prevalence of anxiety ranging from 32 to 45% and of depression from 29 to 31% among medical students (Adhakari et al., 2017:1; Kunwar et al., 2016:22).

Rates of burnout were very high. Nine out of ten respondents were disengaged and seven out of ten were exhausted (Kafle et al., 2021:4). Another Nepalese study showed almost 50% of medical students had burnout syndrome (Pokhrel et al., 2020:18). Burnout and mental health problems were more prevalent in female than male students (Jafari et al., 2012:107). This may be the result of underreporting of symptoms by men, compared to the female gender

(Noorbala et al., 2004:70). Depression seen in female medical students has been found to be linked with personality traits (Hojat et al., 1999:342), gender inequality, and stigma (Bleakley, 2014:111). Cannabis abuse was also found in where 15% students had used cannabis during medical studies. Previous studies in Nepal have reported a similar distribution of alcohol and cannabis abuse, which is aided by the relatively easy availability of cannabis.

Mental health problems are high among Nepalese medical students. Failure to identify these problems leads to increased psychological illness with undesirable effects throughout careers and lives. This study will help stakeholders, including local policy makers, to make further strategic plans to alleviate the mental health problems of students. These strategies could include training to medical students for the early identification of stress and its management and making the academic curriculum more 'student friendly'. Further research is needed to delineate and categorize the factors associated with psychological distress in medical students globally, in order to appropriately inform policy at local, national, and international levels.

Policies Regarding Student Wellbeing

The version of the 2020 National Mental Health Strategy and Action Plan is to improve the mental and psychosocial health of the people of Nepal, enabling them to live productive and quality lives. The guiding principles of the plan are to ensure easy and equal access to high-quality mental health services; integrate mental health services into primary healthcare; maintain participation, cooperation, and partnership between government, non-government, and private sectors; and provide an evidence-based and comprehensive mental health service that is rights-based, participatory and inclusive. Its strategies include managing the necessary resources, workforce, and delivery of mental and psychosocial services; conducting awareness campaigns to remove superstitions and myths related to mental illness and promote mental health; protecting human rights of people with mental illness and psychosocial disability; and promoting research by integration of mental health service-related information into the current information system. It also mentions monitoring and evaluation of programme implementation at all three government tiers—central, provincial, and local.

The components of this plan seem to be positive but the existence of only one psychiatric hospital in Nepal hinders accomplishing its goals. Although there are other referral hospitals providing psychiatric services, most are located in urban areas and lack adequate human resources (Mishra &Khanal, 2018:4) The idea of integrating mental healthcare into the primary healthcare system has already been promoted by the 1996 Mental Health Policy and Nepal Health Sector Programme-II, but a lack of mental health governance mechanisms at national and district levels has not allowed the policy provisions to be put into practice (Upadhaya et al., 2017:12) Moreover, healthcare workers are already overstretched and this integration of services could further burden them. Despite these various barriers, integration can be achievable based on different enabling factors, such as constitutional provision for health as a human right, inclusion of mental health in the national five-year health plan, and inclusion of mental healthcare in the Multisectoral Action Plan for the Prevention and Control of Non-Communicable Diseases.

CMC-Nepal is implementing a school mental health programmein close collaboration with the Ministry of Education, Science and Technology (MoEST) centrally and with (rural) municipalities at a local level. This programme promotes the psychosocial wellbeing of children and adolescents in school, and develops access to psychosocial support for those who have emotional and behavioural problems, learning difficulties, and developmental delays which can impede learning. It mainly focuses on improving classroom behavioural management, empowering parents and other stakeholders involved in school activities, employing a positive disciplinary approach, and managing a student listening unit (school counselling). This programme also encourages referral service mechanism in government hospital for advanced cases from the schools. On the other hand, it is also collaborating and closely working with Centre for Education and Human Resource Development (CEHRD), Ministry of Education and Ministry of Social Development of the concerned provinces for policy advocacy in mainstreaming school mental health components in school education system through development of in teachers' training packages and its delivery at school level. However, there is no policies specific to mental health wellbeing of medical students.

Conclusion

The higher level of psychiatric morbidity depression, anxiety and stress among medical students warrants needs for strategic plans to alleviate depression anxiety and the stressors right from the time they join medical school and has to be continued untilthey finish the course. Various solutions to reduce stress like creating a nurturing learning environment, identifying, and assisting students, teaching skills for stress management and promoting self-awareness as a part of medical education with special focus on preclinical students may improve mental health.

References

United Nations, Department of Economic and Social Affairs, Population Division (2019). World Population; 2019.

Upadhyaya, K.D .(2015). 'Mental health & community mental health in Nepal: major milestones in the development of modern mental health care'. J Psychiatrists' AssocNepal *4*(1):60–67.

Upadhaya, N., Luitel, N.P., Koirala, S., Adhikari, R.P., Gurung, D., Shrestha, P., Tol, W.A., Kohrt, B.A., &Jordans, M.J. (2014). 'The role of mental health and psychosocial support nongovernmental organisations: reflections from post conflict Nepal'. Intervention *12*(Supplement 1):113–128.

Jha, A.K., Ojha, S.P., Dahal, S., Rajendra Kumar, B., Jha, B.K., Pradhan, A., Labh, S., & Dhimal, M. (2018). A Report on Pilot Study of National Mental Health Survey. Kathmandu, Nepal: Nepal Health Research Council.

Shyangwa, P.M., &Jha, A. (2008). 'Nepal: trying to reach out to the community'. Int Psychiatry *5*(2):36–38.

Shankar, P.R. (2011). 'Undergraduate medical education in Nepal: one size fits all?'. J Educ Eval Health Prof *8*: 9.

Dhami, D.B., Singh, A., &Shah, G.J. (2018). 'Prevalence of depression and use of antidepressant in basic medical sciences students of Nepalgunj medical college, Chisapani, *Nepal*'. J Nepalgunj Med Coll *16*(1):32–36.

Adhikari, A., Dutta, A., Sapkota, S., Chapagain, A., Aryal, A., &Pradhan, A. (2017). 'Prevalence of poor mental health among medical students in Nepal: a cross-sectional study'. BMC MedEduc *17*(1):1–7.

Kunwar, D., Risal, A., &Koirala, S. (2016). 'Study of depression, anxiety and stress among the medical students in two medical colleges of Nepal'. Kathmandu Univ Med J *14*(53):22–26.

Carson, A.J., Dias, S., Johnston, A., McLoughlin, M.A., O'connor, M., Robinson, B.L., Sellar, R.S., Trewavas, J.J.C., &Wojcik, W. (2000). 'Mental health in medical students a case control study using the 60 item general health questionnaire'. ScotMedJ *45*(4):115–116.

Dyrbye, L.N., Thomas, M.R., &Shanafelt, T.D. (2005). 'Medical student distress: causes, consequences, and proposed solutions'.Mayo Clin Proc *80*(12):1613–1622.

Levey, R.E. (2001). 'Sources of stress for residents and recommendations for programs to assist them'. AcadMed *76*(2):142–150.

Combes, M.C., Andrzejewski, S., Anthony, F., Bertrand, B., Rovelli, P., Graziosi, G., &Lashermes, P. (2000). 'Characterization of microsatellite loci in Coffea arabica and related coffee species'. MolEcol *9*(8):1178–1180.

Tyssen, R., Vaglum, P., Grønvold, N.T., &Ekeberg, Ø. (2001). 'Suicidal ideation among medical students and young physicians: a nationwide and prospective study of prevalence and predictors'. JAffectDis *64*(1):69–79.

Mandal, A., Ghosh, A., Sengupta, G., Bera, T., Das, N., &Mukherjee, S. (2012). 'Factors affecting the performance of undergraduate medical students: a perspective'. Indian JCommunity Med *37*(2): 126.

Lins, L., Carvalho, F.M., Menezes, M.S., Porto-Silva, L., &Damasceno, H. (2015). 'Health-related quality of life of students from a private medical school in Brazil'. Int J Med Educ *6*:149.

Kafle, B., Bagale, Y., Kadhum, M., &Molodynski, A. (2021). 'Mental health and burnout in Nepalese medical students: an observational study'. Middle East Curr Psychiatry *28*(1):1–4.

Pokhrel, N.B., Khadayat, R., &Tulachan, P. (2020). 'Depression, anxiety, and burnout among medical students and residents of a medical school in Nepal: a cross-sectional study'. BMC Psychiatry *20*(1):1–18.

Jafari, N., Loghmani, A., &Montazeri, A. (2012). 'Mental health of medical students in different levels of training'. IntJPrevMed *3*(Suppl1):107.

Noorbala, A.A., Yazdi, S.B., Yasamy, M.T., &Mohammad, K. (2004). 'Mental health survey of the adult population in Iran'. Br J Psychiatry *184*(1):70–73.

Hojat, M., Glaser, K., Xu, G., Veloski, J.J., &Christian, E.B. (1999). 'Gender comparisons of medical students' psychosocial profiles'. MedEduc *33*(5):342–349.

Bleakley, A., Bleakley A. *Gender matters in medical education. Patient-Centred Medicine in Transition: The Heart of the Matter*. 2014:111–126.

Mishra, S.R., Khanal, P., &Khanal, V. (2018). 'Sustained neglect in mental health during Nepal's crises'. Health Prospect*17*(1):4–7.

Upadhaya, N., Jordans, M.J., Pokhrel, R., Gurung, D., Adhikari, R.P., Petersen, I., & Komproe, I.H.(2017). 'Current situations and future directions for mental health system governance in Nepal: findings from a qualitative study'. IntJMentHealth Syst*11*(1):1–12.

19

New Zealand

The Power of Connection: Perspectives on Medical Student Wellbeing in New Zealand

Fiona Moir, Kristy Usher, and Hamish Wilson

Introduction

We start with this chapter with a summary of Aotearoa New Zealand's historical and cultural context, then provide a brief overview of the health and wellbeing of medical students in New Zealand (NZ), drawing on local, Australasian, and international evidence. As expected, the situation here is largely the same as for students in other countries, with concerning levels of psychological distress. We then report on recent progress in New Zealand medical schools in enhancing wellbeing, including changes in curricula, and support services.

However, we believe that simply 'tweaking' the medical curriculum or augmenting support systems will be insufficient if we are to produce doctors who are energized, robust, and proactive about their own health and wellbeing. Accordingly, we also consider some of the more challenging features of medical training in the twentieth and twenty-first centuries. Medical students experience more distress as training progresses, and it is likely that the social and institutional cultures of medicine are significant contributors. In considering how to mitigate deleterious environmental factors, we suggest that *connection* is one of the keys to students' wellbeing and professional satisfaction. By connection, we are referring to their interactions and relationships with patients, as well as their sense of belonging to the profession; in other words, their professional identity must be nurtured and developed carefully during their journey through medical school.

In the second half of this chapter, we therefore explore the significance of students' connection with patients, with colleagues and other staff, and with the profession more generally. We argue that within their training, medical students can experience a significant sense of disconnection, arising in part to dissonance between their prior expectations and their observations of clinical reality. We also suggest that medical students are faced with a conceptual dilemma: instinctively, they wish to engage and connect with patients, peers, and colleagues, but we believe that currently, they are given insufficient role-modelling, opportunities, and/or specific training in how to do so judiciously and effectively.

We will outline possible pathways between moral distress and burnout as key concepts in student wellbeing, demonstrating how these pathways could also lead to specific faculty initiatives and curriculum design for wellbeing. We suggest that if the factors contributing to dissonance and moral distress are identified and addressed more directly, then students may feel more supported and included within the profession and their wellbeing may improve.

Fiona Moir, Kristy Usher, and Hamish Wilson, *New Zealand* In: *The Mental Health of Medical Students*. Edited by: Andrew Molodynski, Sarah Marie Farrell, and Dinesh Bhugra, Oxford University Press. © Oxford University Press 2024. DOI: 10.1093/oso/9780192864871.003.0019

This section also outlines the benefits of structured reflective activities; provided carefully, these activities can help students in wide variety of ways. Finally, we touch on the benefits of small acts of kindness within clinical care, both for the student (or doctor) as well as for the patient.

Part 1: An Overview of New Zealand Medical Students' Wellbeing

Medical Training in New Zealand

With a population of 5 million, New Zealand has just two medical schools; one at the University of Auckland and another at the University of Otago (based primarily in Dunedin, South Island). Each year, these schools admit approximately 550-580 new students between them from a range of backgrounds including school leavers, postgraduates, international students and 'other' categories, designed to address equity concerns and increase Māori and Pacifica health professionals in the NZ workforce (Curtis et al., 2012). Medical training takes 5 years, and similar to medical education in the US and UK, is largely divided into pre-clinical (medical theory, case-based learning, communication and examination skills) and clinical phases (primary and secondary care attachments around the country) (Perez et al., 2009). In the final apprenticeship year as 'Trainee Interns', students have supervised clinical responsibilities and receive a small stipend.

The New Zealand Social Context

New Zealand is a bicultural society, with Māori and non-Māori in a partnership underpinned by a foundational treaty (Te Tiriti O Waitangi) which acknowledges that Māori are tangata whenua (the people of the land). Therefore, Māori concepts of health are central to any discussion of wellbeing in New Zealand, although in stating this we acknowledge that complexities of the Māori perspective are beyond the scope of this writing. Te Whare Tapa Wha is a holistic model of Māori health (Durie, 1985), with the dimensions of wellbeing depicted as the base and walls of a house. At the foundation is 'whenua', signifying connection to land and roots, with the walls being the constructs of health: Te Taha Wairua (spiritual), Te Taha Tinana (physical), Te Taha Whānau (family and social groups), and Te Taha Hinengaro (mental and emotional) dimensions. All these aspects work together to support the wellbeing of persons or groups of people. Similarities can be found when looking at wellbeing beliefs underlying the Pacific Island communities living in New Zealand (Pulotu-Endemann & Faleafa, 2017).

One of the main differences when comparing these beliefs to the standard biomedical model in Western society is that of connection (often referred to as 'whakawhanaungatanga'—building meaningful connections with others). In Māori models and across many eastern philosophies, there is more emphasis on connection with others, with all the parts of yourself as one, and with the land. The Māori word, whenua, means both 'land' and 'placenta', and it is common after birth for the placenta to be buried in land with ancestral significance, reinforcing the concept of 'coming from the land and returning to the land', with the living generation being regarded as the land's temporary guardians.

With respect to wellbeing, the 'Meihana' model incorporates such wider cultural and social impacts on personal and cultural health (Pitama et al., 2014). In this model, spirituality, family support, physical health, and so on are visualized as parts of a canoe on the ocean. Wider influences of the ocean currents or weather (representing racism, migration, and colonization) may impact the canoe and its journey towards wellbeing. Acknowledging the historical context that impacts on human experience has facilitated institutional initiatives towards individual and collective wellbeing (Huria et al., 2017).

The deep sense of belonging coming from these beliefs contrasts with the often individualistic nature of Western culture, where an emphasis on individualism and self-reliance can also lead to more loneliness and separation. Connection is one of the principal components in Maslow's hierarchy of needs (Hale et al., 2019), and depth of social connection is a positive predictor of psychological wellbeing (Salles et al., 2019).

The importance of connection and prioritizing a sense of community in New Zealand became apparent during the COVID-19 pandemic when the country was invited to be united as a 'team of five million'. The emphasis was on being kind and helping one another through the social and economic pressures. Biculturalism and themes of connection have influenced the mental health of all New Zealanders, including medical students, and is now an integrated feature of undergraduate training at both schools (Huria et al., 2017).

New Zealand Medical Student Wellbeing

Medical students' health and wellbeing have been thoroughly researched around the world, with their mental health continuing to be of concern (Rotenstein et al., 2016). Students suffer from higher rates of psychological difficulties, burnout, and substance misuse than those in the general population (Dyrbye et al., 2014; Maser et al., 2019; Moir et al., 2022). Although specific issues may be more prevalent in certain countries (Molodynski et al., 2021), the causes of student distress and the consequences arising from such distress are consistently similar. We attribute this observation to the remarkable uniformity of biomedical training; the key factor is being socialized into medical culture, a transitional and enculturation process with particular challenges (Hafferty, 1991; Slavin, 2016).

Local research has confirmed that the mental wellbeing of NZ students is similar to those in medical schools in other countries, with high rates of depression (Moir et al., 2018b), substance abuse (cannabis and alcohol) and burnout (Farrell et al., 2019). Mental distress and burnout appear to increase in the clinical phase of training (Dyrbye et al., 2005; Moir et al., 2022). A 2019 consensus statement from educators in both New Zealand and Australia noted the worsening statistics on the health and wellbeing of local students (Kemp et al., 2019), despite Australian Medical Council recommendations to address these issues more directly.

In terms of research into students' 'quality of life', low scores have been associated with high levels of verbal or covert harassment, while higher scores have been associated with higher levels of perceived social support (Henning et al., 2022). Medical students may also feel considerable stigma if they acknowledge or demonstrate personal distress (Lyons et al., 2015). International students appear to be more prone to negative stigma and are less likely to have their own GP. Stigma and concerns about confidentiality appear to increase the barriers to seeking help (Clement et al., 2015).

Minority student groups are also at higher risk of psychological adjustment, isolation, and mental ill-health (Henning et al., 2012). In the last 2 years, COVID-19 has further impacted tertiary students' engagement and learning (Dodd et al., 2021), with over two-thirds of medical students reporting that the pandemic had impacted negatively on their mental wellbeing, particularly in terms of 'social connectedness' (Lyons et al., 2020). These findings are congruent with our own observations of students who have felt more isolated, demotivated, and insufficiently supported during the pandemic.

Medical School Initiatives

In recent years, both medical schools have noted increasing numbers of medical students presenting for help with academic or health issues. However, it is not clear if these numbers are due to an increased prevalence of problems, enhanced student awareness, more willingness to seek help (Moir et al., 2022) or a growing confidence amongst the student body in the confidentiality or perceived usefulness of support processes.

Support services have been strengthened within each medical school and at student health and counselling services, including improved access to online counselling. Both universities provide online wellbeing resources and easy-to-find information about how to seek support as well as additional support networks for specific student sub-groups. There are also many student-led initiatives such as peer mentoring, tutoring programmes, and student wellbeing events. Junior doctors often speak at such events, which normalizes 'wellbeing' conversations and provides healthy role-modelling.

Support for pastoral and academic issues is provided by trained faculty and staff with well-defined roles. These support processes are clearly separated from assessment procedures, grades, or fitness-to-practice issues. As needed, students are offered regular confidential support and/or referral options, and staff can act in advocacy roles at end-of-year board reviews as required.

The impact of faculty interactions on student wellbeing cannot be underestimated, as negative interactions (verbal or written), can engender a feeling of persecution and mistrust by students towards the school (Byrnes et al., 2020). Students are then less likely to acknowledge or report on personal or professional difficulties.

Alongside the provision of adequate support, both New Zealand medical schools now include curricular content aiming to improve student wellbeing. Auckland initiated a definitive and longitudinal 'Health and Wellbeing Curriculum' in 2013 within the Personal and Professional Skills Domain (Yielder & Moir, 2016), including Cultural Safety (Curtis et al., 2019). This curriculum is based on a framework known as 'SAFE-DRS' (Self-care skills, Accessing help, Focused attention, Emotional intelligence, Doctor as patient and colleague, Reflective practice, and Stress resistance) (Moir et al., 2018a). Attendance and engagement in the SAFE-DRS curriculum is compulsory and includes examinable components, a reflective portfolio and observation by clinicians of how students are managing their stress on the wards (Yielder and Moir, 2016).

A longitudinal study was conducted during the staggered implementation of this curriculum, demonstrating that the more students were exposed to the SAFE-DRS wellbeing curriculum, the more they were able to recognize distress, be non-drinkers, undertake positive coping mechanisms like mindfulness, and be registered with a GP (Moir et al., 2022). Students are encouraged to consider how the content in SAFE-DRS is relevant for themselves as well as for patients. For example, students' level of physical activity increases the probability of discussing the benefits of exercise with their patients (Moir et al., 2022). This evidence-based curriculum highlights the links between clinicians' personal practices of wellbeing and patients' health (Frank et al., 2000).

To date, Otago has not initiated a distinct health and wellbeing module, led perhaps by an identified faculty member who could further 'champion' these issues within the curriculum. However similar topics to Auckland are included now in tutorials within the pre-clinical phase of training. Wellbeing content includes mindfulness training, mental health first aid, and awareness of issues such as perfectionism and imposter syndrome.

Because the transition to the clinical phase of training is one of the major hurdles in a medical career (Godefrooij et al., 2010; Malau-Aduli et al., 2020; Palmer et al., 2009; Soo et al., 2015), there has been an increased focus in both schools on better preparation for the challenges of clinical practice.

There are now well-developed vertical modules on topics such as palliative care (Heath et al., 2022), including complex concepts like death anxiety (Mannix, 2017) and how to hold conversations about death and dying. Otago includes small group interviews with patients who have been bereaved within the previous year, and since 2008, junior students work as assistant caregivers in nursing homes to gain an initial appreciation of the complexity of clinical environments (Wilson et al., 2019). Pre-clinical attachments such as this may reduce students' anxiety and uncertainty prior to clinical training.

Auckland has developed a specific multimedia suicide prevention resource, which is introduced to students as part of small group teaching and lectures in Year 2 and is available until graduation. This culturally safe series of podcasts and videos includes how to have conversations about suicide, including with a peer (Ng et al., 2022a).

Similarly, pre-clinical teaching on patient safety now includes learning about the inevitability of adverse outcomes and the emerging roles of apology and open disclosure (Leape, 2021). Students evaluate these modules highly, as they are instinctively apprehensive about how to talk to someone with cancer or who is dying, and they dread the idea of harming patients.

Other challenging topics, such as diagnostic uncertainty (Joyce et al., 2018) are covered in order to increase students' confidence in identifying and managing symptoms when no biomedical cause is clear (Aamland et al., 2017; Stone, 2014). Students are also asked to reflect on their own mind-body interactions when considering these topics.

The two schools have also developed a joint 'Student Code of Professional Conduct', which lists the importance of self-care within a medical career. Teaching about professionalism is starting to develop in both schools. Otago provides lectures on 'unprofessionalism', drawing on local incidences of student misbehaviour (e.g. sharing examination details between cohorts, dishonest reporting from electives). Providing students with a better understanding of categories of unprofessional behaviour may help them become more self-aware of stressors and temptations (Mak-van der Vossen et al., 2017; Mak-van der Vossen et al., 2020). These initiatives may initially seem unrelated to wellbeing; however unprofessional behaviour can be a marker of distress within training, noting that student perceptions about what is 'unprofessional' can differ markedly from that of faculty (Reddy et al., 2007).

Within clinical training, both universities provide occasional reflective groups, in Otago as part of the Professional Development module (Wilson et al., 2003), and in Auckland as part of primary care rotations (Lack et al., 2019). Student participation in reflective groups has been shown to improve collaborative skills, increase students' ability for self-reflection and capacity for empathy (Gold et al., 2019). Reflective groups can also enable students to talk honestly about their observations and experiences of clinical practice and workplace culture including negative role-modelling, disruptive clinician behaviours (Villafranca et al., 2017) and observations of adverse clinical outcomes, thereby addressing the 'no talk' rule within medical practice (Noort et al., 2019) about uncomfortable professional issues.

However, neither school has systematically embraced reflective practice or embedded such an approach to student learning and support within their curricular structures as an integrated feature of clinical training.

Both schools have also been tackling wider systemic factors known to impact on student wellbeing, such as moving towards programmatic assessment and pass/fail gradings (Van Der Vleuten et al., 2015; Yielder et al., 2017). Auckland has also implemented an anonymous reporting system known as 'HOTSPOTS', an award-winning initiative[1] which motivates clinical and academic leaders to address bullying, harassment, discrimination, and lack of inclusion or respect of medical students in their clinical placements (Moir, 2021). Implemented in 2019, HOTSPOTS is proving successful in identifying placements which are 'outliers' to expected learning environments. The HOTSPOTS system enables action to be taken where concerns are identified as well as highlighting excellent (safe and inclusive) teaching practices.

Even in this initiative, the power of 'connection to others' is highlighted, as students are urged to report unprofessional behaviours they have experienced themselves or have *witnessed* towards other students. In this way, HOTSPOTS trains students not to be bystanders, but to consider the wellbeing of their peers' alongside their own (Moir, 2021).

A Workplace Wellbeing Framework

As medical student wellbeing can also be considered a 'workplace wellness' issue, a useful approach is to take an established mental health guideline and apply it to the medical school context. For example, *Developing a Workplace Mental Health Strategy: A How-to Guide for Organisations* (2019) has been developed by Beyond Blue, Australia's foremost mental health organization. Guidelines recommend that institutions develop an integrated strategy of initiatives focused on three areas: Promotion, Protection, and Support. This includes the promotion of positive processes in the workplace, 'protection' of those in the workplace (by minimizing risk factors), and provision of and access to support.

Protection and promotion involve early intervention, for instance, by creating an environment that supports good mental health and healthy lifestyles. Initiatives may target specific groups of people, can be applied at certain points during a programme, and may highlight opportunities to recognize and build on strengths and targeting areas of risk. Support should

---

[1] https://safeguard.co.nz/awards/

be available at a variety of levels, as a proactive measure to pre-empt issues, and for those experiencing psychological difficulties.

Beyond Blue recommends seven actions to create a mentally healthy workplace: promote positive mental health, improve understanding, help prevent suicide, combat stigma, address risks and protective factors, foster an anti-bullying culture, and support those with mental health conditions. Some of these are already in place now in New Zealand. These recommendations could be used to map further wellbeing initiatives within a medical programme, including curricular content, extracurricular events, and support services.

In considering the goal of a mentally healthy workplace, it is important to include the wider context of training, as environmental factors may impact on initiatives designed to improve medical students' mental health. These wider factors could be global (e.g. the COVID-19 pandemic), national (e.g. New Zealand's Health and Safety at Work Act 2015) or institutional (policies or procedures within the university or training placement organizations). The clinician wellbeing literature provides mounting evidence that these contextual and organizational factors, including workplace culture (Sheehan & Wilkinson, 2022), need to be addressed alongside upskilling individual faculty and clinical teachers (Dyrbye & Shanafelt, 2016).

Having outlined key issues and highlighted our ongoing concerns about student wellbeing and current initiatives at both medical schools, Part 2 of this chapter will now focus on more conceptual challenges; namely, that of moral distress associated with enculturation into medical training and clinical workforce and how this might be addressed more proactively.

Part 2: The Value of Meaningful Connections in Medical Training

In the second part of this chapter, we explore what we believe is a central issue in wellbeing: how moral distress can contribute to student burnout. We will discuss the importance for students of meaningful work, the power of connection within the student–patient relationship and the value of reflective practice as an antidote to loss of meaning and burnout.

Burnout is a sentinel marker of student wellbeing. In our view, contextual factors that may contribute to student burnout include feeling overwhelmed by the high cognitive load and time demands, not feeling like they can connect with patients adequately, worrying if they have the right attitudes towards patients or aptitude for medical work, or feeling that despite their study, they will never match up to the clinicians who teach them or whom they observe in clinical settings. Self-doubt as described, has clear links to self-criticism, anxiety, and perfectionistic traits, all of which may interact in a vicious cycle (Moir et al., 2020). This adds weight to the argument that burnout may be related to imposter syndrome (Khan, 2021, Parkman, 2016), as it may contribute to a 'low sense of personal accomplishment', one of the three original constructs of burnout (Maslach & Jackson, 1981).

There is still debate about the definition and causes of burnout (Demerouti et al., 2021), although more recently, *moral distress* has been identified one of its' key contributors (Dzeng & Wachter, 2019). While originally described in war veterans, moral distress is an emerging theme in healthcare (AlQahtani et al., 2021; Whitehead et al., 2015), arising especially in the clinical experience of feeling powerless to help. As Dzeng suggests, moral distress results from *'physicians' inability to act in accord with their individual and professional ethical values, due to institutional and societal constraints'* (Dzeng & Wachter, 2019). In the COVID-19 pandemic, moral distress increased as health services and treatments were rationed due to limits of resources.

The consequences of moral distress are extensive, with associated feelings of shame, guilt, damaged self-worth and identity, lack of self-forgiveness, questioning of moral beliefs, and an increase in mental health diagnoses. Negative coping mechanisms such as substance abuse and avoidance of others are common. Self-perceptions can be affected, for instance questioning career choices or losing trust in the institution. It can also negatively impact on medical culture as a whole by increasing cynicism, damaging relationships and reducing spontaneous initiatives or acts of kindness (Dzeng & Wachter, 2019).

Medical students entering clinical placements may experience many forms of moral challenge, as the theory of clinical practice as espoused in the pre-clinical phase may not match with the complexities of the modern health system (Dzeng & Wachter, 2019). In other words, the 'disconcerting reality' of clinical work may create dissonance between their prior expectations and their observations and clinical experiences (Warmington & McColl, 2017).

Furthermore, if what they observe contrasts with their internal values, students may feel complicit by association. Commonly, they do not feel empowered to speak up (Dyrbye et al., 2005), as resisting embedded hierarchical structures can be very challenging (Shaw et al., 2018). Student observations that may contribute to dissonance include patient factors (e.g. patients who cannot be helped (Smith-Han et al., 2016) or who are harmed by healthcare (Vohra et al., 2007), and doctor factors, such as an apparent lack of empathy towards those who are suffering. Students may also witness poor intradisciplinary teamwork, rivalry (Lempp and Seale, 2004) or unprofessional behaviour such as discrimination or bullying. These observations may cause internalized shame (Bynum IV et al., 2020), personal alienation from medical culture and marginalization, especially for minority students (Romanski et al., 2020).

Similarly, Shanafelt and colleagues have drawn attention to 'incongruence' between the espoused values of medicine and some of the tasks and behaviours that are required of practising clinicians (Shanafelt et al., 2019). For example, while 'self-care' of doctors is promoted, doctors' work rosters and lack of sleep or opportunities for exercise reveal that self-care does *not* in fact appear to be valued by their institutions; instead, physicians are expected to be 'superhuman' and their personal health is not considered to be important, despite the well-established links to patient outcomes (Wallace et al., 2009).

In summary, discrepancies between students' prior expectations, the professions' espoused values, and the reality of clinical work can be unsettling, even profoundly disturbing for students (Gaufberg et al., 2010). Figure 19.1 illustrates the pathways from dissonance, to moral distress, to burnout.

Addressing Moral Distress Through Meaningful Contributions to Patient Care

When students first enter the clinical phase of their training, they mainly observe the work of others in hospital, alongside practising their communication and examination skills

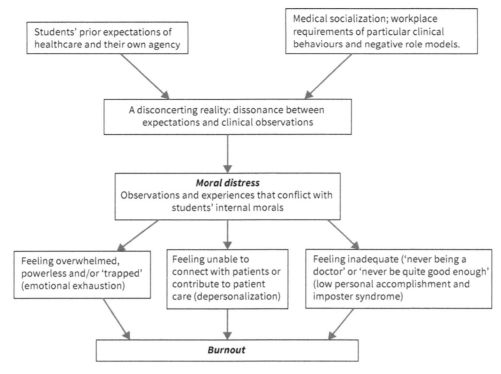

Explanation: *Students' initial clinical experiences can be unsettling, especially if they cannot reconcile what they observe of clinical practice with their prior expectations or values. Feelings of dissonance may match onto constructs of burnout.*

Figure 19.1 Medical students: from moral distress to burnout.

with patients. However because they are unable to contribute directly to patient care, they may feel ambivalence over 'using' patients for their own learning (Warmington & McColl, 2017), and some may even feel alienated from their intended goal of helping people who are suffering.

Medical students are not authorized to make medical decisions about patient care, but some of their learning activities can be specifically designed to enhance their contributions to patient welfare. Authentic and meaningful roles for students, appropriate to their stage of training and professional development, are in fact quite varied (Curry, 2014; Grumbach et al., 2014). In the pre-clinical phase, the value of early clinical experience and 'service learning' is now well-established (Yardley et al., 2013), based not on delivery of medical care, but on learning about patients-as-persons, the illness experience, and patients' journeys through the health system (Helmich et al., 2010; Warmington et al., 2022). Junior students can even contribute to end-of-life care, learning opportunities that they find both powerful and extraordinarily helpful (Wilson & Gilbert-Obrart, 2021).

In the clinical phase of training, there are many opportunities for students to contribute to healthcare that may facilitate an emerging sense of being part of the profession. As Gonzalo et al. suggest, *'value-added learning roles are designed to provide students with opportunities to … [add] value to the healthcare system by legitimately contributing to patient care'* (Gonzalo et al., 2018).

For example, patient navigation clinics enable students to help patients access care through addressing various barriers (Freeman and Rodriguez, 2011). Such clinics help students better understand the patient's perspective and ongoing medical narrative, consistent with patient-centred models of care (Gonzalo et al., 2018). Students can also be trained in motivational interviewing and then engage with patients as health coaches, whether this takes places within hospital centres or in special student clinics. Similarly 'longitudinal integrated clerkships' describe year-long part-time attachments so groups of students can work with a defined cohort of patients with chronic disease or multimorbidity (Norris et al., 2009).

Undertaking such activities can enable students to learn to work directly with patients in an authentic manner within safely defined roles appropriate to their year of training. These activities may provide an antidote to early burnout, as engaging in tasks related to their career choice and having a clear sense of purpose and helpfulness will assist identity formation, while also directly addressing depersonalization, feelings of inadequacy, or 'not belonging' (Cruess et al., 2014).

'Working directly with patients' implies that students are part of a significant relationship; however, to date, the student–patient relationship has not been well theorized in medical education. For example, encouraging students to observe their capacity for engagement (or not) with patients is relatively unusual (Kind et al., 2009). Discussion about the progression of the student–patient relationship to the doctor–patient relationship is beyond the scope of this chapter, although focused reflective activities can help both doctors and students review and enhance their therapeutic relationships, as outlined next.

Reflective Practice

The idea that doctors need to be 'reflective practitioners' is now strongly endorsed by medical councils around the world. During training, most students will mull over or discuss their learning experiences with friends, family, and colleagues. While these informal methods of reflection are helpful, medical schools have increasingly adopted more formal reflective activities within the curriculum over the last 20 years (Sandars, 2009). Reviewing key learning experiences can help students to disentangle their observations of complex interactions within clinical situations, which may drive further learning and self-development. Through experiencing the benefits of reflection, students may embrace habits of reflective practice as a lifelong approach, with advantages for themselves and for patients.

Medical schools now promote reflection in various ways, including reflective writing (Wilson & Ayers, 2004; Yielder & Moir, 2016), small group discussions about student experiences, and individual or group mentoring (Uygur et al., 2019). Reflection needs to be cognizant of student safety and confidentiality in order to support open expression of feelings, responses, dilemmas, and ambivalence about medical training or clinical work. Facilitators of reflective groups must not be involved in grading or assessment of students, as this dual role creates a conflict of interest which can affect students' trust in the process.

The intermediate outcomes from shared reflective discussion can lead to significant clinical and professional outcomes, as outlined in Figure 19.2.

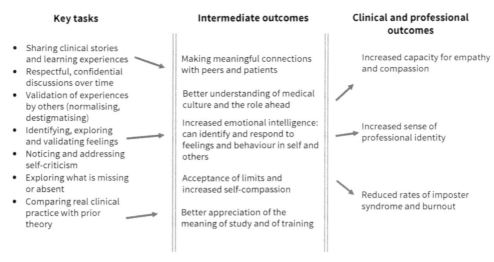

Figure 19.2 Pathways from reflective discussion to clinical and professional outcomes.

Explanation: Well-structured and facilitated reflective groups enable students to share their clinical stories and experiences safely, without fear of being criticized, judged, or of their disclosures impacting on academic grades. Groups need to validate students' experiences (Benitez et al., 2022) *and to identify hidden feelings that may not have been expressed. It is often useful to identify what may have been missing in the clinical environment, such as the patient's perspective or other approaches to the medical issue.*

Group reflection can increase students' sense of being socially connected (Gold et al., 2019) *on a shared journey together, which may reduce feelings of imposter syndrome and destigmatize and normalize experiences. Through multiple shared discussions about challenging clinical situations (e.g. death and dying, unexplained symptoms, negative medical culture), students gain a better understanding of the culture that they are entering* (Gaufberg et al., 2010) *and how to find ways to engage and work within it. Having higher emotional intelligence* (Lindeman et al., 2017) *is helpful, both clinically with patients and with other staff. Empathy is negatively correlated with burnout, i.e. that as the presence of empathy increases, the incidence of burnout decreases* (Wilkinson et al., 2017). *This process can enhance students' sense of autonomy and control, social support, meaning in work, and engagement with organizational culture and values, all of which are known factors in burnout prevention* (Dyrbye & Shanafelt, 2016).

Through these intermediate outcomes, students gain an increased capacity for empathy with other students and their struggles and are more likely to prioritize and feel more comfortable with attempting to understand patients. Cultivating self-compassion is associated with the ability to be more compassionate towards others, going beyond empathy to also include the motivation to act (Neff, 2011).

In brief, regular reflective work increases empathy and compassion, and helps students gain a better sense of who they are in medicine (Sharpless et al., 2015). *An enhanced sense of purpose and identity may also reduce the risk of burnout.*

We believe however, that reflective activities are still underutilized in medical training, including in New Zealand. This observation may also mirror the relatively low uptake of formal reflection by clinicians more generally, who, for example, have low use of regular supportive supervision compared to other health professional groups (Wallbank, 2010). In New Zealand, almost all GPs are members of peer groups, a powerful form of both support and professional development through shared discussion about the challenges of clinical practice (Wilson, 2015), but this is unusual internationally.

Reflective discussion can be usefully focused directly on the doctor– or student–patient relationship. Internationally, the most well-known method is that of 'Balint groups', named after Dr Michael Balint from the UK, who promoted clinical reflective groups after World War II (Balint, 1957). This quite structured approach focuses on challenges in clinical relationships, largely through conjecture and in-depth discussion about the thoughts, feelings and behaviours of doctor and patient in relation to each other (Wilson & Hawken, 2021). Rather than adopting a medical problem-solving approach, participants are encouraged to explore the background to and motivations within significant clinical interactions.

There is increasing evidence that Balint groups are an antidote to burnout (Benson & Magraith, 2005; Monk et al., 2018; Yazdankhahfard et al., 2019) As participants can gain a sense of shared purpose when they have opportunities to discuss the meaning of their work, this outcome may occur with other well-structured methods of group reflection. Moreover, the relief of being authentic, being able to admit to uncertainty and imperfection, and to voice previously unspoken views can reduce feelings of alienation and enhance wellbeing (Kjeldmand & Holmström, 2008).

Balint groups for medical students in the clinical phase of training are now increasingly common in medical schools, especially in the UK and the US. Group leaders or facilitators include GPs, psychiatry registrars, and therapists, usually with supervision from trained Balint leaders. Two recent systematic reviews of research into the outcomes of student Balint groups illustrate how they can help students improve their communication skills and empathy (Yazdankhahfard et al., 2019), become more patient-centred and reduce burnout (Monk et al., 2018).

With respect to the *mechanism of action* within Balint group processes, a recent qualitative analysis of a 5-session student group in Auckland found that it provided students with a 'secure and emotionally resonant experience'. The group appeared to act as 'container' for student vulnerability in their learning, helping them gain a sense of identity within a challenging medical hierarchy (Ng et al., 2022b). In both NZ and Australia however, Balint groups are not provided consistently within training, despite initial promise (O'Neill et al., 2015).

The Role of Meaning and Caring for Others

Returning now to our suggestions about *meaning* as an antidote to student burnout, a key relationship issue for students is how to respond to their own feelings and more powerful emotions, an inevitable feature of healthcare work (McNaughton, 2013). Perhaps this issue is not surprising, given that the foundational principles of modern medicine are based on 'doctor as scientist' or as 'objective observer', implying that students must learn how to 'distance' themselves from patients and to remain 'detached' from their object of study (McWhinney, 1984).

There is insufficient space here to critique the wider implications of the biomedical model (Wilson & Cunningham, 2013), however, these ongoing implicit assumptions contribute to student ambivalence about how to conduct themselves in relation to patients. Students may be torn between wanting to engage on the one hand, versus not wanting to become 'over-involved' on the other (Toon, 2018).

Our contention is that these conceptual tensions can inhibit students from simple acts of kindness towards patients. We are not the first to draw attention to the benefits of compassionate engagement, not just for the patients, but for doctors and medical students themselves. Now supported by modern neuroscience (Goldberg, 2020), being kind and/ or compassionate has proven beneficial outcomes for the giver (Cosley et al., 2010). For example, as Berry et al. suggest, *'the nurturing environment created by extending kindness to others, including co-workers, improves provider wellbeing and can be a potent antidote to physical and emotional exhaustion and burnout'* (Berry et al., 2017).

Others have drawn similar conclusions. Freedy from the US suggests that a *'properly understood and strategically managed doctor–patient relationship promotes patient healing while minimizing physician stress/burnout'* (Freedy, 2021). McKenna et al state that *'the path to enhanced resilience in medical education begins by prioritizing the need for human connection and belonging'* (McKenna et al., 2016). Kind et al assert that *'promoting reflective learning through narrative may help students understand how to make the most of the available resources and ultimately augment their own ability to consistently make connections with families and patients'* (Kind et al., 2009). Finally, Shanafelt states that *'the most sacred and meaningful aspect of medical practice [is] the encounter with the patient and the reward that comes from restoring health and relieving suffering'* (Shanafelt, 2009).

These are consistent messages on the value of engagement, connection, and meaning. The challenge now is to translate these messages into an overall institutional approach to medical training so that students are encouraged to maintain their capacity for kindness and compassion, an approach and an attitude that will be of benefit for themselves as much as for their patients.

Summary

In New Zealand, we have made some progress in identifying the challenges that our medical students encounter, and have attempted to equip students with some initial knowledge and skills. Both schools have well-defined support structures and designated pastoral care staff. However, only one of the schools has an identified faculty champion who leads a carefully designed spiral curriculum that emphasizes the importance of self-care throughout training. This curriculum is mandatory and is assessed, further highlighting the importance that the medical school places on wellbeing. Without such institutional endorsement, however, further progress would be difficult.

Our central message for this chapter is that *meaningful, authentic connection* is one of the keys to enhancing medical students' wellbeing. However at present, we believe there is insufficient role-modelling, opportunities, or specific training on this key feature of training and clinical practice. It would be helpful to focus more on the student–patient relationship and the role of reflective practice, especially in terms of addressing the challenges of training and in gaining a sense of professional identity. Further work is required in terms of overall governance of medical training, curriculum design, and specific learning activities if the next generation of doctors are to optimize their psychological health and quality of life within the culture, demands, and constraints of clinical work.

We began this chapter by highlighting that student wellbeing in New Zealand needs to be viewed from within the wider cultural context. The Māori concept of whakawhanaungatanga is the process of relating well to others by establishing relationships. It encompasses much of what we have discussed—that meaningful connection is at the heart of healing and progress. In building relationships with patients and colleagues, we empower people as partners. This builds trust and respect, enhances roles, legitimacy, expectations, and aspirations, and enables work to be transparent and collaborative. Whakawhanaungatanga reinforces the importance of connection, and is fundamental to the way in which New Zealand graduates approach clinical practice in medical school and beyond.

References

2019. Developing a Workplace Mental Health Strategy: A How-to Guide for Organisations *Heads Up: Better Mental Health in the Workplace*. Melbourne: Beyond Blue.

Aamland, A., Fosse, A., Ree, E., Abildsnes, E., & Malterud, K. (2017). 'Helpful strategies for GPs seeing patients with medically unexplained physical symptoms: a focus group study'. *Brit J Gen Pract* 67: e572–e579.

Alqahtani, R.M., Al Saadon, A., Alarifi, M.I., Muaygil, R., Altaymani, Y.K.M., Elsaid, M.A.M., Alsohime, F., Temsah, M.-H., & Aljerian, K. (2021). 'Moral distress among health care workers in the intensive care unit; a systematic review and meta-analysis'. *J Anesthes Intens Care Emerg Pain Med* 17: 192–202.

Balint, M. (1957). *The Doctor, His Patient, and the Illness*. London: Pitman.

Benitez, C., Howard, K.P., & Cheavens, J.S. (2022). 'The effect of validation and invalidation on positive and negative affective experiences'. *J Pos Psychol* 17: 46–58.

Benson, J. & Magraith, K. (2005). 'Compassion fatigue and burnout: the role of Balint groups'. *Austral Fam Phys* 34: 497–504.

Berry, L.L., Danaher, T.S., Chapman, R.A., & Awdish, R.L. (2017). 'Role of kindness in cancer care'. *J Oncol Pract* 13: 744–750.

Bynum IV, W.E., Varpio, L., Lagoo, J., & Teunissen, P.W. (2020). '"I'm unworthy of being in this space": the origins of shame in medical students'. *Med Educ* 55: 185–197.

Byrnes, C., Ganapathy, V.A., Lam, M., Mogensen, L., & Hu, W. (2020). 'Medical student perceptions of curricular influences on their wellbeing: a qualitative study'. *BMC Med Educ* 20: 1–11.

Clement, S., Schauman, O., Graham, T., Maggioni, F., Evans-Lacko, S., Bezborodovs, N., Morgan, C., Rüsch, N., Brown, J.S., & Thornicroft, G. (2015). 'What is the impact of mental health-related stigma on help-seeking? A systematic review of quantitative and qualitative studies'. *Psychol Med* 45: 11–27.

Cosley, B.J., Mccoy, S.K., Saslow, L.R., & Epel, E.S. (2010). 'Is compassion for others stress buffering? Consequences of compassion and social support for physiological reactivity to stress'. *J Experiment Soc Psychol* 46: 816–823.

Cruess, R.L., Cruess, S.R., Boudreau, J.D., Snell, L., & Steinert, Y. (2014). 'Reframing medical education to support professional identity formation'. *Acad Med* 89: 1446–1451.

Curry, R.H. (2014). 'Meaningful roles for medical students in the provision of longitudinal patient care'. *JAMA* 312: 2335–2336.

Curtis, E., Jones, R., Tipene-Leach, D., Walker, C., Loring, B., Paine, S.-J., & Reid, P. (2019). 'Why cultural safety rather than cultural competency is required to achieve health equity: a literature review and recommended definition'. *Int J Equity Health* 18: 1–17.

Curtis, E., Wikaire, E., Stokes, K., & Reid, P. (2012). 'Addressing indigenous health workforce inequities: a literature review exploring 'best' practice for recruitment into tertiary health programmes'. *Int J Equity Health* 11: 1–15.

Demerouti, E., Bakker, A.B., Peeters, M.C., & Breevaart, K. (2021). 'New directions in burnout research'. *Europ J Work Organizat Psychol* **30**: 686–691.

Dodd, R.H., Dadaczynski, K., Okan, O., Mccaffery, K.J., & Pickles, K. (2021). 'Psychological wellbeing and academic experience of University students in Australia during COVID-19'. *Int J J Environment Res Pub Health* **18**: 866.

Durie, M.H. (1985). 'A Maori perspective of health'. *Soc Sci Med* **20**: 483–486.

Dyrbye, L. & Shanafelt, T. (2016). 'A narrative review on burnout experienced by medical students and residents'. *Med Educ* **50**: 132–149.

Dyrbye, L.N., Thomas, M.R., & Shanafelt, T.D. (2005). 'Medical student distress: causes, consequences, and proposed solutions'. *Mayo Clin Proceed* **80**: 1613–1622.

Dyrbye, L.N., West, C.P., Satele, D., Boone, S., Tan, L., Sloan, J., & Shanafelt, T.D. (2014). 'Burnout among US medical students, residents, and early career physicians relative to the general US population'. *Acad Med* **89**: 443–451.

Dzeng, E. & Wachter, R.M. (2019). 'Ethics in conflict: moral distress as a root cause of burnout'. *JGIM* **35**: 409–411.

Farrell, S.M., Moir, F., Molodynski, A., & Bhugra, D. (2019). 'Psychological wellbeing, burnout and substance use amongst medical students in New Zealand'. *Int Rev Psychiatry* **31**: 630–636.

Frank, E., Breyan, J., & Elon, L. (2000). 'Physician disclosure of healthy personal behaviors improves credibility and ability to motivate'. *Arch Fam Med* **9**: 287.

Freedy, J.R. (2021). 'Relationship integrity and well-being: our shared humanity matters'. *Int J Psychiatry Med* **56**: 131–135.

Freeman, H.P., & Rodriguez, R.L. (2011). 'History and principles of patient navigation'. *Cancer* **117**: 3537–3540.

Gaufberg, E.H., Batalden, M., Sands, R., & Bell, S.K. (2010). 'The hidden curriculum: what can we learn from third-year medical student narrative reflections?'. *Acad Med* **85**: 1709–1716.

Godefrooij, M.B., Diemers, A.D., & Scherpbier, A.J. (2010). 'Students' perceptions about the transition to the clinical phase of a medical curriculum with preclinical patient contacts; a focus group study'. *BMC Med Educ* **10**: 28.

Gold, J.A., Bentzley, J.P., Franciscus, A.M., Forte, C., & De Golia, S.G. (2019). 'An intervention in social connection: medical student reflection groups'. *Acad Psychiatry* **43**: 375–380.

Goldberg, M.J. (2020). 'Compassionate care: making it a priority and the science behind it'. *J Ped Orth* **40**: S4–S7.

Gonzalo, J.D., Wolpaw, D., Graaf, D., & Thompson, B.M. (2018). 'Educating patient-centered, systems-aware physicians: a qualitative analysis of medical student perceptions of value-added clinical systems learning roles'. *BMC Med Educ* **18**: 1–7.

Grumbach, K., Lucey, C.R., & Johnston, S.C. (2014). 'Transforming from centers of learning to learning health systems: the challenge for academic health centers'. *JAMA* **311**: 1109–1110.

Hafferty, F.W. (1991). *Into the Valley: Death and the Socialization of Medical Students*. New Haven: Yale University Press.

Hale, A.J., Ricotta, D.N., Freed, J., Smith, C.C., & Huang, G.C. (2019). 'Adapting Maslow's hierarchy of needs as a framework for resident wellness'. *Teach Learn Med* **31**: 109–118.

Heath, L., Egan, R., Iosua, E., Walker, R., Ross, J., & Macleod, R. (2022). 'Palliative and end of life care in undergraduate medical education: a survey of New Zealand medical schools'. *BMC Med Educ* **22**: 1–8.

Helmich, E., Derksen, E., Prevoo, M., Laan, R., Bolhuis, S., & Koopmans, R. (2010). 'Medical students' professional identity development in an early nursing attachment'. *Med Educ* **44**: 674–682.

Henning, M.A., Krägeloh, C., Moir, F., Doherty, I., & Hawken, S.J. (2012). 'Quality of life: international and domestic students studying medicine in New Zealand'. *Perspect Med Educ* **1**: 129–142.

Henning, M.A., Stonyer, J., Chen, Y., Hove, B.A.-T., Moir, F., Coomber, T., & Webster, C.S. (2022). 'Medical students' quality of life and its association with harassment and social support'. *Med Sci Educ* **32**: 165–174.

Huria, T., Palmer, S., Beckert, L., Lacey, C., & Pitama, S. (2017). 'Indigenous health: designing a clinical orientation program valued by learners'. *BMC Med Educ* **17**: 1–8.

Joyce, E., Cowing, J., Lazarus, C., Smith, C., Zenzuck, V., & Peters, S. (2018). 'Training tomorrow's doctors to explain 'medically unexplained' physical symptoms: an examination of UK medical educators' views of barriers and solutions'. *Pat Educ Couns* **101**: 878–884.

Kemp, S., Hu, W., Bishop, J., Forrest, K., Hudson, J. N., Wilson, I., Teodorczuk, A., Rogers, G.D., Roberts, C., & Wearn, A. (2019). 'Medical student wellbeing–a consensus statement from Australia and New Zealand'. *BMC Med Educ* **19**: 1–8.

Khan, M. (2021). 'Imposter syndrome—a particular problem for medical students'. *BMJ* **375**: n3048.

Kind, T., Everett, V.R., & Ottolini, M. (2009). 'Learning to connect: students' reflections on doctor-patient interactions'. *Pat Educ Couns* **75**: 149–154.

Kjeldmand, D. & Holmström, I. (2008). 'Balint groups as a means to increase job satisfaction and prevent burnout among general practitioners'. *Ann Fam Med* **6**: 138–145.

Lack, L., Yielder, J., & Goodyear-Smith, F. (2019). 'Evaluation of a compulsory reflective group for medical students'. *J Prim Health Care* **11**: 227–234.

Leape, L.L. (2021). *A Conspiracy of Silence: Disclosure Disclosure, Apology Apology, and Restitution*. New York: Springer.

Lempp, H. & Seale, C. (2004). 'The hidden curriculum in undergraduate medical education: qualitative study of medical students' perceptions of teaching'. *BMJ* **329**: 770–773.

Lindeman, B., Petrusa, E., Mckinley, S., Hashimoto, D.A., Gee, D., Smink, D.S., Mullen, J.T., & Phitayakorn, R. (2017). 'Association of burnout with emotional intelligence and personality in surgical residents: can we predict who is most at risk?' *J Surg Educ* **74**: e22–e30.

Lyons, Z., Laugharne, J., Laugharne, R., & Appiah-Poku, J. (2015). 'Stigma towards mental illness among medical students in Australia and Ghana'. *Acad Psychiat* **39**: 305–308.

Lyons, Z., Wilcox, H., Leung, L., & Dearsley, O. (2020). 'COVID-19 and the mental well-being of Australian medical students: impact, concerns and coping strategies used'. *Australas Psychiatry* **28**: 649–652.

Mak-Van Der Vossen, M., Teherani, A., Van Mook, W., Croiset, G., & Kusurkar, R.A. (2020). 'How to identify, address and report students' unprofessional behaviour in medical school'. *Med Teach* **42**: 372–379.

Mak-Van Der Vossen, M., Van Mook, W., Van Der Burgt, S., Kors, J., Ket, J.C., Croiset, G., & Kusurkar, R. (2017). 'Descriptors for unprofessional behaviours of medical students: a systematic review and categorisation'. *BMC Med Educ* **17**: 164.

Malau-Aduli, B.S., Roche, P., Adu, M., Jones, K., Alele, F., & Drovandi, A. (2020). 'Perceptions and processes influencing the transition of medical students from pre-clinical to clinical training'. *BMC Med Educ* **20**: 1–13.

Mannix, K. (2017). *With the End in Mind: Dying, Death, and Wisdom in an Age of Denial*. London: William Collins.

Maser, B., Danilewitz, M., Guérin, E., Findlay, L., & Frank, E. (2019). 'Medical student psychological distress and mental illness relative to the general population: a Canadian cross-sectional survey'. *Acad Med* **94**: 1781–1791.

Maslach, C. & Jackson, S.E. (1981). 'The measurement of experienced burnout'. *J Org Behav* **2**: 99–113.

Mckenna, K.M., Hashimoto, D.A., Maguire, M.S., & Bynum, W.E. (2016). 'The missing link: connection is the key to resilience in medical education'. *Acad Med* **91**: 1197–1199.

Mcnaughton, N. (2013). 'Discourse (s) of emotion within medical education: the ever-present absence'. *Med Educ* **47**: 71–79.

Mcwhinney, I.R. (1984). 'Changing models: the impact of Kuhn's theory on medicine'. *Fam Pract*, **1**, 3–8.

Moir, F. (2021). Hotspots: The Development, Implementation and Outcomes of the First Year of an Anti-Bullying Initiative in the Auckland Medical Programme. *International Conference on Physician Health: A Vision for Humanity in Medicine*. London.

Moir, F., Patten, B., Yielder, J., Sohn, C., Maser, B., & Frank, E. (2022). 'Trends in medical students' health over 5 years: does a wellbeing curriculum make a difference?'. *Int J Soc Psychiat*.

Moir, F., Van Den Brink, R., & Arroll, B. (2020). Self-compassion in primary care: a powerful tool for patients and practitioners. In: Charlton, R. (ed) *New Perspectives in Compassion for Tomorrow's Doctors*. London: SAPC Special Interest Group in Compassion.

Moir, F., Yielder, J., Dixon, H., & Hawken, S. (2018a). 'SAFE-DRS: Health and wellbeing in the curriculum in the Auckland Medical Programme'. *Int J Innovat Creativity Change* 4: 49–64.

Moir, F., Yielder, J., Sanson, J., & Chen, Y. (2018b). 'Depression in medical students: current insights'. *Adv Med Educ Pract* 9: 323.

Molodynski, A., Lewis, T., Kadhum, M., Farrell, S.M., Lemtiri Chelieh, M., Falcão de Almeida, T., Masri, R., Kar, A., Volpe, U., & Moir, F. (2021). 'Cultural variations in wellbeing, burnout and substance use amongst medical students in twelve countries'. *Int Rev Psychiat* 33: 37–42.

Monk, A., Hind, D., & Crimlisk, H. (2018). 'Balint groups in undergraduate medical education: a systematic review'. *Psychoanalytic Psychotherapy* 32: 61–86.

Neff, K.D. (2011). 'Self-compassion, self-esteem, and well-being'. *Soc Pers Psychol Comp* 5: 1–12.

Ng, L., Datt, A., Moir, F., Hakiaha, H., O'Callaghan, A., Lampshire, D., Tennant, G., Henry, J., & Wearn, A. (2022a). 'Medical students' evaluation of a suicide prevention multimedia resource: a focus group study'. *Int J Social Psychiatry,* In Press.

Ng, L., Seu, C., & Cullum, S. (2022b). 'Modelling vulnerability: qualitative study of the Balint process for medical students'. *BMC Med Educ* 22: 1–6.

Noort, M.C., Reader, T.W., & Gillespie, A. (2019). 'Speaking up to prevent harm: A systematic review of the safety voice literature'. *Safety Science* 117: 375–387.

Norris, T., Schaad, D., Dewitt, D., Ogur, B., & Hunt, D. (2009). 'Consortium of Longitudinal Integrated Clerkships. Longitudinal integrated clerkships for medical students: an innovation adopted by medical schools in Australia, Canada, South Africa, and the United States'. *Acad Med* 84: 902–907.

O'Neill, S., Foster, K., & Gilbert-Obrart, A. (2015). The Balint group experience for medical students: a pilot project. *Psychoanalytic Psychotherapy*, 1–13.

Palmer, M., O'Kane, P., & Owens, M. (2009). 'Betwixt spaces: Student accounts of turning point experiences in the first-year transition'. *Stud High Educ* 34: 37–54.

Parkman, A. (2016). 'The imposter phenomenon in higher education: incidence and impact'. *J High Educ Theory Pract* 16: 51.

Perez, D., Rudland, J., & Wilson, H. (2009). 'The revised Early Learning in Medicine curriculum at the University of Otago – focusing on students, patients, and the community'. *NZ Med J* 1292.

Pitama, S., Huria, T., & Lacey, C. (2014). 'Improving Māori health through clinical assessment: Waikare o te Waka o Meihana'. *NZ Med J* 127: 107–119.

Pulotu-Endemann, F.K. & Faleafa, M. (2017). Developing a culturally competent workforce that meets the needs of Pacific people living in New Zealand. In: Smith, M. & Jury, A. (eds) *Workforce Development Theory and Practice in the Mental Health Sector*. New York: IGI Global.

Reddy, S.T., Farnan, J.M., Yoon, J.D., Leo, T., Upadhyay, G.A., Humphrey, H.J., & Arora, V.M. (2007). 'Third-year medical students' participation in and perceptions of unprofessional behaviors'. *Acad Med* 82: S35–S39.

Romanski, P.A., Bartz, D., Pelletier, A., & Johnson, N.R. (2020). 'The "Invisible Student": neglect as a form of medical student mistreatment, a call to action'. *J Surg Educ* 77: 1327–1330.

Rotenstein, L.S., Ramos, M.A., Torre, M., Segal, J.B., Peluso, M.J., Guille, C., Sen, S., & Mata, D.A. (2016). 'Prevalence of depression, depressive symptoms, and suicidal ideation among medical students: a systematic review and meta-analysis'. *JAMA* 316: 2214–2236.

Salles, A., Wright, R.C., Milam, L., Panni, R.Z., Liebert, C.A., Lau, J.N., Lin, D.T., & Mueller, C.M. (2019). 'Social belonging as a predictor of surgical resident well-being and attrition'. *J Surg Educ* 76: 370–377.

Sandars, J. (2009). 'The use of reflection in medical education: AMEE Guide No. 44'. *Med Teach* 31: 685–695.

Shanafelt, T.D. (2009). 'Enhancing meaning in work: a prescription for preventing physician burnout and promoting patient-centered care'. *JAMA* 302: 1338–1340.

Shanafelt, T.D., Schein, E., Minor, L.B., Trockel, M., Schein, P., & Kirch, D. (2019). 'Healing the professional culture of medicine'. *Mayo Clin Proc* 94: 1556–1566.

Sharpless, J., Baldwin, N., Cook, R., Kofman, A., Morley-Fletcher, A., Slotkin, R., & Wald, H.S. (2015). 'The becoming: students' reflections on the process of professional identity formation in medical education'. *Acad Med* 90: 713–717.

Shaw, M.K., Rees, C.E., Andersen, N.B., Black, L.F., & Monrouxe, L.V. (2018). 'Professionalism lapses and hierarchies: a qualitative analysis of medical students' narrated acts of resistance'. *Soc Sci Med* **219**: 45–53.

Sheehan, D. & Wilkinson, T.J. (2022). 'Widening how we see the impact of culture on learning, practice and identity development in clinical environments'. *Med Educ* **56**: 110–116.

Slavin, S.J. (2016). 'Medical student mental health: culture, environment, and the need for change'. *JAMA* **316**: 2195–2196.

Smith-Han, K., Martyn, H., Barrett, A., & Nicholson, H. (2016). '"That's not what you expect to do as a doctor, you know, you don't expect your patients to die." Death as a learning experience for undergraduate medical students'. *BMC Med Educ* **16**: 108.

Soo, J., Brett-Maclean, P., Cave, M.-T., & Oswald, A. (2015). 'At the precipice: a prospective exploration of medical students' expectations of the pre-clerkship to clerkship transition'. *Adv Health Sci Educ*, 1–22.

Stone, L. (2014). 'Blame, shame and hopelessness: medically unexplained symptoms and the 'heartsink' experience'. *Austral Fam Phys* **43**: 191–195.

Toon, P. (2018). Attachment, detachment and indifference in clinical practice. In: Carr, D. (ed) *Cultivating Moral Character and Virtue in Professional Practice*. London: Routledge.

Uygur, J., Stuart, E., De Paor, M., Wallace, E., Duffy, S., O'Shea, M., Smith, S., & Pawlikowska, T. (2019). 'A best evidence in medical education systematic review to determine the most effective teaching methods that develop reflection in medical students: BEME Guide No. 51'. *Med Teach* **41**: 3–16.

Van Der Vleuten, C.P., Schuwirth, L., Driessen, E., Govaerts, M., & Heeneman, S. (2015). 'Twelve tips for programmatic assessment'. *Med Teach* **37**: 641–646.

Villafranca, A., Hamlin, C., Enns, S., & Jacobsohn, E. (2017). 'Disruptive behaviour in the perioperative setting: a contemporary review'. *Can J Anesth* **64**: 128–140.

Vohra, P.D., Johnson, J.K., Daugherty, C.K., Wen, M., & Barach, P. (2007). 'Housestaff and medical student attitudes toward medical errors and adverse events'. *Jt Comm J Qual Patient Saf* **33**: 493–501.

Wallace, J.E., Lemaire, J.B., & Ghali, W.A. (2009). 'Physician wellness: a missing quality indicator'. *Lancet* **374**: 1714–1721.

Wallbank, S. (2010). 'Effectiveness of individual clinical supervision for midwives and doctors in stress reduction: findings from a pilot study'. *Evidence Based Midwif* **8**: 65–71.

Warmington, S., Johansen, M.-L., & Wilson, H. (2022). 'Identity construction in medical student stories about experiences of disgust in early nursing home placements: a dialogical narrative analysis'. *BMJ Open* **12**: e051900.

Warmington, S. & Mccoll, G. (2017). 'Medical student stories of participation in patient care-related activities: the construction of relational identity'. *Adv Health Sci Educ* **22**: 147–163.

Whitehead, P.B., Herbertson, R.K., Hamric, A.B., Epstein, E.G., & Fisher, J.M. (2015). 'Moral distress among healthcare professionals: report of an institution-wide survey'. *J Nurs Schol* **47**: 117–125.

Wilkinson, H., Whittington, R., Perry, L., & Eames, C. (2017). 'Examining the relationship between burnout and empathy in healthcare professionals: a systematic review'. *Burnout Res* **6**: 18–29.

Wilson, H. (2015). 'Challenges in the doctor–patient relationship: 12 tips for more effective peer group discussion'. *J Prim Health Care* **7**: 260–263.

Wilson, H. & Cunningham, W. (2013). *Being a Doctor: Understanding Medical Practice*, Dunedin: Otago University Press.

Wilson, H., Egan, T., & Friend, R. (2003). 'Teaching professional development in undergraduate medical education'. *Med Educ* **37**: 482–483.

Wilson, H. & Gilbert-Obrart, A. (2021). Into the darkness: medical student essays on first experiences of the dying patient. *J Prim Health Care* **13**: 293–301.

Wilson, H. & Hawken, S. (2021). The doctor–patient relationship. In: Morris, K. (ed) *Cole's Medical Practice in New Zealand*, 14th ed. Wellington: Medical Council of New Zealand.

Wilson, H., Warmington, S., & Johansen, M.L. (2019). 'Experience-based learning: junior medical students' reflections on end-of-life care'. *Med Educ* **53**: 687–697.

Wilson, H.J., & Ayers, K.M. (2004). 'Using significant event analysis in dental and medical education'. *J Dent Educ* **68**: 446–453.

Yardley, S., Brosnan, C., & Richardson, J. (2013). 'The consequences of authentic early experience for medical students: creation of mētis'. *Med Educ* **47**: 109–119.

Yazdankhahfard, M., Haghani, F., & Omid, A. (2019). 'The Balint group and its application in medical education: a systematic review'. *J Educ Health Prom*, 8.

Yielder, J., & Moir, F. (2016). 'Assessing the development of medical students' personal and professional skills by portfolio'. *J Med Educ Curric Dev* **3**: JMECD. S30110.

Yielder, J., Wearn, A., Chen, Y., Henning, M. A., Weller, J., Lillis, S., Mogol, V., & Bagg, W. (2017). 'A qualitative exploration of student perceptions of the impact of progress tests on learning and emotional wellbeing'. *BMC Med Educ* **17**: 1–10.

20
Nigeria

Mental Health of Medical Students

Olatunde Ayinde and Oye Gureje

Introduction

It is now widely accepted that the medical profession is one that is fraught with exposure to high levels of work-related stressors, with a significant burden of psychiatric morbidity, including burnout and suicidal behaviour commonly reported among its practitioners (Brooks et al., 2011; Harvey et al., 2021). There are indications that this exposure to occupational stressors and the associated mental health burden may have begun during undergraduate medical training. There is strong evidence for elevated levels of medical training-related stressors and psychiatric morbidity among medical students in both high and low-and-middle-income countries (Dyrbye et al., 2006; Esan et al., 2019; Hope & Henderson, 2014; Kadhum et al., 2022; Molodynski et al., 2021). This has led to calls for action from stakeholders involved at all levels of regulating medical education to reverse the trend (Dyrbye & Shanafelt, 2011; Molodynski et al., 2019).

While interest in the mental health of medical students has been increasing and efforts to institutionalize interventions for this vulnerable population are gaining momentum in high-income countries, the same cannot be said for countries in the Global South. Using Nigeria as an example, while there is a growing body of research on the mental health and wellbeing of medical students in Nigeria (Esan et al., 2019), very little has happened in terms of coordinated institutionalized efforts to address the problem. Responding to the challenge of medical students' mental health would necessitate an understanding of the socioeconomic and health system contexts of medical education, as well as the current state of the mental health of medical students in Nigeria. In this chapter, we attempt to highlight this and examine the current local initiatives geared towards maintaining optimal mental health of medical students. We also discuss how local initiatives align with and measure up to global standard practice, and offer some suggestions for addressing medical students' mental wellbeing in Nigeria.

The Broader Context

Nigeria is a low-middle-income country located on the West Coast of Africa, with a population of about 225 million and real per capita GDP of 4,900 dollars (Central Intelligence Agency, 2021). Important health indicators include: life expectancy of 54.5 years, maternal

Olatunde Ayinde and Oye Gureje, *Nigeria* In: *The Mental Health of Medical Students*. Edited by: Andrew Molodynski, Sarah Marie Farrell, and Dinesh Bhugra, Oxford University Press. © Oxford University Press 2024. DOI: 10.1093/oso/9780192864871.003.0020 mortality ratio of 814 per 100,000, and under-5 mortality rate of 108.8 per 1000 live births (WHO, 2018). Lifetime prevalence of mental disorders is 12.1%, and 80% of Nigerians with severe mental disorders do not receive any treatment in the preceding year (Gureje, 2006; Wang et al., 2007). As at 2014, Nigeria spent only 3.67% of her GDP on health, and only about 3% of this was spent on mental health. Out-of-pocket payment is the predominant mode of payment for health (70% of total health expenditure) (Olanrewaju et al; 2021). Physician, psychiatrist, and psychiatric nurse densities are 0.376, 0.15, and 2.41 per 100,000, respectively, and there are even fewer psychologists, social workers, and occupational therapists (WHO & FMOH, 2006; WHO, 2018). In a nutshell, the Nigerian health system is characterized by unacceptably poor health indices, a large treatment gap for mental disorders and severe general and mental health resource constraints. This has implications for addressing the mental health of medical students.

It is also pertinent to mention two socio-political threats to the health system that have potential implications for medical education and the mental wellbeing of medical students in Nigeria. One of these is the incessant industrial strike action by university teachers and medical doctors, often to protest the deplorable state of the health and education systems in the country. This has the effect of unnecessarily prolonging the duration of medical training and introducing more hardships into an already stressful programme. In addition, the COVID-19 pandemic has also contributed to a major disruption to university education in Nigeria, with a significant impact on medical education and medical students.

The second threat to medical education in the country is the increasing rate of brain drain occurring in the health sector. In recent years, the poor state of the economy, among other factors, has contributed to an unprecedented exodus of medical practitioners out of Nigeria. Of the 80,000 doctors who completed their training and registered to practice in Nigeria, less than half currently practice in the country (Ezigbo, 2022). Nigeria is therefore losing many people who are qualified to serve as medical teachers to well-resourced countries, and this has implications for the resilience and quality of medical education in Nigeria. It is possible that the growing uncertainty in the health sector might be a source of significant worry for medical students who would be joining the sector soon.

Medical School Setting in Nigeria

University-based medical education in Nigeria commenced formally with the establishment of the medical school at the University of Ibadan in the late 1940s (Brown, 1961). With time, other medical schools were established across the country, and as of March 2022 there are about 45 medical and dental schools in Nigeria (MDCN, 2022), graduating between 3,000 and 3,500 doctors every year (Ezigbo, 2022).

In Nigeria, Medicine and Surgery is a straight 6-year undergraduate course resulting in the award of the Bachelor of Medicine and Bachelor of Surgery degree. A typical medical education consists of a pre-medical stage where students take courses in the pure sciences, followed by preclinical stage where students take courses in Anatomy, Physiology, and Biochemistry. Typically, the pre-medical and pre-clinical schools are located within the general university campus while the clinical school is located within the complex of the affiliated teaching hospital. For example, at the University of Ibadan, the pre-medical and preclinical schools are within the larger university campus and the Clinical School is located within the University

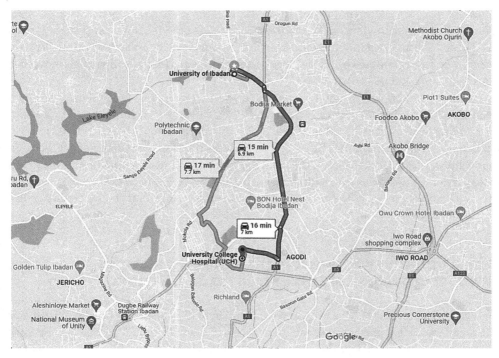

Figure 20.1   University of Ibadan and University College Hospital, Ibadan, Nigeria.

College Hospital (UCH) Complex located about 7 km away (see Figure 20.1). There are student hostels providing accommodation for medical students at both locations.

The State of Medical Students' Mental Health and Wellbeing in Nigeria

There is good evidence that the burden of mental health morbidity among medical students in Nigeria is high. In our recent study among 505 medical students drawn from 25 medical schools in Nigeria, we reported that, prior to entering medical school, 5% of the students had consulted a General Practitioner or other mental health practitioners regarding their mental health, and about 2% of them had received a diagnosis of a mental disorder (Ayinde et al., 2022). Although we found the prevalence of psychological distress of 54.5% among the students, only 5.7% of them admitted to having received a formal mental health diagnosis whilst at medical school, with most of the diagnoses being common mental disorders. Despite this high prevalence of psychological distress, only 4.2% of the students were currently seeing a GP or mental health professional, with 2.6% of them admitting to currently being on psychotropic medications.

Regarding alcohol and substance use, 5% of the students screened positive on the CAGE questionnaire (Ewing, 1984). The only substance, apart from alcohol, that had been used by a sizeable proportion of the students was cannabis (6%). One in seven students reported being worried about their own substance use. Regarding burnout as measured with the Oldenburg

Burnout Inventory (Demerouti et al., 2003), 84.6% of the students met specified case criteria for the disengagement domain, and 77.0% met specified criteria for the exhaustion domain of the tool. The most commonly reported sources of significant stress among the medical students were study (reported by 75.6%), money (52.3%), relationships (intimate/family, such as missing them), and housing (7.1%).

A systematic review of studies conducted in Nigeria (Esan et al., 2019) showed a similar pattern of elevated levels of stressors, perceived stress, psychiatric morbidity, and substance use among medical students. This pattern is also similar to what has been observed in other countries, across different income categories. There is therefore little doubt about the commonality of the burden. However, though there are global similarities in the pattern of risks and psychiatric morbidity across different settings, there are also peculiarities in context and resource availability in different settings. Hence, interventions must be tailored to reflect these differences.

Local Initiatives Addressing the Mental Health and Wellbeing of Medical Students in Ibadan, Nigeria

It is difficult to make sweeping general statements about the initiatives in all medical schools in Nigeria to address medical students' mental health and wellbeing. A convenient approach therefore would be to adopt one medical school in Nigeria to illustrate what obtains in a typical medical school in the country. For this exercise, we choose the University of Ibadan owing to our familiarity with its medical school.

There is no mental health policy for students generally at the University of Ibadan, neither is there for medical students specifically. However, there are two policies in existence that have some bearing on mental health: the gender policy and sexual harassment policy (University of Ibadan, 2022). The first policy seeks to create a gender-sensitive university environment where staff and students are not disadvantaged or discriminated against as a result of their gender, while the other seeks to protect members of the university community from sexual harassment and related issues. However, students' wellbeing features prominently in activities of the university at large and the College of Medicine. For example, the yearly orientation ceremony of new students at the university now includes a mental health talk. Among the stressors reported by medical and dental students in our study and previous studies, financial problems, and accommodation feature prominently. In response to the problem associated with students' accommodation and as part of its overall vision for infrastructural development, the college of medicine recently embarked on a massive fund-raising drive to construct new hostels to ease accommodation problems. Similarly, the college Sponsor-a-Student programme solicits for financial help, mainly from alumni and friends of the college, to support students in need for the entire duration of their undergraduate years. In addition, the college has been liaising with alumni of the college to help with the continued maintenance of hostel and learning facilities over the years. Recently, the alumni of the university collaborated with the college management to organize a community-wide open discussion of one of the common problems in the medical school: students' maltreatment and bullying. Finally, a students' mentoring programme exists within the college, where students are assigned to faculty mentors who can serve as the first port of call for students undergoing difficulties in their student life.

Another emerging area of attention in the college is curriculum design. Although mental health promotion and prevention is not one of its stated objectives, it is now being advocated that the MBBS curriculum revision exercise at the college should take place in 5-year cycles, with plans included to integrate learning across the clinical and preclinical schools, reduce work burden and duplication, as well as improve students' learning experience (Omigbodun, 2020).

A youth-friendly centre being run by the Department of Guidance and Counselling exists within the larger University campus to address students' problems in their personal and academic life. A more structured version of this service exists at the Clinical School. The counselling unit of the College of Medicine in Ibadan was established in 2021 to cater for the wellbeing of students at the college, including medical students. Currently, the unit is being run on a day-to-day basis by a full-time member of staff with a Masters' degree in Child and Adolescent Mental Health. Specialists such as psychiatrists, psychologists, social workers, and other allied professionals in mental health can be called upon at short notice to provide care when needed. The design and operation of the centre are based on the needs of the staff and student community as demonstrated by formative research conducted before commencing operations. Services provided range from addressing psychosocial and emotional problems as well as referral of persons with overt psychopathology to appropriate services when indicated. The unit also maintains a helpline where students can call in or send in distress messages via emails or via social media when they need emergency help. By a special arrangement between the unit and the department of psychiatry at the hospital, students can also call the psychiatry registrar on call directly in cases of emergencies such as a suicide attempt. The unit organizes community-wide mental health promotional and preventive activities, including webinars and mental health promotional messages on student dominated social media, routinely and during times of shared community stress such as during examinations and other widespread events (e.g. at the height of the COVID-19 pandemic in Nigeria), and organizes group counselling in times of community losses (e.g. loss of a student).

A staff clinic situated within the university complex caters to the health of both staff and students of the university, including medical students. It offers mainly primary care, but patients can be referred to the teaching hospital or other peripheral facilities, for specialist care, if the need arises. There is insurance coverage for every student at the university that covers both primary care and more advanced care. A mental health clinic is run on a weekly basis at the staff clinic, where students can consult a resident doctor in psychiatry on an outpatient basis. Students requiring inpatient care are offered one on the psychiatry wards of the Department of Psychiatry, UCH. Students with mental health difficulties are also offered additional support such as establishing communication between the staff clinic and the academic departments of such students to consider and grant special needs such as allowing affected students to sit for examinations while on inpatient care without compromising university examination standards. The university health services also liaise with academic departments to assist students requiring time off from academic work, due to mental health problems, to do so without difficulty and to integrate them back into the academic environment when they return from such leave.

To complement efforts of the university system, there are non-profit organizations operating within the university that offer mental health support services. One prominent one is the ASIDO foundation, a '*Not-for-Profit* Mental Health Advocacy Charity'. The youth wing of the organization, ASIDO Campus Network, is 'a student led mental health promoting club … dedicated to ensuring optimal mental health for every student on campus through awareness creation, advocacy, peer-to-peer counselling and support, youth mental health, drug abuse prevention, outreaches and research' (ASIDO Foundation, 2021).

How Local Initiatives Align with and Measure up to Global Standards: Suggested Future Directions for Interventions for Medical Students' Wellbeing in Nigeria

In appraising the local initiatives for addressing the mental health of students in our setting, and making recommendations going forward, it is important to bear in mind the context in which medical schools operate and the available resources in the health and the university systems.

In our previous work (Ayinde et al., 2022), we laid out a broad outline of what effective interventions for medical students' mental wellbeing might comprise of in Nigeria. In a nutshell, we advocated for political will and leadership to drive the discourse and the process for improving medical students' mental health and wellbeing in our medical schools, with roles for policymakers, medical practice and medical education regulators, professional medical associations, universities, and medical schools. Further, we advocated that school-specific interventions should be well thought out, be firmly embedded within the organizational structures of medical schools and be designed to be sustainable and be well-publicised. Third, we suggested that interventions should target risk factors within medical school structure, culture, and processes, as stressors are often situated within the learning environment and the academic culture of medical schools. Fourth, in recognition of the multiple layers of interacting risk factors, spanning personal (some predating entry into medical school) and medical school environmental factors, interventions should be multilevel and multipronged, and should address building resilience, teach personal reflection and self-care skills. Finally, we advocated that service should be accessible, to facilitate help-seeking, address confidentiality, and reduce stigma.

We turn now to a roadmap for implementing these broad recommendations in a low resource setting such as ours. A concrete step in moving a medical student mental health and wellbeing agenda forward is the development of a national student mental health policy, with particular attention to the mental wellbeing of medical students, since they are recognized as a vulnerable subgroup in this population. This policy can then be adapted by and be domiciled in individual Nigerian universities and medical schools to suit their local needs. To our knowledge, there is currently no national student mental health or university-specific mental health policy in any university in Nigeria. This is likely to be the situation in most universities in sub-Saharan Africa. Notable exceptions are some universities in South Africa (Kaminer & Shabalala, 2019). Alternatives to a stand-alone student mental health policy (e.g. University of Cape Town, 2022) is a university-wide mental health policy (e.g. Stellenbosch University, 2022; University of Western Australia, 2022b).

At the minimum, a university- or medical school-specific mental health policy should reflect the commitment of the institution to providing an environment that promotes and supports the mental wellbeing of students, as well as providing specialized services that cater to the mental health of students in need. It should secure resources for services and coordinate actions across multiple sectors concerned with the mental wellbeing of students within the university. It should also set out procedures and processes for handling mental health crises among students and for making reasonable accommodations for students with mental health difficulties. There are several examples of higher institution-based mental health policy from both high-income (e.g. University of Western Australia, 2022b) and low- and middle-income countries (e.g. Stellenbosch University, 2022; University of Cape Town, 2022) that Universities in Nigeria can draw inspirations from in developing a medical school mental health policy. Kaminer and Shabalala (2019) have described the process employed in developing the student mental health policy for a university in a setting similar to ours. There are also good practice guidelines, such as one provided by University UK (2015) that policy-makers in Nigeria can consult in developing a medical school mental health policy.

As part of a medical school-specific mental health policy, it is important to include an overall framework or strategy for promoting mental wellbeing and preventing mental disorders within the medical school environment. Examples of this exist in some universities in the Global North (e.g. University of Calgary, 2022; University of Western Australia, 2022a). It often documents all resources available for mental health promotion, prevention, and treatment: policies, services, initiatives, personnel, and partnerships with entities outside of the medical school.

While there are identifiable organizational structures and activities in Nigerian universities (using Ibadan Medical School as an example) that appear geared towards mental health promotion and prevention, this is often accidental, and not by design. Mental health support services, although present, are neither well-resourced nor well-developed and operate in silos. In offering a way forward we recommend that medical school leaderships commit to creating an environment that promotes mental health and mental wellbeing by re-orienting, developing and strengthening medical school structures (facilities and learning environment), culture (e.g. bullying, maltreatment, recognition and reward) and processes (e.g. curriculum design, admission and examination procedures), with mental wellbeing in mind, and that these are well spelt out in an overall medical school-specific strategy/framework. Furthermore, there should be a designated unit responsible for leading and coordinating the mental wellbeing effort of the medical school. In some universities, this unit might be the student wellbeing office or the students' affairs office or both. This unit is responsible for initiating policy development, review, and implementation, as well as coordination of mental wellbeing resources within the medical school. The unit also leads and maintains partnerships with the different university sectors and organizations involved in or with bearing on the mental wellbeing of students on campus. It is responsible for leading and coordinating campus mental health literacy efforts, as well other mental wellbeing initiatives such as resilience building, stigma reduction, self-reflection, self-care training, and access to care. Finally, the unit should lead and coordinate the monitoring of trends of risk factors, mental wellbeing indices, and service responsiveness through periodic surveys and bespoke research. In regard to mental wellbeing support services, they should be designed to be responsive to stressors and risk factors, transient mental distress as well as enduring mental illness. Owing to very scarce general and mental health resources in our setting, there is need to build capacity of students and faculty for self-care and to recognize and respond promptly to mental health problems in their community.

Acknowledgement

We are grateful to Drs Tolulope Bella-Awusah, Jibril Abdulmalik, and Alero Adegbolagun for sharing with us information on the local initiatives at Ibadan Medical School.

References

ASIDO Foundation (2021). About Us. In: *asido foundation*. https://asidofoundation.com/about-us/ (Accessed 29 August 2022).

Ayinde, O.O., Akinnuoye, E.R., Molodynski, A., Battrick, O., & Gureje, O. (2022). 'A descriptive study of mental health and burnout among Nigerian medical students'. *Int J Soc Psychiatry* **68**(6): 1223–1231.

Brooks, S.K., Gerada, C., & Chalder, T. (2011). 'Review of literature on the mental health of doctors: are specialist services needed?' *J Ment Health* **20**(2): 146–156.

Brown, A. (1961). 'Medical education in Nigeria'. *Acad Med* **36**(9): 1036–1041.

Central Intelligence Agency (2021). Nigeria. *The World Factbook*. Central Intelligence Agency. https://www.cia.gov/the-world-factbook/countries/nigeria/ (Accessed 4 August 2021).

Demerouti, E., Bakker, A.B., Vardakou, I., & Kantas, A. (2003). 'The convergent validity of two burnout instruments: a multitrait-multimethod analysis'. *Eur J Psychol Assess* **19**(1): 12–23.

Dyrbye, L. & Shanafelt, T.D. (2011). 'Commentary: medical student distress: a call to action'. *Acad Med* **86**(7): 801–803.

Dyrbye, L., Thomas, M.R., & Shanafelt, T.D. (2006). 'Systematic review of depression, anxiety, and other indicators of psychological distress among U.S. and Canadian medical students'. *Acad Med* **81**(4): 354–373.

Esan, O., Esan, A., Folasire, A., & Oluwajulugbe, P. (2019). 'Mental health and wellbeing of medical students in Nigeria: a systematic review'. *Int Rev Psychiatry* **31**(7–8): 661–672.

Ewing, J.A. (1984). 'Detecting alcoholism: the CAGE questionnaire'. *JAMA* **252**(14): 1905–1907.

Ezigbo, O. (2022). Nigeria Loses 40,000 Registered Doctors to Foreign Nations—THISDAYLIVE. https://www.thisdaylive.com/index.php/2021/11/28/nigeria-loses-40000-registered-doctors-to-foreign-nations/ (Accessed 28 August 2022).

Gureje, O. (2006). 'Lifetime and 12-month prevalence of mental disorders in the Nigerian Survey of Mental Health and Well-Being'. *Br J Psychiatry* **188**(5): 465–471.

Harvey, S.B., Epstein, R.M., Glozier, N., Petrie, K., Strudwick, J., Gayed, A., Dean, K., & Henderson, M. (2021). 'Mental illness and suicide among physicians'. *Lancet* **398**(10303): 920–930.

Hope, V. & Henderson, M. (2014). 'Medical student depression, anxiety and distress outside North America: a systematic review'. *Med Educ* **48**(10): 963–979

Kadhum, M., Ayinde, O.O., Wilkes, C., Chumakov, E., Dahanayake, D., Ashrafi, A., Kafle, B., Lili, R., Farrell, S., Bhugra, D., & Molodysnki, A. (2022). 'Wellbeing, burnout and substance use amongst medical students: a summary of results from nine countries'. *Int J Soc Psychiatry* **68**(6): 1218–1222.

Kaminer, D. & Shabalala, N. (2019). 'Developing a student mental health policy for a South African university: consultation, contestation and compromise'. *S Afr J High Educ* **5**: 196–212.

Medical and Dental Council of Nigeria (2022). Accredited Medical and Dental Schools in Nigeria. https://www.mdcn.gov.ng/page/education/accredited-medical-and-dental-schools-in-nigeria-as-at-march-2022 (Accessed 31 August 2022).

Molodynski, A., Lewis, T., Kadhum, M., Farrell, S.M., Lemtiri Chelieh, M., Falcão De Almeida, T., Masri, R., Kar, A., Volpe, U., Moir, F., Torales, J., Castaldelli-Maia, J.M., Chau, S.W.H., Wilkes, C., & Bhugra, D. (2021). 'Cultural variations in wellbeing, burnout and substance use amongst medical students in twelve countries'. *Int Rev Psychiatry* **33**(1–2): 37–42.

Molodynski, A., Ventriglio, A., & Bhugra, D. (2019). 'A crisis brewing for the healthcare system and a crisis already happening for our students'. *Int Rev Psychiatry* **31**(7–8): 545–547.

Olanrewaju Azeez, Y., Olalekan Babatunde, Y., Babatunde, D., Olasupo, J., Alabi, E., Bakare, P., & Oluwakorede, A.J. (2021). 'Towards universal health coverage: an analysis of the health insurance coverage in Nigeria'. *Int J Health Life Sci* 7(3): 3.

Omigbodun, A. (2020). 'Improving undergraduate medical education in Nigeria: insight into the past'. *Trop J Obstet Gynaecol* 37(1): 3.

Stellenbosch University (2022). *Staff and Student Mental Health Policy*. https://www.google.com/url?sa=t&rct=j&q=&esrc=s&source=web&cd=&cad=rja&uact=8&ved=2ahUKEwiK5_7u4Oj5AhUIhM4BHdZQDAoQFnoECB0QAQ&url=http%3A%2F%2Fwww.sun.ac.za%2Fenglish%2Flearning-teaching%2Fstudent-affairs%2Fcscd%2FDocuments%2FMental%2520Health%2520Policy%2520Final%2520for%2520Consultation.pdf&usg=AOvVaw2ikHpQIADt3H0Jt3w322IH (Accessed 1 September 2022).

Universities UK (2015). *Student Mental Wellbeing in Higher Education: Good Practice Guide*. https://www.m25lib.ac.uk/wp-content/uploads/2021/02/student-mental-wellbeing-in-he.pdf (Accessed 30 August 2022).

University of Calgary (2022). *The Campus Mental Health Strategy*. https://www.ucalgary.ca/mentalhealth/strategy (Accessed 30 August 2022).

University of Cape Town (2022). *Student Mental Health Policy*. https://www.google.com/url?sa=t&rct=j&q=&esrc=s&source=web&cd=&ved=2ahUKEwjtr6y1nOn5AhXD0aQKHUvmCGwQFnoECA0QAQ&url=https%3A%2F%2Fuct.ac.za%2Fsites%2Fdefault%2Ffiles%2Fcontent_migration%2Fuct_ac_za%2F39%2Ffiles%2FStudent-Mental-Health-Policy.pdf&usg=AOvVaw27uu0tSMd2lnRaxrLiJzFe (Accessed 1 September 2022).

University of Ibadan (2022). *University of Ibadan Policy*. https://www.ui.edu.ng/content/university-ibadan-policy (Accessed 31 August 2022).

University of Western Australia (2022a). *Mental Health and Well-being Framework*. https://www.google.com/url?sa=t&rct=j&q=&esrc=s&source=web&cd=&cad=rja&uact=8&ved=2ahUKEwi03NTXzPL5AhVrhc4BHYd_BLsQFnoECAYQAQ&url=https%3A%2F%2Fwww.uwa.edu.au%2Fstudents%2FUWA-Mental-Health-and-Wellbeing-Framework&usg=AOvVaw1GDTboelh619FV24iKd-Qu (Accessed 31 August 2022).

University of Western Australia (2022b). *University of Western Australia Policy Library*. https://www.uwa.edu.au/policy (Accessed 31 August 2022).

Wang, P.S., Aguilar-Gaxiola, S., Alonso, J., Angermeyer, M.C., Borges, G., Bromet, E.J., Bruffaerts, R., de Girolamo, G., de Graaf, R., Gureje, O., Haro, J.M., Karam, E.G., Kessler, R.C., Kovess, V., Lane, M.C., Lee, S., Levinson, D., Ono, Y., Petukhova, M., Posada-Villa, J., Seedat, S., & Wells, J.E. (2007). 'Use of mental health services for anxiety, mood, and substance disorders in 17 countries in the WHO world mental health surveys'. *Lancet* 370(9590): 841–850.

WHO and Federal Ministry of Health, Nigeria (2006). *WHO-AIMS Report on Mental Health System in Nigeria*. https://extranet.who.int/mindbank/item/1303 (Accessed 30 October 2021).

World Health Organization (2018). *WHO: Nigeria: Country Cooperation Agreement*. World Health Organization. https://www.google.com/url?sa=t&rct=j&q=&esrc=s&source=web&cd=&ved=2ahUKEwiNk766zPH5AhWSXvEDHUzuAwwQFnoECAMQAw&url=https%3A%2F%2Fapps.who.int%2Firis%2Fbitstream%2Fhandle%2F10665%2F136785%2Fccsbrief_nga_en.pdf%3Bsequence%3D1&usg=AOvVaw2CZyYrWm_jwXRxQ19cBtcx (Accessed 31 August 2022).

21

Paraguay

The Mental Health of Medical Students: The Case of Paraguay

Julio Torales and Israel González

Background

Paraguay is a landlocked country in the heart of South America. It has an estimated population of over seven million people with a marked predominance of young people, more than half of Paraguayans being 30 years old or younger (Nickson et al., 2021). Until very recently, the number of medical schools in the country was small and consisted mainly of the National University of Asunción and the Catholic University. In the last decade, there was an initial explosion of new medical schools that were opened with little regulatory input. In the last few years, the government has put measures in place to ensure that the quality of education delivered by schools are up to the national standards. There are currently 15 medical schools accredited by the Nacional Agency for Evaluation and Accreditation of Higher Education (ANEAES, by its acronym in Spanish) (ANEAES, 2021). Five of these schools are national (state-funded) and the remainder private. Students in state-funded schools pay a nominal fee during their course, but need to bear the costs of transportation, books, and elective courses. Students in private schools are asked to fund their tuition fees.

Mental health issues continue to be highly stigmatized in Paraguay, not only in the general population, but also within the medical community. A recent survey of 243 medical students at the Universidad Nacional de Asunción about the perceptions of medical students on mental health and barriers to accessing mental healthcare services reported that 81% of students considered stigma or shame to be the most important barrier in accessing mental healthcare services offered by the institution, and that only 37% considered that the school was supportive of students with mental health issues (Amarilla et al., 2021). From our conversations with students and residents, from reading posts of rightfully frustrated students on social media platforms, and even from personal lived experience, we know that students are frequently told that they need to be 'mentally tough' if they want to succeed in the medical field. Applicants with a history of mental health issues may be implicitly considered as 'unsuitable' for certain medical specialties. Often, they can be granted leave due to physical health issues but viewed with suspicion when claiming leave due to symptoms or consequences of a mental disorder. As a consequence of this, many medical students choose to delay or avoid asking for help for their mental health as they are justifiably afraid of being perceived and treated differently by peers and faculty (González-Urbieta et al., 2019).

Julio Torales and Israel González, *Paraguay* In: *The Mental Health of Medical Students*. Edited by: Andrew Molodynski, Sarah Marie Farrell, and Dinesh Bhugra, Oxford University Press. © Oxford University Press 2024. DOI: 10.1093/oso/9780192864871.003.0021

Findings from a 2019 survey

In 2019, Torales et al. conducted a survey as part of a global study to attempt to determine the presence or history of psychiatric distress and disorders, burnout, substance use, and quality of life using validated and standardized instruments (Torales et al., 2019). 180 students from the School of Medical Sciences of the National University of Asunción were surveyed, the students were distributed among different years of education and 69% were female.

Two in ten students had sought help from a mental health professional before entering medical school, 15% were diagnosed with a mental health condition, and 6% of them were prescribed psychotropics. Of the students, 14% consulted regularly with a mental health professional at the time of the survey, and 8% were taking a medication for their mental health. The most common medication was Escitalopram, which is widely prescribed for anxiety and depression in Paraguay. When using the GHQ12 screening tool to assess 'caseness', however, 45% of the students surveyed tested positive. Burnout symptoms were screened for using the Oldenburg Burnout Inventory, with just over 60% of students showing high scores for detachment, and almost all scoring high for exhaustion.

Use of substances, including problematic use of alcohol, was also assessed in this survey. Nearly 40% of the students reported using substances to improve performance at school, with over 10% admitting to the use of the stimulant drug methylphenidate for this purpose. Problematic use of alcohol had a prevalence of 20% as determined by a score of two or more on in the CAGE questionnaire. Illicit substance use for recreational purposes was admitted by 26% of the respondents, with almost 75% of users reporting consuming cannabis at least many times in the last year. Moreover, almost all of the students who admitted to using illicit substances reported that someone had been concerned about their substance use.

The study concluded that the findings uniformly point to a higher prevalence of mental disorders and risk factors contributing to mental illness in medical students. Surveys conducted in different countries showed similar results and added to the established evidence that reflects a worldwide trend that may be linked to negative factors deeply intrenched in the medical culture around the world (Almeida et al., 2019; Castaldelli-Maia et al., 2019; Chau et al., 2019; Esan et al., 2019; Farrell et al., 2019b, 2019a, 2019d, 2019c; Lemtiri Chelieh et al., 2019; Masri et al., 2019; Volpe et al., 2019; Wilkes et al., 2019).

Research

There is a wealth of evidence about the high rate of mental health disorders in medical students and medical professionals. A systematic review of 167 cross-sectional studies by Rotenstein et al. found a prevalence of 27% for depression or depressive symptoms and 11% for suicidal ideation (Rotenstein et al., 2016). Quek et al. conducted a meta-analysis of 69 cross-sectional studies comprising over 40,000 students and found that the global prevalence rate of anxiety in this population was around 34%, which is substantially higher than in the general population (Quek et al., 2019). The prevalence of cannabis use among medical students was estimated by Papazisis et al to be of over 31% in a systematic review and meta-analysis of 38 cross-sectional and cohort studies comprising almost 20,000 participants (Papazisis et al., 2018).

Findings from local research in Paraguay follow the same trend, with multiple surveys showing high levels of depression amongst medical students. A survey of 153 medical students at the University of the Integration of the Americas found a 30% prevalence of clinically diagnosed depression. (Barreto Amarilla et al., 2023). Another cross-sectional survey of 206 medical students in the Universidad Internacional Tres Fronteras, using the Beck Depression Inventory (BDI), found a prevalence of 13% of Borderline clinical depression (a score of 17 or more on the scale), but that number increased to 31% after including those who scored 11 or more (Mild mood disturbance according to BDI scoring) (De Dio et al., 2017). This school is in Ciudad del Este, a city located in the border with Brazil, and this study also found that over 60% of the students lived in the Brazilian side of the border and commuted across it to attend school. The language barrier is another factor adding to the complex struggles medical students face in this region. Another similar survey done with 228 medical students in the Universidad Nacional de Caaguazú found a much higher prevalence of depression (57%), but this number is overrepresented by subjects who scored for intermittent depression (41%) (Rodríguez Castro & Rios-González, 2019). Another study surveyed 103 medical students in the Universidad Nacional de Asuncion using the Goldberg Health Questionnaire and found that 28.2% 'perceived' the presence of psychopathology (Barrios & Torales, 2017).

Suicidal ideation was explored in cross-sectional studies. 259 medical students in the Universidad Nacional del Este responded to a survey using the Scale for Suicide Ideation. The prevalence of suicidal ideation was reported as 15% (Mercado et al., 2018). Another survey using the same scale included 288 students from the Universidad Nacional de Asunción, the study found a much higher prevalence of suicidal ideation (54.9%). Alarmingly, 15.8% reported some level of preparation for suicide, and 5.1% had prepared a suicide note (Amarilla et al., 2018).

The reasons for this phenomenon are manifold. Some factors such as the extreme study overload are inherent to the career. However, many of these are structural issues that are deeply ingrained in the medical field in the country and have been passed on from previous generations. These can include fear-based teaching (including offending students, targeting them, expelling them from classes when they express different opinions, singling them out for their appearance), outdated and ineffective teaching methods, and even cases of sexual harassment or discrimination based on gender, gender identity, or sexual orientation (Diario Ultima Hora, 2021; González-Urbieta et al., 2019).

Other factors contributing to a decline in the mental health of medical students in Paraguay were considered in other observational studies. A survey of 76 students in the Universidad Nacional de Asuncion found significant family dysfunction in 22.4% using the family APGAR scale (Torales et al., 2018). The Pittsburgh Sleep Quality Index was used to survey 248 medical students in the Universidad Católica Nuestra Señora de la Asunción, they considered a cut-off of 5 points or higher across the scale to determine the quality of 'bad sleepers', this resulted in almost 74% of the respondents qualifying as bad sleepers. Interestingly, over 75% of the bad sleepers subjectively reported having a very good sleep quality, suggesting that students may not be aware of their true quality of sleep (Adorno Nuñez et al., 2021). A similar survey using the same scale in 199 medical students in the Universidad Nacional de Caaguazú also estimated the number of bad sleepers to be above 70% (Ortiz Sandoval, 2019).

Burnout syndrome has been evaluated in a number of studies. 120 medical students from the Universidad Internacional Tres Fronteras were surveyed using the Maslach Burnout Inventory—Student Survey. They found that approximately 55% showed some level of

Burnout, and that 40% were at risk of developing it (González-Escobar et al., 2020). In a similar survey including 157 medical students of the Universidad Nacional de Asuncion, approximately 45% of the students met the criteria for Burnout Syndrome using the same scale as in the previous study (González-Urbieta et al., 2020).

Low self-esteem can have a negative effect on the behaviour of students and be a factor involved in their ability to adapt to the environment in their personal and social spheres, as well as an influence on academic performance. 75 medical students in the Universidad Nacional de Asuncion were surveyed using the Rosenberg Self-Esteem Scale: it found a prevalence of 33% of low self-esteem in the sample (Torales et al., 2016). A replication study with 78 studies in the Santa Rosa del Aguaray Branch of the medical school at the Universidad Nacional de Asuncion found a lower prevalence of low self-esteem (24%), but with an important gender gap, as the rate of low self-esteem in females was almost double that of their male counterparts (Camacho Santa Cruz & Vera-Ovelar, 2019).

Interventions

As an example of an intervention designed to improve the mental health of students, The authors were involved in the creation of the Department of Mental Health at the medical school at the Universidad Nacional de Asuncion, which is a service tailored specifically to the needs of the students, residents, and other personnel working in the school.

The service has characteristics that make it particularly effective in addressing the needs of this population. One of the issues that we found in our interaction with the students was that they were concerned about their privacy when using our regular psychiatry and psychology clinics, as the medical records were routinely examined by peers and seniors for investigation purposes. The new department has a separate archive from our regular clinics and the records are therefore unavailable for access by students, residents, or attendings at the school. Protocols are being designed to find ways to analyse the data without affecting the privacy and confidentiality of the consultations. Another strength of the department is that the time for consultations is protected and does not affect the attendance rate of the students. Finally, clinicians in the team are uniquely equipped, due to their clinical experience gained by working in this specialized service and by the empowerment from the school authorities, to interact with school faculty to facilitate adaptations and adjustment required for students struggling with mental health issues.

Conclusions

Medical students are at higher risk of developing mental health issues, including depression, suicidality, and substance use disorders. This is not an issue that is isolated to a particular school, country, or even region. There are multiple factors contributing to this phenomenon, and many result from an entrenched culture in the medical field of overworking students and undervaluing the significance of developing a healthy study-life balance. These issues are clearly prevalent in Paraguay and have been documented in multiple surveys with medical students around the country. Efforts such as the creation of the Mental Health Department in medical school at the Universidad Nacional de Asuncion can be improved upon and replicated in other medical schools in the country, but they only act as secondary and tertiary prevention measures once mental health issues have already been established. Systemic efforts to address the risk factors at the structural level are required and can have an incredible impact in improving the mental health of medical students.

References

Adorno Nuñez, I.D.R., Gatti Pineda, L.D., Gómez Páez, L.L., Mereles Noguera, L.M., Segovia Abreu, J.M., Segovia Abreu, J.A., Castillo, A., 2021. [Calidad del Sueño en Estudiantes de Medicina de la Universidad Católica de Asunción]. Cienc. E Investig. Medico Estud. Latinoam. 21(6), 5–8.

Almeida, T., Kadhum, M., Farrell, S.M., Ventriglio, A., Molodynski, A., 2019. A descriptive study of mental health and wellbeing among medical students in Portugal. Int. Rev. Psychiatry 31, 574–578.

Amarilla, D., Cacace-Vely, C., Fretes-Fariña, R., Hiebl-Espinoza, A., Huang-Liao, M., Liñan-Leguizamón, A., López-González, M., Vera-Gómez, P., Villalba-Quiñónez, J., Barrios, I., Torales, J.C., 2021. National University of Asunción medical students' perceptions on mental health and on the barriers to accessing mental healthcare services offered by the institution. An. Fac. Cienc. Médicas Asunción 54, 109–124.

Amarilla, J., Barrios, F., Bogado, F., Centurión, R., Careaga, D., Cardozo, J., Guillén, W., Ferreira, Y., Trinidad, A., Maggi, C., Arce, A., 2018. Suicidal ideation in Medical Students of the National University of Asunción. Med. Clínica Soc. 2, 13–24.

ANEAES, 2021. Carreras de Grado Acreditadas en el Modelo Nacional - Vigentes [WWW Document]. Agencia Nac. Eval. Acreditación Educ. Super. URL http://www.aneaes.gov.py/v2/programas-acreditados (Accessed 15 September 2021).

Báez, C.M.M., Colmán, B.M.J., 2017. [Prevalencia de Depresion en Estudiantes de Medicina de la Unida; Asuncion - Paraguay; Año 2016]. Rev. Unida Científica 1.

Barreto Amarilla, E.A., Cardozo, K.S., Inchausti Loncharich, O.I., Jiménez Aponte, G.M., Kawecki Gomes, L.R., Marín Mareco, M.C.S., 2023. [Análisis de la depresión postpandemia de COVID-19 en los estudiantes de medicina hasta el quinto año de la Universidad de la Integración de las Américas, en el período 2021-2022]. UNIDA Salud. 2(2), 6–11.

Barrios, I., Torales, J., 2017. Salud mental y calidad de vida autopercibida en estudiantes de medicina de Paraguay. Rev. Científica Cienc. Médica 20, 5–10.

Camacho Santa Cruz, C., Vera-Ovelar, F., 2019. Self-esteem Levels in Medical Students of Santa Rosa del Aguaray. Med. Clínica Soc. 3, 5–8.

Castaldelli-Maia, J.M., Lewis, T., Marques dos Santos, N., Picon, F., Kadhum, M., Farrell, S.M., Molodynski, A., Ventriglio, A., 2019. Stressors, psychological distress, and mental health problems amongst Brazilian medical students. Int. Rev. Psychiatry 31, 603–607.

Chau, S.W.H., Lewis, T., Ng, R., Chen, J.Y., Farrell, S.M., Molodynski, A., Bhugra, D., 2019. Wellbeing and mental health amongst medical students from Hong Kong. Int. Rev. Psychiatry 31, 626–629.

De Dio, S., Ramírez Soto, A.B., Rocha, B.C.E., Mezzomo da Fonseca, K., Ottoni, L., Chamorro, R.C., Handam, Y., Espínola, V.H., Ramos, P., 2017. [Depressive disorders in students of medicine of the Universidad International Tres Fronteras "Uninter", Ciudad del Este, Paraguay (2016)]. Rev. Nac. Itaugua 9, 20–31.

Diario Ultima Hora, 2021. UNA: Tras cinco años, docente admite acoso y coacción sexual. D. Ultima Hora.

Esan, O., Esan, A., Folasire, A., Oluwajulugbe, P., 2019. Mental health and wellbeing of medical students in Nigeria: a systematic review. Int. Rev. Psychiatry 31, 661–672.

Farrell, S.M., Kadhum, M., Lewis, T., Singh, G., Penzenstadler, L., Molodynski, A., 2019a. Wellbeing and burnout amongst medical students in England. Int. Rev. Psychiatry 31, 579–583.

Farrell, S.M., Kar, A., Valsraj, K., Mukherjee, S., Kunheri, B., Molodynski, A., George, S., 2019b. Wellbeing and burnout in medical students in India; a large scale survey. Int. Rev. Psychiatry 31, 555–562.

Farrell, S.M., Moir, F., Molodynski, A., Bhugra, D., 2019c. Psychological wellbeing, burnout and substance use amongst medical students in New Zealand. Int. Rev. Psychiatry 31, 630–636.

Farrell, S.M., Molodynski, A., Cohen, D., Grant, A.J., Rees, S., Wullshleger, A., Lewis, T., Kadhum, M., 2019d. Wellbeing and burnout among medical students in Wales. Int. Rev. Psychiatry 31, 613–618.

González-Escobar, J.M., Ramos-Franco Netto, R.O., de Almeida Rodrigues-Franco Netto, J., Flores, B.H., Borges Andreo, S., Coronel-de Bobadilla, B., 2020. Prevalence of Burnout Syndrome in Medical Students. Rev. Inst. Med. Trop. 15, 13–18.

González-Urbieta, I., Alfonzo, A., Aranda, J., Cámeron, S., Chávez, D., Duré, N., Pino, A., Penner, D., Ocampo, S., Villalba, S., Torales, J., 2020. Burnout Syndrome and Alcohol Dependence in Medical Students. Med. Clínica Soc. 4, 52–59.

Gonzalez-Urbieta, I., Almiron, M., Torales, J., 2019. Are we doing enough to address self-esteem issues in medical and other health sciences students? Med. Clínica Soc. 3, 2–3.

Lemtiri Chelieh, M., Kadhum, M., Lewis, T., Molodynski, A., Abouqal, R., Belayachi, J., Bhugra, D., 2019. Mental health and wellbeing among Moroccan medical students: a descriptive study. Int. Rev. Psychiatry 31, 608–612.

Masri, R., Kadhum, M., Farrell, S.M., Khamees, A., Al-Taiar, H., Molodynski, A., 2019. Wellbeing and mental health amongst medical students in Jordan: a descriptive study. Int. Rev. Psychiatry 31, 619–625.

Mercado, C.Y.A., Viveros, E.C.C., Santander, K.E.D., Barboza, M.T.G., Cabrera, C.F., 2018. Frecuencia de los trastornos depresivos y de la ideación suicida en estudiantes de la Facultad de Ciencias de la Salud de la Universidad Nacional del Este. Rev. CIENTÍFICA UNE 3, 40–50.

Nickson, R.A., Painter, J.E., Service, E.R., Butland, G.J., Williams, J.H., 2021. Paraguay. Encycl. Brittannica.

Ortiz Sandoval, M.H., 2019. [Calidad del sueño en estudiantes de medicina de la Universidad Nacional del Caaguazú, Coronel Oviedo-Paraguay, año 2019.] (Thesis). FCM-UNCA.

Papazisis, G., Siafis, S., Tsakiridis, I., Koulas, I., Dagklis, T., Kouvelas, D., 2018. Prevalence of Cannabis Use Among Medical Students: A Systematic Review and Meta-analysis. Subst. Abuse Res. Treat. 12, 1178221818805977.

Quek, T.T.-C., Tam, W.W.-S., Tran, B.X., Zhang, M., Zhang, Z., Ho, C.S.-H., Ho, R.C.-M., 2019. The Global Prevalence of Anxiety Among Medical Students: A Meta-Analysis. Int. J. Environ. Res. Public. Health 16, E2735.

Rodríguez Castro, A.I., Rios-González, C.M., 2019. Frequency of depression in medical students of the National University of Caaguazú, 2017. Med. Clínica Soc. 2, 128–135.

Rotenstein, L.S., Ramos, M.A., Torre, M., Segal, J.B., Peluso, M.J., Guille, C., Sen, S., Mata, D.A., 2016. Prevalence of Depression, Depressive Symptoms, and Suicidal Ideation Among Medical Students: A Systematic Review and Meta-Analysis. JAMA 316, 2214–2236.

Torales, J., Barrios, I., Samudio, A., Samudio, M., 2018. Apoyo social autopercibido en estudiantes de medicina de la Universidad Nacional de Asunción (Paraguay). Educ. Médica 19, 313–317.

Torales, J., Kadhum, M., Zárate, G., Barrios, I., González, I., Farrell, S.M., Ventriglio, A., Arce, A., 2019. Wellbeing and mental health among medical students in Paraguay. Int. Rev. Psychiatry Abingdon Engl. 31, 598–602.

Torales, J.C., Barrios, I., Piris, A., Viola, L., 2016. [Autoestima en Estudiantes de Medicina de la Universidad Nacional de Asuncion, Paraguay.]. An. Fac. Cienc. Médicas 49, 27–32.

Volpe, U., Ventriglio, A., Bellomo, A., Kadhum, M., Lewis, T., Molodynski, A., Sampogna, G., & Fiorillo, A. (2019). Mental health and wellbeing among Italian medical students: a descriptive study. Int. Rev. Psychiatry 31, 569–573.

Wilkes, C., Lewis, T., Brager, N., Bulloch, A., MacMaster, F., Paget, M., Holm, J., Farrell, S.M., Ventriglio, A., 2019. Wellbeing and mental health amongst medical students in Canada. Int. Rev. Psychiatry 31, 584–587.

22
Portugal

The Mental Health of Medical Students in Portugal

Telma Almeida

Background

Portugal is a country located in Southwestern Europe with 10 344 802 inhabitants (Censos, 2021).

Its territory also includes the Atlantic archipelagos of the Azores and Madeira.

There are ten public/state medical schools around the country:

Faculty of Medicine of University of Coimbra (FMUC, Portugal),
Faculty of Medicine of University of Lisbon (FMUL, Portugal)
Beira Interior Institute (UBI, Portugal)
Abel Salazar Biomedical Sciences Institute—University of Porto (ICBAS, Portugal)
Faculty of Medicine of University of Oporto, (FMUP, Portugal)
Faculty of Medicine of University of Algarve (DCBM-UAlg, Portugal)
Faculty of Medicine of Nova University of Lisbon (FCM|NMS, Portugal)
Faculty of Medicine of University of Minho (FMUM, Portugal)
Faculty of Medicine of University of Azores (UA, Portugal)
Faculty of Medicine of University of Madeira (UM, Portugal).

In addition, a private medical school, the Faculty of Medicine of Catholic University of Portugal (UCP, Portugal), opened in 2021.

In both public and private medical schools, students are required to pay a tuition fee which does not include transportation, accommodation, and/or study materials.

The Integrated Master's in Medicine course in Portugal takes six years to finish. The first three years are more theoretical and cover a Basic Health Sciences Degree. The other years include a Master's in Medicine and are more practically and clinically focused.

To gain admission students are ranked according to their application grade, which depends on a combination of the final average of high school and the classifications obtained in the application exams specific to each faculty that are provided by the Portuguese Ministry of Health. Until very recently, medicine had the highest admission grades in the country and nowadays it is still one of the most desirable ones. This ranking process and the high grades are in themselves a stress factor right from even before the start of the degree.

Medical students' mental health has been widely studied. The evidence suggests that medical students face great psychological pressure during graduation, which makes them more

Telma Almeida, *Portugal* In: *The Mental Health of Medical Students*. Edited by: Andrew Molodynski, Sarah Marie Farrell, and Dinesh Bhugra, Oxford University Press. © Oxford University Press 2024. DOI: 10.1093/oso/9780192864871.003.0022 vulnerable to psychiatric disorders, burnout, and poor mental wellbeing (Bhugra et al., 2019; Molodynski et al., 2021; Volpe et al., 2019; Wilson et al., 2019). The prevalence of stress and depressive symptoms among medical students has been found to be higher than among other students in Portugal (Moreira de Sousa et al., 2019).

Medical students in Portugal face numerous stressors that can affect their wellbeing (Loureiro et al., 2008; Roberto & Almeida, 2011). The first years of medical school can generate significant stress, due to their theoretical nature and rigorous academic pace. On the other hand, it can lead to some frustration due to the expectation of a more practical approach and about what they had idealized about being a doctor. Length of courses, the financial burden, lack of leisure time, work relationships, and career choices are identified as other causes of stress. There are other factors pointed to, such as workload, conflict, low focus on quality of care, and reduced professional autonomy (Lee et al., 2013).

A systematic review (Coentre & Figueira, 2015) revealed a prevalence of depression in medical students internationally from 2.9% to 38.2%, suicidal ideation from 4.4% to 23.1% and suicidal attempts from 0.0% to 6.4%. Studies suggest that the prevalence of depression is higher in female medical students, younger students, and in earlier years in medical schools (Coentre & Figueira, 2015; Puthran et al., 2016; Loureiro et al., 2008; Roberto & Alemida, 2011).

One study (Silva et al., 2017) suggested that personal factors (anxiety traits, medicine choice factors, relationship patterns and academic burnout) are relevant for the persistence of high levels of Beck Depression Inventory during medical training.

A meta-analysis (Rotenstein et al., 2016) found an estimated worldwide prevalence of 27.2% of depressive symptoms and/or depression in medical students, while the prevalence found among European studies was between 12.8% and 21.9%.

Medical students themselves tend toward certain characteristics of personality and high levels of trait-anxiety that places them at increased risk of stress, with maladaptive perfectionism leading to excessive concerns about academic performance (Silva et al., 2017). In this study medical students reported more relationship issues, cynicism, and decreased satisfaction with social activities.

Having a stable and supportive family or being married were found to be protective factors (Tyssen et al., 2000).

Our Findings

In 2019, as part of a wider global initiative, a large descriptive study of Portuguese medical students was performed to clarify their current state of wellbeing (Almeida et al., 2019). Specifically, it aimed to quantify and characterize difficulties medical students faced regarding stressors, psychological distress, and psychiatric morbidity. We used standardized reliable and validated instruments.

A total of 622 medical students participated in the study (Table 22.1).

Among the 622 respondents, 26% reported visiting a general practitioner, psychologist, psychiatrist, or psychotherapist specifically for their mental health prior to medical school (Table 22.2).

These consultations were noted to be due to feelings of sadness, stress, anxiety, mania, eating disorders, or obsessional behaviour. Results indicated that 8% of Portuguese medical

Table 22.1 Sociodemographic characteristics of the medical students (*n* = 622)

Characteristics	*n*	%
Total number of participants:	622	100
Gender:		
Female	452	73
Male	167	27
Other	3	<1
University of Participant:		
Faculty of Medicine of University of Coimbra, FMUC	124	20
Faculty of Medicine of University of Lisbon, FMUL	303	49
Beira Interior Institute, UBI	1	<1
Abel Salazar Biomedical Sciences Institute—University of Porto, ICBAS	194	31
Year of study in medical school:		
1st	109	18
2nd	129	21
3rd	99	16
4th	91	15
5th	93	15
6th	95	15

Reproduced with permission from Almeida T, Kadhum M, Farrell SM, Ventriglio A, Molodynski A. A descriptive study of mental health and wellbeing among medical students in Portugal. *Int Rev Psychiatry.* 2019 Nov-Dec;31(7–8):574–578.

students were formally diagnosed with mental ill health before starting medical school, with 15% being diagnosed during medical school.

The reported diagnoses before starting medical school were: 4% depressive disorders, 2% anxiety disorders, 1% attention deficit hyperactivity disorder (ADHD) or autism, 1% obsessive compulsive disorder, and 0.2% eating disorders. Regarding psychotropic medication, 88 (14%) students reported being prescribed medication for their mental health (including depression, anxiety, psychosis, and ADHD). Specifically, 40 (6%) had antidepressants, 32 (5%) had benzodiazepines, 5 (1%) antipsychotics, and 4 (1%) stimulants (Table 22.2).

Specific diagnoses during medical school were: 7% anxiety disorders, 6% depressive disorders, 1% eating disorders, 0.3% ADHD or autism. Nearly one in five respondents (n = 111; 18%) reported currently seeing a general practitioner, psychologist, psychiatrist, or psychotherapist. 81 students (13%) were taking medication for their mental health. 48 (8%) were taking antidepressants, 12 (2%) benzodiazepines, 8 (1%) other drugs, and 4 (1%) stimulants (n 1⁄4 4; 0.64%).

Various stressors were identified. Of note, 446 (72%) students noted money, 77 (12%) housing, 41 (7%) studying and 293 (47%) relationships as key stressors in their life.

Table 22.2 Mental health of respondents (*n* = 622)

Mental health	*n (%)*
Prior to medical school:	
Students with existing contact with healthcare professionals regarding mental health	160(26)
Psychiatric diagnosis	47(8)
Depressive disorders	22(4)
Anxiety disorders	15(2)
ADHD or autism	7(1)
OCD	4(1)
Eating disorders	3(<1)
Psychotropics	88(14)
Antidepressants	40(6)
Benzodiazepines	32(5)
Antipsychotics	5(1)
Stimulants	4(1)
Whilst at medical school	
New contact with healthcare professional regarding mental health	111(18)
Psychiatric diagnosis	
Anxiety disorders	94(15)
Depressive disorders	44(7)
Eating disorders	40(6)
ADHD or autism	5(1)
OCD	2(<1)
BPD	1(<1)
Burnout	1(<1)
Psychotropic	81(13)
Antidepressants	48(8)
Benzodiazepines	12(2)
Other drugs	8(1)
Stimulants	4

Reproduced with permission from Almeida T, Kadhum M, Farrell SM, Ventriglio A, Molodynski A. A descriptive study of mental health and wellbeing among medical students in Portugal. *Int Rev Psychiatry* 2019 Nov–Dec;31(7–8):574–578.

The CAGE questionnaire (Saitz et al., 1999) was administered to identify problematic drinking. In total, 10% students were identified as being at risk of alcohol-related health problems. In addition, 8% students reported taking a non-prescription substance or prescription medication outside of its intended use to feel better or uplift their mood, including multivitamins (12%), methylphenidate (2%), benzodiazepines (1.5%), propranolol (1.1%) and modafinil (0.2%).

The GHQ-12 (El-Metwally et al., 2018) was used to assess non-psychotic 'minor psychiatric disorders' among medical students. The mean score of the whole sample was 5.77. 565 (91%) of students scored 2 or more and therefore flagged positive as a case. The OLBI was used to ascertain rates of burnout. For burnout, disengagement was found in 81% and exhaustion in 89% of respondents.

The major stressors identified by the students were interpersonal relationships and financial difficulties. Problem drinking, as identified through the CAGE questionnaire, was seen in 10% of students. Cannabis use was reported in 79% of the participants, a much higher rate than in other countries. Cannabis remains the most commonly used substance in Portugal, with an average of 10% regular use across the Portuguese population (World Health Organization, 2009). Whilst regular cannabis use may be in line with the national average, the high stress environment and academic adaptation required in medical school combined with cannabis use may lead to detrimental effects on mental wellbeing. 91% of respondents reached 'caseness' on the GHQ12 questionnaire, which appears to indicate widespread 'mild' mental distress in this cohort.

Previous studies in Portugal investigating psychological wellbeing and psychiatric illness in medical students, namely anxiety and depression, revealed varied results ranging from 6% to 21.5% (Moreira de Sousa et al., 2018; Roberto, 2009). These results are considerably lower than in this study, but distinct differences exist in the instruments and cut-offs used that could at least in part explain such variance. For example, these studies used the Hospital Anxiety and Depression Scale (HADS), which is limited towards anxiety and depression and disregards other conditions (Moreira de Sousa et al., 2018). Burnout has previously been investigated by one study in Portugal (Pereira et al., 2014). Through use of the Maslach Burnout Inventory, the authors observed high levels of emotional exhaustion, disbelief, and professional efficacy similar to our findings. Previous studies investigating problem drinking in Portuguese students reveal similar results to our study, identifying 9% of respondents as cases (Gonçalves & Carvalho, 2017).

Results in Portugal are consistent with global trends (Bhugra et al., 2019; Chau et al., 2019; Farrell et al., 2019b, 2019a, 2019c; Lemtiri Chelieh et al., 2019; Masri et al., 2019; Molodynski et al., 2021; Volpe et al., 2019; Wilkes et al., 2019; World Health Organization, 2009) and as such helps to further characterize medical students as a unique population requiring more support, safeguarding, and interventions.

Policies Regarding Student Wellbeing

High levels of psychological distress in medical students can lead to lower quality of care offered to the patients in future. Despite high levels of psychological distress, studies show that only 8% to 15% of medical students seek psychological support during their training (Shaw et al., 2006). Of those who seek, around 22-40% have a mood disorder, usually depression (Shaw et al., 2006).

To tackle the consequences of poor mental health and wellbeing, burnout, and mental ill-health in medical students and junior doctors, the medical community has been more active recently in recognizing the degree of the problem and showing motivation to appropriately investigate and generate solutions (BMA, 2019).

Presently, Portugal is the European country with the second highest rate of psychiatric disorders, mainly because of its high rate of anxiety disorders.

The fear of failure can trigger psychological disturbances in students. A study with medical students of the Universidade da Beira Interior reveal that clinical year students, especially fourth year students, had more feelings of psychological wellbeing and less distress when compared to third year peers (Roberto & Almeida, 2011). This fact may be related to the decrease in stress factors existing in the basic years and with the self-esteem that the beginning of regular clinical practice and contact with patients can bring them.

The actual Portuguese National Mental Health Programme aims to increase by 30% the number of initiatives for mental health promotion and the prevention of mental illness in general population.

Mental wellbeing and mental ill health have been linked to detrimental effects on physical health (including alcohol and drug misuse and suicidal ideation) and reduced academic success (Dyrbye & Shanafelt, 2011). During the late 1990s, Portugal suffered from very high levels of alcohol and substance misuse in the general population (World Health Organization, 2009). By 2000, a new strategy was introduced focusing on a public health approach to controlling substance misuse, rather than a criminal justice approach (World Health Organization, 2009). Of particular importance, distress amongst medical students can damage professional performance, with detrimental effects on empathy, ethical conduct, and professionalism (Dyrbye & Shanafelt, 2011).

Copping strategies like support from family and friends, exercise, recreational activities, and spirituality are all reported to promote a greater sense of wellbeing. A study of 140 medical students at Hong Kong University found that optimism and a positive outlook had the strongest negative correlations with depression and anxiety (Verna, 2005).

Research, Innovation, and Interventions

Access to appropriate psychiatric care for Portuguese medical students remains limited, with low numbers seeking help due to complex reasons. The majority of students indicated concerns about confidentiality and the potential impact of having stress-related issues appear on their academic record. Many students may refuse help or may not recognize the importance of seeking professional help, whilst others express financial difficulties and time constraints (Moreira de Sousa et al., 2018). Stigma surrounding mental health remains prominent in Portugal and extends into the medical student population (Korszun et al., 2012; Rodrigues-Silva et al., 2017; Telles-Correia et al., 2015; Schwenk et al., 2010).

This indicates the need for intensified support for Portuguese medical students and awareness campaigns.

Some steps that have already been taken in Portugal regarding to psychological support to medical students (Table 22.3).

Despite increasing awareness, there is still a long way to go in the fight against stigma. On the other hand, these services are not as effective as they could be due to the lack of resources

Table 22.3 Psychological support to medical students in the main Portuguese medical schools

Faculty	Consultations	Intervention Areas
Faculty of Medicine of the University of Porto (FMUP)	• Provided by a psychological consultation service in partnership with the Hospital of S. João Psychiatry Service • Carried out by psychology professionals • In person and by video call	• Consultations cover various situations that require psychological and psychotherapeutic support or counselling (frequent problems: anxiety, phobias, depression, grief, life transition phases, difficulties in interpersonal relationships, eating disorders, stress, difficulties in managing time ...)
University of Coimbra (FMUC)	• Provides a general psychological support office for all university students, including medical students • Carried out by education and psychology professionals	• Consultations ensure psychological support, psychopedagogical support, career counselling, guidance, and socioeducational intervention service, and counselling in the area of sexuality
Abel Salazar Biomedical Sciences Institute— University of Porto (ICBAS)	• Provided by a student support office • Carried out by a team of psychologists • Presential and online appointments	• Their areas of intervention are: • psychological support and counselling • psychopedagogical support • support for the adaptation and integration of new students • support for students with special educational needs • career management and transition to the professional world • promotion of 'soft skills' • prevention and promotion of psychological health • assessment, prevention, and intervention in psychosocial risks • intervention in crisis and emergency situations.
Faculty of Medicine of University of Lisbon (FMUL)	• Space S department (joint initiative by the Board of the Students Association of FMUL and the Board of the FMUL, support by the Psychiatry and Mental Health Service of the Northern Lisbon University Hospital Centre-SMH) • Carried out by two Clinical Psychologists with no teaching link to FMUL • Video conference sessions and one day a week of personal assistance	• Provides psychological support to FMUL Students and promotes Mental Health at the Faculty • The space S is intended to be an independent place that allows safeguarding the confidentiality for all who wish to be received
Beira Interior Institute (UBI)	• Provided by UBI Medical and Sport Support Centre and with the collaboration of a company specialized in these services • Offer medical and sport services to students and all the other members of the academic community	• Physiotherapy appointments

Table 22.3 Continued

Faculty	Consultations	Intervention Areas
Faculty of Medicine of Nova University of Lisbon (FCM|NMS)	• Student support offices	• Their mission is to integrate and support students during their academic career and to focus on their satisfaction and wellbeing • It aims, at the student's request, to support and promote the design of appropriate and personalized solutions to students' problematic situations • It aims to promote the monitoring and resolution of these situations, through close articulation with other Services, internal or external, of NMS

in the national health system, which is overcrowded. Some of the students' complaints are that the appointments are too short in time and too infrequent. This often leads people to resort to the private system of health for those who have the ability to do so.

Actions should be taken to encourage medical students to seek help for psychological problems and to provide adequate facilities.

Targeted interventions that promote psychological wellbeing during medical education, teaching students to recognize and deal with symptoms of distress and help them to understand when they need support, may be an effective way of dealing with this problem.

The promotion of mental health by medical schools can be achieved through personal stress management techniques, mindfulness techniques (Erogul et al., 2014), support groups, workshops, and retreats, wellbeing committees, and other psychosocial support.

Conclusions

Portuguese medical students report high levels of burnout and mental ill health, higher than other students. Financial and interpersonal stressors are identified as key difficulties throughout medical school. Future research is needed to confirm and compare these results globally, understand causality, monitor future trends and crucially to determine evidence-based interventions to tackle burnout and psychiatric illness and improve mental wellbeing in medical students.

In Portugal, students tend not to seek help from the support services available to them. Barriers to access include lack of time, fear of lack of confidentiality, the stigma associated with the use of mental health services, cost, fear of documentation in academic records, and fear of unwanted intervention.

Early intervention, through university-wide campaigns, support groups, and education of medical staff and tutors, with activities to promote psychological wellbeing and health (such as self-help, meditation, or mindfulness), may be crucial to safeguard future generations of doctors.

Helping students in psychological distress promotes the resilience necessary for future medical professionals and their personal fulfilment, in addition to improving professionalism and patient care.

References

Almeida, T., Kadhum, M., Farrell, S.M., Ventriglio, A., & Molodynski, A., (2019). 'A descriptive study of mental health and wellbeing among medical students in Portugal'. *Int Rev Psychiatry* 31: 574–578.

Bhugra, D., Sauerteig, S.-O., Bland, D., Lloyd-Kendall, A., Wijesuriya, J., Singh, G., . . . Ventriglio, A. (2019). 'A descriptive study of mental health and wellbeing of doctors and medical students in the UK'. International Review of Psychiatry. Advance online publication. doi:10. 1080/09540261.2019.1648621

BMA (2019). Supporting the mental health of doctors and medical students. Retrieved from https://www.bma.org.uk/ collective-voice/policy-and-research/education-training-and- workforce/supporting-the-mental-health-of-doctors-in-the- workforce

Censos 2021, INE, https://www.pordata.pt/censos/resultados/emdestaque-portugal-361, data from 11th February

Chau, S.W.H., Lewis, T., Ng, R., Chen, J.Y., Farrell, S.M., Molodynski, A., & Bhugra, D. (2019). 'Wellbeing and mental health amongst medical students from Hong Kong'. *Int Rev Psychiatry* 31: 626–629.

Coentre, R. & Figueira, M. (2015). 'Depression and suicidal behavior in medical students: a systematic review'. Current Psychiatry Reviews,

Dyrbye, L.N. & Shanafelt, T.D. (2011). 'Commentary: medical student distress: a call to action. *Acad Med* 86(7): 801–803.

El-Metwally, A., Javed, S., Razzak, H. A., Aldossari, K. K., Aldiab, A., Al-Ghamdi, S. H. Al-Zahrani, J. M. (2018). 'The factor structure of the general health questionnaire (GHQ12) in Saudi Arabia'. *BMC Health Services Research* 18(1): 595. doi:10.1186/s12913-018-3381-6

Erogul, M., Singer, G., McIntyre, T., & Stefanov, D.G. (2014). 'Abridged mindfulness intervention to support wellness in first-year medical students'. *Teach Learn Med* 26(4): 350–356.

Farrell, S.M., Kadhum, M., Lewis, T., Singh, G., Penzenstadler, L., & Molodynski, A. (2019a). 'Wellbeing and burnout amongst medical students in England'. *Int Rev Psychiatry* 31: 579–583.

Farrell, S.M., Kar, A., Valsraj, K., Mukherjee, S., Kunheri, B., Molodynski, A., & George, S. (2019b). 'Wellbeing and burnout in medical students in India; a large scale survey'. *Int Rev Psychiatry* 31: 555–562.

Farrell, S.M., Molodynski, A., Cohen, D., Grant, A.J., Rees, S., Wullshleger, A., Lewis, T., & Kadhum, M. (2019c). 'Wellbeing and burnout among medical students in Wales'. *Int Rev Psychiatry* 31: 613–618.

Gonçalves, I. A., & Carvalho, A. A. D S. (2017). 'Pattern of Alcohol Consumption by Young People from North Eastern Portugal'. *Open Medicine (Medicine)*, 12: 494–500. doi:10.1515/med-2017-0068

Korszun, A., Dinos, S., Ahmed, K., & Bhui, K. (2012). 'Medical student attitudes about mental illness: Does medical-school education reduce stigma?' *Academic Psychiatry* 36(3): 197. doi:10.1176/appi.ap.10110159

Lee, R.T., Seo, B., Hladkyj, S., Lovell, B.L., & Schwartzmann, C. (2013). 'Correlates of physician burnout across regions and specialties: a meta-analysis'. *Hum Resour Health* 11(1): 48.

Lemtiri Chelieh, M., Kadhum, M., Lewis, T., Molodynski, A., Abouqal, R., Belayachi, J., & Bhugra, D. (2019). 'Mental health and wellbeing among Moroccan medical students: a descriptive study'. *Int Rev Psychiatry* 31: 608–612.

Loureiro, E., Mcintyre, T., Mota-Cardoso, R., & Ferreira, A. (2008). 'The relationship between stress and lifestyle of students at the Faculty of Medicine of Oporto'. *Acta Med Por* 21(3): 209–214.

Masri, R., Kadhum, M., Farrell, S.M., Khamees, A., Al-Taiar, H., & Molodynski, A. (2019). Wellbeing and mental health amongst medical students in Jordan: a descriptive study. *Int Rev Psychiatry* 31: 619–625.

Molodynski, A., Lewis, T., Kadhum, M., Farrel, S., Chelieh, M., Falcão-Almeida, T., Masri, R., Kar, A., Volpe, U., Moir, F., Torales, J., Castaldelli-Maia, J., Chau, W., & Bhugra, D. (2021). 'Cultural variations in wellbeing, burnout and substance use amongst medical students in twelve countries'. *Int Rev Psychiatry* 33(1–2): 37–42.

Moreira de Sousa, J., Moreira, C., & Telles-Correia, D. (2018). 'Anxiety, depression and academic performance: a study amongst Portuguese medical students versus non-medical students'. *Acta Med Port* 31(9): 454–462.

Pereira, H., Fernandes, M., Costa, V., Amorim, L., La-Rizza, F., & Hermenegildo, R. (2014). 'Burnout in Portuguese medical students: Coping strategies as a mediating variable'. *Journal of Community Medicine and Health Education* **04**(04): 1–6. doi:10.4172/21610711.1000306

Puthran, R., Zhang, M., Tam, W., & Ho, R. (2016). 'Prevalence of depression amongst medical students: a meta-analysis'. *Med Educ* **50**(4): 456–468.

Roberto, A. R. (2009). 'A saúde mental dos estudantes de medicina da Universidade da Beira Interior'. Retrieved from https://ubibliorum.ubi.pt/handle/10400.6/1025

Roberto, A. & Almeida, A. (2011). 'Mental health of students of medicine: explorative study in the Universidade da Beira Interior'. *Acta Med Port* **24**(S2): 279–286

Rodrigues-Silva, N., Falcão de Almeida, T., Araujo, F., Molodynski, A., Venâncio, A., & Bouça, J. (2017). 'Use of the word schizophrenia in Portuguese newspapers'. *J Ment Health* **26**(5): 426–430.

Rotenstein, L., Ramos, M.A., Torre, M., Segal, J.B., Peluso, M.J., Guille, C., Sen, S., & Mata, D.A. (2016). 'Prevalence of depression, depressive symptoms, and suicidal ideation among medical students: a systematic review and meta-analysis'. *JAMA* **316**: 2214–2236.

Saitz, R., Lepore, M. F., Sullivan, L. M., Amaro, H., & Samet, J. H. (1999a). 'Alcohol misuse and dependence in latinos living in the United States'. *Archives of Internal Medicine* **159**(7): 718. doi:10.1001/archinte.159.7.718

Schwenk, T., Davis, L., & Wimsatt, L. (2010). 'Depression, stigma, and suicidal ideation in medical students'. *JAMA* **304**(11): 1181–1190.

Shaw, D., Wedding, D., Zeldow, P., & Diehl, N. (2006). Special problems of medical students: cap 6. In Wedding, D. (eds) *Behavior & Medicine*. Göttingen: Hogrefe Publishing, pp. 67–79.

Silva, V., Costa, P., Pereira, I., Faria, R., Salgueira, A., Costa, M., Sousa, N., Cerqueira, J., & Morgado, P. (2017). 'Depression in medical students: insights from a longitudinal study'. *BMC Med Educ* **17**(1): 184.

Telles-Correia, D., Gama Marques, J., Gramaça, J., Sampaio, D., & Sampaio, D. (2015). 'Stigma and attitudes towards psychiatric patients in portuguese medical students'. *Acta Medica Portuguesa* **28**(6): 715. doi:10.20344/amp.6231

Tyssen R., Vaglum P., Gronvold T., & Ekeberg O. (2000). 'The impact of job stress and working conditions on mental health problems among junior house officers. A nationwide Norwegian prospective cohort study'. *Med Educ* **34**:374–384,

Verna, Y. (2005). 'Supporting the well-being of medical students'. *CMAJ* **172**(7): 889–890.

Volpe, U., Ventriglio, A., Bellomo, A., Kadhum, M., Lewis, T., Molodynski, A., Sampogna, G., & Fiorillo, A. (2019). 'Mental health and wellbeing among Italian medical students: a descriptive study'. *Int Rev Psychiatry* **31**: 569–573.

Wilkes, C., Lewis, T., Brager, N., Bulloch, A., MacMaster, F., Paget, M., Holm, J., Farrell, S.M., & Ventriglio, A. (2019). 'Wellbeing and mental health amongst medical students in Canada'. *Int Rev Psychiatry* **31**: 584–587.

Wilson, T., Kenneth, L., & Pacheco, J. (2019). Prevalence of depressive symptoms among medical students: overview of systematic reviews. *Med Educ* **53**(4): 345–354.

World Health Organization. (2009). Effective and Humane Mental Health Treatment and Care for All. Retrieved from https://www.who.int/mental_health/policy/country/Portugal_CountrySummaryFINAL_MOH.pdf

23
Russia

The Mental Health of Medical Students in Russia

Egor Chumakov, Nataliia Petrova, and Ivan Pchelin

Introduction

Physicians and medical students work and study in a system that significantly affects their mental wellbeing and ability to provide the best care for patients. The training period is the peak period for the occurrence of mental health issues among physicians, with stress, mental disorders and burnout being more common among physicians than among their peers in other specialties at each stage of their training (medical school, residency, early career physicians) (Dyrbye et al., 2014). Medical students and junior physicians have the highest rate of diagnosed mental disorders, which may be due to the fact that the age of medical students and junior physicians corresponds to the vulnerable age group at which mental health disorders begin to develop (Bhugra et al., 2019). As future physicians, medical students today require significant emotional and financial investment. Therefore, it is imperative that faculty and administrators understand the needs of the student community by providing the necessary skills to these future physicians in an unstigmatized manner (Watson et al., 2020). Constantly increasing volume of information assimilation required, high nervous-emotional stress during exam sessions, and some destructive features of lifestyle (alcohol, drug use, smoking) not only distinguish the student community from other social groups, but also create a favourable ground for the formation of chronic mental disorders (Kobylatskaya et al., 2015). Although worldwide much attention is paid to issues of screening, diagnosis, and timely assistance to medical students (Kadhum et al., 2022; Molodynski et al., 2021), in Russia there are limited reports considering the topic of medical students' mental health with a slight increase in research attention to this area in recent years (Bukhanovskaya & Demcheva, 2019; Chritinin et al., 2016; Chumakov et al., 2021).

The System of Education in Medical Universities in Russia

The first medical educational institution—the Apothecary's Decree—appeared in Russia in the 17th century. Currently, the organizational system of training specialists with higher medical education in the Russian Federation includes 90 state educational organizations under the jurisdiction of various Ministries: 46 educational organizations of the Ministry of Health, 36 educational organizations of the Ministry of Education and Science of Russia

Egor Chumakov, Nataliia Petrova, and Ivan Pchelin, *Russia* The Mental Health of Medical Students in Russia In: *The Mental Health of Medical Students*. Edited by: Andrew Molodynski, Sarah Marie Farrell, and Dinesh Bhugra, Oxford University Press.
© Oxford University Press 2024. DOI: 10.1093/oso/9780192864871.003.0023

(medical faculties of universities), two educational organizations of the Russian Government, two educational organizations of the Ministry of Sports of Russia, and four regional educational organizations. There are also 43 research institutes in Russia that provide training in a number of educational programmes of higher education. Only eight educational organizations for training specialists with higher medical education are non-state. Higher medical education in Russia can be obtained only by full-time education at a higher educational institution. There is no distance medical education in Russia.

It is possible to enter medical universities in Russia right after high school. Universities offer programmes in Russian and English. The system for training medical personnel in the country is based on the principles of continuous lifelong learning. The following algorithm is in place: (i) early career guidance (specialized classes, colleges, pre-university schools); (ii) formation of knowledge, abilities, skills, and training within the framework of a specialty (six years of medical school); (iii) specialty training (2 years of residency); (iv) continuous professional education throughout life. The goals of higher medical education are related to the formation of the personality of the future doctor, competent and responsible, able to provide assistance, and a person of mercy and compassion.

Stress and Stress Factors of Medical School Education

Medical students report pressure from their professional environment and academic studies as the main source of stress (Chumakov et al., 2021). Due to the high educational load, chronic stress is more widespread among medical students than in the general population, which leads to increased anxiety, decreased performance, sleep disorders (Ruzhenkova, 2020; Turovaya et al., 2014). Significant triggers of deterioration in Russian medical students are fear for their future, lack of desire to learn, the need to meet the expectations of relatives (Korshunova & Mukhina, 2014), and/or satisfaction with learning outcomes (Bukhanovskaya & Demcheva, 2020). Among other reasons contributing to the development of educational stress in medical students, the following have been highlighted: a large number of absences and related academic debts, poor performance, conflicts with teachers, lack of educational material, dissatisfaction with the assessment received and disappointment of chosen profession (Torshina et al., 2016). Contacts with terminally ill patients in clinical departments and the feeling of helplessness in the face of illness and death are also specific sources of stress for medical students (Khan et al., 2013). All this leads to high perceived stress among medical students in Russia, as demonstrated by Drachev et al. (2020): 26.0%, 69.1%, and 4.9% of medical students reported low, moderate, and high perceived stress, respectively.

Mental Disorders in Medical Students

Over the past decade, screening studies of mental disorders among medical students in Russia have shown high rates of minor mental disorders, with variations by region. Thus, a longitudinal study of mental disorders among medical students from Moscow revealed clinically distinct non-psychotic mental disorders in 34.2% of first-year medical students and 33% of sixth-year medical students, including high levels of neurotic reactions (43.2%) and neurotic disorders (13.7%). They also reported rates of 4.6% recorded personality disorders and 7.95%—behavioural abnormalities (Minnibaev et al., 2012). According to research in Rostov-on-Don, the prevalence of neurotic disorders in medical students was 14.8%. Most often these were neurasthenic and hypochondriacal disorders as well as adjustment disorders accompanied by anxiety and decreased mood (Bukhanovskaya & Demcheva, 2019). A survey of medical students from Belgorod revealed mental disorders in 24.4% of senior students and 16.2% of junior students (Ruzhenkova, 2020). In 18.8% of cases, non-pathological subthreshold reactions were registered. Stress-related and somatoform disorders were found in 8.5% of students, personality disorders in 3.7%, and mood disorders in 2.7%.

Depression and Anxiety

Anxiety and depression are among the most common mental disorders in medical students, as confirmed by several studies in Russia. Thus, the survey of medical students from Nizhny Novgorod revealed symptoms of depression in 33.6% of respondents (according to the Beck Depression Inventory) (Kasimova et al., 2018). Subclinical levels of depression (according to HADS) during the study period were registered in 35.8%, and clinically severe in 18.9% of medical students from Ulan-Ude. During exams, these rates increased to 38.1% and 31.7%, respectively (Tumutova et al., 2008). The following risk factors for depression in medical students have been established: family burden with mental disorders, periods of maladjustment in childhood, chronic somatic diseases, low physical activity, concomitant anxiety, and sleep disorders (Kasimova et al., 2018). In another study of first- and fifth-year medical students from Krasnodar, the prevalence of anxiety-depressive disorders was 6.8% in the first year and 11.5% in the fifth with a predominance of clinically pronounced anxiety in the first year and a significant predominance of clinically pronounced depression in the fifth year (Strizhev et al., 2016). Clinically significant symptoms of social phobia and generalized anxiety were found in 16% of medical students from Belgorod, while symptoms of depression (according to the Depression Anxiety Stress Scale-21) were observed in 34% of medical students (Ruzhenkova et al., 2018). The incidence of depression and anxiety in this sample was four and six times higher than in other students. Clinically significant anxiety was observed in 14.3% of medical students from Ulan-Ude during the study period and increased up to 31.7% during the exams (Tumutova et al., 2008). In another study of sixth-year students from Tomsk, anxiety was revealed more often among female (48.3%) than male (26.1%) (Ukraintsev et al., 2019).

Suicidality

The data on suicide among medical students is alarming. A narrative review of suicide and suicidal behaviour in medical students showed the role of social and environmental factors, including medical school systems (curriculum, housing, social support and academic pressure), interpersonal factors (social isolation, the competitive nature of training, and being away from home at an early age), and endemic factors typical only for medical training (simulation training, work with cadavers and observation of pathologies of patients) in increasing suicide risk (Watson et al., 2020). According to national data, 26.5% of surveyed Rostov-on-Don medical students were at high risk of developing suicidal behaviour (Soldatkin et al., 2012), and in a study in Moscow, 40.7% of medical students reported having suicidal thoughts in the present or past (Chritinin et al., 2016). Students with suicidal thoughts were characterized by mistrustfulness, anxiety, neatness, high expression of insecurity, and/or emotional distress.

Addictions and Addictive Behaviours

Substance abuse and addictive behaviours are among other common mental disorders in medical students, but at the same time can be perceived as a form of self-help for medical students. Thus, 11.5% of medical students from Rostov-on-Don had experience of psychoactive substance use, 30.8% were at risk of Internet addiction and 4.8% had already formed it (Soldatkin et al., 2012). Among medical students from Cheboksary 78% consumed alcohol and 7.4% of students (among whom men predominated) were classified as a risk group for developing alcohol addiction (Golenkov et al., 2009). The survey of senior medical students from Belgorod revealed alcohol abuse-related problems in 13% of cases, and addictive behaviour in 11.2% of students (14.8% of male and 9.9% of female), including alcohol addiction in 6.6% of young males and 1.2% of females (Lukyantseva et al., 2018). It has been shown that with an increase in the frequency of alcohol consumption by students, the level of trauma increases: up to 10.5% of students were injured due to alcohol consumption, 12% were beaten or assaulted by another student drinking alcohol, and 2% were victims of sexual violence (assault or date rape). This in turn increases the risk of negative effects on the mental state of students (Ruzhenkov & Lukyantseva, 2016). Individuals with addictive behaviour and dependence were characterized by high levels of social frustration and aggressiveness, low levels of self-motivation, inability to control emotions, low levels of responsibility, tolerance, and negative thinking, a higher frequency of asthenia, anxiety, and depression, as well as obsessive-compulsive symptoms, sociophobia, and dysmorphophobia. These created additional difficulties in social adaptation. Neurotic, stress-related, somatoform disorders, and personality disorders were predominant (Lukyantseva et al., 2018).

COVID-19 and Medical Students' Wellbeing

Specific conditions associated with the COVID-19 pandemic significantly affected the psychological wellbeing of medical students around the world (Essangri et al., 2021), with an increased need for psychological (emotional) support (Popova et al., 2021). It is already known that young people have been particularly exposed to psychological stress during the period of social isolation in Russia (Sorokin et al., 2020). Not surprisingly, research at the beginning of the pandemic has confirmed that lockdowns led to emotional disturbance, depression, irritability, insomnia, anger, and/or emotional exhaustion in medical students in Russia (Gritsenko et al., 2021). Another study conducted during the COVID-19 pandemic in Saratov revealed high levels of depression symptoms (73.6%) in medical students, with a moderate level of depressive symptoms observed in 12.5%, and 6.3% and 3.3% of respondents showed severe and extremely severe levels of depressive symptoms, respectively (Belyaeva et al., 2021). More than half (53%) of students from Chelyabinsk surveyed experienced intense anxiety because of COVID-19 restrictions and 69.4% of respondents recognized the COVID-19 pandemic and restrictions as new sources of stress (Avilov & Galiulina, 2020).

Several studies have demonstrated a high level of fear among medical students in Russia during the new coronavirus pandemic, the leading ones being concern for relatives' life and health, and fear for their own health (Avilov & Galiulina, 2020; Sudakov et al., 2021). It also has been shown that an additional source of anxiety and depression among medical students during the pandemic was remote learning and difficulties with homework (Belyaeva et al., 2021), accompanied by fear of missing clinical practical skills because of COVID-19 restrictions (Sudakov et al., 2021).

Results of Our Own Research

In 2020, we conducted our own research as part of an international initiative aimed at screening for minor psychiatric disorders, burnout, problematic alcohol use, and quantify the psychological issues and stress among a sample of medical students (n = 165 from all years of study; 80% females) in St. Petersburg, Russia (Chumakov et al., 2021). The survey was conducted in Russian; minor psychiatric disorders were identified through the Short General Health Questionnaire (GHQ-12); Oldenburg Burnout Inventory (OLBI) was used to identify burnout, whilst problem alcohol use was identified using the CAGE (Cut-down; Annoyed; Guilty; Eye-opener) questionnaire.

   We found a high incidence of self-reported mental health disorders in the sample: ten individuals (6%) being diagnosed before entering university and twenty-five students (15%) during their own training. Our data confirm the academic stress and the pressure of the professional environment were rated as the leading source of stress (89% of respondents). Other sources of stress included social relationships (intimate or family; 50.9%), financial wellbeing (38.2%), work (32.1%), and housing problems (20.6%). Screening with the CAGE* tool identified alcohol problems in 33 students (20.0%). According to the GHQ-12**, 140 students (84.8%) had a total score of 2 or higher, indicating a high risk of minor mental disorders in the sample. The mean value of the total GHQ-12 score in the study group was 5.05±3.04. Screening for burnout using the OLBI*** showed positive scores in 121 (73.3%) students for disengagement and 132 (80.0%) students for exhaustion. No differences were found in the frequency of positive screening of the survey's techniques when dividing respondents by gender.

   * For the CAGE questionnaire, a score of ≥ 2 was considered as the cut-off for problem drinking.
   ** For the GHQ-12, the bimodal GHQ scoring method (0-0-1-1) was used, and a score of two was considered as the cut-off to identify cases.
   *** For the OLBI, burnout was detected by combining the mean score of 2.25 for *exhaustion* and 2.10 for *disengagement*.

Psychological and Psychiatric Care and Prevention Programmes for Medical Students in Russia

Given the high prevalence of mental disorders among medical students, medical schools should implement programmes to identify students at risk of developing mental disorders and provide them with easy access to specialized psychiatric care (Kasimova et al., 2018). At the same time, the low awareness among medical students about how to get psychological help or support is alarming (Bhugra et al., 2019). Therefore, it is important to develop and implement active screening and identification programmes for students with signs of mental distress in order to provide them with psychological and psychiatric care in a timely manner.

Another important aspect of assistance programmes is prevention. Academic schedules and burdens of medical students should be balanced to prevent educational stress, anxiety, and depression (Ruzhenkova et al., 2018). Russian researchers have developed and tested 'Stress management' training aimed at teaching medical students constructive ways to combat stress and reduce anxiety and depression (Ruzhenkova, 2020). This training includes a cycle of lectures and practical sessions on topics that deal with the concept of crisis and crisis situations, stress, conflict, psychological defence mechanisms, mental trauma, addictive and suicidal behaviours, stigmatization, and issues of emergency psychological aid in crisis situations. It is recommended for use in the primary and secondary prevention of mental disorders during university education, but so far there is no data on how often and effectively it is used. Other programmes of psycho-prevention could also be used, such as dialogue forms of joint work between a teacher and a student and/or, support of contacts in a social network.

Academic authorities also develop their own programmes to provide psychological assistance to students. For example, St. Petersburg State University (SPbU) has a separate subdivision, the Psychological Assistance Service. This was created in 2012 to provide assistance and support in solving a variety of psychological problems and overcoming difficult life situations. The main mission of the Service is to provide free psychological assistance to SPbU students and employees. The subject of counselling is anxiety or depression. The Service is staffed by professors from the Faculty of Psychology at St. Petersburg State University who are trained and experienced in the field of psychological counselling. Consultations are conducted jointly with undergraduate and graduate students of the Faculty of Psychology at St. Petersburg State University who have received special training. The duration of the consultation is 50 minutes, and the client can receive up to five psychological consultations.

Conclusions

This chapter provided an overview of research on the psychological wellbeing of medical students in Russia, as well as shedding light on some of the programmes available for implementation for prevention and early help to those in need. A review of the literature revealed a lack of multicentre studies on the topic of the chapter, which greatly limits the systematization of the data. It is also problematic to compare various studies in Russia because the socioeconomic situation in the regions is very different. Since the country is multinational, the characteristics of individual peoples (genetic, cultural, religious) can have a significant impact on the challenges faced by medical students. However, data from cross-sectional studies conducted in recent years substantiate the importance and relevance of continuing work on the mental state of medical students and the risk factors for mental disorders in this population. In the authors' opinion, it is also important to expand the work on the publication of research results in international peer-reviewed journals in order to increase the availability of data on the research topic for the scientific international community. Of most importance is to obtain practical data on the effectiveness and degree of implementation of the developed programmes for the prevention of mental disorders in medical students in Russia.

References

Avilov, O.V. & Galiulina, K.Y. (2020). 'Stress among medical students caused by COVID-19 restrictions'. *Psychophysiology News* 4: 73–83. (In Russ.)

Belyaeva, Y.N., Shemetova, G.N., Baboshkina, L.S., & Gaydarova, D.S. (2021). 'Dynamics of the psychological status of medical university students in remote vocational training in the context of the coronavirus pandemic'. *Modern Problems of Science and Education* 1: 59–59. (In Russ.)

Bhugra, D., Sauerteig, S.-O., Bland, D., Lloyd-Kendall, A., Wijesuriya, J., Singh, G., Kochhar, A., Molodynski, A., & Ventriglio, A. (2019). 'A descriptive study of mental health and wellbeing of doctors and medical students in the UK'. *Int Rev Psychiatry* 31(7–8): 563–568.

Bukhanovskaya, O.A. & Demcheva. N.K. (2019). 'Psychopathological characteristics of neurotic, stress-related and somatoform disorders among medical students'. *Bull Neurol Psych Neurosurg* 9: 20–33. (In Russ.)

Bukhanovskaya, O.A. & Demcheva. N.K. (2020). 'Relationship between satisfaction with learning outcomes and mental health of medical and technical students'. *Bull Neurol Psych Neurosurg* 1: 70–78.

Chritinin, D.F., Sumarokova, M.A., Esin, A.V., Samokhin, D.V., & Shchukina, E.P. (2016). 'Conditions of suicidal behavior formation among medical college students'. *Suicidology* 2(23): 49–54. (In Russ.)

Chumakov, E., Petrova, N., Mamatkhodjaeva, T., Ventriglio, A., Bhugra, D., & Molodynski, A. (2021). 'Screening of minor psychiatric disorders and burnout among a sample of medical students in St. Petersburg. Russia: a descriptive study'. *Middle East Curr Psychiatry* 28(1): 38.

Drachev, S., Stangvaltaite-Mouhat, L., Bolstad, N.L., Johnsen, J.A., Yushmanova, T., & Trovik, T. (2020). 'Perceived stress and associated factors in Russian medical and dental students: a cross-sectional study in north-west Russia'. *Int J Environ Res Public Health* 17(15): 5390. (In Russ.)

Dyrbye, L.N., West, C.P., Satele, D., Boone, S., Tan, L., Sloan, J., Shanafelt, T.D. (2014). 'Burnout among U.S. medical students, residents, and early career physicians relative to the general U.S. population'. *Acad Med* 89(3): 443–451.

Essangri, H., Sabir, M., Benkabbou, A., Majbar, M.A., Amrani, L., Ghannam, A., Lekehal, B., Mohsine, R., & Souadka, A. (2021). 'Predictive factors for impaired mental health among medical students during the early stage of the COVID-19 pandemic in Morocco'. *Am J Trop Med Hyg* 104(1): 95–102.

Golenkov, A.V., Andreeva, A.P., & Bulygina, I.E. (2009). 'Quantitative and qualitative measures and motives for alcohol use in medical students'. *Narcology* 10: 25–29. (In Russ.)

Gritsenko, V., Skugarevsky, O., Konstantinov, V., Khamenka, N., Marinova, T., Reznik, A., & Isralowitz, R. (2021). 'COVID 19 fear, stress, anxiety, and substance use among Russian and Belarusian University students'. *Int J Ment Health Addiction* 19: 2362–2368.

Kadhum, M., Ayinde, O.O., Wilkes, C., Chumakov, E., Dahanayake, D., Ashrafi, A., Kafle, B., Lili, R., Farrell, S., Bhugra, D., & Molodysnki, A. (2022). 'Wellbeing, burnout and substance use amongst medical students: a summary of results from nine countries'. *Int J Soc Psychiatry* 68(6): 1218–1222.

Kasimova, L.N., Svyatogor, M.V., & Smirensky, E.A. (2018). 'Socio-demographic and clinical risk factors for depressive disorders development in medical students'. *Medical Almanac*, 5(56): 185–188. (In Russ.)

Khan, J.M., Altaf, S., & Kausar, H. (2013). 'Effect of perceived academic stress on students' performance'. *FWU Journal of Social Sciences* 7(2): 146–151.

Kobyliatskaya, I.A., Osykina, A.S., & Shkatova, E.Y. (2015). 'The state of health of student youth'. *Advances in Modern Natural Science* 5: 74–75. (In Russ.)

Korshunova, A.N., & Mukhina, T.K. (2014). 'Socio-psychological features of stress in adolescents'. *Young Scientist* 18: 749–752. (In Russ.)

Lukyantseva, I.S., Ruzhenkov, V.A., & Ponomarenko, D.O. (2018). 'Addictive behavior and alcoholism in medical students of senior courses (prevalence, comorbidity and treatment)'. *I.P. Pavlov Russian Medical Biological Herald* 26(3): 380–387. (In Russ.)

Minnibaev, T.Sh., Timoshenko, K.T., & Goncharova, G.A. (2012). 'Time budget, progress, and adaptation in school-university profile class pupils'. *Hygiene and Sanitation* **91**(2): 67–69. (In Russ.)

Molodynski, A., Lewis, T., Kadhum, M., Farrell, S.M., Lemtiri Chelieh, M., Falcão De Almeida, T., Masri, R., Kar, A., Volpe, U., Moir, F., Torales, J., Castaldelli-Maia, J.M., Chau, S.W.H., Wilkes, C., & Bhugra, D. (2021). 'Cultural variations in wellbeing, burnout and substance use amongst medical students in twelve countries'. *Int Rev Psychiatry* **33**(1–2): 37–42.

Popova, D.A., Davletgildeev, E.R., Yerlanova, E.E., & Abikulova, A.K. (2021). 'Psychoemotional state of KazNMU students during COVID-19 pandemic'. *Vestnik KazNMU* **2**: 309–314. (In Russ.)

Ruzhenkov, V.A., & Lukyantseva, I.S. (2016). 'Prevalence of addictive behavior among medical students'. *Bull Neurol Psych Neurosurg* **9**: 14–19. (In Russ.)

Ruzhenkova, V., Tarabaeva, V., Ruzhenkov, V., & Lukyantseva, I. (2018). 'Medical and psychological characteristics of the 1st year students of medical and pedagogical institutes and their features of educational adaptation'. *Drug Invention Today* **10**: 3240–3246. (In Russ.)

Ruzhenkova, V.V. (2020). 'The prevalence and clinical structure of mental disorders in medical students (problems of primary and secondary psychoprophylaxis)'. *Res Results Biomed* **6**(1): 135–153. (In Russ.)

Soldatkin, V.A., Dyachenko, A.V., & Merkureva, K.S. (2012). 'The study of suicidological and addictological situation among students of Rostov-on-Don'. *Suicidology* **3**(4): 60–64. (In Russ.)

Sorokin, M., Kasyanov, E., Rukavishnikov, G., Makarevich, O., Neznanov, N., Lutova, N., Mazo, G.E. (2020). 'Structure of anxiety associated with the COVID-19 pandemic in the Russian-speaking sample: results from on-line survey'. *Bulletin of Russian State Medical University* **3**: 70–76.

Strizhev, V.A., Boyko, E.O., Lozhnikova, L.E., & Zaitceva, O.G. (2016). 'Anxiety and depressive disorders in medical students'. *Kuban Scientific Medical Bulletin* **2**: 126–131. (In Russ.)

Sudakov, D.V., Sudakov, O.V., Yakusheva, N.V., Shevtsov, A.N., & Belov, E.V. (2021). On the psychological adaptation of medical students to the distance learning process during the new coronavirus infection pandemic. In Barashkina, S.B. (ed) *Actual Questions of Pedagogy and Psychology: A Monograph*. Russia: Sreda, pp. 133–144 (In Russ.)

Torshina, T.I., Zueva, A.A., & Drobysheva, O.M. (2016). 'Psychodiagnostics of stress in medical students'. *Int J Appl Fund Res* **11**(4): 806–807. (In Russ.)

Tumutova, E.Ch., Durinova, A.B., & Strambovskaya, N.N. (2008). 'Anxiety-depressive disorders in medical students of BSU'. *Bulletin of East-Siberian Scientific Center of Siberian Branch of Russian Academy of Medical Sciences* **3**(61): 147–148. (In Russ.)

Turovaya, A.Y., Kade, A.H., Velichko, M.A., Uvarov, A.V., & Plotnikova, A.O. (2014). 'Manifestations of psycho-emotional stress in medical students depending on performance during sessions'. *Int J Appl Fund Res* **5**: 145–146. (In Russ.)

Ukraintsev, I.I., Schastnyy, E.D., & Bokhan, N.A. (2019). 'Incidence rate of anxiety and personality disorders and their interrelationship in senior-year students of the medical university'. *Bull Siber Med* **18**(4): 143–149. (In Russ.)

Watson, C., Ventriglio, A., & Bhugra, D. (2020). 'A narrative review of suicide and suicidal behavior in medical students'. *Indian J Psychiatry* **62**(3): 250–256.

24
Sri Lanka

The Mental Health of Medical Students: Supporting Wellbeing in Medical Education in Sri Lanka

Dulangi Dahanayake and Anuprabha Wickramasinghe

The Development of Medical Undergraduate Training in Sri Lanka

Sri Lanka is an island nation with a population of approximately 22 million people. The healthcare needs are largely met by allopathic practitioners and Sri Lanka has achieved relatively high standards in terms of healthcare indices (Rajapaksa et al., 2021). This has come in the wake of the free education policy of 1944 and the delivery of free healthcare since 1951 by the Sri Lankan government (Alawattegam, 2020; Rajapaksa et al., 2021).

The training of Sri Lankans in allopathic medical practices was initially done abroad. The Colombo Medical School was established in 1870 during the British colonial era and the Diploma of Licentiate of Medicine and Surgery (LMS) granted by the institution was accepted as qualifying for registration with the General Medical Council of the United Kingdom. The language of instruction was English since the establishment of the initial course. In 1892, women were given the opportunity to enter Colombo Medical School and in 1942 Diploma of LMS was elevated to the MBBS degree. In 1962, a second medical school was founded in Peradeniya and this was followed by the establishment of medical faculties in the Universities of Ruhuna, Jaffna, Sri Jayewardenepura, Kelaniya, Rajarata, Eastern University, Wayamba, Sabaragamuwa and, in 2020, at Moratuwa. In addition, a Faculty of Medicine was established in 2009 at the General Sir John Kotelawela Defence University; this is the only national military medical institution for higher education in Sri Lanka.

Sri Lanka is one of the few countries in the world which provides education free of charge to all. This extends to undergraduate education, including medical education. Despite the country having established private post-secondary education institutions, attempts to initiate private medical schools have been met with resistance.

The Higher Education Act (No. 20 of 1966) led to the establishment of the National Council of Higher Education; the forerunner of the University Grants Commission (UGC) established in 1978. UGC, which is under the higher education sector of the Ministry of Education, is involved in planning, administration, allocation of funds, maintaining academic standards, and the regulation of admissions to universities.

Entrance to the MBBS course is through the highly competitive General Certificate of Examination (Advanced Level), with the average age at entrance around 20 years. There are no pathways for lateral entrance. The selection of students for the MBBS degree following the

Dulangi Dahanayake and Anuprabha Wickramasinghe, *Sri Lanka* In: *The Mental Health of Medical Students.*
Edited by: Andrew Molodynski, Sarah Marie Farrell, and Dinesh Bhugra, Oxford University Press. © Oxford University Press 2024.
DOI: 10.1093/oso/9780192864871.003.0024

aforementioned examination is as follows; 40% on an all-island merit basis, 55% on a district quota system, and 5% from 16 districts identified as disadvantaged. In addition, a few foreign students and children of diplomatic/foreign/state service personnel as well as a small number of students with national level achievements in fields such as sports are given admission (National Education Commission Sri Lanka, 2019).

The medical curriculum and models of teaching in Sri Lanka have evolved in keeping with global trends. In 1995, the Faculty of Medicine, Colombo introduced a new curriculum aimed at being more integrated and student-centred, with system-based modules, early contact with clinical and community-based learning and a behavioural sciences stream. There has been a move towards similar changes in other medical faculties. Programme reviews by the Quality Assurance Council of the UGC are conducted regularly. In 2015, the UGC introduced the Sri Lanka Qualifications Framework (SLQF) staging the higher education qualifications and the MBBS degree requires a minimum of 150 credits and a minimum student workload of 7500 notional learning hours, encompassing professional practice. Online teaching-learning has developed and gained prominence, especially during the COVID-19 pandemic, with learning management systems and Zoom accounts created for academics through the Lanka Education And Research Network (LEARN), which exempted students from data charges.

Psychological Wellbeing of Medical Undergraduates in Sri Lanka

Progress has been made in the arena of student welfare and wellbeing under the direction of the UGC, acknowledging the importance of mental wellbeing among students. There are no published studies on the indicators of mental wellbeing in Sri Lankan medical undergraduates, and existing studies have used tools developed in western countries (Dahanayake et al., 2022; Wimberly et al., 2022). In a collectivist culture, such as that in Sri Lanka, there is low prominence given to self-expression, self-promotion, and pursuing self-chosen paths to satisfaction. Traditionally, equality is promoted within the university subculture, in keeping with the political influence of leftist parties. Thus, the experience of psychological wellbeing among medical students in Sri Lanka is likely to be qualitatively different from their counterparts in Western countries.

The readiness of medical students for independent living and decision-making, as well as parental encouragement to do so, is low. A majority rely on their parents for finances and lodging, with students having adequate access to resources having less psychological stress (Dahanayake et al., 2022). Education is given a high value in society due to cultural as well as economic reasons, and high achievements in examinations, including receiving classes, distinctions, and other awards are a positive influence on mental wellbeing. English language proficiency is widely viewed as a measure of social status and students who view themselves as proficient in the language have shown better results at examinations (Wijesundara et al., 2018). The importance of fulfilling social relationships and the ability to integrate well with the larger student body are also important for mental wellbeing. This is facilitated by new entrants being free of fears related to violence and ragging.

In summary, medical undergraduate training in Sri Lanka continues to evolve to keep up with the changing healthcare needs of the population and global trends in medical education. For the medical undergraduate in this setting, mental wellbeing is a construct of myriad factors, including personal attributes, cultural values, and economic as well as political influences. In Sri Lanka, as in the global tableau, despite its pivotal role in an individual's life, the definition and measurement of mental wellbeing remain a challenge.

Psychological Problems Among Medical Undergraduates in Sri Lanka

Medical students in Sri Lanka are faced with psychological problems, including stress, burnout, depression, anxiety, suicidal ideation, other severe mental health conditions, substance use, internet and gaming addictions, personality problems, and poor quality of life.

Stress and Burnout

Medical undergraduate programmes are intellectually demanding and may make students feel overwhelmed. Burnout is a common phenomenon among medical students, resulting from chronic stress that has not been successfully managed. A recent study involving 1097 students from all years from several medical schools in Sri Lanka revealed 93% to have disengagement and 79% to have exhaustion on the Oldenburg Burnout Inventory (OLBI), indicating a high prevalence of burnout (Dahanayake et al., 2022). In another study, medical students in Jaffna showed a high (83.7%) prevalence of burnout as per OLBI (Weerasinghe et al., 2020). A study looking at students in Ruhuna which used the Kessler-10 psychological distress scale showed that 40.4% of medical students were suffering from severe psychological distress (Wimberly et al., 2022).

In a study conducted at the University of Sri Jayewardenepura comparing final-year medical undergraduates with parallel non-medical undergraduates using the General Health Questionnaire (GHQ-30), 63% of medical undergraduates showed psychological distress as opposed to 56% in the other group (Liyanage, 2017). Studies that compared medical undergraduates in different academic years of training have reported that psychological distress and burnout are more common among final-year medical students (Wimberly et al., 2022; Weerasinghe et al., 2020) while others did not find such a clear relationship with the year of study (Dahanayake et al., 2022). With regard to gender, one study showed that female students suffered from burnout more than male students (Wimberly et al., 2022), while others failed to demonstrate such a relationship (Dahanayake et al., 2022; Liyanage, 2017; Weerasinghe et al., 2020).

Psychological distress and burnout appear to be common among Sri Lankan medical students. Failure to address stress and burnout can lead to devastating consequences such as poor quality of life and mental health problems like depression and suicide (Ishak et al., 2013), addictive behaviours and reduced academic performance among medical students (Dyrbye et al., 2005; Ruzhenkova et al., 2018).

Depression

Medical undergraduates in Sri Lanka show a high prevalence of depressive symptoms (19%) (Torabi & Perera, 2006), with major depression in 9.9% (Amarasuriya et al., 2015b). Depressive symptoms are commoner (76%) among first years than their non-medical peers (Perera, 2011), as well as compared to medical students in later years of training (Wickramasinghe et al., 2019). Students from the final year of training were the next most vulnerable group (Wickramasinghe et al., 2019).

Depression can lead to other negative outcomes such as suicide and poor academic achievements and thus calls for active case finding and management. One recent Sri Lankan study showed medical undergraduates were no more ready to seek treatment for depression compared to non-medical undergraduates (Amarasuriya et al., 2015a).

Anxiety Disorders

Studies have shown high rates of caseness using the GHQ (which assesses anxiety and somatic concerns) among Sri Lankan medical students (Dahanayake et al., 2022). Experience indicates that social anxiety disorder, obsessive compulsive disorder, health anxiety, trait anxiety, and perfectionism are common among Sri Lankan medical students. Anxiety may have a negative impact on academic grades, mental health, physical health, and quality of experience. Affected students may consider anxiety as their character flaw or moral weakness rather than seeking help.

Severe and Enduring Mental Illness

There is a lack of research regarding schizophrenia and bipolar disorder among Sri Lankan medical students. Students suffering from serious mental illnesses are at risk of failing examinations and taking a longer time to complete the course or dropping out.

Suicide and Self-harm

Several suicides have occurred among medical students over the last decade, but there is no data available apart from newspaper articles to quantify or recognize trends in this important area of concern. Depression, academic stress, lack of administrative support, suboptimal student counselling and mentoring services, break up of romantic relationships and other relationship disputes have been informally quoted as contributory factors. Students have requested higher transparency regarding data on suicides. Research outside Sri Lanka also demands better transparency in such data (Laitman & Muller, 2019).

Personality Disorders

Although anecdotal evidence suggests personality disorders as an important issue among Sri Lankan medical students, there is a notable lack of research evidence exposing these trends.

Substance Use Among Medical Undergraduates

In a large sample of medical undergraduates across six medical colleges in Sri Lanka (Dahanayake et al., 2022), 7% reported having used at least one form of substance other than alcohol in their lifetime. Five per cent of students were found to be at risk of alcohol-related health problems, as shown in the screening using CAGE questionnaire. Males used alcohol and other substances significantly more than females.

Reduced Quality of Life (QoL)

In one interesting Sri Lankan study, 78 fourth-year medical students were screened using the World Health Organization Quality of Life (WHOQOL-BREF) questionnaire, prior to and a few weeks after their main examination (Hettiarachchi et al., 2014). Results showed that the mean QoL was significantly lower during the period before the examination when compared to the period afterwards. Higher QoL was associated with better grades at the examinations and a better profile of stress biochemical parameters (Hettiarachchi et al., 2014).

Internet Addiction

Internet addiction and addiction to gaming are seen among medical undergraduates, but their prevalence in Sri Lankan medical undergraduates has not been studied. Internet addiction gives rise to poor QoL scores, and poor academic performance, and the COVID-19 pandemic worsened the situation among students.

Factors Contributing to Psychological Problems

The psychological wellbeing of a student is affected by different factors that can be broadly divided into characteristics of the individual, medical education, and contemporary society.

The Individual

The selection process to medical faculties in Sri Lanka consists of one summative theory examination after two years of training in biology, chemistry, and physics. The choice by the individual student to follow biology stream and his or her ability to obtain a high mark in this examination are the only qualifying criteria, which may be proxy indicators of student's commitment, intelligence, work ethics, time management, and resilience. However, other aspects like communication and language skills, personality attributes, social skills, and so-called soft skills, ethical and moral standards, emotional intelligence, unhelpful habits, and financial commitment are not tested in the selection process. Although it is inevitable that even the most stringent selection criteria leave space for a mismatch between the student profiles and course requirements, the current selection criteria in Sri Lanka are seen as widening this gap. Studies have shown this examination to be a poor predictor of performance as a medical undergraduate (de Silva et al., 2006).

Only a handful of studies have looked at contributory individual characteristics in the Sri Lankan context. Higher emotional intelligence (Ranasinghe et al., 2017) was shown to be protective against stress and burnout among medical students in Sri Lanka. Participation in extracurricular activities showed a protective effect against depressive symptoms (Wickramasinghe et al., 2019).

On the other hand, several factors have been shown to be associated with development of depression such as living in hostels, exposure to threatening life events, deaths in the family, relationship break-ups, problems with close associates and academic difficulties (Amarasuriya et al., 2015b). Increased depressive symptoms were shown to be associated with a sedentary lifestyle, sexual inactivity, and/or poverty (Perera, 2011).

The Medical Faculty and the Course

Possible overloading of the undergraduate curriculum was a point raised at programme reviews conducted by the University Grants Commission of Sri Lanka (*Programme review report, MBBS programme, Faculty of Medicine, University of Colombo*, 2019). There is concern that this may place unhealthy pressure on medical students. The difficulty in monitoring workload due to lack of attention to the credit system and notional hours may be contributing to the problem. There is little evidence that our medical undergraduate programmes incorporate student feedback to make adjustments to the curriculum, teaching-learning processes, and assessments.

Secondary education is mainly conducted in the Sinhala or Tamil medium, and limited English language proficiency creates a disadvantage for students, especially those from rural backgrounds. This can affect the social confidence of the students as well as their grades (Chandradasa, 2017; Wijesundara et al., 2018). Academic pressure caused by frequent assessments, clinical training, and interactions with hospital consultants has been recognized as one of the main reasons for stress (Liyanage, 2017). High student numbers in medical faculties are a hindrance to small-group teaching and adequate student engagement in activities.

In Sri Lanka, the teacher-student gap remains wide, which is different to present practices in the West. Jayasinghe et al. in 2011 examined sources of student anxiety from a group of new graduates and found that a significant number have experienced punitive measures such as getting scolded, group punishments, and negative remarks on English language skills. An authoritarian learning environment is generally felt to be counterproductive for adult (or indeed any!) learners (Jayasinghe et al., 2004).

The limited income generation by medical faculties in Sri Lanka forces them to rely on government financing. The current economic struggles lead to difficulties in developing the necessary infrastructure, facilities, and human resources in medical faculties. Retaining academic staff in medical schools is problematic, causing challenges in meeting the desired student-teacher ratio.

Wider Society and Culture

Ensuring student safety from potential risks that exist in society is considered a priority, which puts serious restrictions to socializing, night life, leisure, and sports. This is further enhanced by the adherence to male and female roles expected from the society. Student hostels are traditionally arranged separately for male and female students. Students are discouraged by society from engaging in premarital sexual activity and sometimes even romantic relationships. Students have a poor understanding of contraception and the stigma on pre-marital sexual activity further hinders the use of contraception. There is no research data available on sexual activity and contraception in this population.

There is an expectation from society that medical students will take responsibility when a family member falls unwell. This can put them under a lot of strain.

The lack of an established system of student loan facilities places some students in significant financial hardship. It is very rare for a student to do a part-time job during medical undergraduate courses in Sri Lanka, mainly because of the lack of work opportunities and the expectations from society in relation to a budding doctor.

Ragging, in the form of verbal, physical, or sexual insults, used to be rife in the Sri Lankan university subculture. Many students have been harmed, and such incidents have led to death due to physical exhaustion or suicide. Scientific studies are lacking in this field but one such study on dental undergraduates showed that 50% had experienced some form of mistreatment, and verbal and emotional abuse were more common than physical or sexual abuse (Premadasa et al., 2011). Although overt ragging may not be present in medical undergraduate courses, several restrictions are put by senior student groups for new entrants that includes a stricter dress code, and prohibition of using common facilities like the library, canteen, and student common rooms.

External social and political movements often seep into the universities. A communist movement in 1971, riots against establishing private medical schools in 1986 and 2017, anti-government movement during 1988–89, and the riots of 2022 led to significant disruptions in student lives and medical education.

Other divisions can be more subtle and more generic. Students belonging to some ethnic groups tend to isolate themselves from others, which can lead to stigma. Students with different social class backgrounds generally mix well, but there can be occasional polarization between students who communicate in English and students speaking their mother tongue, which is stressful for some students.

In summary, medical undergraduates in Sri Lanka face significant mental health problems including stress, burnout, anxiety, and depression. These adverse impacts on mental wellbeing are determined by various factors, including (but not limited to) characteristics of individuals, the medical course, and the wider sociocultural, economic, and political landscape.

Interventions in the Sri Lankan Settings to Enhance the Mental Wellbeing of Medical Students

There are established methods, both formal and informal, that are utilized by the university system and individual students in Sri Lanka to overcome negative influences on their mental wellbeing and emphasize positive influences.

In terms of managing issues related to individual students, the UGC has introduced a student support and welfare system (UGC Circ 933, 1998). This encompasses six areas including student services, accommodation and cafeteria, healthcare service and facilities for sports and recreational activities, student welfare and counselling, career guidance, and security services.

There are established financial assistance schemes (Mahapola scholarship, bursaries, and endowed scholarships) and programmes at individual university and faculty levels, funded by alumni and well-wishers. The UGC has partnered with state banks to set up a loan scheme for students to acquire laptop computers. Residential facilities or hostels are provided free of charge, depending upon the financial situation of the family and the distance from home. Cafeterias provide meals and snacks at extreme concessionary rates. Free library facilities, including access to e-libraries and free Wi-Fi facilities within university premises are provided.

Facilities for sports and recreation exist, and annual sports and cultural events within and between different universities and faculties are held, with the participation of academic staff. These events serve to develop a sense of community and wellbeing in the student fraternity.

Formal programmes for student mentoring are established in the medical faculties and academic staff members are allocated mentees. In addition, counselling services, with the appointment of senior student counsellors, are available. These include helplines for students. There are hostel wardens supporting students. The University Medical Officer offers help for physical as well as mental health issues and facilitates referrals to specialist services where necessary.

The 'Prohibition of ragging and other forms of violence in educational institutes act' by the government of Sri Lanka in 1998, was a measure taken to endow suitable punishment against those who engage in ragging (Universities Act, 1978). The ragging complaints portal of the UGC is available for victims and in 2017, a 24-hour hotline was established for students and staff to report ragging.

Delayed age at graduation, which impacts adversely on mental wellbeing, has led to proposals to optimize the age of graduation of MBBS graduates following discussions with the Ministries of Health and Education.

Policies and practices have been adopted by the UGC and individual universities to optimize curricula, examination procedures, lecturer-student ratios, research opportunities, and improved access to medical literature for students. The UGC has appointed a Standing Committee, which submits recommendations regarding proposals by universities for curricular reforms and promotes new initiatives to improve the quality and relevance of MBBS degree programmes (Universities Act, 1978). At individual university and medical faculty level, internal quality assurance cell (IQAC) and curriculum development committees ensure that curricula are updated and reviewed regularly. Quality assurance programmes have actively investigated improving assessment methods, both to enhance the capturing of knowledge, skills, and attitudes and to reduce the stress related to summative assessments.

In exceptional circumstances when a student fails to fulfil requirements for the MBBS degree, the UGC circular on fall-back qualifications will enable them to receive a qualification at a lower SLQF level and to follow an alternative career path.

The UGC has recommended that for the MBBS degree the lecturer to student ratio should be one to seven. This goal has been challenging, especially for those medical faculties situated away from the commercial capital of Colombo and there are financial incentives offered by some universities to attract academic staff. In relation to staff development, there are established staff development centres which conduct compulsory induction programmes and continuing professional development programmes.

Enhancing 'soft skills' among medical students, in aspects such as language, learning methods, time management, stress management, problem-solving, teamwork, ethics, and moral values are addressed through the behavioural sciences stream, the community sciences stream, and through student-centred and group activities. Medical faculties have established

Language Units and facilitate improving English language skills in medical students through intensive English language courses at the start of the MBBS programme and throughout the programme for those who request it.

In addition to these formal support measures, informal support systems exist that help enhance mental wellbeing. Within the university system of Sri Lanka, a subculture exists where equality is valued and students refer to each other in Sinhala or Tamil terms indicating brotherhood, in keeping with socialist and communist political influences. This creates a sense of belonging and community, with students sharing food, books, and other possessions as well as supporting students who have failed at examinations. A type of coaching, given free of charge, variably termed 'kuppi' or 'bats', is a form of peer-assisted learning which has gained popularity among medical students. Within this subculture, there is also a support system for female medical students, with male students accompanying them when they travel between the campus or hospital and their hostels at night-time. Furthermore, student societies and clubs such as the Golden Z club and Rotaract club have organized programmes to enhance mental health literacy and support the mental wellbeing of students.

Future Directions for Supporting Mental Wellbeing of Medical Students in Sri Lanka

Despite the availability of aforementioned support systems for medical students in Sri Lanka, there are areas which need further attention. The most striking is the lack of research on the mental wellbeing of medical undergraduates in Sri Lanka. There is a knowledge gap related not only to the prevalence of mental health issues, but also in relation to underlying factors that impact positively and negatively on the mental wellbeing of medical students. This is a barrier to identifying suitable measures to enhance psychological wellbeing in this population, and further studies, which are integrated into the university system, are needed.

Exposure to stressful and traumatic clinical material and events, such as witnessing deaths and patients with severe injuries, have been associated with adverse impacts on mental wellbeing. However, formal measures to help students to handle these stressors are scarce. Student support systems, for both academic matters and mental health issues, with the possibility of online modes of delivery are areas that need to be actively considered. The available support for emerging issues such as internet addiction also appears to be inadequate.

Although monitoring systems are in place to assess the learning environment and related issues, there is a lack of integration between university teachers and the extended faculty, which includes Consultants of the Ministry of Health working in teaching hospitals. Encouraging active participation of the extended faculty in curriculum development and planning of teaching-learning activities will be helpful.

Student inclusion needs more attention. Despite provision for student inclusion in the administrative processes, their contribution to the system is still limited. Formal recognition of student unions and involvement of academic staff in providing guidance when needed, are possible measures to support students to make decisions that will impact positively on their future and wellbeing, while allowing for self-expression and upholding their rights.

In conclusion, there is an established system in place within the Sri Lankan university structure to support the mental wellbeing of medical undergraduates. There is a need to adopt methods to keep up with the changing needs of this population and to make help more accessible to all.

References

Alawattegam, K.K. (2020). 'Free education policy and its emerging challenges in Sri Lanka'. *Eur J Educ Sci* **7**(1): 1–14.

Amarasuriya, S.D., Jorm, A.F., & Reavley, N.J. (2015a). 'Perceptions and intentions relating to seeking help for depression among medical undergraduates in Sri Lanka: A cross-sectional comparison with non-medical undergraduates'. *BMC Med Educ* **15**(1): 1–10.

Amarasuriya, S.D., Jorm, A.F., & Reavley, N.J. (2015b). 'Prevalence of depression and its correlates among undergraduates in Sri Lanka'. *Asian J Psychiatr* **15**: 32–37.

Chandradasa, S.J.D. (2017). 'The impact of the university subculture on learning English as a second language'. *PEOPLE: Int J Soc Sci* **3**(2): 1029–1048.

Dahanayake, D., Rajapakse, H., Wickramasinghe, A., Chandradasa, M., Rohanachandra, Y., Perera, S., Nillo, A.M., & Molodynski, A. (2022). 'Psychological wellbeing and mental health amongst medical undergraduates: a descriptive study assessing more than 1,000 medical students in Sri Lanka'. *Int J Soc Psychiatry* **68**(6): 1263–1269.

Dyrbye, L.N., Thomas, M.R., & Shanafelt, T.D. (2005). 'Medical student distress: causes, consequences, and proposed solutions'. *Mayo Clin Proc* **80**(12): 1613–1622.

Hettiarachchi, M., Fonseka, C.L., Gunasekara, P., Jayasinghe, P., & Maduranga, D. (2014). 'How does the quality of life and the underlying biochemical indicators correlate with the performance in academic examinations in a group of medical students of Sri Lanka?'. *Med Educ Online* **19**(1): 1–6.

Ishak, W., Nikravesh, R., Lederer, S., Perry, R., Ogunyemi, D., & Bernstein, C. (2013). 'Burnout in medical students: a systematic review'. *Clin Teach* **10**(4): 242–245.

Jayasinghe, S., de Silva, P., & de Silva, D. (2004). 'Unacceptable teacher behaviour or medical student abuse?'. *Ceylon Med J* **49**(2): 69.

Laitman, B.M. & Muller, D. (2019). 'Medical student deaths by suicide: the importance of transparency'. *Acad Med* **94**(4): 466–468.

Liyanage, G. (2017). 'Psychological distress among final year medical undergraduates in a Sri Lankan university'. *Int J Comm Med Public Health* **4**(11): 3952.

National Education Commission Sri Lanka (2019). *National Policy Proposals on Higher Education December 2019, Higher Education Commission.*

Perera, B. (2011). 'Are medical undergraduates more vulnerable than their non-medical peers to develop depressive symptoms?'. *Galle Med J* **16**(1): 1.

Premadasa, I.G., Wanigasooriya, N.C., Thalib, L., & Ellepola, A.N. (2011). 'Harassment of newly admitted undergraduates by senior students in a Faculty of Dentistry in Sri Lanka'. *Med Teach* **33**(10): e556–563.

Programme Review Report, MBBS programme, Faculty of Medicine, University of Colombo (2019).

Rajapaksa, L., De Silva, P., Abeykoon, A., Somatunga, L., Sathasivam, S., & Perera, S. (2021). Sri Lanka Health System Review, World Health Organization Regional Office for South-East Asia. https://apo.who.int/publications/i/item/sri-lanka-health-system-review.

Ranasinghe, P., Wathurapatha, W.S., Mathangasinghe, Y. G., & Ponnamperuma. (2017). Emotional intelligence, perceived stress and academic performance of Sri Lankan medical undergraduates. *BMC Med Educ* **17**, 41. https://doi.org/10.1186/s12909-017-0884-5

Ruzhenkova, V.V., Ruzhenkov, V.A., Lukyantseva, I.S., & Anisimova, N.A. (2018). 'Academic stress and its effect on medical students' mental health status'. *Drug Invention Today* **10**(7): 1171–1174.

Torabi, M.R., & Perera, B. (2006). 'A study of depressive symptomatology, its behavioral correlates and anxiety among undergraduates in Sri Lanka'. In M.V. Landow (ed) College *Students: Mental Health And Coping Strategies*. New York: Nova Science Publishers, pp. 133–151.

UGC Circ 933 (1998). *Commission Circular No 933, University Grants Commission, Sri Lanka.*

Universities Act (1978). *Standing committee on Medical and Dental Sciences, Universities Act, No. 16 of 1978*, Sri Lanka.

Weerasinghe, R.H.M. *et al.* (2020). 'Burnout syndrome, associated factors and coping strategies of jaffna medical students'. *Jaffna Med J* **32**(1): 12.

Wickramasinghe, P., Almeida, D., & Samarasekera, D. (2019). 'Depression and stressful life events among medical students during undergraduate career: Findings from a medical school in South Asia'. *The Asia Pacific Scholar* **4**(1): 42–47.

Wijesundara, M., Wijerathna, C., Wijerathna, K., Wijerathna, R., Wijethunga, S., Wijewardana, A., Wickramasinghe, A., & Rathish, D. (2018). 'A significant association between examination results and self-satisfaction with English language proficiency: preliminary findings among pre-clinical undergraduates'. *BMC Res Notes* **11**(1): 4–9.

Wimberly, C.E., Rajapakse, H., Park, L.P., Price, A., Proeschold-Bell, R.J., & Østbye, T. (2022). 'Mental well-being in Sri Lankan medical students: a cross-sectional study'. *Psychol Health Med* **27**(6): 1213–1226.

25
Regional Themes

Andrew Molodynski and Sarah Marie Farrell

Over the preceding chapters, levels of stress, burnout, mental ill health, and substance misuse in 20 countries across five continents have been laid bare. These specific years as a student are worth our focus as they underpin a large aspect of when new doctors are trained and are also known to be a vulnerable time for mental health difficulties (Auerbach, Mortier et al., 2019). Comparison allows us to highlight similarities, pinpoint differences, highlight areas that may need safeguarding in particular countries, and most importantly to share best practice for intervention.

No country had an acceptable level of wellbeing amongst medical students when surveyed using general health questionnaires and burnout scoring (see Figure 25.1 for overall weighted country averages). One exception may be the lower scores on the GHQ12 in Georgia, mentioned next, though low sample size limits our ability to interpret this data (n = 41) and in any case burnout levels are still high in the region. In most other countries over 50% of students are classified as a 'case' (see earlier chapters for methodology), with the majority of countries scoring percentages in the 70s and 80s. Burnout levels are even more shocking. The mean average across all countries surveyed is 84% (range 61–95) for burnout disengagement and 86% (range 65–99) for burnout exhaustion. Summary scores across countries can be found in Table 25.1.

These results are in line with the rest of the literature. The British Medical Association (BMA) conducted an online survey in 2019 of over 4,300 doctors and medical students in the UK. It reported high rates of stress and burnout among both junior doctors and medical students. 27% of the sample reported diagnosed psychiatric disorders. Medical student hazing (or ragging) and mistreatment have been reported in many countries (Cook et al., 2014; Wiebe, 2007). Indeed, previous work has demonstrated that students display high levels of stress, anxiety, depressive disorders, and burnout compared to the general population (Dyrbye, Thomas et al., 2006; Schwenk, Davis et al., 2010; Stecker, 2004). The stigma of mental illness can delay help-seeking behaviours, as can lack of awareness of the problem. Limited resources for outreach can compound matters further. It is also possible that high rates of substance misuse in this age group in general pose an additional threat.

There are certainly generalized reasons as to why medical students are under increased pressure. These apply internationally. A medical degree is significantly longer than a normal three-year degree and with that comes financial pressure, delayed gratification, and mental fatigue. It is extremely competitive at entry. It is not a course offered at every higher education centre and many students do not have the option of living local to their family home. The factual content is heavy, as are the practical commitments on top of the theoretical learning. Students are required to rotate through placements, facing new environments, often residing

Andrew Molodynski and Sarah Marie Farrell, *Regional Themes* In: *The Mental Health of Medical Students*.
Edited by: Andrew Molodynski, Sarah Marie Farrell, and Dinesh Bhugra, Oxford University Press. © Oxford University Press 2024.
DOI: 10.1093/oso/9780192864871.003.0025

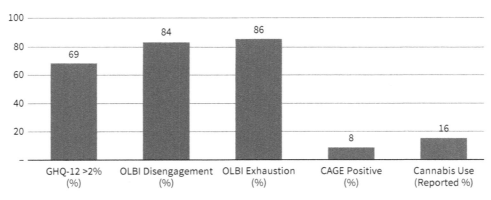

Figure 25.1 Overall positive rate on key measures, n = 9,681.
Source: data from: Kadhum, M., et al. 2022. Wellbeing, burnout and substance use amongst medical students: A summary of results from nine countries. *International Journal of Social Psychiatry*, 68(6), pp.1218-1222; and Molodynski, et al. 2021. Cultural variations in wellbeing, burnout and substance use amongst medical students in twelve countries. *International Review of Psychiatry*, 33(1–2), pp. 37–42.

in poor quality accommodation. The psychological pressures of 'their life in our hands' is unique to medicine. The step-up required is rapid and can be overwhelming.

In addition, each country has its own specific cultural or socioeconomic factors that add to the pressures of medical student life. For example, the authors of Chapter 13 (India) stress that social prestige and financial stability are particularly important reasons for attending medical school in India, but their privately run institutions can cost three times as much as in many other countries. Additionally, selection pressures arising in the bottleneck between undergraduate and postgraduate medicine mean that only one in five trainees will progress to postgraduate level. Chapter 7 (Canada) highlights the vast expansive geography of its landscape as an exacerbating factor in feelings of loneliness and isolation amongst Canadian students. Chapter 10 (Egypt) details a recent system change in Egypt that adds an extra year to the medical degree, which may well impact wellbeing (be it positively or negatively). Chapter 20 (Nigeria) reports that as a low middle-income country life expectancy is only 54.5 years, and maternal and infant mortality are high (WHO, 2018). It would be reasonable to infer that this increases the trauma they witness as students and exacerbates the feeling of pressure and responsibility when thinking ahead to their life as part of the medical workforce. They also highlight a 'pertinent socio-political threat' as a disruptive force, that of incessant industrial strike action by university teachers and medical doctors, often to protest about the state of the country's health and education systems.

In some cases, a country-specific reason can be seen to account for a given particular variation apparent when looking across the descriptive statistics. We have inferred from our data and from the chapters of this book that there is some clear variation between countries on all measures. GHQ-12 scores are substantially lower in Morocco, New Zealand, Nigeria, and Nepal, and at a very low level in Georgia. Paraguay had the highest proportion of students who were 'cases' in the GHQ-12 as used in our survey, at 95%, with Hong Kong close behind at 87%. Rates of exhaustion and disengagement as measured by the Oldenburg Burnout Inventory (OLBI) had highest combined rates in Hong Kong (95%), though it is also worth pointing out that 99% of the students in Paraguay were 'cases' for the exhaustion component of OLBI. The lowest rates were seen in Canada and New Zealand. The CAGE questionnaire,

Table 25.1 Number of responses and scores of 'caseness' on GHQ12, OLBI disengagement, and OLBI exhaustion, by country

Country	Sample size	GHQ-12 >2% (%)	OLBI disengagement (%)	OLBI exhaustion (%)	Key stressors			
					Money %	Relationships %	Studies %	Housing %
Indonesia	1,729	74	93	95	28	45	68	1
Sri Lanka	1,097	62	93	79	31	46	82	9
Denmark	647	68	70	70	33	43	83	6
Morocco	637	47	68	93	37	42	90	13
Portugal	622	81	81	89	72	47	7	12
India	597	62	88	81	18	6	69	42
Egypt	547	64	92	94	7	23	59	1
Nigeria	505	55	85	77	52	30	76	7
Jordan	479	83	87	91	68	52	15	10
UAE	385	75	81	95	25	2	27	13
Italy	360	74	79	84	76	49	17	11
India II	341	70	86	80	26	52	70	14
Wales	266	89	84	87	52	23	85	59
New Zealand	220	53	68	77	51	15	81	51
Paraguay	180	95	61	99	24	28	41	8
Iran	179	77	86	79	44	44	65	10
Russia	174	85	73	80	38	51	89	21
Nepal	169	50	85	65	29	34	64	7
Brazil	129	73	82	88	43	57	85	12
Hong Kong	123	87	95	95	27	47	98	12
Canada II	101	74	61	75	34	62	81	9
England	84	77	82	85	52	24	83	59
Canada	69	75	64	70	46	64	83	19
Georgia	41	8	80	83	71	51	82	92
Overall	9,681	69	84	86	37	38	64	13

n.b. India and Canada had two rounds of surveys in subsequent years and therefore are represented twice in this table. Numbers rounded to nearest integer.

Source: data from: Kadhum, M., et al. 2022. Well-being, burnout and substance use amongst medical students: A summary of results from nine countries. *International Journal of Social Psychiatry*, 68(6), pp. 1218–1222; and Molodynski, et al., 2021. Cultural variations in well-being, burnout, and substance use amongst medical students in twelve countries. *International Review of Psychiatry*, 33(1–2), pp. 37–42.

used in our international survey and mentioned in many chapters (identifying problematic alcohol consumption), demonstrates that 10% of students screened positive, disguising substantial variability from 1% in Indonesia to 20% in Russia. In terms of recreational drug use, cannabis was found to be the most used substance amongst medical students, with rates of up to 79% reported in Portuguese students and 39% in Canada. See Table 25.2.

If this variation in scores is true at a population level, there must be reasons. Identifying a reason for a problem is the first step to ameliorating it. Our authors speak to possible reasons for these variations. Some of these are perhaps obvious. In Canada the government legalized and regulated access to cannabis in 2018, perhaps relaxing the public mindset as to its appropriateness. The even higher cannabis rates among students in Portugal are also in keeping with the decriminalization of possession and consumption of it in 2000. These high levels may make more sense when compared to relatively high national average use. As to whether this benefits the wellbeing of students, the GHQ-12 and OLBI scores remain high, though interestingly Portugal does show a particularly low percentage of students marking their studies as a potential source of stress (7% compared to the overall weighted country score of 64%). The author of Chapter 22 (Portugal) interprets the high cannabis usage to be detrimental when combined with the high stress environment. Meanwhile, low levels of alcohol in Indonesia and UAE (<1%) are explained by disapproval on religious, social, and in some cases legal grounds. The 8% 'caseness' of GHQ12 in Georgia, despite high levels of burnout and similar 'stressor' scores when compared to other countries, could be due to the stigma surrounding mental illness mentioned in Chapter 11 (Georgia). This could potentially encourage medical students from this region to be wary of how they respond. Alternatively, students could be benefiting from targeted strategies, e.g. some universities have started to provide accommodation directly. However, 95% of medical students from Georgia reported housing to be a stressor. This particular problem for Georgia is highlighted by the authors of this chapter, who explain that as a lower-middle-income country there is economic instability and political turmoil, and a large number of international students who have further hurdles of finding accommodation and adjusting in a new country.

The comparatively lower levels of burnout in New Zealand (although still high), might be impacted by factors specific to the culture of the region, as detailed by the authors in Chapter 19 (New Zealand). The Maori influence on concepts of wellbeing, for example 'whakawhanaungatanga', may encourage a sense of connection and prioritize a sense of community in New Zealand. It is possible this has proved somewhat protective for students, even those who are non-Maori. By contrast, the high levels of burnout in Hong Kong could be explained not only by the political unrest noted in Chapter 12 (Hong Kong) but by a series of studies evaluating the temperament, psychology, and cultural leanings of the region in which the authors noted that Hong Kong medical students reported lower levels of protective qualities such as grit and resilience compared to their USA counterparts (Miller-Matero, Martinez et al., 2018) and also exhibited higher levels of power distance, i.e. acceptance of hierarchical order. This may create barriers to challenging authority or asking questions. Coupled with this, the students scored high for the masculinity dimension (Monrouxe, Chandratilake et al., 2021), meaning that failure was viewed as weakness. The authors of this chapter also highlighted the Chinese family-orientated culture valuing family over the individual and suggested that revealing personal distress may shame the family and might prevent students from seeking help.

Table 25.2 Rates of positive CAGE questionnaire and cannabis use, by country

Country	Sample size	CAGE positive (%)	Cannabis use (reported %)
Indonesia	1,729	1	1
Sri Lanka	1097	5	2
Denmark	647	13	16
Morocco	637	5	28
Portugal	622	10	79
India	597	8	15
Egypt	547	9	2
Nigeria	505	5	6
Jordan	479	8	3
UAE	385	1	1
Italy	360	9	21
India II	341	14	12
Wales	266	24	23
New Zealand	220	18	35
Paraguay	180	20	26
!ran	179	6	8
Russia	174	20	22
Nepal	169	14	9
Brazil	129	28	50
Hong Kong	123	14	11
Canada II	**101**	13	39
England	84	18	29
Canada	69	22	36
Georgia	41	12	10*
Overall	**9,681**	**8**	**16**

*For illicit drug use. Scores for cannabis alone not provided.

n.b. India and Canada had two rounds of surveys in subsequent years and therefore are represented twice in this table Numbers rounded to nearest integer.

Source: data from: Kadhum, M., et al. 2022. Well-being, burnout and, substance use amongst medical students: A summary of results from nine countries. *International Journal of Social Psychiatry*, 68(6), pp. 1218–1222; and Molodynski, et al. 2021. Cultural variations in wellbeing, burnout, and substance use amongst medical students in twelve countries. *International Review of Psychiatry*, 33(1–2), pp. 37–42.

Despite the worrying findings laid out in this book, we see many countries pushing forward to create solutions. There are examples from multiple countries developing their own specific strategies to help improve the wellbeing of their medical students. In Hong Kong, to target the less active role of Chinese students in help-seeking, an outreach programme seeks to normalize this through the delivery of psychoeducation using social and informal group formats. The use of separate spaces for wellness services as compared to the learning space and flexibility in time and location are tactics used to increase the uptake of help from the students. Specific approaches such as special events on World Mental Health Day and the use of a resident therapy dog have also become popular. In Canada there is a dedicated Canadian Organization of Undergraduate Psychiatric Education (COUPE) that meets regularly to support wellness and address the lack thereof in medical education. The use of mentors has enhanced feelings of community, and the development of a 'Forum on failure' has worked to normalize conversations surrounding difficulties. In Egypt, 2019 saw the development of a student psychiatric and mental health support service to support the students at Ain Shams University. Similarly, in Nigeria, the University of Ibidan provide a talk on mental health during the yearly induction process to highlight its importance from day one. There is also a weekly mental health clinic that can be accessed on campus, as well as not-for-profit student-run mental health clubs. Perhaps the most definitive example of incorporating conscious connection to wellbeing during medical school is Auckland's incorporation of a 'Health and Wellbeing Curriculum' into medical school life. As outlined in Chapter 19 (New Zealand), the curriculum teaches 'SAFE-DRS' (Self-care skills, Accessing help, Focused attention, Emotional intelligence, Doctor as patient and colleague, Reflective practice, and Stress resistance). The curriculum has been monitored since its inception in 2013 and research shows that the more that students were exposed to the SAFE-DRS wellbeing curriculum, the more they were able to recognize distress, be non-drinkers, undertake positive coping mechanisms like mindfulness and be registered with a GP (Moir, Patten et al., 2023).

Conclusion

The very low levels of wellbeing amongst medical students is a pressing global issue. Levels of stress, burnout, and substance misuse vary across countries, with different areas highlighting different key stressors, but problems are present in all. Variations may be influenced by cultural, religious, and socioeconomic factors, and we have seen representatives from different countries speak to this.

Being a medical student has probably always been a demanding experience, and it may be that now we are just more aware. Even if true, this is not a good enough reason to ignore the issue. Even if the problem has always been present, it still needs solving. However, there is enough evidence that points towards increased pressures on the medical workforce, whether that be globalization and the increased spread of disease, longer lifespans and increased multiple comorbidities, increased availability of testing and treatments, rises in public expectations of what health services should provide, and of course with that, the availability of legal action should a patient be unhappy.

Looking after our future medical workforce is crucial to the health of current and future populations. Taking the first steps to recognize and document this global problem, where bright and motivated students are suffering, achieves two key inroads:

1. Students and institutions can encourage the conversation to continue without feeling shame
2. It creates the pressure in which the next steps become funded and materialize.

Further research is imperative to delineate key factors in both the individuals and their environment, including how these interact and the role of this in creating wellbeing problems. Assessment and audit are necessary to evaluate interventions and their efficacy. Intervention is in its infancy and varies not just from country to country, but within regions of the same country. Perhaps one of the biggest impacts this book can have is a greater awareness of solutions, allowing the exchange and borrowing of ideas within this arena.

References

Auerbach, R.P., Mortier, P., Bruffaerts, R., Alonso, J., Benjet, C., Cuijpers, P., Demyttenaere, K., Ebert, D.D., Green, J.G., Hasking, P., Lee, S., Lochner, C., McLafferty, M., Nock, M.K., Petukhova, M.V., Pinder-Amaker, S., Rosellini, A.J., Sampson, N.A., Vilagut, G., Zaslavsky, A.M., Kessler, R.C., & W.W.-I. Collaborators (2019). 'Mental disorder comorbidity and suicidal thoughts and behaviors in the World Health Organization World Mental Health Surveys International College Student initiative'. *Int J Methods Psychiatr Res* **28**(2): e1752.
Cook, A.F., Arora, V.M., Rasinski, K.A., Curlin, F.A., & Yoon, J.D. (2014). 'The prevalence of medical student mistreatment and its association with burnout'. *Academic Medicine: Journal of the Association of American Medical Colleges* **89**(5): 749.
Dyrbye, L.N., Thomas, M.R., & Shanafelt, T.D. (2006). 'Systematic review of depression, anxiety, and other indicators of psychological distress among U.S. and Canadian medical students'. *Acad Med* **81**(4): 354–373.
Kadhum, M., Ayinde, O.O., Wilkes, C., Chumakov, E., Dahanayake, D., Ashrafi, A., Kafle, B., Lili, R., Farrell, S., Bhugra, D., & Molodysnki, A. (2022). 'Wellbeing, burnout and substance use amongst medical students: A summary of results from nine countries'. *Int J Soc Psychiatry* **68**(6): 1218–1222.
Miller-Matero, L.R., Martinez, S., MacLean, L., Yaremchuk, K., & Ko, A.B. (2018). 'Grit: A predictor of medical student performance'. *Educ Health (Abingdon)* **31**(2): 109–113.
Moir, F., Patten, B., Yielder, J., Sohn, C.S., Maser, B., & Frank, E. (2023). 'Trends in medical students' health over 5 years: Does a wellbeing curriculum make a difference?' *Int J Soc Psychiatry* **69**(3): 675–688.
Molodynski, A., Lewis, T., Kadhum, M., Farrell, S.M., Lemtiri Chelieh, M., Falcão De Almeida, T., Masri, R., Kar, A., Volpe, U., Moir, F., &Torales, J. (2021). 'Cultural variations in wellbeing, burnout and substance use amongst medical students in twelve countries'. *Int Rev Psychiatry* **33**(1–2): 37–42.
Monrouxe, L.V., Chandratilake, M., Chen, J., Chhabra, S., Zheng, L., Costa, P.S., Lee, Y. M., Karnieli-Miller, O., Nishigori, H., Ogden, K., Pawlikowska, T., Riquelme, A., Sethi, A., Soemantri, D., Wearn, A., Wolvaardt, L., Yusoff, M.S.B., & Yau, S.Y. (2021). 'Medical students' and trainees' country-by-gender profiles: Hofstede's cultural dimensions across sixteen diverse countries'. *Front Med (Lausanne)* **8**: 746288.
Schwenk, T.L., Davis, L., & Wimsatt, L.A. (2010). 'Depression, stigma, and suicidal ideation in medical students'. *JAMA* **304**(11): 1181–1190.
Stecker, T. (2004). 'Well-being in an academic environment'. *Med Educ* **38**(5): 465–478.
Wiebe, C. (2007). 'Medical student "hazing" is unhealthy and unproductive'. *Medscape General Medicine* **9**(2): 60.
World Health Organization. (2018). *WHO country cooperation strategy at a glance: Nigeria (No. WHO/CCU/18.02/Nigeria)*. World Health Organization.

PART 3

26

Medical Student Reflections

Sarah Marie Farrell, Amy Schranz, Sharad Philip, Hannah Koury, Harmani Daler, and Nabila Ananda Kloping

Introduction

What is it really like being a medical student in today's world? We must avoid making the age-old mistake of claiming 'it was harder in our day'. If we wish to comment, we must first listen. Countless studies gather quantifiable data, but this can never capture complex individual emotions and difficulties. We include a series of reflections that lift the lid on several students' ideas, concerns, and expectations. Each student organically found their way into our consciousness during various points of editing this book and have been selected for their unsolicited passion for the issues we explore. Here they give us their considerations of the difficulties of life as a medical student.

Amy Schranz, University College Dublin, Ireland

When I first started writing this piece, I didn't entirely know where to start. I thought about everything I had learned in the past 3 years of Medical School—and everything I had tried to learn and forgotten, then learned again, and then forgotten again … I thought about all the embarrassing moments on the wards and in surgery where I had to answer a question with 'I don't know'. The shame, the anger, the anxiety, the exhaustion—all moulded into a particular emotion I can't quite name. So, like any other clever student, I turned to Google. After casually browsing some articles on medical student burnout, there was one fact I kept coming across; apparently burnout peaks in the first clinical year of medical programmes, aka the year I am currently in. Ahhh, so that's what that vague sense of impending doom is in the back of my head—it makes a lot of sense.

I'm a Canadian studying graduate entry medicine abroad in Dublin, in my third year of a four-year programme. That means it's my first year spending all my time in the hospital on different rotations. It's also the year I spend prepping for my residency applications. That means USMLE Step 2 studying, Canadian MCCQE and NAC exams, chasing down Consultants and Registrars to fill out the 'comment section' of my attendance sheet for my MSPE, working on audits, taking on any extracurricular that comes my way—all in the hopes that I build up a good enough application that Canada takes me back. Ironically enough, as I write this piece, I am currently sitting in a window sill across from theatre, waiting for a surgeon to finish operating for the evening so that we can go through my presentation on a

Sarah Marie Farrell, Amy Schranz, Sharad Philip, Hannah Koury, Harmani Daler, and Nabila Ananda Kloping, *Medical Student Reflections*
In: *The Mental Health of Medical Students*. Edited by: Andrew Molodynski, Sarah Marie Farrell, and Dinesh Bhugra, Oxford University Press.
© Oxford University Press 2024. DOI: 10.1093/oso/9780192864871.003.0026

surgical case for next week. It's Friday night and all I can think about is the Chinese food that's waiting for me at home.

When I first started in the hospital, I think something that genuinely surprised me was that there were no changing rooms for medical students. Instead, we have a break room with an entire wall of windows—no blinds—where we drop our pants and don our scrubs for the world to see. And if that's too public for you, there's some bathrooms across the hall, but staff come in and get angry if you're hogging the stalls. We also attend rounds at 7 am and then have lectures 4–6 pm, and for those 8 hours in-between we are expected to remain in the hospital. If there's nothing for you to do, then you should be studying in the library. But the library only seats 20 people and some weeks there's 90 students on rotation in the hospital. I'm not saying I have a solution, I know healthcare is notoriously underfunded and it has been especially frustrating these past 2 years globally—but there is clearly room for improvement, and I can't help but wonder where tuition goes if not to develop the needed facilities for the students' programme.

As if stressing about finding a quiet corner to study most days isn't enough, there's still this frustration of inequity we are constantly fighting within medicine. For example, the hospital has a rugby team made up of (male) medical students and consultants, which play against other hospitals, giving the boys in the class an unfair advantage in building rapport from the first year. When I reached out to the class to gauge female interest in putting together a sports team, a boy in the class thought the issue was that women don't play rugby in Ireland, opposed to the reality of institutional sexism. I remember thinking 'wow, ignorance really is bliss'. And the cherry on top is the kickback from admin I am currently getting with trying to find a way to advertise building a sports team to the female consultants in the hospital.

Believe it or not, it's not the lack of change rooms or encounters of sexism that keep me up at night anymore. What keeps me up is knowing that Residency Application deadlines are coming (said in an ominous winter is coming tone). As an IMG student trying to get back to Canada, we have fewer residency positions allocated to us compared to Canadians studying in Canada. And to top it all off, the American match date is now before the Canadian match, meaning if I match to a residency in America, my application is withdrawn from Canada. So, I don't even have the option to make America my plan B anymore. I've really struggled with this over the past year. The advice we get from the medical school is to apply as broadly as possible—to America and Canada, and apply to Family Medicine as backup, and Intern Year in Ireland, and while you're at it maybe toss in some applications for the fast food joint down the street. Okay, so not that last point, but everything else is true. But thinking about this logistically—I want to do Radiology, that's a 5-year residency programme. When I graduate I'm going to be 30. That means, somewhere in those 5 years, odds are I start a family (if that's what I want). But do I want to have a kid in America? Did you read about the last school shooting? The potential Trump comeback that's looming over the horizon? The vaccination rates? Yet the programme seems to imply none of these things matter, all that matters is you get a residency position no matter the cost.

I miss my family and friends. My best friend of 10 years had her first baby while I was completing my first 6-week Surgery rotation—I was 5,247 km away in a different time zone. I hadn't been home to visit since the start of the pandemic. Maybe it's because we've been in a global pandemic for the last 3 years—but I want to go home. But I also equally want to study Radiology—The school tells me if I want to go home, then apply to Family medicine, and if I want Radiology, then apply to America. But there are Radiology positions for IMGs in Canada—why can't I prioritize this as my first option? Why is the system set up this way?

I think burnout isn't just about medical school, it's the fact that life outside of medicine goes on. We have all these tabs open in our heads, much like the Chrome browser on our laptops. School is one tab. Making sure the dog is walked and fed before ward rounds is another tab. Then there's do laundry, boil diva cup, vacuum, figure out who's going to write a letter of recommendation for residency applications, call parents, cry about the consultant making fun of your Canadian accent, check on your brother, work on the audit … I have so many different tabs open in my head at one given moment. But have you ever noticed how Chrome crashes when you have too many tabs open?

Sharad Philip, All-India Institute of Medical Sciences, India

Should you really be here? This is the question I've always had to grapple with—by 'here', I mean my entry and subsequent practice as a medical professional. What is so wrong with me that others enquire thus? I am visually impaired—I have an eye condition called Retinitis Pigmentosa. It's one of the most common inherited retinal disorders—a progressive condition afflicting 1.1 to 2.6 million people worldwide. The most common variant affects peripheral vision first, progressing to leave limited central vision.

For me, becoming a medical professional was my dream. I ticked all the right boxes—read the Robin Cook novels, was a biology whiz, and was the most active in all medical knowledge clubs. Struggling to read the fine print from large books, I trudged on because I did not want to let some eye problem determine what I would do or be for the rest of my life. For this, I must be found within the top 10% of all aspirants in my country—a whopping 1.5 million yearly!

I made it into a prestigious medical school way back in 2005. As a time point, the first iPhone was released only in 2007. Soon the entire college got to know there's a partially blind guy here trying to become a doctor. I at first attempted my best to satisfy their curiosity. Questions such as—'Can you see me?' 'Can you tell me how far I am from you?' Later it became clearer I was not dealing with curiosity alone—questions such as 'How will you be able to do surgery or suture wounds?' And then came the not-so-subtle line of questioning—'Should you really be here?'

India has a shortage of well-trained doctors—if you are not going to be a fully functioning one, then you have cost another their opportunity to serve the nation and deprive the needy of essential healthcare services! That was when I began withdrawing into my shell. People around me could only see my deficient vision as if I was a pair of floating malfunctioning eyes bereft of any other humanoid features. What else could I do? There was no help out here for me.

Very soon, I developed a fear of letting others down and, in the process, of letting myself down, an anxiety that I would be adjudged unable or unworthy to continue my dream career, and an overwhelming sense of inadequacy. Every task became a do-or-die mission. This was my mountain—it may look insurmountable to others, but I had to prove them wrong.

CRASH! I flunked my anatomy papers! The feedback I got was that I had not drawn enough diagrams and figures to illustrate how well I had learnt. I was also told my writing had become difficult to read. My eyesight had diminished further. What dawned on me now was a dreadful possibility—what if my vision deteriorated further till there wasn't any left? So, it wasn't really my effort that would lose me my dream career—it was what I had lost earlier that would now lose me more! The cruelty and injustice of it all was staggering for me.

I found in my classmates some wonderful friends who soon became my allies. Hours poring over books with tearing eyes became hours spent next to caring and empowering friends who either read out aloud as they read themselves or others who looked for me to re-vise what they had read already. This arrangement soon became tenuous for many reasons. Firstly, I felt extremely dependent on my friends and help. Secondly, I felt tremendously in-debted to them for every instance of their help. Thirdly, I became extremely aware and cau-tious of ensuring I had everyone's goodwill. Something inside began gnawing away—it was the same sense of overwhelming inadequacy; only now, there was a sense of being a burden. I had to find a way I could fill in the gaps.

I tried scanning and printing all my books in large fonts and tried reading using some screen narration software. All these things flopped. I began withdrawing into my safe shell. My friends' help felt like heavy burdens or loans I could never repay. My visual acuity had dipped further with blemished and useless patches of visual field. Ironically, I could draw parallels here with my life—I was now useless for many things. Through these times, I looked for a mentor or a confidante, or at least a sounding board. There were so many great people around me but all of them were clueless about what I was going through. Most of their opin-ions were outlandish to me—they were talking about how I could pursue hospital admin-istration, become a teacher in non-clinical fields, or take up psychiatry. Another faculty recounted to me the utility of getting chorionic villus sampling for any children I was plan-ning to have and check for this same genetic error and carefully consider pregnancy. All this seemed too heady a mix for a 23-year-old guy going blind.

And then CRASH! I had not cleared the exams for internal medicine. I remember crying myself to sleep on many nights, shorted on all my dreams and goals. The sense of failure was so great. I had a further 12 months ahead after I cleared one subject to get my degree. Ice cream time soon became personal reflection time. Now I wondered why I had equated excel-lence with clearing exams and being independent. Probably it was because I so desperately wanted to blend in. This impediment was my shame—my personal flaw. I must excel so much that those noticing me must remark that I am more than a pair of malfunctioning eyes.

Resuming studies in earnest, I found out I could no longer make out what I had just written—there were blind spots in my vision. I found out, however, that I could make out grossly where I had written using my peripheral vision on the left side. Determined to find a solution, I began practising writing while seeming to look away. This time I resolved I would do whatever it takes. So, there I was, in the peak of summer, sitting away from everyone else being blazed by the sun so that I could write my exams. Looking at preserved specimens of organs, histology slides, and the lines or boxes on electrocardiography reports were im-possible, so I worked out a system with the examiners to be tested extra on other areas. This helped greatly. I cleared that last subject exam and finally made the customary trip to get myself registered. Through my rotations in psychiatry, I was selected to complete my service commitment in the department. This was a far cry from the orthopaedist I had envisioned myself to be barely a decade earlier. But I was here.

Looking back, a lot of the distress and self-loathing I went through could have been avoided had there been mentorship and support available. I could have been spared the gnawing sense of being an anomaly had I known and understood what I do today about disability accommodations. I have since moved on to empower other doctors with disabilities. And just for reference, Apple is going to release its newest shiniest version of the iPhone soon.

Hannah Koury, University of Calgary, Canada

Canada is home to 17 medical schools spread across our geographically large country. The majority of the medical schools are four years long. However, two schools (the University of CalgaryCumming School of Medicine and McMaster University Medical School) are condensed 3-year programmes. These condensed programmes have the same curricular hours without the summer breaks. During the last year of medical school, all students across the country apply to residency programmes, which range from 2 to 5 years in length. Canadian students enter medical school after completing part or all of an undergraduate degree or a Master's or PhD graduate degree. The diversity in the educational background upon entering medical school creates an exciting mix of students at the outset of their medical degrees. Some first-year medical students have three years of undergraduate education completed. In comparison, others have had seven years of postgraduate education total under their belts.

I am a third-year medical student from the University of Calgary. For the past three years, I have been fortunate to serve as the Vice President of Student Advising and Wellness for my class, the Class of 2022. I was keen to apply for this role because of my interest in student wellness. This interest stemmed during my Master's degree when I was a Co-President of a new Student Health Promotion Committee. In this role, I learned how to survey students on their health and wellness needs and categorize them into the three areas of wellness, nutrition, physical exercise, and mental health. Based on these needs, goals and Campus Health Improvement Plans to meet these goals were created. Through this work, I found my passion for supporting my colleagues. I have been very fortunate to continue fostering this passion with my medical school class. My philosophy is to best take care of others, you need to take care of yourself. Additionally, I wanted to make medical school easier by creating a supportive environment that fosters celebrating accomplishments, sharing and overcoming setbacks, and promoting balance.

Over the past three years, I have observed and reflected on common themes relating to medical student wellness that I will share in chronological order. Pre-clerkship is the era of imposter syndrome and the stress associated with figuring out how to be a medical student. The transition to a virtual environment demonstrated the importance of social support and how isolating school can be without it. Finally, clerkship represents adjusting to the reality of a physician's schedule demands. I should preface my discussion on these topics. While these stressors were a real challenge, there were many rewarding and enjoyable memories from medical training that I know I will cherish for a lifetime. I vividly remember during our first week of medical school, I was sitting in the first case-based learning session on biostatistics in the Population Health course. I left the room thinking, 'What in the world did I get myself into?! I am SO not smart enough for this!'. I later found out that there was a name for this feeling, just like everything in medicine: imposter syndrome. According to the Oxford Dictionary, imposter syndrome is the persistent inability to believe one's successes are deserved or have been legitimately achieved as a result of one's own efforts or skills. Meeting 160 other high-achieving individuals, some of whom have done more in their 20-something years than I could imagine doing in a lifetime, makes that one medal in a dance competition irrelevant. The constant comparison to others resulted in feeling inadequate, and this happened almost every day as you slowly met the rest of your classmates. It turned out that many of my classmates shared similar feelings. We are so fortunate to have a school community where it was 'okay' to talk about these common sentiments without fear of impacting how others see us. Once those conversations started happening, the tension began to decrease, and students began to settle into their new role as medical students, with the support of their new peer group within the class. Imposter syndrome never truly disappears because medicine is one profession where you constantly meet incredible people. However, I found that shifting your mindset from 'I'm not good enough' to 'what inspiration or learning can I take from this person' is one cure for the syndrome. Reflecting on our first year, I was very inspired to watch the energy go from nervous to calm and more confident. Little did we know another big curveball was headed our way ...

The beginning of the pandemic coincided with the start of the second year of pre-clerkship. That calm, confident energy we had just found was replaced with the uncertainty of the future of our medical education in a matter of days. I would argue the most challenging part of transitioning online was the lack of connection with our peers and mentors. Previously, it was so easy to vent and share experiences between lectures and labs, which was incredibly validating. Now, we had to navigate adjusting to the new normal of living with the pandemic restrictions and being incredibly self-disciplined and motivated to stay on top of our podcast material. Many early clinical exposures that are crucial for career exploration were now cancelled. This would be the second-largest stressor for us during that time, especially in a three-year programme. Finally, the feelings of guilt surrounded by setbacks of our upper-year classmates and not being able to be on the front lines added to the uncomfortable feelings. Nevertheless, just like our first year of in-person pre-clerkship, my resilient classmates found a way to adjust to the new normal through things like online socials and study groups and finding the silver linings of the new flexibility of our online schedule.

Finishing pre-clerkship was a celebratory milestone in our education. However, the nervous energy returned with the clerkship on the horizon (the third time is the charm, right?). I found the nervous energy quickly turned into excitement and motivation, and adjustments were made even quicker than in pre-clerkship. This is because, and I believe most of my classmates would agree, that clerkship is the better part of medical school training. The hands-on experiences are incomparable to reading the textbook or sitting in front of Zoom. It was refreshing to be back in the clinical environment and working with a team to better the health and care of patients. The novelty of clerkship, however, can and does wear off. Starting a new rotation every 2–4 weeks with a new teaching team at a new hospital or clinic can be exhausting, especially with a rotation you are not keen on. When not working, your free time is consumed with the pressures of studying, completing research, or other scholarly activities, career exploring, or simply worrying about the future. And when you are not doing that, you are tired. This fatigue can begin to impact your personal life. Burnout in clerkship is common and is potentially made worse by the element of isolation. Part of overcoming these challenges begins with realizing this schedule and learning environment are similar to what residency will be like and even more demanding! It was healthy to start adjusting the activities you once relied on to keep yourself balanced to the new rigours and demands. In addition, it is helpful to remember clerkship is a marathon, not a sprint. Learn where it is important to put in what extra gas in the tank you have to protect yourself from completely burning out.

I am now almost at the end of this journey, and I can confidently say that I would not have changed much (aside from, you know, the whole global pandemic). Observing myself and my classmates' ability to navigate these stressors and uncertainties faced during different parts of our training has truly been inspiring. I believe our adaptability and resiliency are more robust than when we entered, but even more so than had we not faced these unique challenges. I am proud of my class and school community for handling it with grace and determination. As I think about all my peers who are completing residency interviews now, I know that the future of medicine is bright. The culture will continue to improve to promote healthy, resilient, and happy physicians.

Harmani Daler, University of Lancaster, England

From the beginning, entry to medical school demands a degree of excellence both within academic and personal pursuits, thus producing an intake of students who strive for the best in all that they do—many of whom may come from privileged backgrounds financially and academically. This culture of attainment can facilitate a sense of competitiveness within the social environment of medical school. Pressure for success, combined with the high work-load from a combination of placement and university-based work, can cause students to burnout and feel disillusioned with their work.

In the first year of medical school, the pressures appeared less obvious to me, and I felt like a normal university student—going to lectures, studying for exams, and being able to attend societies and events on campus. After this year, it became obvious how important time management skills were for success in medical school as we were required to balance clinical requirements and university study to successfully complete our training. The difficulty here comes in finding time for oneself, in order to recover from the stress of daily work and the expectation to succeed. As medical school progressed, the pressure to achieve increased, alongside longer placement hours; it was not uncommon for students to need moments to recover or to cry from the stress, nor for us to experience self-doubt in our ability as future medics. The increased time pressure resulted in sacrificing social activities and hobbies for time completing clinical requirements, with work–life balance becoming a greater struggle than the studies themselves. Support from fellow medical students became paramount here, where splitting study and work between colleagues allowed for university content to be covered in sufficient detail while balancing clinical commitments. However, the competitive nature of medical school can lead to difficulty in co-operation between some students, particularly due to the ranking system acting as a factor in deciding location for our immediate future.

For minority students studying in a less diverse locale or who have struggled with discrimination, there is an added pressure to perform so that they may be accepted to competitive regions with more diversity. However, due to their minority status within medical school, they may further struggle in socializing and finding a peer support group willing to engage in collaborative study, compounding the burden of expectations for these students. Students from less privileged backgrounds may also require a part-time job to fund the latter years of their studies, as the NHS bursary and student finance may not adequately cover their rent and study costs—this will affect whether they are able to fund electives, travel to placements, as well as the significant impact on time spent studying and therefore ranking and exam performance. Thus, these students may struggle with attainment due to factors beyond their control and find themselves burnt out.

In my personal situation, an added burden to this was my diagnosis of a long-term mental health condition during my first year of university. Fortunately, my medical school were very supportive of the diagnosis, and facilitated a period of absence for my recovery; there was a dedicated student support service that offered referral to a clinical psychologist, which proved invaluable upon my return. The psychotherapy offered improved my coping skills when it came to perceptions of self-worth and emotional regulation, allowing me to rediscover sources of enjoyment both within and outside of medicine. One particular lecture proved particularly memorable, with a doctor disclosing her story of a mental health crisis during medical school; witnessing vulnerability from a senior provided a sense of validity and acceptance of my own struggles.

Experiences of discrimination on placement were also not uncommonly discussed between minority students, and provided further questions around our future careers; would this behaviour persist as another struggle we had to cope with, alongside a heavy workload and high expectations? In these moments, support from both peers and medical school with addressing discriminatory behaviour in any of its forms proved extremely important, as it provided recognition of our experiences and hope for future change. This was done at my medical school through open forums with medical school staff on discussing incidents of discrimination, online forms for anonymous reporting, and referrals to student support services. Meeting students and mentors of a similar background provided safe spaces for discussion of the added stresses that discrimination places upon practitioners, and empathy for shared experiences.

Nabila Ananda Kloping, Universitas Airlangga, Surabaya, Indonesia

Printed or not, there are numerous evidence-based articles with the know-hows and tricks to overcome and avoid burnout. But here in this section of this paper, I would like to give a little bit of that personal human flavour that seemed to be missing from scientific articles. My experiences and opinion cannot represent all medical students of Indonesia. This however may provide insight for those dealing with similar instances.

Ever since high school, being a medical student has always been seen as the 'difficult major' or 'you won't have a life outside of school' kind of programme. For me personally, the first semester was the most exhausting. Not only adapting to new people and the system, but the subjects were absolutely demanding. The stress was there before we became a medical student, and it slowly piles up more along the years. Moreover, external factors outside of academics such as personal relationships, families, and financial problems are some of many things weighing a student's mind—particularly in the case of Indonesia, where there is a mandatory national exam at the end of the programme needed to fully receive the title of Medical Doctor. This puts an immense weight on students as their hard work for five and a half years will be judged on their performance in a CBT (computer-based test) and OSCE (objective structured clinical examination), which lasts only a few hours.

In recent years the pandemic caused a major shift in course. Classes were conducted online for a year and a half. One full year of pre-clinical and half a year of clinical courses were all taught from digital devices in the comfort of our homes. We were so worried about what kind of medical doctors we would be if we never studied and had the chance to learn directly from a patient themselves. However, we were so grateful that now we could learn medicine properly again.

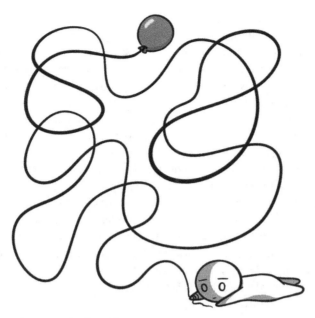

Figure 26.1 What a 'burnout' feels to me.
Illustration by Nabila Ananda Kloping.

At one point during the pandemic, I realized I was undergoing burnout after my friends mentioned that I constantly sound tired or that I do not seem to enjoy the things I do anymore. I might have been in denial most of the time, trying to convince myself that I was just lacking sleep. However, I noticed I was experiencing burnout when I woke up in bed, saw a message from my professor about revisions regarding a research project, cried for several minutes, and went back to sleep.

To me burnout is the feeling of helplessness, your mind shutting down, and physically not being able to function the way you want it to. The tasks you should be doing suddenly felt as if it is punishing instead (Figure 26.1).

I do not think that we can avoid burnout entirely. There will be times where we prioritize our tasks more than ourselves. The most important thing is to realize that some things can be overwhelming. A potential solution we could do is to dissect the roots of our problems into things within our control and issues outside of our hands. This would differ among students for sure, and sometimes it is okay to not put academic tasks as our first priority.

At the end of the day, putting our wellbeing first and being more kind to ourselves is important and should be regularly reminded to all medical students around the world.

Summary

In these narratives we hear about the pressures of medical school, and far more than this, the pressure of representing a vocation, a morality, and an ideology. Such pressures are exacerbated by the restrictive systems in which they arise, with competitive entry points and limited funding.

Our students deal with a multitude of psychological phenomena, including imposter syndrome, feelings of worthlessness, and sometimes specific physical or mental health issues. They are not always (or indeed often) provided with resources that would be expected in a normal workplace. Additionally, societal issues each have their own place in medicine: sexism, ablism, race, class, and isolation during a global pandemic. This clearly weighs on the basal stresses of educational placements and exams.

Despite their deep understanding of the pressure of studying medicine and despite having been hit hard by the process, for the most part our students are positive about the outlook going forward, showing a commendable resilience and strength. They identify their needs, spot flaws in the system, and where possible try and create their own tools to navigate their way through. This might involve finding social support groups, identifying like-minded mentors, consciously adjusting previously acquired 'tools' to fit new demands, and learning to prioritize day-to-day non-medical tasks with an understanding that 'life goes on'.

It is important we do these deep dives on medical students' mental states to try to get an understanding of the wide-ranging issues they face. Only then can we focus on what tools could help them endure, and ultimately transcend. We look at what can be changed to support students better towards the end of this book. What is clear is that there will not be a one size fits all panacea; rather it is more likely to comprise multiple individualized measures through which students can self-create their own box of tools.

27

Considering the Needs of Those Studying Medicine Abroad

Sapna Agrawal

Introduction

Global health is a rapidly growing field focusing on advancing international and interdisciplinary healthcare. What has become evident since the onset of pandemics such as COVID-19 is that in the modern era, health issues transcend borders and national governments, which helps healthcare professionals understand global issues to improve healthcare delivery worldwide (Khan, 2020). What has also changed in the modern era is that migration between countries is much easier (Holst, 2020), and medical students can travel to complete or participate in medical studies in a country different from where they were born or raised. This may be due to the lack of medical education facilities in their own country or a perceived idea that medical education in certain institutes or countries is better/more accessible.

There are about 2,600 medical schools worldwide. The countries with the most significant number of schools are India (n = 304), Brazil (n = 182), the USA (n = 173), China (n = 147), and Pakistan (n = 86). A third of all medical schools are in five countries, and nearly half are in 10 countries. Of 207 independent states, 24 have no medical schools, and 50 have only one (Duvivier et al., 2014).

It is understandable why many students seek their medical education abroad. The International Federation of Medical Students Association states that each year 14,000 medical students embark on a journey to explore healthcare delivery and health systems in different cultural and social settings.

Globally many students strive to learn in centres of excellence, their ambitions limited by opportunities and economic factors. The United Kingdom, Australia, Germany, and France account for nearly half of the most sought-after places to study; in contrast, most international students come from China, India, and South Korea. Asian students represent more than 50% of international students studying abroad, with European countries (38%) at the forefront of preferred study locations, followed by North America (23%). More recently, more students from Africa and Asia have sought to study in China. Table 27.1 lists the currently ranked global top 10 medical schools.

Many international medical students (IMSs) return to their country of origin upon completing their studies, but even more, adopt their country of education and settle there, bringing their ideas and culture to the host country. With the global shortage of health workers, some work in countries where there is demand and opportunity for them to progress further in their careers and thus become International medical graduates. International

Sapna Agrawal, *Considering the Needs of Those Studying Medicine Abroad* In: *The Mental Health of Medical Students*.
Edited by: Andrew Molodynski, Sarah Marie Farrell, and Dinesh Bhugra, Oxford University Press. © Oxford University Press 2024.
DOI: 10.1093/oso/9780192864871.003.0027

Table 27.1 Global Medical School Rankings

Rank	Medical School	Country
1	University of Oxford	UK
2	University of Cambridge	UK
3	Harvard University	USA
4	Imperial College London	UK
5	Tsinghua University	China
6	Stanford University	USA
7	University of Toronto	Canada
8	UCL	UK
9	Yale University	USA
10	King's College London	UK

Source: Times Higher Education's World University Rankings 2023 data

medical graduates (IMGs) refer to all doctors who obtained their primary qualification outside their country of origin or those whose primary medical qualification was received outside of the country where they are now practising medicine.

Motivation for Studying Abroad and Decisive Factors for Choosing a Medical School

For most students, the expectation of excellent levels of teaching not necessarily available in their own country is a big motivation to come and study abroad. Many other factors also come into play. Some students want to study overseas to establish their autonomy and independence while experiencing a sense of adventure in a new environment. Others migrate with a long-term plan to broaden their horizons and settle in a foreign country where there are better job opportunities and remuneration (Goel et al., 2018).

Many reasons may be listed for why a student chooses a particular medical school; however, the most relevant and apparent reason is the international reputation of a specific school. Secondary factors that may come into play include a prior connection to the country or school through relatives or friends, which may reassure the student and their families that the education they will receive will be of a particular standard but also the reassurance that there is someone to lean on or ask for help in times of difficulty.

Economic factors are critical when choosing a medical school abroad. The students, or, in many cases, their parents, need to consider not only the tuition fees but also living expenses and stable exchange rates before deciding on a place of study. A lot will also consider the opportunities for local jobs and the progression of their careers within the host country or how valued the degree is globally.

Other essential factors to consider include the age at which admission into medical school is accepted. For example, American medical schools require completion of a four-year pre-medical undergraduate degree before starting the medical degree. In the UK, students only need to complete an A-level or equivalent qualification and generally start at 18, a much younger age. As English is a globally recognized language, English-based universities are always popular.

For some medical students, however, it is only a question of which medical school they can get into, and they happily accept wherever they are offered a place. For example, medical schools in the UK are capped in the proportion of international students they can admit in a year at around 7.5% (The Royal College of Physicians, 2021). This makes entry into medical schools for international students very competitive.

General Challenges

Anyone travelling to a new country will face the everyday challenges of finding suitable accommodation and means of transport. For example, in England, they may need to gain a new driver's licence and learn to drive on the left side of the road. They will need initial funding to open a bank account and register with a doctor. They will likely suffer from homesickness and loneliness initially as they will have left family and friends behind with no one to support them or lean on in periods of difficulty. Even basics in entertainment, such as missing a favourite TV programme or not having sports partners to train or play with, are important. IMSs may not be around people from similar religious backgrounds to celebrate religious or cultural events. Culture shock is a common experience for people who have moved from one country or cultural environment to another. It can lead to disorientation when experiencing an unfamiliar way of life (Al-Saadi et al., 2020).

All these factors may lead to isolation and a sense of loneliness. Where studies are concerned, a lack of feedback and pointers from peers from similar backgrounds can hinder success in examinations and careers.

Students and their families may have underestimated living costs in the host country. Such financial difficulties may result in depression for international students as they may not even have enough money to pay for basics such as food and heating. In contrast, many may have lived very comfortably in their home country.

Language difficulties may lead to challenges in both being understood and understanding others. Language difficulties may also lead to isolation with difficulty in making friends. It is often seen that international students make friends with other international students who are experiencing similar problems or are fortunate enough to find students from similar backgrounds. However, this leads to problems of not integrating with the local population and learning from them.

IMSs have the additional stress of visa applications and the possibility of being deported if the visas are not approved or are no longer valid, leading to a lack of security that can harm their mental health.

As alluded to before, many IMSs begin their medical journey relatively young and inexperienced in handling things themselves. Many have, in the past, been accustomed to being catered for by their families. Suddenly having to fend for themselves without their family supporting them can lead to problems in a foreign land.

Many choose to come to the UK or other international medical schools because of the perceived high education standards. Those that do succeed, therefore, sometimes come with unreasonably high expectations. Many are disappointed, expecting more precise guidance in their studies rather than the self-directed study expected of medical students in some medical schools. International students' expectations to succeed are also greater from their families, who will have sacrificed much to get them to study abroad. This extra academic and financial pressure, along with the perceived social exclusion and accultur-ative stress, results in increased depressive symptoms, lower life satisfaction among inter-national students, and, consequently, lower academic performance levels. Medical schools have a higher proportion of students suffering from depression when compared to students in other specialties or the general population. The recorded prevalence in American med-ical schools was 14.3% (Schwenk et al., 2010). Many believe this underestimates the true prevalence due to commonly held perceptions about lack of confidentiality or perceptions of symptoms being seen as a failure or weakness. It was further shown that depression was more prevalent in women and that more students got depressed as they progressed through their academic years. The problem is likely to be magnified in international students who may avoid or delay seeking help due to their cultural beliefs on mental health. It may also be secondary to not knowing where to seek help. Differences in differential attainment may continue to persist following graduation leading to large socioeconomic gaps between IMSs and local graduates.

Looking into mental health and wellbeing, eight key factors have been universally recog-nized, regardless of background, as impacting health and social care staff's wellbeing, flour-ishing, and work engagement, aligned across these three core needs (see Figure 27.1) (West et al., 2020).

Medical schools have been making extra efforts to recruit trainees from more diverse backgrounds, but this does not necessarily mean that inclusion for IMSs is now a given. There needs to be more clarity in understanding the complex and nuanced interaction be-tween inclusion and acculturation/adaptation. The tension between encouraging accultur-ation to British values and practice while retaining fidelity to one's culture and identity is often replaced with a simplistic model of encouraging everyone to adopt rather than adapt to their host culture. This can be pretty damaging as international students are encour-aged to bridge the gaps in their communication skills and cultural knowledge of their host

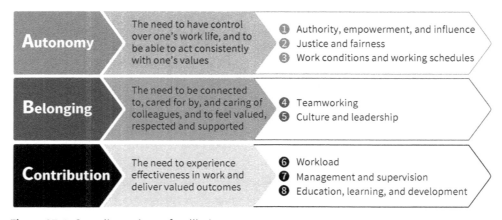

Figure 27.1 Core dimensions of wellbeing.
Reproduced with permission from West, M. et al. (2020). The courage of compassion: Supporting Nurses and midwives to deliver high-quality care. The King's Fund.

country rather than a strength-based model that values the strengths that the diverse group of IMSs bring to the learning environment and to learn from them instead of educating them to change.

Attrition rates in medical schools have shown a solid correlation to poor academic performance (Wright et al., 2008). Unfortunately, poor academic performance has been demonstrated in a higher proportion of IMSs, more of whom abandon their training in the first year. The reason for these failures is multifactorial. Some of the possible factors include those already listed.

Inclusion

One of the most significant or reported factors for dissatisfaction amongst IMSs was the lack of a sense of inclusion, with IMSs not having relatable role models or peer groups.

What do we mean by inclusion? The sense of being' comfortable in your skin' and not having to pretend to be something you are not, alongside feeling that you are part of something and not getting excluded. Achieving that balance between individuality and community can be tricky for IMSs who are expected to perform in an unfamiliar and potentially hostile environment. Add to that the loss of social capital occasioned by migration and lack of intrinsic knowledge of local systems and practices, both in personal and professional domains.

Various groups have recently done much work on inclusion at the undergraduate and graduate levels. It is still variable though, relying on the goodwill of individuals rather than being a coordinated response from the universities or the National Health Service. At the end of this chapter, we make key recommendations for employers and local, regional, and national education providers to address the issue.

Communication

Being a good doctor demands not only mastery of assessment, diagnosis, and treatment but the ability to communicate effectively with your patients. When a doctor arrives from abroad to work in the UK, they must pass the International English Language Test (IELT) and the Professional and Linguistic Assessments Board (PLAB) examination set by the General Medical Council (GMC). No such formal arrangements are made for medical students. Language difficulties can hinder their progress at medical school and later in their careers. Even if IMSs superficially master the language of their host country, there will be nuances of body language and local colloquial phrases that local students will have grown up with that are not easily acquired by IMSs, leading to barriers between colleagues, lecturers, and even patients on placements. Significant language and cultural variations exist in the UK, so any induction programme, including a national communication package, should be adapted locally to include regional colloquialisms. IMSs should have special classes to incorporate language and cultural lessons to help them integrate. Some Non-English universities already do this. Therefore, these cultural and geographical differences within the United Kingdom can add extra pressure on international students on what is required to acculturate on arrival to the local medical schools.

This point was reinforced in a 2019 study led by the Medical Advisor, Workforce Race Equality Strategy (WRES) Implementation Team, and NHS England, in which IMGs reported communication, including understanding colloquial English, with patients, the public, and colleagues as the most encountered challenge (Rao et al., 2022). The researchers could not find any trust induction to assist new doctors in improving language and oral and written communication competence. Communication difficulties are an obvious potential source of misunderstanding and patient dissatisfaction, and an introductory programme including these aspects for both international graduates and IMSs could prevent many problems from arising in the future and hopefully decrease referral rates to the GMC if they choose to continue working in a foreign country after graduating.

Impact of Medical Migration

We have already discussed that while IMGs are instrumental in helping relieve the workforce crisis in the NHS, they face a range of short-term and long-term personal and professional issues. However, the impact of medical migration goes beyond individual IMGs; there has been significant debate about the adverse effects of medical immigration and 'brain drain', leading to a severe workforce crisis in underdeveloped and under-resourced areas of the world. For example, despite having 11% of the world's population and 24% of the global disease burden, sub-Saharan Africa has only 3% of the world's healthcare workers (Wright et al., 2008). Many global workforce experts believe that countries that recruit the most IMGs have longstanding patterns of under-investment in medical education and advocate for these countries to become more self-sufficient by adopting education policies to train a physician workforce close to the size of the demand for medical care in practice in their own countries. While self-sufficiency is ideal, some others argue that medical graduates in a global economy should be allowed the freedom of movement amongst countries, but this should be on the proviso that they are given the same opportunities in training and be allowed to contribute somewhat to their new places of work. They must not be seen as a cheap workforce to fulfil the host country's needs and prop up their deficiencies in healthcare.

Higher-income countries have a responsibility to address issues of 'brain drain' by providing resources to less developed countries so that they can educate, train, and retain medical personnel and ensure adequate healthcare delivery to their citizens and, at the same time, not rely solely on IMGs to solve their shortages in the healthcare workforce crisis (Zerehi, 2008).

Refugee doctors and students must also be considered as a particular group of international medical graduates/students who merit additional comments. They are doctors who have had to flee their home countries under exceptional circumstances to escape, in some cases, persecution or threats. They will have experienced some form of trauma and, in most cases, have financial difficulties. Additional difficulties include having less certainty regarding visas leading to more isolation. Refugee doctors might not have all the required documents for registration as they will have had to flee their homes rapidly. In some cases, the documentation may be unretrievable, thus complicating the ability to fulfil GMC requirements and leading to the potential exploitation in less-than-ideal jobs and lack of progress with regard to careers and training if they are allowed to work in the first place (Cohn et al., 2006). More importantly, however, they may be suffering from additional mental health issues such as post-traumatic stress disorder, and microaggressions may lead to further deterioration in their mental health.

Interventions for Improvement

In recent years the Royal Colleges, Health Education England (HEE), and the Medical Education Committees (MECs) have been looking at interventions to improve support and inclusiveness for international learners and to attempt to bridge the gap in attainment between the different groups. It is helpful to consider some suggested and implemented strategies under the following headings.

- Interventions supporting learners.
- Interventions supporting educators.
- Interventions developing and implementing curricula and assessment.
- Interventions to change educational governance and leadership.

Interventions at the Student Level

The following steps are of utmost importance in successfully initiating medical students and trainees to the country. Providing a welcoming and valuing international medical student or graduate induction programme including cultural competence, consultation skills, and social and linguistic support. Where required, coaching on language, accent, and role plays, with verbal and non-verbal cues guidance, could be helpful. A settling-in package includes information on housing, finances, and a guide to local supermarkets and shops. Induction periods should be long enough to have a period of shadowing and administrative and IT education.

Attempts should be made to pair up or match the international candidates with a mentoring or buddying programme, ideally with people from a similar background and who are between one to two years difference in training levels.

Students should be encouraged to seek out colleagues in similar positions and learn together where possible. They should be encouraged to ask for help and find a mentor for support and guidance. They should also be encouraged to give feedback to trainers and educators so that improvements can be made.

As much information as possible should be provided to the IMSs about the university and course, i.e. the campus map, lecture timetable, and what books and equipment are required. Also, the expected placements, available resources, and some information about the area or city, ideally well in advance, so they can arrange things beforehand if necessary.

Practical information on things like how much money may be required in the first month must be included. They should also be briefed about the need to register with a GP and be given helpful information on lists of nearby GPs and how to register or be directed to a university GP for students if there is one.

Also, in earlier placements, where possible, consider whether the student may or may not have a driving licence and whether earlier placements for IMSs should be close to the campus while they are still acclimatizing and where public transport is readily available and affordable.

Any biases should be identified and addressed, for example, any real or perceived dismissal of IMSs questions or concerns in class. Any differences in opportunities, such as promotion to committees or different grades amongst other student groups, should be monitored and addressed. Is there less complimentary language, encouragement, or letters of recommendation when addressing IMSs? Is there an attainment and award gap? Can measures be taken to address this if one is identified?

For graduates coming to England, much work has been done recently. Some GMC initiatives have been put in place to address the differential attainment; these include the optional 'Welcome to UK Practice' workshop, which according to a recent report, is highly valued by doctors and their supervisors, improving knowledge on ethical issues, GMC guidance, and UK practice in general, as well as communication and a focus on patient-centredness. It provides opportunities to meet colleagues, share learning, and gain support, but the report also suggested that IMGs still felt a general lack of support once they began working.

The British Medical Association (BMA) website also has a section focusing on IMGs, including life and work in the UK; the BMA has also set up an IMG newsletter focused on essential news and information relevant to IMGs.

No single training package can ever provide support for all students' needs. Instead, it is hoped that students are supported to identify their individual learning needs and that tutors, after discussion with their students, can aid them in developing bespoke plans for themselves, with the guidance and support of their seniors as required.

Interventions at Educator/Trainer Level

Educators and trainers must be recruited in fair and transparent processes to ensure a diversity of mentors and advisors. There is a need to develop educators who promote fairness and diversity in medical education.

Any identified differential attainment should be addressed by collecting data on ethnicity and analysing against performance. Educational Supervisors need to be provided with school-level progression data about international students compared to local graduates to address any identified issues.

There should be awareness of cultural differences and sensitivity when dealing with international students. All trainers must receive unconscious bias training and promote cultural competence.

Tutors should identify skills and encourage further development in those areas while supporting areas of weakness identified in IMSs.

When arranging small group teaching, the groups should include a mix of students from different backgrounds to promote better learning and integration.

Attempts should be made to identify problems earlier (from the very beginning of courses) to allow time to intervene and support students.

Tutors should be good at giving effective feedback (which is supportive), role modelling, coaching, and mentoring.

Tutors should know how to offer guidance and signpost trainees to the available resources.

They should consider extra supervision time for IMSs and not just consider educational needs but have a more holistic approach to their academic supervision, i.e. trying to develop a rapport with their students, asking about their wellbeing, and offering support where possible.

They should recognize diversity and avoid treating all trainees as a homogeneous group.

Address any differences in the ethical frameworks of the IMS's country of training and the host country.

It should be emphasized to all IMSs that the national governing body guidelines for doctors set out their professional values, shared knowledge, skills, and behaviours expected of all doctors studying or working in the host country and are a requirement rather than 'best practice'.

Trainers should aim to promote fairness and diversity in medical education and provide equal opportunities to all their students, addressing any complaints of bullying, harassment, and discrimination within their department either to or from their students or other staff and escalating concerns where necessary. Ideally, there should be an identifiable anti-bullying or harassment guardian or champion who has had training in managing these issues, can identify any inconsistencies, prioritize the findings, and initiate the implementation to change them to improve.

Educators may require special training to deal with refugee students who may have undergone post-traumatic stress disorder.

Interventions in Developing and Implementing Curricula and Assessments

Over the past few years, health inequalities have been exposed by pandemics such as the coronavirus. Many believe a more diverse and inclusive learning environment needs to be developed in medical schools to help reduce these inequalities by including a more thorough discussion of race in the medical curriculum.

This should include standard modules on anti-racism, microaggressions, unconscious bias, and bystander training early in the curriculum, possibly in year 1 or 2 of training. Unconscious biases can stem from medical school education. Stereotypes are reinforced by examination questions such as bone pain in an African Caribbean always indicates sickle cell disease or chest symptoms in an Asian indicate tuberculosis. This stereotyping can lead to severe mistakes in diagnosis, and medical students should be diligently taught to include sensible differentials and exclude options on a scientific basis rather than simple algorithms.

The concept of decolonizing the curriculum first appeared in the 1990s and aims to reflect on how we discuss and present race within medical teaching; it is essential to evaluate the language of medicine and how there is a lack of representation of how a disease presents in people from different ethnic groups. For example, skin conditions in skin types III-VI are poorly taught visually and in terms of text, resulting in poor and delayed diagnosis of these conditions in more pigmented skin types. A stated example of this is a delayed diagnosis of Lyme's disease at the arthritic stage in skin types V–VI (Khan, 2020).

Medical students should graduate with the ability to understand intersectionality, racial justice, and social issues that impact patient populations and how to ensure their practice can be ethical and inclusive.

All trainees and learners should know how to access and have equitable access to the curriculum. It should be presented in a format that is easy to comprehend.

Any assessments and examinations should be fair, reliable, and valid. There should be regular analysis of the outcomes to identify if specific cohorts are failing out of proportion to their demographic. If such differentials in attainment are identified, then steps should be taken to rectify any potential problems that may result in disadvantages for international students.

The appointment of assessors should be fair and equitable with appropriate consideration of protected characteristics. It is worth bearing in mind that while IMS status is not a protected characteristic in UK law, given that it mediates the most significant effect size in attainment gaps, IMGs must also be considered in recruiting trainers and examiners. It is essential to provide adequate training on assessing a candidate so that all assessments are uniform and objective.

Additional training and support should be provided for learners, when necessary, especially about written assessments, and negative feedback should be given in a sensitive but constructive manner.

With the increasing migration of health workers between countries and continents, developing global health modules and learning from managing health problems in different countries is becoming increasingly important. Apart from the apparent learning, this also helps build respect for other cultures and their management of specific issues. This became very relevant during the Covid pandemic of 2019-2020.

Interventions to Change Educational Governance and Leadership

In modern patient-centred healthcare systems, doctors must be good clinicians and also possess good communication and leadership skills to efficiently negotiate and use their resources to manage healthcare services. Students would therefore benefit from management training at medical schools, but this is limited by an already packed curriculum requirement stretching over five years. However, medical schools should allow students to participate in leadership roles and meetings when possible. Good leadership leads to good outcomes in healthcare, and it is therefore essential that students are exposed to these concepts early on in their training. Many students also show a keen interest in learning management skills professionally.[3] Most students, however, need to be aware of opportunities in leadership when they are advertised. IMSs will be even more unaware of any advertised posts by word of mouth if they need more communication skills. However, before altering the entire medical curriculum, one must consider whether management would be best taught to everyone or select a few interested.

Systems for selecting leadership roles must be fair and transparent, including equality, diversity, and inclusion training. Job advertisements for these positions should be well publicized before appointments, giving doctors from all backgrounds a chance to apply.

HEE quality frameworks should be used to raise concerns around education and training.

There should be a zero-tolerance policy towards bullying and harassment with definitive action taken against it.

A system should be developed to ensure fairness in incident reporting and complaints investigation. It should be blame-free and with a focus on learning and not punishment.

Surveys should be carried out 4-6 weeks within posts to identify trainees who may need extra support, for example, through mentorship.

Summary

Given the central role of doctors in delivering healthcare, the challenges presented by the migration of healthcare workers, and questions concerning the adequacy of existing medical schools to meet global healthcare needs in terms of quality and numbers to prevent global shortages in doctors, it is essential to monitor existing schools and their graduates and help where possible to standardize the curriculum and assessments delivered in medical schools globally.

It is also essential that international students are supported correctly to ensure they develop their full potential into happy and valuable physicians.

To ensure this, the following steps will be helpful:

Every effort is made to support equality and diversity in education and the workforce.

Empathy for IMSs at the trainer and systems level.

Individualized learning agreements based on trainees' strengths and learning needs.

Appropriate induction and early diagnosis and intervention.

Systems level data and monitoring, standing item on school agenda.

Tailored support with good debriefing and feedback for those failing exams or other attainment gaps.

Practical solutions can go a long way to improve the IMS journey. Still, kindness, compassion, and simple steps such as inviting an IMS to dinner, making friends with them, or other activities such as going to the cinema can further make them feel welcome and included.

References

Al-Saadi, Hatem. et al. (2020). "Home and Away" a look at Gulf Medical Students' influencing factors, challenges and attitudes for studying medicine abroad. European Journal of Medical and Health Sciences 2(4). July 2020.

Baker, C. (2021). 'NHS staff from overseas: statistics. House of Commons Library. Number 7783.

Bhanot R. (2018) Improving leadership and management education in medical school. Adv Med Educ Pract. 9: 305–306

Cohn, S. et al. (2006). Experiences and expectations of refugee doctors: Qualitative study. The British Journal of Psychiatry. 189(1): 74–78.

Dave, S. et al. (2020). A scoping review of differential attainment in undergraduate medicine: Bridging the gap—Thematic series on tackling differential attainment in medical profession 2020. Sushruta Journal of Health Policy & Opinion 13(3): 1–10.

Dawnay, G. (2019) Doctor suicide – How many more? BMJ Opinion 13 June 2019

Duvivier RJ, Boulet JR, Opalek A, van Zanten M, Norcini J. Overview of the world's medical schools: an update. Med Educ. 2014 Sep;48(9):860–869.

Fraser, R.C. (1991). 'Undergraduate medical education: present state and future needs. BMJ 1991;303, pp 41–43

General Medical Council (2013). Good medical practice available at: www.gmc-uk.org/gmp

General Medical Council (2015). Promoting excellence: standards for medical education and training.

General Medical Council (2021). The state of medical education and practice in the UK

General Medical Council (2022). The GMC publishes figures on death during investigations.

Goel, S., Angeli, F., Dhirar, N. et al. What motivates medical students to select medical studies: a systematic literature review. BMC Med Educ 18, 16 (2018).

Hawkridge, A., et al (2021). 'Differential attainment case study. How Health Education Northwest (HEE NW) has improved exam re-sit outcomes for GP trainees who have had their GP programme training time extended.' GMC

Holst, J. Global Health – emergence, hegemonic trends and biomedical reductionism. *Global Health* 16, 42 (2020). https://doi.org/10.1186/s12992-020-00573-4

Jalal, M. (2019). Overseas doctors of the NHS: migration, transition, challenges and towards resolution. *Future Healthcare Journal* 6(1): 76–81

Khan, S. (2020) Racism and medical education. *The Lancet* 20(9): P1009, September 01.

Lagunes-Cordoba, E. et al (2020). International medical graduates: how can UK psychiatry do better? British Journal Psychiatry Bulletin.

Mountford-Zimdars, A.S. et al. (2015). Causes of differences in student outcomes. Higher Education Funding council for England.

Patel, M. (2019). 'Narrowing the gap of Differential Attainment by getting the best out of everyone.' Speaking at the Northwest PGMDEL Conference, 19th September 2019.

Quiney, G.S. (2021) Retaining the doctors we train. BMJ 2021;374: n1998

Rao, M., et al. (2022). 'Welcoming and Valuing International Medical Graduates A guide to induction for IMGs recruited to the NHS.' Workforce Race Equality Strategy, NHS England 2022

Scarborough, N. (2020) Differential Attainment case study. How Health Education East Midlands (HEE EM) are using early performance indicators to provide tailored support for GP trainees. General Medical Council.

Schwenk, T.L. et al (2010). Depression, Stigma, and Suicidal Ideation in Medical Students. JAMA 304(11): 1181–1190.

Slowther, A. et al. (2012). Experiences of non-UK-qualified doctors working within the UK regulatory framework: a qualitative study. Journal of the Royal Society of Medicine 105(4).

The Royal College of Physicians (2021) Double or quits: a blueprint for expanding medical school places. (Report)

UK House of Commons health committee. (2011) 4th report. Revalidation of doctors. London: House of Commons.

UK national patient safety agency. (2011) National clinical assessment service. Concerns about professional practise and associations with age, gender, place of qualification and ethnicity-2009/10 data. London NCAS.

West, M. et al. (2020). The courage of compassion: Supporting Nurses and midwives to deliver high-quality care. The King's Fund.

Woolf, K. et al. (2016). Fair Training Pathways for All: Understanding Experiences of Progression. General Medical Council

World Health Organization (2006) The global shortage of health workers and its impact.

Wright D, Flis N, Gupta M. (2008). The 'Brain Drain' of physicians: historical antecedents to an ethical debate, c. 1960-79. Philos Ethics Humanit Med. Nov 10; 3:24.

Zerehi, M.R. (2008) 'The Role of International Medical Graduates in the U.S. Physician Workforce. A Policy Monograph. American College of Physicians.

28

Supporting the Wellbeing of Medical Students with Disabilities and Long-Term Health Conditions

Hannah S. Barham-Brown

'As a medical student, I am more than my grades'

—M, Medical Student, Scotland

Over recent years, medical professional bodies in the UK have increasingly considered the needs of students and doctors with disabilities and long-term health conditions (LTHC), for example, *Welcomed and Valued, Supporting Disabled Learners in Education and Training* (General Medical Council, 2019)—a report offering advice on how medical schools and postgraduate educators can support these cohorts. Whilst there is no data available to confirm that there are increasing numbers of disabled students attending medical schools (partly due to limited reporting of disability by the students themselves), anecdotally, the author would suggest that we are seeing not only a greater number of students with a wide variety of conditions applying for medical schools, but a growing awareness of their presence in the profession more widely. This anecdotal understanding is backed up by an increasing number of events and organizations set up both for and by this cohort such as 'Wonky Teacups', a support group for all Allied Health Professionals with disabilities or LTHC (Barham-Brown, 2017a), and the Disabled Doctors Network (Disabled Doctors Network, 2022). These conversations also continue on social media using various hashtags, such as #DisabledDocs, #DocsWithDisabilities and #DisabledMedTwitter. Indeed, many of us would argue that the increasing representation of disability within this population is of considerable benefit to the patients who will be cared for by these doctors (Barham-Brown, 2017b).

For clarity, when considering 'disability', I shall be utilizing the Social Model of Disability, a concept first conceived in 1975 by the Union of the Physically Impaired Against Segregation (Finkelstein & Davis, 1975) and formally developed and popularized by Prof Mike Oliver in his 1983 book, *Social Work with Disabled People* (Oliver, 1983) . Whilst this is the most commonly used 'model' of disability in the UK, it is not above criticism, as highlighted in *The Social Model of Disability* (Shakespeare, 2010). However the principle that individuals with physical impairments are disabled by a society designed without them in mind is one that many disabled people in the UK passionately uphold.

Utilizing case studies from disabled medical students and junior doctors alongside data from the BMA Disability Report (British Medical Association, 2020), we shall consider how

Hannah S. Barham-Brown, *Supporting the Wellbeing of Medical Students with Disabilities and Long-term Health Conditions* In: *The Mental Health of Medical Students*. Edited by: Andrew Molodynski, Sarah Marie Farrell, and Dinesh Bhugra, Oxford University Press.

the additional psychological load of negotiating training with a disability or LTHC impacts on the wellbeing of these students.

In Great Britain (i.e. not Northern Ireland), the rights of disabled people are encapsulated in the Equality Act 2010, which states, 'You're disabled under the Equality Act 2010 if you have a physical or mental impairment that has a 'substantial' and 'long-term' negative effect on your ability to do normal daily activities' (UK Government, 2010). If an individual is disabled under this definition, the Equality Act entitles them to 'reasonable adjustments' in their workplace or place of education. As we will later explore however, many students and doctors find that these reasonable adjustments do not come to fruition—and if they do appear, many have struggled on for a considerable period before receiving them.

In 2020, prior to the COVID-19 pandemic, the British Medical Association carried out the first Disability Survey of medical students and doctors with disabilities and LTHCs (British Medical Association, 2020). As a wheelchair-using, neurodivergent doctor assisting with this work, I felt I would be able to predict much of what our respondents would highlight in both the qualitative and quantitative elements of this project. In reality, the results, particularly from the newer members of our profession, horrified me. When preparing this chapter, I was hugely grateful for the input of my five 'case studies'—medical students and newly-qualified UK Drs with a range of disabilities and LTHCs, from mental health conditions to physical impairments, and a range of neurodivergent diagnoses. The feedback that I received from E, B, M, L and J shone a light on a system that not only fails in its duty of care to these students, but in some cases actively discriminates against them to such a degree that I can only describe it as an abusive relationship.

Medical School is hard. No one going into it truly believes that it will be a walk in the park, however academically talented an individual may be. The range of ways in which students are taught, tested, and observed, from theoretical to clinical skills, communication assessments, and the unpredictable nature of placements, means that no one student can possibly excel in every area. This is to be expected, but amidst the pressures all students experience—practical, financial, and academic—those who have disabilities and LTHCs have a whole range of additional challenges to tackle as a result of the system having been designed without them in mind—and as I will show, the impact of this additional burden affects their mental and physical health, not just their grades.

In 2012, university fees increased substantially, with most, if not all, medical students paying £9,000 per year for their education (or at least taking substantial student loans to cover these costs)—and this increased to £9,250 in 2017 (Fazackerley, 2022). Alongside this, the funding available is significantly limited: 'Student doctors in the penultimate two years of their training are only permitted to borrow a maximum of £6,458 to live on annually (this is a combination of Student Finance Loan (maximum £1,975) and NHS bursary (maximum £2,643 means-tested, £1,000 non-means-tested, plus £84 for 10 extra weeks—based on a 40-week term, living away from home, outside of London)' (Doctor's Association UK, 2022). We know that many students have to take on jobs alongside what is supposed to be a 'full time' course with placements—to the extent that the NHS specifically makes suggestions of part time roles within the organization that may also be useful in terms of experience for medical students (NHS Careers, 2015).

If one is a student with a disability however, the course alone may be a physical and psychological struggle (as I will discuss later)—let alone taking on a part time job alongside it. This leaves disabled students in an impossible situation—and doesn't take into account the additional costs they may face. Scope, a UK disability charity, calculated the 'average additional monthly income a disabled person would need in order to enjoy the same standard of living as a non-disabled person' in their Disability Price Tag report (John et al., 2019). This came to the startling sum of £583 per month.

Looking to our case studies, money featured heavily in the responses of several. J specifically listed 'Financial, travel, and exams' as key elements causing a negative impact on her wellbeing at medical school—'the last couple of years were very difficult financially as NHS bursary funding is less than student finance and I had accumulated debts while I had taken time off the course due to my health as all student finance payments stopped but I still had to pay my rent/bills, etc'. More worryingly, she struggled with getting to placements because she 'couldn't really afford taxis' but would often come into contact with cigarette smoke on public transport, which for her is a 'major asthma trigger'.

B also listed money as having a negative impact on her wellbeing, stating that she had to in fact take on extra shifts of her part time job specifically because of the 'additional costs incurred which in turn messed with pacing'. Pacing is a key part of disability management for many people, and not being able to manage symptoms in this way would likely increase the strain of an impairment (Abonie et al., 2020).

He describes funding, and the systems around it as 'the biggest barrier for me … particularly through issues with the NHS bursary'. She has 'to take taxis to placements as I am unable to drive due to my sleep disorder and unable to take public transport due to sensory overload. At the end of each month I have to submit my receipts for my taxis and I'll be reimbursed the majority of the cost'. Except in practice, this doesn't happen in a timely manner. 'Between October 2021 and the start of March 2022 I had to battle to get my money back, having spent over £800 on travel and being owed £600—this amount was the same as my entire student loan for the same period of time, leaving me very little to live on'. She describes this situation and the £20/week that she gets from the NHS bursary as leading to 'so much distress for both me, my husband, and our families'.

The NHS bursary provides funding for medical students and dentists, with a selection of tuition fee contributions, a non-means-tested grant of £1,000 per academic year, and a means-tested bursary which is based on the household income of the student in question (NHS Business Services Authority, 2022a). There are also 'Extra Allowances' available within the scheme, including Childcare Allowance (CCA), an NHS Bursary Hardship Grant, Travel and Dual Accommodation Expenses (TDAE) and Disabled Student Allowances (DSAs). The DSAs constitute four different parts that students can apply for. These are Specialist Equipment Allowance, Non-Medical Helper Allowance, General Allowance, and Travel Allowance. Travel Allowance covers only 'excess travel costs', which are worked out as the excess between public transport costs and the type of travel used due to someone's disability (NHS Business Services Authority, 2022b). These generally require students to keep receipts and process these within the system, which E finds quite a time-consuming process, particularly on top of placements and study.

Examination methods and their apparently immovable nature raised a wide variety of issues for my case studies. The General Medical Council (GMC) expect medical schools to assess against specific outcomes, but they don't stipulate how these assessments should be carried out (General Medical Council, 2003)—so if an individual school wished to change their assessment methods, that would be acceptable as long as the new method met the GMC's quality assurance (General Medical Council, 2009).This gives medical schools a degree of flexibility in terms of potential methodologies for examination—and yet this flexibility seems to be rarely experienced by medical students who need reasonable adjustments. B, a profoundly deaf medical student, found written exams 'fine', but highlighted that OSCEs were particularly challenging for her, as she wrangled a combination of 'hearing aids, adapted stethoscope, and radio aid alongside auditory processing, to get everything done in the same time as everyone else'. She describes these experiences as 'quite stressful' (which sounds somewhat of an understatement), but also reports that when asking for reasonable adjustments throughout medical school (to which she is legally entitled (UK Government, 2010)), these were not only declined, despite being recommended by 'other doctors and occupational health', but that she was 'made to feel guilty for asking for adaptations, resulting in a lot of anxiety'.

Some elements which students struggle with would be relatively simple to fix, such as feedback on exams to better focus or address areas of particular 'weakness'—as raised by M, a medical student with mental health diagnoses.

Others would prove more challenging, but not impossible. L, a student with multiple diagnoses, including attention deficit hyperactivity disorder (ADHD) and Dyslexia, has found exam methods to be her biggest barrier to graduating. She raises the very legitimate question of 'why we are examined by memory testing in isolation when the same practice ... is entirely unrepresentative of how we actually practice medicine as FY1s'. She considers 'the format of multiple-choice questions (MCQs) as a sight unseen, time bound memory test in isolation and without normal resources is archaic, and discriminatory to those with additional leaning needs'. As she puts it, 'asking me to select one correct answer from four almost identical options is literally asking the fish to climb the proverbial tree', and she has failed 3 MCQ exams by <10% each time, despite performing well in every other area of assessment. Unfortunately for her, the school doesn't average her marks across the year, and so due to this exam method, she is at risk of 'getting kicked out of med school'. Alongside the challenges she faces with the format of the exams, she was also let down by the services that were meant to support her through the process; 'I was given the wrong information about length of exam by disability services. I was told the exam would be two hours standard but it was three hours standard. This meant that with additional time and breaks, I was facing a five-hour exam which my body would never have managed. I highlighted this in November, and still didn't get it resolved until after I'd already failed my January exam. They would not entertain any other option for me, other than sit the five-hour exam or declare myself not fit to sit and resit in the summer. At this point, I was also threatened in a Zoom meeting with FTP [Fitness to Practice] if I chose to sit as scheduled inappropriately, as this would demonstrate a lack of insight into my conditions/capabilities'. Eventually, she was able to get the changes she needed; 'They "fixed" it for June and August exams by separating the exams into two halves ... They've now done this for ALL students ironically, so some good has come out of it for others I suppose'.

This final point is incredibly important when considering the support we provide for disabled medical students. When we get it right, when sufficient provision is in place, it often benefits non-disabled students too, whether that be in terms of examinations, mental health support, or funding. If anything, it could be argued that this particular group of students should be seen as the canaries in the mine of medical training, often going above and beyond what should be reasonably expected of them in terms of self-advocacy, in order to be able to study as effectively as their non-disabled colleagues.

'I feel the support in medical school has been very superficial—as soon as you need genuine help and advocacy, it feels like you're left alone'.
    E—Medical student, Midlands

By interviewing a range of students from different medical schools across the UK, I was able to see the huge disparities that there were in terms of support for this cohort, and the challenges different services had in empowering them. One of the systemic issues that many had to overcome was accessing support that understood how medical courses work. The structure of many medical schools is that they exist within a wider university structure, and it is the university who often take responsibility for support services such as counselling and Disabled Student support. As J states, these 'often didn't have a great understanding about the specific challenges of a medical degree'.

M reported that her university had psychological and counselling services that are technically available to medical students. Unfortunately, she reports that 'these have waiting lists of over a year', and often aren't accessible to those on placement. As someone with an eating disorder and diagnosed with depression, she found that these 'don't accept students with more specialized or complex issues'. Fortunately, her medical school does have a 'welfare service—a liaison psychiatrist who works two afternoons a week'. However she expands that this one doctor covers 'all welfare issues affecting a medical school of over 1,500 students. As you can imagine, waiting times are long'. She describes this medical welfare service as feeling 'tokenistic', as if it 'exists more to cover their own backs ... if you manage studies alongside health issues they aren't very helpful'.

She was allotted an 'Advisor of Studies', and despite having been warned against divulging her mental health issues to her medical school by her previous GP; 'I decided I would be open ... and mention what was going on for me. When I spoke of the eating disorder, however, he simply responded, 'Don't worry, you don't look like it; you'll be fine.''

J reported specific issues as a result of the disconnect between medical school and university; having requested to train Less Than Full Time (LTFT)—a concept I shall discuss in more depth later—she was informed that whilst the medical school were 'investigating' the option, 'it was denied by the university'. For L, the separation of service provision leads to a 'lack of transparency'—'the medical school policies seem to supersede all university policies, meaning the SU [Student Union] can't support you, and often, neither can the disability services as they don't have insight (or even access!) to the medical school policies'. The chasm between services has meant significant delays for E in accessing a 'Reasonable Adjustments Plan' (RAP) from the university—'I applied ... straight away, and by the time exams came, I still had not been able to get my RAP and therefore adjustments in place'. She goes on to clarify that this had meant a wait of nearly 4 months to get the plan in place.

Reasonable Adjustments were a key topic of the BMA Disability Report (British Medical Association, 2020). Only 55% of the doctors and medical students who responded reported receiving reasonable adjustments, despite these being a legal requirement (UK Government, 2010) and when asked about their priorities for improving the circumstances of disabled doctors and medical students, 69% reported that accessing reasonable adjustments was a priority for them. As the authors outlined, 'Difficulties securing adjustments included: lengthy and complex processes, slow or only partial implementation, lack of engagement in the process by employers and schools, perceived costs and impacts on others, and fears about asking in case of negative career consequences'(British Medical Association, 2020) . Respondents to the BMA Disability Report have, in some cases, indicated that they have funded their own adjustments, despite the law being clear that they should not have to (British Medical Association, 2020).

It is important to acknowledge that disability never exists in a vacuum for these students. One must acknowledge the intersectional nature of discrimination that many of them experience, be that linked to race, gender, sexuality, or other protected characteristics. This intersectionality was raised by M, who stated 'The toxic culture, hierarchies, and competitiveness have always made me feel inadequate and out of place, this is also amplified as a queer woman not originally from the UK'.

These students may also have children or family members to care for or support, with the additional time and financial implications of this—though that was not the case for any of our case studies.

Whilst the impact of the pandemic on these students could make up an entire PhD thesis of its own, there were some (unpleasant) surprises amongst my case studies that are important to note as medical education recovers and 'normalizes' following the pandemic, in the hope that there can be some positive outcomes for this cohort. Many had hopes that the move to online lectures (something that had been requested by disabled medical students for many years, and almost always declined until a pandemic came along), would increase accessibility going forwards. However, for some, these not only did not continue, but made things worse. B, a deaf medical student found that the lack of cohesion between university's disability services and the medical school meant her requirements weren't enforced, and so for over a year, she was unable to hear any of the online lectures, and transcripts were never provided. Similarly, closed captions did not exist on Zoom, which was used to host most meetings for a great deal of the pandemic, so she was 'also struggling to follow'. A year's worth of paid tuition simply didn't exist for her as a result, with no acknowledgement from her medical school. It is hard to conceive of the additional mental load placed on a student in this situation during a global pandemic.

Having found online lectures incredibly helpful when managing early morning and late afternoon 'flares' of her idiopathic hypersomnia, E asked after the first wave of COVID-19 if she could keep joining these specific lectures from home virtually—attending others but utilizing the technology that the university had been using for months for all students. She was told, 'this wasn't possible, and I had to be there in person otherwise my attendance would be flagged. Just weeks later, in advance of the second wave … all teaching that wasn't clinical was moved online because we had to be 'safe' … I guess it just wasn't possible for someone with a disability. It was difficult to see adjustments that people like me have been begging for, suddenly be so easily implemented'. So even when the technology is available, it is the somewhat archaic attendance checking systems that seem to disadvantage this group—it is not the computer that 'says no' in this situation.

Lectures were not the only area in which COVID-19 disproportionately impacted our case studies. Placements were also affected. For example, E found that 'when social spaces were closed in our hospital … I no longer had a safe space to take my rest breaks when needed, which I relied on. I ended up having to sneak out to my car … and have a nap in the car just to be able to get through the day'.

One of the case study students, J, was classed as 'Clinically Extremely Vulnerable' (CEV), meaning access to placements during the pandemic was not an option for her—but she reports that her medical school was 'very supportive of my desire to remain on the course during the COVID pandemic'. Whilst there is as yet no published research on the impact of the pandemic on the training of CEV medical students, the effects of shielding on junior doctors has been researched; and this shows that the support given to these trainees was lacking, if present at all (Martin, 2022).

There are many things that the world of medical education can and should do to support these students, who are often left feeling incredibly isolated amidst their peers. It is clear that there needs to be an attitudinal change across the whole profession towards disability. The 'Superhero' narrative that surround healthcare staff, particularly at times of crisis such as war or pandemic, can be incredibly damaging through its erasure of the humanity and vulnerability of these workers, on whom the pressure to perform can take a terrible, and in some cases fatal, toll (McAllister et al., 2020).For those who have disabilities and LTHCs, this pressure can manifest in negative internal and external experiences as they feel unable to match up to their peers and are judged by seniors before they've even had a chance to try. E, a medical student who has an interest in emergency medicine, on mentioning this to a consultant from a different specialty, was told that she 'wouldn't want to cause a problem for the specialty'. She reports that experiences such as this have 'made me wonder if I'm even valuable to the profession at all—I have nearly left a number of times'. The issues around culture were raised by other students. In response to the question 'What about the medical school environment negatively impacted your wellbeing?' J answered 'I think mainly the unspoken view that people in medicine can't get ill. It was really hard to find people who understood the situation I was in when I suddenly found myself being admitted to hospital acutely unwell every few weeks. So I ended up keeping a lot of it to myself and I think my mental health definitely suffered as a result ... Additionally at times my health was brought up as a potential professionalism issue. While I do understand that it could potentially be an issue, I felt like it was brought up before there were any problems and made me feel quite guilty and wary about being too open with issues'.

For M, the challenges accessing support started before she'd even had her first day at medical school. She describes going to see her GP at the age of 15 about her eating disorder; 'I remember her responding "Didn't I want to apply to medical school?" and commenting that I should snap out of what are essentially silly "teenage girl behaviours", if I wanted to be successful in applying, alluding to me not being suited to medical school if I couldn't handle school'. This response led to her feeling she had to hide how much she was struggling for 'the next few years'. Sadly for her, the attitudes of clinicians to mental health issues in the profession didn't improve for her when she did try to inform people; 'When I got into medical school, we were given an occupational health form to fill out which needed to be signed by our GP. At this point, I wanted to be open about and disclose what was going on as I knew that being honest with the world and therefore myself was key to my getting well. My GP actually made me cross out where I wrote this on the form, telling me it would look bad ... this set me up to start medical school already convinced my poor mental health made me lesser'. It would have been understandable if she'd continued to believe this and hidden her problems from her medical school. This would ultimately have left her at risk of a GMC referral, as the Disabled Doctors Network highlights; 'you as a professional also have an obligation to be honest and open about your condition, abilities, and limitations. Whilst not obliged to disclose the nature of your condition to everyone, you must share adequate information to key relevant people in order that they can decide how to provide you with the support required to meet the required professional competencies' (Disabled Doctors Network, 2022).

If there was one change medical schools and universities could make for students with disabilities and LTHCs to improve their mental load and overall wellbeing, this author would suggest that it should be the implementation of Less Than Full-Time study options. This is an option throughout postgraduate medical training, with disabled trainees entitled to Category 1 LTFT training (Health Careers NHS, 2022). As such, students with disabilities and LTHCs are almost guaranteed the option to work LTFT once they qualify—but this is rarely an option during medical school, when they are expected to attend placement and study at the same rate as their non-disabled colleagues, often at the detriment of their mental and physical health, as well as having financial implications—whilst many of their colleagues have part-time jobs to manage the deficit between bursary provision and living costs, those who struggle to manage full-time study and placement do not have the capacity for additional work on top. Some of our case study students have actively sought out LTFT options, but none have yet succeeded. E was told by her course that the GMC 'would not allow it'—but on a review of GMC policies, this is clearly not the case—indeed, the GMC themselves state 'We do not object to students completing a medical course in part-time/less than full-time mode as a potential reasonable adjustment, as long as the medical school is assured the above requirements. This would be a decision for the medical school to take for an individual student'. However they go on to say, 'There are no part-time medical courses in the UK at the moment' (General Medical Council, 2022). He goes on to explain 'I asked about the possibility of splitting my fourth year over two calendar years, on the basis that upon graduation I could immediately train less than full time (potentially down to 50%) and that it was ridiculous to have that option once you got to being a doctor but not during the training to get to be a doctor'. Given that LTFT training is an option for trainees to keep people working when full-time training would not be a practical option for them (Health Education England, 2022), it seems incredibly impractical not to offer this option to medical students that we would (and sadly do) otherwise lose. It is unclear whether any medical schools in the UK are actively looking into creating Less than Full-Time medical courses, which the GMC have clarified would 'need to go through our approval process for new programmes' (General Medical Council, 2022) .

In the spirit of 'Nothing About Us Without Us', a phrase adopted for the disabled community by disability rights activist James Charlton in the 1990s (Overdorff, 2022), I asked each of my case studies what three things they would change for someone else with their condition applying to medical school today.

One student specifically named LTFT study, though a few of the case studies had highlighted their desire to study this way elsewhere in the interviews. Another suggestion was improving funding for disabled students, who experience considerable extra costs and financial challenges through their degrees, as we have seen in the case of E.

The overriding theme amidst the requests was support. The form this should take varied between the respondents, with some wanting specific disability advisors or services, one was keen for support tailored around foundation job applications, and another highlighted the importance of this support being provided from as early a stage as possible. There was a clear demand however that any support was specifically for the medical school and disabled medical students in particular. This would suggest that the university-based support they had all experienced, despite being at different schools, clearly wasn't working for any of them.

Few of the suggestions the students had were particularly challenging to fulfil, bar an overhaul of funding for these students, and redesigning exam methods to be more accessible for students who feel that they currently they are 'literally asking the fish to climb the proverbial tree', as E puts it. Other requests involved increased training for staff and awareness of disability in medicine, access to other disabled doctors to speak to, and maintaining access to the online lectures and teaching that was brought in for the pandemic.

It is a testament to the characters of these students that despite the incredibly hard situations they have found themselves battling through medical school, they all highlighted someone who had helped them, whether their peers, Occupational Health doctors, pastoral support teams, or others. M concludes by emphasizing that whilst 'formal support is entirely lacking, I want to highlight that so many individuals have been nothing but wonderful and genuinely helpful and supportive and that I am so grateful for this. Without that handful of tutors, lecturers, etc. who noticed and on (sic) their own accord, gave me space and time to help navigate things, I genuinely don't think I would still be in medical school'.

The potential options available to better support disabled students and those with LTHCs are broad—and the myriad ways in which having them in the profession could benefit the patients they will care for are being discussed across health and social care. It is vitally important that we work with this cohort to make medicine an accessible profession which values the wellbeing of those applying to be a part of it.

'I always felt that in the right environment and with the right support, I was as capable as anyone else and could be a perfectly good doctor, and maybe even excel in something.'

—E, medical student, Midlands

References

Abonie, U.S., Sandercock, G.R.H., Heesterbeek, M., & Hettinga, F.J. (2020). Disability and Rehabilitation 42, 613–622.

Barham-Brown, H. (2017a). *Wonky Teacups*. Facebook. https://www.facebook.com/groups/175242942 5069687 (Accessed 28 July 2022).

Barham-Brown, H. (2017b). Doctoring with a disability. *British Medical Journal*. https://blogs.bmj.com/ bmj/2017/02/09/hannah-barham-brown-doctoring-with-a-disability/ (Accessed 27 June 2022).

British Medical Association (2020). Disability in the medical profession.

Disabled Doctors Network (2022). Disabled Doctors Network [WWW Document]. https://www.dis ableddoctorsnetwork.com/ (Accessed 28 July 22).

Doctor's Association UK (2022). *A Liveable NHS Bursary*. Doctor's Association UK. https://www.dauk. org/elementor-6416/ (accessed 7 October 2022).

Fazackerley, A. (2022). The Guardian.

Finkelstein, V. & Davis, K. (1975). *The Union of The Physically Impaired Against Segregation and The Disability Alliance discuss Fundamental Principles of Disability*.

General Medical Council (2003). *Tomorrow's Doctors*. https://www.educacionmedica.net/pdf/doc umentos/modelos/tomorrowdoc.pdf (Accessed 7 October 2022).

General Medical Council (2009). *Assessment in Undergraduate Medical Education*. https://www.gmc-uk.org/-/media/documents/Assessment_in_undergraduate_medical_education___guidance_0 815.pdf_56439668.pdf (Accessed 7 October 2022).

General Medical Council (2019). *Welcomed and Valued*. General Medical Council. https://www.gmc-uk.org/education/standards-guidance-and-curricula/guidance/welcomed-and-valued (Accessed 27 June 2022).

General Medical Council (2022). *Studying medicine and graduating with a primary medical qualification*. https://www.gmc-uk.org/education/standards-guidance-and-curricula/guidance/welcomed-and-valued/our-involvement-as-a-professional-regulator/studying-medicine-and-graduating-with-a-primary-medical-qualification (Accessed 7 November 2022).

Health Careers NHS (2022). *Less than full-time training for doctors.* Health Careers NHS. URL https://www.healthcareers.nhs.uk/explore-roles/doctors/career-opportunities-doctors/less-full-time-training-doctors (Accessed 28 July 2022).

Health Education England (2022). *Less Than Full Time Training.* https://london.hee.nhs.uk/medical-training/trainee-resources/less-full-time-training (accessed 7 October 2022).

John, E., Thomas, G., & Touchet, A. (2019). *The Disability Price Tag 2019 Policy Report.*

Martin, A. (2022). Exploring the experiences of junior doctors who were 'shielding' during the COVID-19 Pandemic (Master's Dissertation). University Of Glasgow.

McAllister, M., Lee Brien, D., & Dean, S. (2020). Contemporary Nurse 56, 199–203.

NHS Business Services Authority (2022a). *NHS Bursary Students.* NHS Business Services Authority Webpage. https://www.nhsbsa.nhs.uk/nhs-bursary-students (Accessed 28 July 2022).

NHS Business Services Authority (2022b). *Disabled Student Allowances (DSAs.* NHS Business Services Authority Webpage. https://www.nhsbsa.nhs.uk/nhs-bursary-students/disabled-student-allowances-dsas (Accessed 28 July 2022).

NHS Careers (2015). *Summer Jobs and Part-Time Work While at Medical School.* NHS Careers. https://www.healthcareers.nhs.uk/explore-roles/doctors/medical-school/summer-jobs-and-part-time-work-while-medical-school (Accessed 7 October 2022).

Oliver, M. (1983). *Social Work with Disabled People.* London: Macmillan Education UK.

Overdorff, N. (2022). *Nothing About Us Without Us: Input from People With Disabilities.* Equidox PDF Accessibility Solutions. https://equidox.co/blog/nothing-about-us-without-us-input-from-people-with-disabilities/ (Accessed 7 November 2022).

Shakespeare, T. (2010). *The Social Model of Disability.*

UK Government (2010). *Equality Act 2010.* https://www.legislation.gov.uk/ukpga/2010/15/enacted/data.pdf (accessed 27 June 2022).

29

Substance Misuse Amongst Medical Students

Kate Irvine, Christopher Mohan, Eimear O'Neill, and Mary Cannon

1. licit—alcohol, nicotine, caffeine;
2. purely illicit—cannabis, hallucinogens, and inhalants;
3. and prescribed and also illicit substances—stimulants (including prescription stimulants, cocaine, ecstasy, ketamine), opioids (including opiates), and hypnotics.

Background

Interest in substance use among medical students and physicians dates back as far as 1896 (Paget [1869] as cited in Baldisseri, 2007). Interest is driven by the high prevalence and potential consequences of substance misuse. Of particular concern is the association of substance use and the decreased ability to detect, treat, and educate patients against SUD (Baldwin et al., 1991; Birch et al., 1998; McAuliffe et al., 1984; Papazisis et al., 2017; Roncero et al., 2014; Weissberg et al., 2006). Further risks include the tendency of drug dependant physicians to over-prescribe addictive substances and their impaired judgement. This is often preceded by increased absenteeism and increased exam failure by medical students (Gignon et al., 2015; Weissberg et al., 2006; Westermeyer, 1991).

Medical students have a higher prevalence of substance misuse than the general adult population yet share similar figures with their peers and other students (Bourbon et al., 2019; MacLean et al., 2016; Papazisis et al., 2018a; Papazisis et al., 2018b; Webb et al., 1998). Experimentation and use of illicit substances have increased over the past five decades, matching trends in society (United Nations Office on Drugs and Crime [UNODC], 2011; European Monitoring Centre for Drugs and Drug Addiction [EMCDDA], 2021). Medical student use of substances was estimated at 13% in the 1970s, increasing to between 24.7% (Greece) and 33.1% (United Kingdom [UK]) in the 2000s. Despite the increasing prevalence, not all substances are used by medical students, and there is a nuanced relationship between medical students and substances that could explain why previously medical students were thought to use fewer substances than the general population (Roncero et al., 2015; Westermeyer, 1991).

There are different patterns of substance use dependent upon country and culture, and studies have been analysed by geographical area (McAuliffe et al., 1984; Molodynski et al., 2021; Papazisis et al., 2018b; Roncero et al., 2015). Boland and colleagues (2006) found in a 30-year study that students from westernized cultures had a higher lifetime prevalence of

Kate Irvine, Christopher Mohan, Eimear O'Neill, and Mary Cannon, *Substance Misuse Amongst Medical Students* In: *The Mental Health of Medical Students*. Edited by: Andrew Molodynski, Sarah Marie Farrell, and Dinesh Bhugra, Oxford University Press.
© Oxford University Press 2024. DOI: 10.1093/oso/9780192864871.003.0029

being offered and taking drugs compared with non-western students. Substance selection by medical students follows societal trends, for example, in the 1960s in the United States of America, cannabis, LSD, and hallucinogens were favoured, whereas MDMA and cocaine became substances of choice in the 1980s among western society (McAuliffe et al., 1984).

Chapter Overview

Apart from variations between countries and cultures, studies have examined the types of substances, levels of misuse, and changes over time. This chapter examines these differences substance by substance. Table 29.1 shows an overview of prevalence per study, and geographical region. Nine substances were consistently found relevant to medical students, divided equally into three broad categories:

1. licit—alcohol, nicotine, caffeine;
2. purely illicit—cannabis (including cannabinoid products, marijuana/hashish), hallucinogens (including LSD and hallucinogenic mushrooms) and inhalants;
3. both illicit and prescribed—stimulants (including prescription stimulants, cocaine, ecstasy, ketamine, opioids—including opiates) and hypnotics and anxiolytics.

The latter category includes non-medical use of prescription drugs (NMUP) which is a facet of substance misuse unique to medics and shall be discussed later in greater detail. There are other substances, such as synthetic drugs (e.g. spice, K2, 'bath salts') or anabolic steroids, which are not covered in detail as medical students do not tend to use these drugs (Merlo et al., 2017).

Licit Substances

Alcohol

Research indicates that students enrolled in demanding university courses which lead to responsibility-laden careers tend to suffer from increased alcohol misuse compared with peers. A cross-sectional survey of 889 medical students in the UK found that 33.9% to 43.8% engage in hazardous use of alcohol, 0.8% to 8.9% in harmful use, and 1.2% to 7.9% suffer from alcohol dependency (Bogowicz et al., 2018). Studies completed in other countries have equally high numbers, with 50% to 60% of medical students scoring positivity on the CAGE screening tool (Akvardar et al., 2004; Boland et al., 2006). Studies across the USA and Europe, show that 13% to 24% of participants engaged in high-risk drinking, with highest misuse seen in the UK, Germany, and Spain, at levels exceeding the general population (Roncero et al., 2015). Medical students attending western universities tend to misuse alcohol more often, and there is a concerning upward trend of binge and hazardous use of alcohol, with numbers utilizing alcohol in a harmful manner increasing dramatically in the past 30 years (Boland et al., 2006; Goel et al., 2015; Ketoja et al., 2013).

The primary reasons given for alcohol misuse are experimentation, recreation, and control of stress related to increasing workloads and college demands, personal expectations, and

Table 29.1 List of journals from a literature search of substance abuse by medical students, highlighting the country where the study was completed, study type, sample size, the substance(s), and percentage prevalence

Author	Year	Journal	Country	Study type	Sample size	Substance	Prevalence %
Acosta	2019	*Puerto Rico Health Sciences Journal*	Puerto Rico	Web survey	152	ADHD medication	47.6 males
						* no breakdown d-amphetamine or methylphenidate	46.0 females
Akvardar et al.	2004	*Social Psychiatry and Psychiatric Epidemiology*	Turkey	Questionnaire	173	Alcohol	62.3–71.2
						Cigarettes	39.8–55.8
						Sedatives/hypnotics	0–3.8
Almutham et al.	2019	*Journal of Family Medicine and Primary Care*	Saudi Arabia	Cross-sectional questionnaire	256	E-cigarettes	10.6
Amin-Esmaeili et al.	2013	*Medical Journal of the Islamic Republic of Iran*	Iran	Questionnaires	1,568–1,761	Cigarettes	10.5–12.9
Aslam et al.	2013	*Archives of Public Health*	Pakistan	Cross-sectional and observational survey	866	Energy drinks	40.4
						Tea	29.1
						Coffee	9.5
						Cola drinks	7.2
						Cigarettes	2.9
						Heroin	2.5
						Alcohol	2.7

(continued)

Table 29.1 Continued

Author	Year	Journal	Country	Study type	Sample size	Substance	Prevalence %
Baldisseri	2007	*Critical Care Medicine*	USA	Literature review	2000	Alcohol	87.5
						Marijuana	10
						Benzodiazepines	3.7
						Cocaine	2.8
						Tranquilizers	2.3
						Opioids	1.1
Baldwin et al.	1991	*JAMA (Journal of the American Medical Association)*	USA	Survey questionnaire	2000	Alcohol	98.1
						Marijuana	66.4
						Tobacco	55.3
						Cocaine	32.5
						Amphetamines	22.8
						Tranquilizers	19.6
						Psychedelics	18.3
						LSD	11.8
						Opiates	9.4
						Barbiturates	7.3
						Heroin	0.9
Balogh et al.	2018	*BMC Public Health*	Germany and Hungary	Multicentre cross-sectional survey	2,935	Cigarettes	18
						Waterpipe smoking	4.8
						E-cigarettes	0.9–4.5

Author	Year	Journal	Country	Study type	Sample size	Substance	Prevalence (%)
Balough et al.	2020	*Substance Use and Abuse*	Germany and Hungary	Multicentre cross-sectional survey	1,514	E-cigarettes	8.0
Banimustafa et al.	2018	*The Arab Journal of Psychiatry*	Jordan	Cross-sectional study	385	Caffeinated drinks	98.4
						Tea	84.7
						Coffee	80
						Soft drinks	69.1
						Energy drinks	15.1
Basu.	2011	*Journal of Pharmacy and Bioallied Sciences*	India	Cross-sectional questionnaire	182	Cigarettes	30
Bazin et al.	2021	*Substance Use & Misuse*	France	Cross-sectional study	592	MDMA	21.5
Bin Abdulrahman et al.	2021	*International Journal of Environmental Research and Public Health*	Saudi Arabia	Survey	675	Coffee	91.4
Birch et al.	1998	*The Lancet*	UK	Survey questionnaire	90	Alcohol	93
						Cannabis	19–35
						Hallucinogenic mushrooms, LSD, ecstasy, cocaine, amphetamines, amyl nitrite.	1–13
Bogowicz et al.	2018	*BMJ (British Medical Journal)*	UK	Cross-sectional questionnaire	1,242	Alcohol	53.1–59.7 (AUDIT positive)
Boland et al.	2006	*Alcohol and Drug Dependence*	Ireland	Questionnaire survey in 1973, 1990, 2002	537	Alcohol	71.2
						Cigarettes	9.5
Bossaer et al.	2013	*Academic Medicine*	US	Online survey	786	Non-medical use of prescription stimulants	11.3

(continued)

Table 29.1 Continued

Author	Year	Journal	Country	Study type	Sample size	Substance	Prevalence %
Bourbon et al.	2018	*Progress in Neuropsychopharmacology and Biological Psychiatry*	France	Internet questionnaire	10,985	Cigarettes	18.9
Castaldelli-Maia et al.	2019	*International Review of Psychiatry*	Brazil	Survey	129	Non-prescribed medication	13.2
Cattaruzza, West	2013	*European Journal of Public Health*	Europe	Literature review	Based on general population	Cigarettes	35
Choi et al.	2013	*Academic Psychiatry*	US	Online survey	301	Non-medical prescription stimulant	5
Cohen et al.	2015	*Journal of Neurosciences in Rural Practice*	Israel	Questionnaire	229	Methylphenidate	17.0
Conard et al.	1989	*American Journal of Psychiatry*	USA	Questionnaire	589	Cocaine	36
De Bruyn	2019	*Substance Use & Misuse*	Belgium	Questionnaire	1,095	Stimulants *no breakdown of methylphenidate, modafinil or (dextro)amphetamine	8.7
Duroy et al.	2017	*Encephale*	France	Cross-sectional study, questionnaire	302	Alcohol	74.8 (binge drinking)
Emmanuel et al.	2013	*Journal of General Internal Medicine*	US	Web based questionnaire	1,115	Psychostimulants	18
Fallah et al.	2018	*Caspian Journal of Internal Medicine*	Iran	Questionnaire	444	Stimulants	11
						Methylphenidate	6.5
						Amphetamine	2.5

Author	Year	Journal	Country	Study type	N	Drug	%
Farrell et al.	2019	International Review of Psychiatry	New Zealand	Cross-sectional electronic survey	220	Cannabis	35
						Ecstasy	12
						Other-Khat, LSD	6
						Cocaine	5
						Opiates	4
						Amphetamines	3
						Ketamine	1
Finger et al.	2013	Revista da Associacao Medica Brasileira		Systematic review		Methylphenidate	8.3–9
Flaherty et al.	1993	The Psychiatric Clinics of North America	USA	Survey	143	Alcohol	20.3 (abuse/dependence)
Fond et al.	2016	Medicine	France	Cross-sectional questionnaire	1,681	Psychostimulants	33
Fond et al.	2018	Journal of Affective Disorders	France	Descriptive cross-sectional observational epidemiological national survey	10,985	Ecstasy	12.5
						Cocaine	7.4
						Codeine	8.6
						Mushrooms	6.7
						Amphetamine	3.9
						LSD	2.2
						Ketamine	1.6
						Heroin	0.2

(continued)

Table 29.1 Continued

Author	Year	Journal	Country	Study type	Sample size	Substance	Prevalence %
Fond et al.	2020	*European Archives of Psychiatry and Clinical Neuroscience*	France	Cross-sectional survey	10,985	Cannabis	47.3–52.7
						Alcohol	27.5–69.7
						Anxiolytic	5.4–6.8
						Antidepressant	2.8–3.0
						Hypnotic	1.9–3.2
						Mood stabilizer	0.4–0.6
						Antipsychotic	0.4–0.6
Gignon et al.	2015	*Workplace Health and Safety*	France	Cross-sectional survey	225	Alcohol	97
						Cigarettes	16–21
						Cannabis	77
						Alkyl, cyclic, or aliphatic nitrites	93
						Hallucinogenic mushrooms	14
						LSD	12
						Cocaine	12
						Prescription medications	9
						Ecstasy	6
						Heroin	3
Giri et al.	2013	*Annals of Medical and Health Sciences Research*	India	Cross-sectional questionnaire	150	Coffee	67.3
						Smoking	18.7
						Alcohol	24

Author	Year	Journal	Country	Method	Sample size	Substance	%
Goel et al.	2015	Central Asian Journal of Global Health	India	Questionnaire	150	Alcohol	16.6
						Tobacco	8
Heradstveit et al.	2020	Frontiers in Psychiatry	Norway	From Students' Health and Wellbeing Study cross-sectional survey	44,818	Cannabis	15.2
						MDMA	4.0
						Cocaine	3.0
						LSD/psilocybin	2.1
Horowitz et al.	2008	Journal of Addictive Diseases	United States	Questionnaire	340	'Club drugs'	16.8
						MDMA	11.8
						Cocaine	5.9
						LSD	4.1
						Methamphetamine	2.2
Jackson et al.	2016	Academic Medicine	USA	National survey	4,402	Alcohol	32.4 (abuse/dependence)
Jain et al.	2017	The South African Journal of Psychiatry	South Africa	Questionnaire	541	Methylphenidate	11
Jebrini et al.	2021	Frontiers in Psychiatry	Germany	Online survey	1,159	Neuroenhancement drugs	90.1
						Coffee	78.8
						Energy drinks	45.7
						Caffeine tablets	24.3
						Methylphenidate	5.2
						Illicit amphetamines	2.0
						Cocaine	1.7

(continued)

Table 29.1 Continued

Author	Year	Journal	Country	Study type	Sample size	Substance	Prevalence %
Ketoja et al.	2013	*Addictive Behaviours*	Korea	Questionnaire using cluster sampling	465	Alcohol	33 (Risky use)
Kudlow et al.	2013	*Journal of Psychoactive Drugs*	Canada	Online survey	326	Caffeine	92
						High caffeine products	52
						Natural supplements	30
						Tobacco, decongestants	12
						Off-label stimulants	15
						Methylphenidate	7
						Modafinil	6
						Dextroamphetamine	3
						Dextro/levoamphetamine	3
						Adrafinil	2
						Piracetam	2
Kusturica et al.	2019	*Acta Medica Academica*	Bosnia and Herzegovina	Questionnaire	214	Coffee	72.9
						Energy drinks	58.4
						Nicotine	37.8
						Alcohol	24.7
						Marijuana	19.0
Lengvenyte et al.	2016	*Nordic Studies on Alcohol and Drugs*	Lithuania	Survey	579	Cognitive enhancers	8.1

Author	Year	Journal	Country	Method	Sample size	Drug	Percentage
McAuliffe et al.	1986	*New England Journal of Medicine*	USA	Survey	504	Marijuana	32–76
						Cocaine	20–39
						Hallucinogens	2–19
						Stimulants	2–17
						Sedatives	0–16
						Analgesics	0–10
						Tranquillizers	1–28
						Opiates	2–37
McAuliffe et al.	1984	*Journal of Health and Social Behaviour*	USA	Survey	360-364	Marijuana	44–61
						Tranquillizers	6–48
						Amptamines	3–17
						Sedatives	3–25
						Hallucinogens	3–16
						Cocaine	10–49
						Opiates	3–36
McKay et al.	1973	*BMJ (British Medical Journal)*	UK	Questionnaire survey	786	Nicotine	16–30.1
						Marijuana	80.8 (Tried)
							30 (Regular use)

(continued)

Table 29.1 Continued

Author	Year	Journal	Country	Study type	Sample size	Substance	Prevalence %
Merlo et al.	2017	*Substance Abuse*	USA	Online questionnaire	1,141	Alcohol	70 (Binge use)
					414	Marijuana	22.7
					241	Nicotine	26.9
					65	E-cigarettes	7.3
					252	Prescription stimulants	28.7
					79	Prescription opioids	9.1
					94	Ecstasy	10.8
					83	Hallucinogens	9.6
					60	Cocaine/methamphetamine/speed	6.9
					35	Inhalants	4
					30	Synthetic substances (spice, K2)	3.5
					21	Non-prescription opioids (heroin, opium)	2.4
					3	Anabolic steroids	0.4
Miranda & Barbosa	2021	*Acta Medica Portuguesa*	Portugal	Questionnaire	1,573	Methylphenidate	35.1
						Modafinil	10.4
						Citicoline	3.9
						Idebenone	2.6

Author	Year	Journal	Country	Method	Sample size	Substance	Value
Molodynski et al.	2021	*International Review of Psychiatry*	Morocco, Portugal, India, Jordan, Italy, Wales, New Zealand, Paraguay, Brazil, Hong Kong, England, Canada	Questionnaire	3,766	Alcohol	11.5–28 (Harmful use)
						Cannabis	25.6
Newbury-Birch et al.	2001	*Drug and Alcohol Dependence*	UK	Longitudinal survey	110	Alcohol	94
						Cannabis	65.5
						LSD	12.7
						Amphetamines	19.1
						Ecstasy	13.6
						Amyl/butyl nitrate	16.4
						Hallucinogenic mushrooms	15.5
						Cocaine/crack	6.4
						Temazepam/diazepam	8.2
						Opium/morphine/heroin	1.8
						Steroids	0.9
Papazisis et al.	2018	*Substance Abuse: Research and Treatment*	Europe, central and southern America, USA	Systematic review and metanalysis	110–2,308	Cannabis	0.93–74

(continued)

Table 29.1 Continued

Author	Year	Journal	Country	Study type	Sample size	Substance	Prevalence %
Papazisis et al.	2017	*Hippokratia*	Greece	Online survey and questionnaire	591	Cannabis	22.2
						Alcohol	22.7 (Binge drinking) 6.4 (CAGE+)
						Nicotine	19.6
Papazisis et al.	2018	*Substance Abuse: Research and Treatment*	Greece	Online survey	591	Prescribed opioids	19.3
						Temazepam, triazolam, and Z-drugs, e.g. zolpidem, zopiclone	14.7
						Tranquillizers	7.3
						Stimulants	1.4
						LSD, ecstasy, cocaine, amphetamine, shisha, ketamine, mephedrone, mushrooms, or inhalants	1.5-3
						Heroin, crack, methadone	0.5
Pandejpong et al.	2014	*Journal of the Medical Association of Thailand*	Thailand	Survey	494	Caffeinated beverage	83.8
						- Tea	87.5
						- Cocoa	82
						- Soda	70.9
						- Coffee	60.4
						- Energy drinks	11.1

Author	Year	Journal	Country	Method	Sample size	Substance	%
Pickard et al.	2000	*Medical Education*	UK	Questionnaire	136	Alcohol	86
						Cannabis	84.6–93.8
						Amphetamines	4.3–6.7
						LSD	2.2–3.3
						Ecstasy	2.2–3.3
						Amyl/butyl nitrate	2.2
						Hallucinogenic mushrooms	3.3–4.3
Rai et al.	2008	*National Medical Journal of India*	India	National cross-sectional survey	2,135	Alcohol	7.1
						Tobacco	6.1
Ram et al.	2016	*Drug and Alcohol Review*	New Zealand	Questionnaire	442	Cognitive enhancers	6.6
Retief & Verster	2016	*The South African Journal of Psychiatry*	South Africa	Questionnaire	251	Sympathomimetics	17.5
Rezaei Kalat et al.	2021	*Journal of Substance Use*	Iran	Questionnaire	301	Methylphenidate	46.5
						Modafinil	3.0
						Bupropion	0.7
						Methylphenidate and modafinil	0.3
						Novartis	0.3
						Methylphenidate and caffeine	0.3
						Citalopram	0.3
						Modafinil and fluoxetine	0.3
						Methylphenidate and zolpidem	0.3

(continued)

Table 29.1 Continued

Author	Year	Journal	Country	Study type	Sample size	Substance	Prevalence %
Roncero et al.	2015	*Actas Españolas de Psiquiatría*	America and Europe	Literature review over twenty-five year period	88,413	Alcohol	24
						Tobacco	17.2
						Cannabis	11.8
						Hypnotics and sedatives	9.9
						Stimulants	7.7
						Cocaine	2.1
						Opiates	0.4
Samaha et al.	2019	*Data in Brief*	Lebanon	Cross-sectional questionnaire	596	Caffeine	74.8
Sapkota et al.	2021	*Journal of the Nepal Medical Association*	Nepal	Cross-sectional study	226	Psychoactive substances	42.0
						Alcohol	38.5
						Smoking	17.3
						Cannabis	11.9
						Cocaine	0.9
						Benzodiazepines	0.9
						Opioids	0.9
Silveira et al.	2014	*Trends in Psychiatry and Psychotherapy*	Brazil	Cross-sectional study	152	Non-medical use of methylphenidate (5th year students)	13.15
						Non-medical use of methylphenidate (6th year students)	32.89

Author	Year	Journal	Country	Method	N	Substance	%
Singh et al.	2014	PloS One	UK and Ireland	Survey	861	Caffeine pills	24.3
						Modafinil	6.2
						Methylphenidate	4
						Adderall	2
Sreeramareddy et al.	2018	BMJ Open (British Medical Journal)	America and Europe	Survey of each WHO region	107,527	Cigarettes	20–23
Usman et al.	2015	The Journal of Pakistan Medical Association	Pakistan	Cross-sectional study	233	Energy drinks	51.9
Van der Veer et al.	2011	PLoS One	Holland	Online survey	902	Alcohol	46 (excessive use)
						Nicotine	6
Voight et al.	2009	BMC Health Services Research	Germany	Questionnaire	940	Alcohol	75
						Cigarettes	21.5
Vorster et al.	2019	Health SA Gesondheid	South Africa	Cross-sectional questionnaire (2nd / 3rd year)	171	Magic mushrooms	2.7 / 1.8
						Cocaine	1.8 / 5.2
						Ecstasy	1.8 / 1.7
						Methamphetamine	0.9 / 3.5
						LSD	0 / 5.2
						'Crack'	0 / 3.5

(continued)

Table 29.1 Continued

Author	Year	Journal	Country	Study type	Sample size	Substance	Prevalence %
Webb et al.	1998	*Medical Education*	UK	Questionnaire	785	Alcohol	86 (exceeded weekly limits)
							19 (high risk levels)
						Amphetamines	8
						LSD	7
						Ecstasy	4
						Amyl/butyl nitrate	10
						Hallucinogenic mushrooms	7
						Cigarettes	31.7 (regular use)
						Cannabis	20.6 (regular use)
						Cocaine/crack	2.2
						Steroids	1.0
						Barbiturates	1.9
						Opioids	2
						Prescribed tranquilizers, anti-depressants, sleeping tablets	5.3
Westermeyer	1991	*JAMA (Journal of the American Medical Association)*	USA	Questionnaire survey		Marijuana	18.8

financial difficulties (Boland et al., 2006; Jackson et al., 2016). Most students misuse more alcohol in their first two years of medical school, with reducing amounts towards the final year. Studies indicate that males in their early twenties, from middle to upper-class backgrounds, abuse alcohol most frequently (Boland et al., 2006). Female medical students show a worrying pattern of binge drinking and harmful use of alcohol over time, using increased volumes more frequently (Akvardar et al., 2004).

Stress is a major risk factor for alcohol misuse in physicians, given their high levels of work stress, burnout, and unhealthy lifestyle habits (Jackson et al., 2016). The pattern of using alcohol to manage stress may start before medical school as most report a binge drinking pattern developing prior to enrolment (Bogowicz et al., 2018), risking later dependency or substance misuse when practising clinicians (Flaherty & Richman, 1993; Papazisis et al., 2017).

Stress is also a risk factor resulting in medical students' overuse of alcohol, as well as demographics, stage in training, family history, difficult familial relationships, and perfectionist personality types (Akvardar et al., 2004; Flaherty & Richman, 1993). There is an association between alcohol use as a coping mechanism and the strain of performance in medical school, with high expectations being well known (Bogowicz et al., 2018).

There is a correlation between increased misuse of alcohol in medical schools and reduced work-lifestyle balance. The accessibility, affordability, and likely social acceptability of alcohol all contribute to higher use (Boland et al., 2006).

The significance of such high rates of alcohol misuse by medical students is obviated by the need for them to become knowledgeable, mature, and reliable role models within society and responsible for the treatment of patients. Doctors who misuse alcohol are less likely to make objective decisions on patient care and recognize the abuse of alcohol in their patients (Duroy et al., 2017). Additional consequences include increased illness, relationship difficulties, deterioration in coursework, risky behaviours, and drug misuse (Duroy et al., 2017).

Access to training in self-care and educational modules within the medical school curriculum are considered the best way to address harmful use in medical students (Cape et al., 2006).

Nicotine

Nicotine use has significantly decreased for all students over recent decades, but medical student use worldwide ranged between 3.8% to 29.2% in a 2017 survey and cigarette use remains high in low and middle-income group countries and in some European countries such as Italy and Spain (Cattaruzza & West, 2013; Sreeramareddy et al., 2018). A paper written in 1999 showed rates of smoking between zero and 56.9% depending on the country, with lower rates of smoking among medical students in the UK and USA compared to Asia and Turkey (Richmond, 1999). Higher numbers and levels of smoking are observed among males, students above the age of twenty-five years, in the latter years of their medical education, and among students from the Middle East or Asia—most smoking ten to 20 cigarettes daily (Bogowicz et al., 2018; Balogh et al., 2018). Female medical students in Asia and Middle Eastern countries had lower rates of smoking compared to males, which is likely reflective of cultural tendencies (Richmond, 1999).

As with alcohol, cigarette smoking tended to pre-date medical school entry and increased the likelihood of ongoing use and difficulties with stopping after medical school. Indeed historically, cigarette smoking was closely linked to alcohol use, but medical students no longer pair alcohol and cigarette (Boland et al., 2006). There are however associations with addiction to other substances, peer influence and parental cigarette use (Basu et al., 2011) work-related stress and exposure to stress coping mechanisms amongst peers (Amin-Esmaeili et al., 2013). Easy availability and social acceptability increase the risk of cigarette use to alleviate stress and aid in coping with adversity.

E-cigarettes have become an attractive alternative to cigarettes for young people worldwide (prevalence 0.9% to 3.5%), with perceived lower levels of nicotine and attractive marketing. E-cigarettes are popular in medical schools too, with a doubling in use from 4.5% to 8% in Eastern Europe in 2018 (Balogh et al., 2020). A proportion of medical students using e-cigarettes were not smokers previously (from 2% to 2.5%) (Balogh et al., 2020), with one in ten students reporting trying e-cigarettes in university for the first time (Almutham et al., 2019).

Public health advice and media campaigns have been successful in highlighting the health effects of tobacco use, and medical students should be aware of the latest research and health policy advice (Richmond, 1999). However, there is a lack of public knowledge about the dangers of e-cigarettes, and 28% of participants in a USA survey believed that they are a safe alternative to cigarettes (Almutham et al., 2019). Medical schools worldwide tend not to contain modules on smoking and smoking cessation in their curriculum (Richmond, 1999). This educational gap, along with the impact of personal use of nicotine, could mean that future clinicians may struggle to advise patients on healthy lifestyle choices as they may not identify smoking as harmful.

Caffeine

Consumption of caffeine containing beverages including coffee, tea, energy drinks, or soft drinks amongst medical students ranges from 29.7% to 98.4%. Tea and coffee are most commonly consumed; however, energy drinks can surpass this as shown in a study from Pakistan. There was little consistency in frequency or amounts of consumption, and trends between genders vary greatly between nations (Alabbad et al., 2019; Aslam et al., 2013; Banimustafa et al., 2018; Bin Abdulrahman et al., 202; Fond et al., 2016; Giri et al., 2013; Kudlow et al., 2013; Pandejpong et al., 2014; Samaha et al., 2019; Usman et al., 2015).

The most common reasons which medical students reported for increased caffeine consumption were to increase energy and alertness, and to aid in study for exams. With associations found between caffeinated energy drink consumption and studying (53.3%), stress (33.1%), and increased use in the week prior to exams. There is also an association between daily caffeine intake and time spent online, which may have implications as medical courses move to more online based teaching (Aslam et al., 2013; Kusturica et al., 2019; Pandejpong et al., 2014; Samaha et al., 2019; Singh et al., 2014; Usman et al., 2015).

There is a lack of knowledge regarding appropriate levels of caffeine use, with up to 94.4% of students not knowing how much caffeine is contained in energy drinks (Usman et al., 2015). Medical students should be informed of the effects of caffeine, including the common side effects of excessive caffeine use: restlessness (53.81%), nervousness (47.08%), and anxiety (33.84%). Withdrawal symptoms include fatigue (39.01%), headaches (33.18%), and caffeine craving (31.83%) (Samaha et al., 2019), as well as the risk of dependency which increases when used for stimulation and with the amount consumed (Pandejpong et al., 2014).

Illicit Substances

Cannabis

Cannabis remains the most prevalently used illicit substance by medical students, across all nations, over the last five decades, accounting for approximately 80% of all illicit substances used (see Table 29.1) (Boland et al., 2006; Bore et al., 2016; Gignon et al., 2015; McKay et al., 1973; Newbury-Birch et al., 2001; Papazisis et al., 2017; Papazisis et al., 2018a; Papazisis et al., 2018c; Pickard et al., 2000; Roncero et al., 2015). Cannabis use has increased in students, medical students, and the general population over the past 10 years (Baldwin et al., 1991; UNODC, 2011).

Meta-analysis of twenty-eight studies on medical student use found a pooled international lifetime prevalence of 31.4%, with 17.2% past-year use and 8.8% current users (Papazisis et al., 2018b), giving a 5% higher lifetime prevalence than adults at that time (EMCDDA, 2017). Studies on medical students from Europe show an even higher lifetime prevalence of 66% of students trying cannabis at least once (Gignon et al., 2015; Newbury-Birch et al., 2001; Papazisis et al., 2017). Molodynski et al. (2021), found more overall cannabis use than harmful alcohol use, with one in four medical students using cannabis, ranging from the highest frequency of 79% in Portugal and the lowest in Jordan at 3%. Of note, Portugal had the lowest impact of 'study stress' at 7%, compared to the majority of students rating study stress at above 80%. Comparison of the meta-analysis by Papazisis et al. (2018b) and the previous literature review from 1988 to 2013 (Roncero et al., 2015), demonstrates increases from 20% past year use in Europe, 16.5% in North America and 10% in Latin America (Gignon et al., 2015; MacLean et al., 2016; Newbury-Birch et al., 2001; Papazisis et al., 2017; Roncero et al., 2015). Asia shows the lowest prevalence figures however these are increasing. There is little data on medical student cannabis use from Oceania (Bore et al., 2016), with the average past year use in the general adult population for this region at 12.1%, and this was found in an ageing population of users (UNODC, 2011).

France has one of the highest rates of cannabis use among medical students in western Europe, with studies showing high rates of prevalence at 77% for the past year and 66% monthly use (Gignon et al., 2015), much higher than the 21.8% of peer group in general population (EMCDDA, 2017). They report 7% use once a day, 14% several times a week and 12% several times a month (Gignon et al., 2015). Another French study by Fond and colleagues (2021b) found 15.6% of medical students are current users, which is nearly twice the pooled world figure of 8.8% (Papazisis et al., 2018b), with 6.1% classified as Cannabis Use Disorder (using the diagnostic tool CAST). They also report that 30% started use during their medical studies, with 50% of these during their second year. The European Drug Report 2021 (EMCDDA, 2021) shows lifetime use of cannabis in adults in France to be considerably higher than other countries at 45%.

Medical students in North America and the US report high and increasing prevalence rates with 48.1% yearly use, but lower use than both the general and university population (Merlo et al., 2017). Merlo and colleagues (2017) found 22.7% reported marijuana use during medical school with 12.2% increasing their use. The UNODC (2011) reports an increase in cannabis use in North America of three times the global average, possibly explained by legalization in some states. Canada has even higher figures at 25% past year use, with even higher figures in the 20-24 age group.

Cannabis has become more potent, especially in North America and Europe, but evidence shows that adolescents perceive cannabis as a less harmful drug. There is an association between a lower perception of risk and higher use of cannabis (UNODC, 2011). A range of psychological factors suggests that cannabis may be used as self-treatment by students (Fond et al., 2021b). Stressful events, and the use of hypnotics, were associated with Cannabis Use Disorder (CUD), with men three times more at risk of having CUD, although gender differences in cannabis consumption behaviour were considered a complex interaction between sociocultural and neurobiological factors (Fond et al., 2018; 2021b).

Hallucinogens

This category broadly refers to LSD (lysergic acid diethylamide) and hallucinogenic or 'magic' mushrooms, which are used 'occasionally' by medical students and often along with other substances like cannabis or amphetamines (Fond et al., 2018; McAuliffe et al., 1984; McKay et al., 1973). Approximately 1–3% of students have experimented with LSD and 2-4% have tried magic mushrooms (Newbury-Birch et al., 2001; Papazisis et al., 2017; Papazisis et al., 2018a; Pickard et al., 2000; Roncero et al., 2015). Ecstasy and ketamine are also partially hallucinogenic, while having further desirable effects including stimulant action in ecstasy and anaesthesia via ketamine use. Lifetime prevalence figures of hallucinogen experimentation are as high as 10–20%. Studies often do not differentiate between specific hallucinogens used and figures may involve newer synthetic forms such as phencyclidine (PCP) (Baldwin et al., 1991; Gignon et al., 2015; Merlo et al., 2017).

Inhalants

The highest levels of inhalant use in medical students have been observed amongst male students in Brazil, with a lifetime prevalence of 14–18.4%, reflecting an equal prevalence in its general population (Lambert Passos et al., 2006; Roncero et al., 2015). Inhalants include a variety of vasodilating substances including Amyl Butyl Nitrate (ABN), commonly known as 'poppers', and Gamma-Hydroxybutyrate (GHB), which outside of the Brazilian population are used by 0.2–4% of students and are observed as being largely confined to the male population. The majority (57.7%) of medical students decreased use during university, with 11.5% reporting increased use (Merlo et al., 2017; Newbury-Birch et al., 2001; Papazisis et al., 2017; Pickard et al., 2000).

In a French study by Gignon et al. (2015), poppers (alkyl, cyclic, or aliphatic nitrites) were the most commonly used illegal substance after cannabis with 23% of students experimenting over the previous 12 months, 2% used several times a week, 12% several times a month and 78% once a month or less.

The European and World Drug reports do not mention inhalants specifically but include a section on novel substances. There were few published studies outlining inhalant use in medical students.

Illicit and Prescribed Substances

Stimulants

The use of cognitive-enhancing substances which are not prescribed for treatment is an increasing cause of concern. Prevalence rates for the misuse of prescription stimulants in medical students range from 0% to 52.2%, with methylphenidate the most frequently misused (Acosta et al., 2019; Alrakaf et al., 2020; Bossaer et al., 2013; Choi et al., 2013; Cohen et al., 2015; De Bruyn et al., 2019; Emanuel et al., 2013; Fallah et al., 2018; Finger et al., 2013; Fond et al., 2016; Kudlow et al., 2013; Kusturica et al., 2019; Lengvenyte et al., 2016; Miranda and Barbosa, 2021; Retief and Verster, 2016; Rezaei Kalat et al., 2021; Roncero et al., 2015; Silveira et al., 2014). Not all countries report high prevalence of non-prescribed stimulants in medical students, for example a Canadian study reported just 4% past-year use, and a systematic review reported lifetime use at 3–16% for methylphenidate (Finger et al., 2013; Kudlow et al., 2013). This may reflect improved detection of Attention Deficit and Hyperactivity disorder (ADHD) and subsequent treatment and prescribing.

The majority of medical students still report their first use of methylphenidate in college, confirmed at 65.2% by systematic review (Alrakaf et al., 2020; Finger et al., 2013; Fond et al., 2016; Jain et al., 2017; Retief & Verster, 2016; Silveira et al., 2014), with increasing risk of misuse at increasing academic levels (Erasmus & Kotzé, 2020; Fallah et al., 2018; Kudlow et al., 2013; Silveira et al., 2014). In South Africa, 80% of medical students believed that the academic performance of people without a diagnosis of ADHD could be improved with methylphenidate (Erasmus & Kotzé, 2020) and a study of the whole student populations in Ireland and the UK reported that 41.5% identified methylphenidate as a cognitive enhancer (Singh et al., 2014). Most (62.5% to 96.6%) students who have used stimulants illicitly tend to do so repetitively (Alrakaf et al., 2020; Cohen et al., 2015; De Bruyn et al., 2019).

Medical students report the main reasons for prescribed and non-prescribed stimulant use were to improve attention and concentration, to facilitate improvement in learning, and to improve academic results (Acosta et al., 2019; Bossaer et al., 2013; Fallah et al., 2018; Fond et al., 2016; Jain et al., 2017; Lengvenyte et al., 2016; Miranda and Barbosa, 2021; Ram et al., 2016; Retief & Verster, 2016; Rezaei Kalat et al., 2021; Silveira et al., 2014). Users of methylphenidate were more likely to give lower estimates for their grades (Cohen et al., 2015). A study by Lempp and Seale (2004) found that half of medical students found medical school a competitive rather than a collaborative experience. The highly competitive nature of medical school has been associated with the misuse of stimulants to enhance study performance during perceived periods of academic stress, and increased academic demand (De Bruyn et al., 2019; Jain et al., 2017; Roncero et al., 2015). This was highlighted by a US study which found that medical students assigned a class rank were significantly more likely to report psychostimulant use than those attending schools that did not assign class rank (Emanuel et al., 2013).

Medical students may use cognitive-enhancing substances for non-academic reasons including anxiety related to examinations, to increase energy, improve mood, and for recreational use including having an active lifestyle, and/or for experimentation (Fallah et al., 2018; Fond et al., 2016; Haas et al., 2019; Kusturica et al., 2019; Retief & Verster, 2016). The consequences of abuse of cognitive-enhancing substances can lead to addiction issues (Franke et al., 2013), and the pressure to succeed can lead to the ongoing use of cognitive-enhancing substances in later employment (De Bruyn et al., 2019). Psychoeducation regarding the risks of stimulant misuse, and the availability of alternative interventions, e.g. non-pharmaceutical methods to manage stress, should begin in medical school and continue into employment (De Bruyn et al., 2019).

Cocaine

The prevalence of cocaine use in medical students ranges from 1.3% to 7.4% (Fond et al., 2018; Jebrini et al., 2021; Roncero et al., 2015; Sapkota et al., 2021; Vorster et al., 2019). The varying prevalence of cocaine use worldwide may relate to access, legal, or moral reasons. A Sudanese study found that 79.3% of students reported having knowledge regarding co-caine but that 92.6% disagreed with cocaine use and 93.1% thought it would be either diffi-cult or impossible for them to access cocaine (Ibn Auf & Alnor, 2020). A French study found the top three reasons for psychostimulant use, including cocaine, by medical students were recreational (82.0%), pleasure-seeking (78.3%), and novelty-seeking (52.9%). More males re-ported these reasons, whereas females more frequently used psychostimulants to aid in re-ducing anxiety and stress prior to exams (Fond et al., 2016). More males than females (5.0% vs. 2.1%, respectively) reported the use of cocaine in the past year amongst higher education students in Norway (Heradstveit et al., 2020).

Ecstasy

Ecstasy (methylenedioxy-methylamphetamine, MDMA) use amongst medical students ranges from 1.8% to 21.5%. The main reasons reported for MDMA use are a desire for eu-phoria, novelty seeking, and recreational use in social settings (Bazin et al., 2021; Castaldelli-Maia et al., 2019; Fond et al., 2016; Fond et al., 2018; Horowitz et al., 2008; Vorster et al., 2019). In a study of Parisian medical students (Bazin et al., 2021), students who had not used ecstasy were more likely to consider occasional use as dangerous (83.9% vs. 66.9%). Both users and non-users agreed that regular use was dangerous (86.0% vs. 79.6%, respectively). Similar percentage levels (72.0% vs. 57.0%) were reported by medical students in the USA (Horowitz et al., 2008).

Over 90% of students in the US study disapproved of physicians using 'club drugs' and 20–30% felt that a physician's medical licence should be revoked depending on the type of club drug used. Bazin and colleagues (2021) found that the risk of polysubstance use was high in medical students in Paris using ecstasy, including tobacco (79.9%), alcohol (90.6%), cannabis (42.0%), cocaine (20.5%), and LSD (3.6%).

Opiates and Opioids

Studies consistently show that medical students do not misuse high levels of opiates (heroin, opium, and morphine) with a lifetime prevalence of 0.2 to 0.5%. Students in Iran present as an outlier where 6% have used opiates and 2% have used heroin (Papazisis et al., 2017; Papazisis et al., 2018a; Roncero et al., 2015) and two studies in the USA had lifetime prevalence figures of 0.9% and 2.4% (Baldwin et al., 1991; Merlo et al., 2017). Medical students were more likely than law or nursing students to have tried an opiate with a 7% lifetime prevalence.

Prescription analgesia use by medical students is mostly prescribed legitimately for pain but use in all students has increased from the 1960s onwards (McAuliffe et al., 1984). The study by Merlo and colleagues (2017) found 9.1% of medical students used opiates during medical school, 80% of which were prescribed, and only 9.3% were using unprescribed opiates, with 11.4% using a combination of prescribed and non-prescribed opiates. There were no gender differences in rates or patterns of prescription opioid use or misuse (Westermeyer, 1991). Overall, most opioid formulations such as fentanyl, methadone, or buprenorphine are rarely misused by medical students (Papazisis et al., 2017).

Opioids (synthetic formulations and prescription drugs) are increasingly misused in society. 97% originate from pharmaceutical sources (UNODC, 2011), making divergence and poor prescribing practice of greater importance. The prevalence of opiate and opioid misuse is 1–5% globally, with past-year prevalence of opioid use in Europe in 2019 estimated at 0.7% of the population aged 15–64, with concerningly high and rising numbers of deaths from accidental fentanyl overdose, particularly in North America (UNODC, 2011).

Hypnotics and Anxiolytics

Hypnotic and sedative drugs are used by 2-25% of medical students (Fond et al., 2018; McAuliffe et al., 1984; Roncero et al., 2015) and approximately 3% utilize anxiolytic medications (Baldwin et al., 1991; Newbury-Birch et al., 2001) in the self-treatment of anxiety rather than for recreational use. Twice as many women use hypnotics, sedatives, and anxiolytics. These are the only substances used more by female students than male. Cannabis has sedative properties, which may explain its association with hypnotic consumption (Fond et al., 2020; 2021a), and is likely used to ease anxiety by some students. Barbiturates (which are sedating and anxiolytic) are no longer of focus in research, but studies from the 1980s and 1990s show that they had similar lifetime prevalence to hypnotics and anxiolytics, which have since replaced barbiturates with a prevalence of 7.8% (Baldwin et al., 1991; McKay et al., 1973).

Non-Medical Use of Prescription Drugs (NMUP)

Medics are known to self-prescribe, although this is strongly counselled against. Depending on what is prescribed, it may be against medical ethics and can be considered a breach of licence, particularly for controlled drugs (American Medical Association, 2022; General Medical Council, 2022; Medical Council Ireland, 2019). Its forerunner in medical school is self-treatment where medical students take medications which were not prescribed to them. The main reason for this is for self-treatment rather than recreation, for issues such as insomnia, anxiety, depression, or pain, using hypnotics, anxiolytics, antidepressants, and opiates respectively (Baldwin et al., 1991; Fond et al., 2018; McAuliffe et al., 1984; Newbury-Birch et al., 2001; Papazisis et al., 2017; Webb et al., 1998). This misuse of medications has been shown to increase in the later years of study and is associated with illicit substance use (Papazisis et al., 2018a).

The medications used and the reasons for self-treatment vary but include longer term mental illness, shorter or more acute symptoms of stress, insomnia, and pain. Medical students worry about the impact of known illness, particularly mental illness, on their future careers and report a lack of available or accessible healthcare that takes this into account and that they consider safe and transparent. This results in poor healthcare and self-prescribing as well as creating an additional burden of stress when already unwell. The lifetime prevalence of medical students using medications not prescribed to them was 10.7% for at least one of the four prescription drug classes, whereas 9% utilized multiple medications. The most frequently misused were opioid analgesics (prevalence of lifetime misuse of 19.3%), followed by sedatives (14.7%), tranquilizers (7.3%), and stimulants (1.4%). Apart from anxiolytics, hypnotics, and antidepressants, risk of self-treatment is twice as high for male compared to female students. Female medical students are more likely to seek help for difficulties and follow up with services (Fond et al., 2018; Papazisis et al., 2018a; Roncero et al., 2015; Voigt et al., 2009).

Substances taken by healthy individuals to improve their baseline cognitive functioning (so-called smart-drugs) (Erasmus & Kotzé, 2020; Fond et al., 2016; Kudlow et al., 2013; Kusturica et al., 2019) have become one of the more contentious self-treatment issues. These substances range from over-the-counter products containing caffeine or nicotine to prescribed medications, including methylphenidate, and even on to illicit substances including amphetamines. It is estimated that between 2.9 and 5.8% of university students misuse methylphenidate per year, despite the known risks associated with use (Sussman et al., 2006); and circa 60–75% of the medical students that were not prescribed stimulants, but were using them, obtained them from a friend or relative (Emanuel et al., 2013; Fallah et al., 2018; Kusturica et al., 2019; Merlo et al., 2017; Miranda & Barbosa, 2021; Silveira et al., 2014; Singh et al., 2014).

Risk Factors for Substance Misuse in Medical Students

The reasons for misusing substances include experimentation, peer pressure, and self-treatment. Reports by UNODC (2011) and EMCDDA (2021) indicate that illicit substance use is increasing worldwide. Ease of access to substances and social acceptability should be considered in the misuse of substances by medical students, including alcohol, nicotine, and cannabis (Boland *et al.*, 2006). A defining demographic in substance misuse is gender, with males misusing twice as frequently as females, including cocaine, ecstasy, alcohol, and tobacco, apart from females who use anxiolytics, hypnotics, and antidepressants more frequently (Bazin et al., 2021; Boland et al., 2006; Fond et al., 2018; Heradstveit et al., 2020; Papazisis et al., 2018b; Roncero et al., 2015; Voigt et al., 2009).

Medical students have higher rates of mental illness compared to their peers and to the general population, with 46% reporting at least one mental health concern and a deterioration in mental health with increased time in training. Medical students are 55% less likely to seek or receive treatment for mental illness including SUD (5%), with stigma and career concerns as significant barriers to accessing care. The negative outcomes of increased stress in medical school include dropout, suicidal ideation, and SUD (Bore et al., 2016; Eisenberg et al., 2007; Farrell et al., 2019; Gignon et al., 2015; Lane et al., 2020; MacLean et al., 2016; Molodynski et al., 2021; Roberts et al., 1996; Roberts et al., 2001; Schwenk et al., 2010). There was no association found between SUD and increased mental illness in students. However, studies have shown that students suffering from depression and 'burnout', as well as 50% of physicians who self-prescribe, were more likely to endorse stigma attitudes against mental illness (Dyrbye et al., 2015; Schwenk et al., 2010).

The pressures experienced by medical students have been found to contribute to the development of harmful coping mechanisms, including reliance on substances (Bogowicz et al., 2018). This is exemplified by the misuse of stimulants increasing with academic demand, and increased use of substances in the latter stages of medical school (Aslam et al., 2013; De Bruyn et al., 2019; Erasmus & Kotzé, 2020; Fallah et al., 2018; Jain et al., 2017; Kudlow et al., 2013; Kusturica et al., 2019; McAuliffe et al., 1984; 1986; Newbury-Birch et al., 2001; Papazisis et al., 2018a; Roncero et al., 2015; Silveira et al., 2014).

Use by peers was the most influential factor for the misuse of cognitive enhancers, with up to 23% of medical students prescribed psychostimulants reporting that they shared their prescription on at least one occasion (Emanuel et al., 2013; Lengvenyte et al., 2016; Singh et al., 2014). Also, 48.5% of students reported that a main source of information regarding energy drinks was from a friend (Usman et al., 2015).

The misuse of alcohol and binge drinking patterns increase the risk of using illicit substances by a factor of three, and cigarette use by a factor of five. Students rarely use just one substance, raising concerns about gateway drugs and polysubstance use (Bazin et al., 2021; McKay et al., 1973; Newbury-Birch et al., 2001; Papazisis et al., 2017; 2018a; Pickard et al., 2000; Roncero et al., 2014; Webb et al., 1998). Many medical students with hazardous alcohol use risk later difficulties with alcohol dependency, or substance misuse as qualified clinicians (Flaherty & Richman, 1993; Papazisis et al., 2017). Misuse of cognitive-enhancing substances can result in subsequent addiction issues (De Bruyn et al., 2019; Franke et al., 2013). The ability of doctors who misuse substances to counsel patients with SUDs can be affected, with evidence that drug dependant physicians are more likely to over-prescribe addictive substances (Westermeyer, 1991; Westermeyer *et al.*, 2006).

Conclusion

The majority of medical students have concerns about the professional integrity and health of colleagues using psychoactive substances, and concerns about fairness and academic dishonesty (Bossaer et al., 2013; Erasmus & Kotzé, 2020; Retief & Verster, 2016). There is public concern regarding medical students using substances illicitly and then becoming future practising professionals (Fallah et al., 2018; Horowitz et al., 2008; Kudlow et al., 2013; Silveira et al., 2014; Vorster et al., 2019). It is concerning that substance misuse increases during medical school despite students acquiring increasing knowledge regarding substances during their training (Jain et al., 2017). This emphasizes the importance of medical programme coordinators, including education regarding illicit substances, and that possession and use has legal and professional consequences.

Whilst medical students may benefit from explicit curricula on appropriate prescribing practices, and how professional impairment threatens quality of care (Dyrbye et al., 2015), they also need adequate confidential mental health services and support for their known increased risk of mental illness, in particular anxiety and depression. Medical schools need to implement transparent regulations and policies that protect the student and eliminate any undue concern that diagnosis and treatment of mental illness can threaten progress in their careers. Students also need confidential professional supports and treatment for any addiction issues that can be accessed easily and without prejudice, so that addiction is addressed early. These could be modelled on the proven early intervention and impairment prevention programmes implemented for physicians (Baldwin et al., 1991). Enhanced social supports and high emotional resilience are key factors in minimizing and managing psychological distress and enhancing wellbeing (Bore et al., 2016) and should be encouraged.

Medical students tend to be naturally competitive and have perfectionist personalities which can increase success (Rai et al., 2008). Medical professionals are vulnerable to work stress, burnout, and unhealthy lifestyle habits (Jackson et al., 2016), and there are known correlations between work or study stress, managing expectations, financial difficulty, and mental health difficulties in medical students (Morgan et al., 2020). This stress can lead to unhealthy lifestyle habits (Jackson et al., 2016), including self-medicating for stress (Baldwin et al., 1991; Fond et al., 2018; McAuliffe et al., 1984; Newbury-Birch et al., 2001; Papazisis et al., 2017; Webb et al., 1998). Given that medical students have a higher lifetime prevalence of using any substance compared to the general population (Bourbon et al., 2019; MacLean et al., 2016; Papazisis et al., 2018a; Papazisis et al., 2018b; Webb et al., 1998), risk factors for stress and substance misuse need to be highlighted for these students who are not considered vulnerable by society and yet struggle with many occupational and personal pressures (Stubbing et al., 2019). Other methods to try to succeed academically, including stress management, exercise programmes and study techniques, relaxation techniques, and support groups have been identified as useful by medical students, and could help avoid stimulant misuse (Acosta et al., 2019; De Bruyn et al., 2019).

Public health campaigns (such as those against tobacco use) have been successful in society (Richmond, 1999). Similar health campaigns could be successfully hosted by medical schools, targeting their medical students in a culturally appropriate way, highlighting the physical, psychological, social, and professional risks of misuse of substances. Holistic learning frameworks comprising core elements about drug use, treatment and recovery can result in better patient outcomes (Armaos & Tsiboukli, 2019) and should be encouraged.

There is a longstanding debate, notably in the USA and UK, regarding whether physicians should undergo mandatory drug testing, in line with other professions such as airline pilots (Baldwin et al., 1991; Swani & Miller, 2013). The majority of studies on medical students concluded that integrated education on substance abuse in the curriculum is the best approach (Baldisseri, 2007; BBC News, 1998; BBC News, 2005; Birch et al., 1998; McAuliffe et al., 1984; Newbury-Birch et al., 2001; Pickard et al., 2000). There is an opportunity for the medical faculties to lead in promoting greater student mental health and reducing substance use. Promoting and ensuring the integration of healthy behaviour and appropriate coping mechanisms into the medical school curriculum, that are culturally specific, will have a beneficial effect in supporting healthy healthcare professionals, which will ultimately improve patient care and outcomes.

References

Acosta, D.L., Fair, C.N., Gonzalez, C.M., Iglesias, M., Maldonado, N., Schenkman, N., Valle, S.M., Velez, J.L., & Mejia, L. (2019). 'Nonmedical use of d-amphetamines and methylphenidate in medical students'. *PR Health Sci J* **38**(3): 185–188.

Akvardar, Y., Demiral, Y., Ergor, G., & Ergor, A. (2004). 'Substance use among medical students and physicians in a medical school in Turkey'. *Soc Psychiatry Psychiatr Epidemiol* **39**(6): 502–506.

Alabbad, M.H., AlMussalam, M.Z., AlMusalmi, A.M., Alealiwi, M.M., Alresasy, A.I., Alyaseen, H.N., & Badar, A.(2019). 'Determinants of energy drinks consumption among the students of a Saudi University'. *J Family Community Med* **26**(1): 36–44.

Almutham, A., Altami, M., Sharaf, F., & AlAraj, A. (2019). 'E-cigarette use among medical students at Qassim University: knowledge, perception, and prevalence'. *J Family Med Prim Care* **8**(9): 2921–2926.

Alrakaf, F.A., Binyousef, F.H., Altammami, A.F., Alharbi, A.A., Shadid, A., & Alrahili, N. (2020). 'Illicit stimulant use among medical students in Riyadh, Saudi Arabia'. *Cureus* **12**(1): e6688.

American Medical Association (2022). 'Code of medical ethics: professional self-regulation'. https://www.ama-assn.org/delivering-care/ethics/code-medical-ethics-professional-self-regulation

Amin-Esmaeili, M., Rahimi-Movaghar, A., Yunesian, M., Sahimi-Izadian, E., & Moinolghorabaei, M. (2013). 'Trend of smoking among students of Tehran University of Medical Sciences: Results from four consecutive surveys from 2006 to 2009'. *Med J Islam Repub Iran* **27**(4): 168–178.

Armaos, R., & Tsiboukli, A. (2019). 'Medical students' training needs and attitudes on substance abuse: Implications for medical education in Greece'. *Drugs: Education, Prevention and Policy* **26**(6): 508–516.

Aslam, H.M., Mughal, A., Edhi, M.M., Saleem, S., Rao, M.H., Aftab, A., Hanif, M., Ahmed, A., & Khan, A.M.H. (2013). 'Assessment of pattern for consumption and awareness regarding energy drinks among medical students'. *Arch Pub Health* **71**(1): 31.

Baldisseri, M.R. (2007). 'Impaired healthcare professional'. *Crit Care Med* **35**(2): S106–S116.

Baldwin, D.C., Jr., Hughes, P.H., Conard, S.E., Storr, C.L., & Sheehan, D.V. (1991). 'Substance use among senior medical students. A survey of 23 medical schools'. *JAMA* **265**(16): 2074–2078.

Balogh, E., Faubl, N., Riemenschneider, H., Balázs, P., Bergmann, A., Cseh, K., Horváth, F., Schelling, J., Terebessy, A., Wagner, Z., Voigt, K., Füzesi, Z., & Kiss, I. (2018). 'Cigarette, waterpipe and e-cigarette use among an international sample of medical students. Cross-sectional multicenter study in Germany and Hungary'. *BMC Pub Health* **18**(1): 591.

Balogh, E., Wagner, Z., Faubl, N., Riemenschneider, H., Voigt, K., Terebessy, A., Horváth, F., Füzesi, Z., & Kiss, I. (2020). 'Increasing prevalence of electronic cigarette use among medical students. Repeated cross-sectional multicenter surveys in Germany and Hungary, 2016–2018'. *Subst Use Misuse* **55**(13): 2109–2115.

Banimustafa, R.A., Abuelbeh, I.A., AlBadaineh, M.n.A., Safi, M.M., & Nawaiseh, M.B. (2018). 'Caffeine consumption among the medical students at the University of Jordan'. *Arab J Psychiatry* **29**(2): 117–122.

Basu, M., Das, P., Mitra, S., Ghosh, S., Pal, R., & Bagchi, S. (2011). 'Role of family and peers in the initiation and continuation of smoking behaviour of future physicians'. *J Pharm Bioallied Sci* **3**(3): 407–411.

Bazin, B., Duroy, D., & Lejoyeux, M. (2021). 'MDMA use by Paris medical students: prevalence and characteristics'. *Subst Use Misuse* **56**(1): 67–71.

BBC News (1998). 'Junior doctors "drink heavily and take drugs"'. http://news.bbc.co.uk/1/hi/health/164298.stm

BBC News (2005). 'Intoxication "rife among doctors"'. http://news.bbc.co.uk/1/hi/health/4080424.stm

Bin Abdulrahman, K.A., Khalaf, A.M., Bin Abbas, F.B., & Alanezi, O.T. (2021). 'The lifestyle of Saudi medical students'. *Int J Environ Res Public Health* **18**(15): 7869.

Birch, D., Ashton, H., & Kamali, F. (1998). 'Alcohol, drinking, illicit drug use, and stress in junior house officers in north-east England'. *Lancet* **352**(9130): 785–786.

Bogowicz, P., Ferguson, J., Gilvarry, E., Kamali, F., Kaner, E., & Newbury-Birch, D. (2018). 'Alcohol and other substance use among medical and law students at a UK university: A cross-sectional questionnaire survey'. *Postgrad Med J* **94**(1109): 131–136.

Boland, M., Fitzpatrick, P., Scallan, E., Daly, L., Herity, B., Horgan, J., & Bourke, G. (2006). 'Trends in medical student use of tobacco, alcohol and drugs in an Irish university, 1973–2002'. *Drug Alcohol Depend* **85**(2): 123–128.

Bore, M., Kelly, B., & Nair, B. (2016). 'Potential predictors of psychological distress and well-being in medical students: a cross-sectional pilot study'. *Adv Med Educ Pract* **7**: 125–135.

Bossaer, J.B., Gray, J.A., Miller, S.E., Enck, G., Gaddipati, V.C., & Enck, R.E. (2013). 'The use and misuse of prescription stimulants as 'cognitive enhancers' by students at one academic health sciences centre'. *Acad Med* **88**(7): 967–971.

Bourbon, A., Boyer, L., Auquier, P., Boucekine, M., Barrow, V., Lançon, C., & Fond, G. (2019). 'Anxiolytic consumption is associated with tobacco smoking and severe nicotine dependence Results from the national French medical students (BOURBON) study'. *Prog Neuro-Psychopharmacology Biol Psychiatry*, 94: 109645.

Cape, G., Hannah, A., & Sellman, D. (2006). 'A longitudinal evaluation of medical student knowledge, skills and attitudes to alcohol and drugs'. *Addiction* 101(6): 841–849.

Castaldelli-Maia, J.M., Lewis, T., Marques dos Santos, N., Picon, F., Kadhum, M., Farrell, S.M., Molodynski, A., & Ventriglio, A. (2019). 'Stressors, psychological distress, and mental health problems amongst Brazilian medical students'. *Int Rev Psychiatry* 31(7–8): 603–607.

Cattaruzza, M.S. & West, R. (2013). 'Why do doctors and medical students smoke when they must know how harmful it is?'. *Eur J Public Health* 23(2): 188–189.

Choi, D., Tolova, V., Socha, E., & Samenow, C.P. (2013). 'Substance use and attitudes on professional conduct among medical students: a single-institution study'. *Acad Psychiatry* 37(3): 191–195.

Cohen, Y.G., Segev, R.W., Shlafman, N., Novack, V., & Ifergane, G. (2015). 'Methylphenidate use among medical students at Ben-Gurion University of the Negev'. *J Neurosci Rural Pract* 6(3): 320–325.

De Bruyn, S., Wouters, E., Ponnet, K., & Van Hal, G. (2019). 'Popping smart pills in medical school: Are competition and stress associated with the misuse of prescription stimulants among students?'. *Subst Use Misuse* 54(7): 1191–1202.

Duroy, D., Iglesias, P., Perquier, F., Brahim, N., & Lejoyeux, M. (2017). 'Alcoolisation à risque chez des étudiants en médecine parisiens [Hazardous drinking in Parisian medical students]'. *L'Encephale* 43(4): 334–339.

Dyrbye, L.N., West, C.P., Satele, D., Boone, S., Sloan, J., & Shanafelt, T.D. (2015). 'A national study of medical students' attitudes toward self-prescribing and responsibility to report impaired colleagues'. *Acad Med* 90(4): 485–493.

Eisenberg, D., Gollust, S.E., Golberstein, E., & Hefner, J.L. (2007). 'Prevalence and correlates of depression, anxiety, and suicidality among university students'. *Am J Orthopsychiatry* 77(4): 534–542.

Emanuel, R.M., Frellsen, S.L., Kashima, K.J., Sanguino, S.M., Sierles, F.S., & Lazarus, C.J. (2013). 'Cognitive enhancement drug use among future physicians: Findings from a multi-institutional census of medical students'. *J Gen Intern Med* 28(8): 1028–1034.

Erasmus, N., & Kotzé, C. (2020). 'Medical students' attitudes towards pharmacological cognitive enhancement with methylphenidate'. *Acad Psychiatry* 44(6): 721–726.

European Monitoring Centre for Drugs and Drug Addiction [EMCDDA] (2017). *European Drug Report: Trends and Developments*. https://www.emcdda.europa.eu/publications/edr/trends-devel opments/2017_en

European Monitoring Centre for Drugs and Drug Addiction [EMCDDA] (2021). *European Drug Report: Trends and Developments*. https://www.emcdda.europa.eu/publications/edr/trends-devel opments/2021_en

Fallah, G., Moudi, S., Hamidia, A., & Bijani, A. (2018). 'Stimulant use in medical students and residents requires more careful attention'. *Caspian J Intern Med* 9(1): 87–91.

Farrell, S.M., Moir, F., Molodynski, A., & Bhugra, D. (2019). 'Psychological wellbeing, burnout and substance use amongst medical students in New Zealand'. *Int Rev Psychiatry* 31(7–8): 630–636.

Finger, G., Silva, E.R.d., & Falavigna, A. (2013). 'Use of methylphenidate among medical students: A systematic review'. *Rev Assoc Méd Bras* 59(3): 285–289.

Flaherty, J.A., & Richman, J.A. (1993). 'Substance use and addiction among medical students, residents, and physicians'. *Psychiatr Clin North Am* 16(1): 189–197.

Fond, G., Bourbon, A., Auquier, P., Micoulaud-Franchi, J.A., Lançon, C., & Boyer, L. (2018). 'Venus and Mars on the benches of the faculty: Influence of gender on mental health and behaviour of medical students. Results from the BOURBON national study'. *J Affect Disord* 239: 146–151.

Fond, G., Bourbon, A., Boucekine, M., Messiaen, M., Barrow, V., Auquier, P., Lançon, C., & Boyer, L. (2020). 'First-year French medical students consume antidepressants and anxiolytics while second-years consume non-medical drugs'. *J Affect Disord* 265: 71–76.

Fond, G., Bourbon, A., Picot, A., Boucekine, M., Lançon, C., Auquier, P., & Boyer, L. (2021a). 'Hazardous drinking is associated with hypnotic consumption in medical students in the BOURBON nationwide study: psychological factors explored'. *Eur Arch Psychiatry Clin Neurosci* 271(5): 883–889.

Fond, G., Gavaret, M., Vidal, C., Brunel, L., Riveline, J.-P., Micoulaud-Franchi, J.-A., & Domenech, P. (2016). '(Mis)use of prescribed stimulants in the medical student community: motives and behaviors: a population-based cross-sectional study'. *Medicine* 95(16): 1–8.

Fond, G., Picot, A., Bourbon, A., Boucekine, M., Auquier, P., Lançon, C., & Boyer, L. (2021b). 'Prevalence and associated factors of cannabis consumption in medical students: the BOURBON nationwide study'. *Eur Arch Psychiatry Clin Neurosci* 271(5): 857–864.

Franke, A.G., Bagusat, C., Dietz, P., Hoffmann, I., Simon, P., Ulrich, R., & Lieb, K. (2013). 'Use of illicit and prescription drugs for cognitive or mood enhancement among surgeons'. *BMC Med* 11(1): 102.

General Medical Council (2022). *Ethical Guidance for Doctors.* https://www.gmc-uk.org/ethical-guida nce/ethical-guidance-for-doctors

Gignon, M., Havet, E., Ammirati, C., Traullé, S., Manaouil, C., Balcaen, T., Loas, G., Dubois, G., & Ganry, O. (2015). 'Alcohol, cigarette, and illegal substance consumption among medical students: a cross-sectional survey'. *Workplace Health Saf* 63(2): 54–63.

Giri, P., Baviskar, M., & Phalke, D. (2013). 'Study of sleep habits and sleep problems among medical students of Pravara Institute of Medical Sciences Loni, Western Maharashtra, India'. *Ann Med Health Sci Res* 3(1): 51–54.

Goel, N., Khandelwal, V., Pandya, K., & Kotwal, A. (2015). 'Alcohol and tobacco use among undergraduate and postgraduate medical students in India: A multicentric cross-sectional study'. *Cent Asian J Glob Health* 4(1): 187.

Haas, G.M., Momo, A.C., Dias, T.M., Ayodele, T.A., & Schwarzbold, M.L. (2019). 'Sociodemographic, psychiatric, and personality correlates of non-prescribed use of amphetamine medications for academic performance among medical students'. *Braz J Psychiatry* 41(4): 363–364.

Heradstveit, O., Skogen, J.C., Edland-Gryt, M., Hesse, M., Vallentin-Holbech, L., Lønning, K.-J., & Sivertsen, B. (2020). 'Self-reported illicit drug use among Norwegian university and college students. associations with age, gender, and geography'. *Front Psych* 11: 543507.

Horowitz, A., Galanter, M., Dermatis, H., & Franklin, J. (2008). 'Use of and attitudes toward club drugs by medical students'. *J Addic Dis* 27(4): 35–42.

Ibn Auf, A., & Alnor, M.A. (2020). 'Sudanese medical students' perceptions of psychoactive substance use'. *Addict Health* 12(3): 186–195.

Jackson, E.R., Shanafelt, T.D., Hasan, O., Satele, D.V., & Dyrbye, L.N. (2016). 'Burnout and alcohol abuse/dependence among U.S. medical students'. *Acad Med* 91(9): 1251–1256.

Jain, R., Chang, C.C., Koto, M., Geldenhuys, A., Nichol, R., & Joubert, G. (2017). 'Non-medical use of methylphenidate among medical students of the University of the Free State'. *S Afr J Psychiatr* 23: 1006.

Jebrini, T., Manz, K., Koller, G., Krause, D., Soyka, M., & Franke, A.G. (2021). 'Psychiatric comorbidity and stress in medical students using neuroenhancers'. *Front Psychiatry* 12: 771126.

Ketoja, J., Svidkovski, A.S., Heinälä, P., & Seppä, K. (2013). 'Risky drinking and its detection among medical students'. *Addict Behav* 38(5): 2115–2118.

Kudlow, P.A., Treurnicht Naylor, K., Xie, B., & McIntyre, R.S. (2013). 'Cognitive enhancement in Canadian medical students'. *J Psychoactive Drugs* 45(4): 360–365.

Kusturica, J., Hajdarević, A., Nikšić, H., Skopljak, A., Tafi, Z., & Kulo, A. (2019). 'Neuroenhancing substances use, exam anxiety and academic performance in Bosnian-Herzegovinian first-year university students'. *Acta Med Acad* 48(3): 286–293.

Lambert Passos, S.R., Alvarenga Americano do Brasil, P.E., Borges dos Santos, M.A., & Costa de Aquino, M.T. (2006). 'Prevalence of psychoactive drug use among medical students in Rio de Janeiro'. *Soc Psychiatry Psychiatr Epidemiol* 41(12): 989–996.

Lane, A., McGrath, J., Cleary, E., Guerandel, A., & Malone, K.M. (2020). 'Worried, weary and worn out: mixed-method study of stress and well-being in final-year medical students'. *BMJ Open* 10(12): e040245.

Lempp, H., & Seale, C. (2004). 'The hidden curriculum in undergraduate medical education: qualitative study of medical students' perceptions of teaching'. *BMJ* 329(7469): 770–773.

Lengvenyte, A., Strumila, R., & Grikiniene, J. (2016). 'Use of cognitive enhancers among medical students in Lithuania'. *NAD* 33(2): 173–188.

MacLean, L., Booza, J., & Balon, R. (2016). 'The impact of medical school on student mental health'. *Acad Psychiatry* **40**(1): 89–91.

McAuliffe, W.E., Rohman, M., Fishman, P., Friedman, R., Wechsler, H., Soboroff, S.H., & Toth, D. (1984). 'Psychoactive drug use by young and future physicians'. *J Health Soc Behav* **25**(1): 34–54.

McAuliffe, W.E., Rohman, M., Santangelo, S., Feldman, B., Magnuson, E., Sobol, A., & Weissman, J. (1986). 'Psychoactive drug use among practicing physicians and medical students'. *N Engl J Med* **315**(13): 805–810.

McKay, A.J., Hawthorne, V.M., & McCartney, H.N. (1973). 'Drug taking among medical students at Glasgow university'. *BMJ* **1**(5852): 540–543.

Medical Council Ireland (2019). *Guide to Professional Conduct and Ethics 8th edition*. https://www.medicalcouncil.ie/news-and-publications/reports/guide-to-professional-conduct-ethics-8th-edition.html

Merlo, L.J., Curran, J.S., & Watson, R. (2017). 'Gender differences in substance use and psychiatric distress among medical students: a comprehensive statewide evaluation'. *Subst Abus* **38**(4): 401–406.

Miranda, M., & Barbosa, M. (2021). 'Use of cognitive enhancers by Portuguese medical students: do academic challenges matter?'. *Acta Med Port* **34**(13): 1–8.

Molodynski, A., Lewis, T., Kadhum, M., Farrell, S.M., Lemtiri Chelieh, M., Falcão De Almeida, T., Masri, R., Kar, A., Volpe, U., Moir, F., Torales, J., Castaldelli-Maia, J.M., Chau, S.W.H., Wilkes, C., & Bhugra, D. (2021). 'Cultural variations in wellbeing, burnout and substance use amongst medical students in twelve countries'. *Int Rev Psychiatry* **33**(1-2): 37–42.

Morgan, T.L., McFadden, T., Fortier, M.S., Tomasone, J.R., & Sweet, S.N. (2020). 'Positive mental health and burnout in first to fourth year medical students'. *Health Educ J* **79**(8): 948962.

Newbury-Birch, D., Walshaw, D., & Kamali, F. (2001). 'Drink and drugs: from medical students to doctors'. *Drug Alcohol Depend* **64**(3): 265–270.

Pandejpong, D., Paisansudhi, S., & Udompunthurak, S. (2014). 'Factors associated with consumption of caffeinated-beverage among Siriraj pre-clinical year medical students, a 2-year consecutive survey'. *J Med Assoc Thai* **97**(3): S189–S196.

Papazisis, G., Siafis, S., Tsakiridis, I., Koulas, I., Dagklis, T., & Kouvelas, D. (2018b). 'Prevalence of cannabis use among medical students: a systematic review and meta-analysis'. *Subst Abuse* **12**: 1–9.

Papazisis, G., Tsakiridis, I., Koulas, I., Siafis, S., Dagklis, T., & Kouvelas, D. (2017). 'Prevalence of illicit drug use among medical students in Northern Greece and association with smoking and alcohol use'. *Hippokratia* **21**(1): 13–18.

Papazisis, G., Tsakiridis, I., Pourzitaki, C., Apostolidou, E., Spachos, D., & Kouvelas, D. (2018a). 'Nonmedical use of prescription medications among medical students in Greece: Prevalence of and motivation for use'. *Subst Use Misuse* **53**(1): 77–85.

Papazisis, G., Tsakiridis, I., & Siafis, S. (2018c). 'Nonmedical use of prescription drugs among medical students and the relationship with illicit drug, tobacco, and alcohol use'. *Subst Abuse* **12**: 1–3.

Pickard, M., Bates, L., Dorian, M., Greig, H., & Saint, D. (2000). 'Alcohol and drug use in second-year medical students at the University of Leeds'. *Med Educ* **34**(2): 148–150.

Rai, D., Gaete, J., Girotra, S., Pal, H.R., & Araya, R. (2008). 'Substance use among medical students: time to reignite the debate?'. *Natl Med J India* **21**(2): 75–78.

Ram, S., Hussainy, S., Henning, M., Jensen, M., & Russell, B. (2016). 'Prevalence of cognitive enhancer use among New Zealand tertiary students'. *Drug Alcohol Rev* **35**(3): 345–351.

Retief, M., & Verster, C. (2016). 'Prevalence and correlates of non-medical stimulants and related drug use in a sample of South African undergraduate medical students'. *S Afr J Psychiatr* **22**(1): a795.

Rezaei Kalat, A., Taghavi, A., Askari, E., Parizadeh, S.M., Jafarzadeh Esfehani, A., Rajaei, Z., Jafarzadeh Esfehani, R., & Talaei, A. (2021). 'Medical students and stimulants; they have enough knowledge but they still use non prescribed stimulants'. *J Subst Use* 1–5.

Richmond, R. (1999). 'Teaching medical students about tobacco'. *Thorax* **54**(1): 70–78.

Roberts, L.W., Hardee, J.T., Franchini, G., Stidley, C.A., & Siegler, M. (1996). 'Medical students as patients: a pilot study of their health care needs, practices, and concerns'. *Acad Med* **71**(11): 1225–1232.

Roberts, L.W., Warner, T.D., Lyketsos, C., Frank, E., Ganzini, L., & Carter, D. (2001). 'Perceptions of academic vulnerability associated with personal illness: A study of 1,027 students at nine medical schools'. *Compr Psychiatry* **42**(1): 1–15.

Roncero, C., Egido, A., Rodríguez-Cintas, L., Pérez-Pazos, J., Collazos, F., & Casas, M. (2015). 'Substance use among medical students: a literature review 1988–2013'. *Actas Esp Psiquiatr* **43**(3): 109–121.

Roncero, C., Rodríguez-Cintas, L., Egido, A., Barral, C., Pérez-Pazos, J., Collazos, F., Grau-López, L., & Casas, M. (2014). 'The influence of medical student gender and drug use on the detection of addiction in patients'. *J Addict Dis* **33**(4): 277–288.

Samaha, A., Al Tassi, A., Yahfoufi, N., Gebbawi, M., Rached, M., & Fawaz, M.A. (2019). 'Data on the relationship between caffeine addiction and stress among Lebanese medical students in Lebanon'. *Data Brief* **28**: 104845.

Sapkota, A., Silvanus, V., Shah, P., Gautam, S.C., & Chhetri, A. (2021). 'Psychoactive substance use among second-year and third-year medical students of a medical college: a descriptive cross-sectional study'. *JNMA J Nepal Med Assoc* **59**(238): 571–576.

Schwenk, T.L., Davis, L., & Wimsatt, L.A. (2010). 'Depression, stigma, and suicidal ideation in medical students'. *JAMA* **304**(11): 1181–1190.

Silveira, R.d.R., Lejderman, B., Ferreira, P.E.M.S., & Rocha, G.M.P.d. (2014). 'Patterns of non-medical use of methylphenidate among 5th and 6th year students in a medical school in southern Brazil'. *Trends Psychiatry Psychother* **36**(2): 101–106.

Singh, I., Baxrd, I., & Jackson, J. (2014). 'Robust resilience and substantial interest: A survey of pharmacological cognitive enhancement among university students in the UK and Ireland'. *PloS One* **9**(10): e105969.

Sreeramareddy, C.T., Ramakrishnareddy, N., Rahman, M., & Mir, I.A. (2018). 'Prevalence of tobacco use and perceptions of student health professionals about cessation training: results from global health professions students survey'. *BMJ Open* **8**(5): e017477.

Stubbing, E.A., Helmich, E., & Cleland, J. (2019). 'Medical student views of and responses to expectations of professionalism'. *Med Educ* **53**(10): 1025–1036.

Sussman, S., Pentz, M.A., Spruijt-Metz, D., & Miller, T. (2006). 'Misuse of "study drugs:" prevalence, consequences, and implications for policy'. *Substance Abuse Treatment, Prevention, and Policy* **1**: 15.

Swani, J., & Miller, M.R. (2013). 'Should random drugs testing be applied to the medical profession?'. *Lancet* **382**(9899): 1174.

United Nations Office on Drugs and Crime [UNODC] (2011) *The non-medical use of prescription drugs: Policy direction issues* (Discussion Paper). https://www.unodc.org/documents/drug-prevention-and-treatment/nonmedical-use-prescription-drugs.pdf

Usman, A., Bhombal, S.T., Jawaid, A., & Zaki, S. (2015). 'Energy drinks consumption practices among medical students of a private sector University of Karachi, Pakistan'. *J Pak Med Assoc* **65**(9): 1005–1007.

Voigt, K., Twork, S., Mittag, D., Göbel, A., Voigt, R., Klewer, J., Kugler, J., Bornstein, S. R., & Bergmann, A. (2009). 'Consumption of alcohol, cigarettes and illegal substances among physicians and medical students in Brandenburg and Saxony (Germany)'. *BMC Health Serv Res* **9**: 219.

Vorster, A., Gerber, A.M., van der Merwe, L.J., & van Zyl, S. (2019). 'Second and third year medical students' self-reported alcohol and substance use, smoking habits and academic performance at a South African medical school'. *Health SA* **24**(0): a1041.

Webb, E., Ashton, C.H., Kelly, P., & Kamali, F. (1998). 'An update on British medical students' lifestyles'. *Med Educ* **32**(3): 325–331.

Weissberg, M., Sakai, J.T., Miyoshi, T.J., & Fryer, G.E. (2006). 'Medical student attitudes to risk taking and self-perceived influence on medical practice'. *Med Educ* **40**(8): 722–729.

Westermeyer, J. (1991). 'Substance use rates among medical students and resident physicians'. *JAMA* **265**(16): 2110–2111.

30

How Can Universities and Health Systems Look After Medical Students?

Evie Kemp

Introduction

For the last four years I worked as a lecturer and Director of Medical Student Wellbeing at the Technion American Medical School (TeAMS) in Haifa, northern Israel. TeAMS runs a four-year postgraduate medical programme for North American students who wish to study abroad. The two highlights of the academic year are the White Coat Ceremony at the beginning of the first year, and the Graduation (Commencement) Ceremony at the end of the fourth year. The White Coat Ceremony particularly interested me as a British graduate, as it was not something I had personally experienced (and indeed white coats are no longer worn in England due to infection control protocols). The excited students, dressed in their finest clothes and watched by their proud families and friends, are individually called up on stage where the Dean helps them don their new white coat with their name embossed on the front. The ceremony is a rite of passage that welcomes students to medical practice and marks the beginning of their journey from layperson to physician. It includes an oath that students take in front of family members, medical faculty, and their peers to acknowledge their future obligation to patient care and wellbeing.

However, it is striking that nowhere in the ceremony does the medical school pledge a similar oath to acknowledge its future obligation to *medical student* care and wellbeing. The obligation for the system to provide doctors with appropriate care and wellbeing should also begin on day one of medical school and continue throughout our lives as physicians.

I have spent most of my career as a consultant occupational health physician at the Centre for Occupational Health and Wellbeing at Oxford University Hospitals NHS Foundation Trust in the UK. Occupational medicine is a small medical specialty concerned with the effect of work on health and the effect of health on work. The main remit of our centre was to look after all the staff in the hospital from an occupational health perspective, including a range of pro-active wellbeing and lifestyle medicine activities and education. We also cared for many healthcare students from Oxford Brookes University in fields such as nursing, occupational therapy, and physiotherapy, plus medical students from Oxford University. I developed a special interest in doctors' and medical students' health and wellbeing and many of my patients came from these two groups. My more recent foray into medical education has been a second twilight career. I believe this combination of occupational medicine and medical education has given me a unique perspective regarding the challenges affecting the health and wellbeing of medical students.

Evie Kemp, *How Can Universities and Health Systems Look After Medical Students?* In: *The Mental Health of Medical Students.*
Edited by: Andrew Molodynski, Sarah Marie Farrell, and Dinesh Bhugra, Oxford University Press. © Oxford University Press 2024.
DOI: 10.1093/oso/9780192864871.003.0030

In this chapter I aim to present a practical framework to help universities and healthcare systems approach the topic of wellbeing in medical education.

Three-level Model for Preventing Stress and Improving Resilience

Resilience can be defined as 'how to engage with stressors with minimum negative impact, whilst experiencing personal growth and leading to the development of new coping mechanisms' or in more simple terms 'the ability to bounce back after a setback'.

However, my favourite description of resilience can be found in A.A. Milne's *The House at Pooh Corner* when Tigger says, 'Life is not about how fast you run or how high you climb, but how well you bounce (Milne, A.A. 1928)'.

Is it possible to teach medical students how to bounce, and if yes, is this even a good idea?

Some medical students and doctors are rightly cynical about the wellbeing or resilience training offered to them at their universities or places of work, thinking this is simply a tick box exercise organized by management. Others believe that most medical students and doctors have good levels of resilience anyhow (having navigated the many hurdles to be accepted into medical school) and the aim of making medical students and doctors more resilient just allows them to be further abused by a flawed system.

However, I often saw students a few months after beginning their medical studies, who were already suffering from stress, anxiety, and low mood. They described sleeping poorly, eating junk food, and using alcohol or even drugs as coping mechanisms. How could the initial fresh-faced excitement be replaced so quickly by this level of distress, unhelpful behaviour, and poor coping strategies?

Medical schools have a moral and ethical imperative to look after the health and wellbeing of their students, and indeed some countries have this included in their medical education accreditation standards (Promoting excellence: standards for medical education and training, n.d.; lcme.org, n.d.).

In my opinion, it is possible to reduce stress and improve resilience in medical students but *only* if we consider the issue in an appropriate and holistic manner.

Occupational medicine often utilizes the three-level model of prevention to assess and prevent risks or threats to health in the workplace, utilizing primary, secondary, and tertiary preventative interventions. This model can be readily adapted for use in medical education—the three-level model for preventing/reducing stress and improving resilience in medical schools:

- **Primary prevention** aims to prevent disease or injury before it actually occurs. The medical school would need to identify, eliminate, or reduce risks in the learning environment.
- **Secondary prevention** aims to reduce the impact of a disease or injury that has already occurred. In this case the medical school would need to provide tools and support to modify how a medical student manages or responds to pressures during their medical education.
- **Tertiary prevention** aims to provide timely help and treatment for a disease or injury that has already occurred. The medical school would need to provide early, ideally free, and most importantly, confidential rehabilitation/treatment once mental health problems have arisen in their students.

Too many organizations naively believe that if they provide a secondary prevention intervention e.g. a mindfulness workshop, that they are delivering an appropriate and effective wellbeing activity whilst fulfilling their obligations as an educational provider or employer. However, without the above three-level holistic approach this is akin to putting a bandage on a bleeding artery; it might improve the situation for a very short period of time, but then the problem will burst back with a vengeance. Indeed, sometimes secondary preventative interventions may make the participants feel worse because responsibility for change and action are placed solely on the individual, rather than via joint responsibility with the organization or educational institution. The student may even feel guilty that they are not coping better having participated in the recommended training intervention.

A growing body of opinion suggests that organizations need to employ interventions at all three levels of prevention in order to implement effective change (Kinman & Teoh, 2018).

Wellbeing

Wellbeing is not easy to define and means very different things to different people. When it comes to educational or workplace wellbeing it is appropriate to use a wide definition i.e. 'when individuals have the psychological, social, and physical resources they need to meet a particular psychological, social and/or physical challenge' (Dodge et al., 2012). Wellbeing therefore extends beyond psychological health to include many other areas including nutrition, exercise, relationship management, ergonomics etc.

I am amazed at how many students arrive at medical school with a lack of wellbeing and coping skills. It makes me wonder whether our secondary education system is failing its students by not prioritizing life skills in their curricula. In addition, many medical schools use mainly academic criteria for selecting medical students when emotional intelligence—which has been associated with better stress management—should be considered as well (Ramesar et al., 2009). Indeed, the process of obtaining a place in medical school can be so arduous that some students arrive in a chronically stressed state before they have even started their medical studies (Thorndike, 2022).

Director of Medical School Wellbeing

In 2009 Dr Steve Boorman performed his landmark review on the health and wellbeing of the NHS workforce, and then published a report with 20 recommendations (Boorman, 2009). At that time, I was jointly running the Centre for Occupational Health and Wellbeing with my very experienced nurse manager, and we were part of the team that was tasked with implementing the Boorman Review in the hospital. We wrote the occupational health and wellbeing policy and delivered training, plus an associated toolbox to managers, and additional training and support for staff. Despite the challenges of putting the recommendations into action (especially as the initiative did not come with any associated budget and was supposed to pay for itself via savings from reduced sickness absence) we gained a huge amount of knowledge through both the successes and limitations of the initiative. One of our main learning outcomes was the importance of a simultaneous top-down and bottom-up approach. The health and wellbeing director sat on the hospital board and conveyed ideas and information to and from the senior management team. At the same time the director chaired the hospital health and wellbeing committee, which had representatives from all major hospital divisions and staff groups; ideas were welcomed from every staff member in the organization and could be taken back up to the hospital board.

In a similar way, medical schools should appoint a director of medical school wellbeing/wellbeing executive with operational authority and financial resources to oversee and support all wellbeing activities in the organization. The role should include the wellbeing of the entire faculty and not just the students.

The most important components of the job description should include:

- Creating a culture of wellness and a safe space for open dialogue throughout the medical school
- Reporting to senior leadership/the university management board
- Having authority and adequate funding to deliver change
- Creating and implementing a health and wellbeing policy using the three-level model of prevention
- Forming and leading a health and wellbeing committee to include faculty members and student representatives from each year of the programme
- Supporting the health and wellbeing committee to organize informal events for students e.g. a healthy cooking demonstration
- Measuring student wellbeing on a regular basis to benchmark and follow progress
- Training faculty about their own wellbeing plus how to support and manage the wellbeing of their students
- Implementing and evaluating evidence-based interventions
- Fighting stigma associated with reaching out for help

A more detailed job role could be crafted after reviewing the job descriptions for the American Medical Association Chief Wellness Officer (Ama-assn.org, 2020) and National Health Service Wellbeing Guardians (learninghub.leadershipacademy.nhs.uk, n.d.).

I would like to look at the three levels of prevention in more detail.

Primary Prevention

Primary prevention aims to prevent disease or injury before it actually occurs. The medical school would need to identify, eliminate, or reduce risks in the learning environment.

I have seen and treated many senior doctors who have been suffering from work-related psychological ill-health, ranging from significant chronic stress to severe depression with suicidal ideation. Doctors nearly always present very late, and following occupational health assessment, had often reached a point where they were unfit for work and had to be persuaded to take a short period of sickness absence. This would allow the doctor to stop running on the never-ending hamster wheel of work, and step off to have time to sleep, recover, reflect, brainstorm together, and then plan a way forward. I am trained in cognitive behaviour therapy (CBT) and we usually finished the first consultation by crafting a CBT formulation with a home rehabilitation plan based on a holistic biopsychosocial model of care. Once the doctors had had time to recuperate a little and had started their home rehabilitation plan, we would begin to review their workplace issues in detail, and this would invariably include a workplace stress risk assessment. We would then often arrange a meeting for the doctor, their manager, human resource manager and occupational health physician to review the stress risk assessment and see what positive workplace changes could be accommodated by the organization. There is no point taking an employee out of work, getting them better and then putting them straight back into the same environment that made them sick in the first place. Over the years many reasonable adjustments and changes were put in place by the hospital, allowing the doctors to slowly return and then successfully remain in work.

Workplace stress risk assessments can be performed for an individual, a specific group of employees e.g. junior doctors in Accident and Emergency, or for all the employees in an entire department, and this tool can be used in an educational as well as workplace setting. It is based on the UK Health and Safety Executive management standards which cover six key areas of work design, that if not properly managed, are associated with poor health and wellbeing, lower productivity, and increased levels of sickness absence. In other words, the six management standards cover the primary sources of stress at work (Health and Safety Executive, 2019).

The six areas (demands, control, support, relationships, role and change) can be adapted for use in relation to medical school as follows:

Demands—This includes workload (including the exponential rise in medical knowledge), work patterns, and the educational environment.

i.e. can students cope with the demands of the course?

Aims:
- Curriculum is designed to be within the capabilities of students
- Achievable demands in relation to timetable and personal study
- Students' skills and abilities are matched to educational demands
- Students' concerns about their educational and general environment can be addressed, e.g. finances/loans, housing, administrative support, organization, and travel time to clinical rotations etc.

Examples of interventions include curriculum review and reform, reduction of administrative bureaucracy, financial planning support etc. (Slavin et al., 2014).

Control—This includes student input into how they study, the curriculum and timetable, and personal learning styles.

i.e. do students have a say about the way the educational curriculum and milieu is organized?

Aims:
- Students have a say over the timetable e.g. when breaks are put into the timetable or when exams are scheduled
- The medical school helps each student to understand and develop their personalized study needs and skills
- Where possible, students are then able to study using their preferred learning styles

Examples of interventions include meeting with each student twice per year to review individual study skills, having a day of flexible leave to use for personal reasons, use of flipped classroom e.g. watching pre-recorded lectures in their own time and then attending workshops to embed the learning face to face, or electives where the students have a choice of topics.

Support—This includes encouragement, support, and resources provided by the medical school and other students.

i.e. do students receive adequate information and support from the faculty and their co-students?

Aims:

- Systems are in place to enable/encourage faculty to support their students
- Systems are in place to enable/encourage students to support each other and create community
- Students know what support is available and how and when to access it
- Students receive regular and constructive feedback

Examples include quick and confidential access to educational and psychological support, identifying and meeting students with new or ongoing performance issues, a buddy system where each new first year student is matched with a second- or third-year student for peer support, and faculty training regarding provision of emotional support, supervision, and faculty role modelling.

Relationships—This includes promoting a positive educational environment in order to reduce, manage and ideally avoid conflict, and appropriately dealing with unacceptable behaviour.

i.e. students are not subjected to unacceptable behaviours from other students or Faculty members, e.g. bullying or harassment.

Aims:

- The medical school promotes positive behaviours to avoid conflict and ensure fairness
- The medical school has agreed policies and procedures to prevent or resolve unacceptable behaviour
- The medical school educates students and faculty about these policies and procedures
- Systems are in place to enable/encourage faculty to deal with unacceptable behaviour
- Systems are in place to enable/encourage students to report unacceptable behaviour without fear of a backlash

Examples include writing, advertising, and implementing a policy and procedure for managing bullying, promoting a culture of collaboration for both students and faculty, and moving to pass/fail grading system to reduce competition between students. Several studies have suggested that pass/fail curricula not only reduce stress and burnout but also lower medical school dropout rates (Bloodgood et al., 2009; Reed et al., 2011; Rohe et al., 2006).

Role—This includes whether students have clarity regarding their role and responsibilities as learners.

i.e. do students have a clear idea of what is expected of them in each module/semester/year of the course?

Aims:

- The medical school ensures that, as far as possible, that differing requirements it places upon students are clear and compatible

- The medical school provides information to enable students to understand their role and responsibilities
- Systems are in place to enable students to raise concerns about uncertainties or conflicts they have in their roles and responsibilities without fear of a backlash

Examples include making sure exams are well spaced out and hand in deadlines for work are given in good time and don't conflict with other commitments. In addition, making it clear that responsibility for health and wellbeing is a joint endeavour between the school, its students, and the hospitals and clinics where students take part in their clinical placements.

Change—This includes how organizational change is managed and communicated within the medical school.

i.e. does the medical school engage students regularly when undergoing organizational change?

Aims:
- The medical school provides students with timely and transparent information to enable them to understand the reasons for proposed changes
- The medical school ensures adequate student consultation on changes and provides opportunities for students to influence proposals
- Students are aware of timetables for changes and potential impact on them
- Students have access to relevant support during changes

Examples include student involvement in discussions around curricular and timetable changes and informing students about changes in a timely manner.

So how would a medical school organize a stress risk assessment? It is an easy tool to learn to use and the process is similar to performing an audit cycle which many faculty members will already be familiar with. The students are briefed that the educational stress risk assessment will be taking place and asked to start thinking about the issues they wish to raise. A senior faculty member/s then meet with the students or student representatives, and the group identify potential hazards using the six areas as a framework for discussion. A simple form (see Figure 30.1) can be completed looking at each stressor, existing mitigating factors plus ideas for further action. An action plan can them be agreed with responsibilities and time scales for action.

Type of stressor	Stressors identified in each category	Mitigating factors already in place	Further action to be taken	Who is responsible and review date
Demands				
Control				
Support				
Relationship				
Role				
Change				

Figure 30.1 Stress risk assessment form.

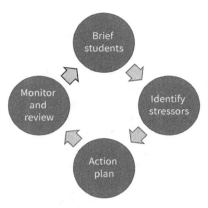

Figure 30.2 Stress risk assessment cycle.

The action plan should be monitored and reviewed at subsequent meetings and then the cycle starts again. (See Figure 30.2)

Ideally a stress risk assessment would be performed at least once, and then reviewed in each semester for each year group.

It goes without saying that different stressors predominate in preclinical and clinical years and will vary significantly between medical schools and their educational curricula. For example, one study published in 2018 looked at stressors facing medical students in the millennial generation. This found that academic workload and financial difficulties were the main stressors in the first year, competition with peers in the second year, time spent commuting to placements, romantic relationship management, and work–life balance in the third year, with exposure to human suffering being the major issue in the final year (Hill et al., 2018).

It is recommended that separate risk assessments are also performed for the faculty team or teams.

Secondary Prevention

Secondary prevention aims to reduce the impact of a disease or injury that has already oc-curred. In this case the medical school would need to provide tools and support to modify how a medical student manages or responds to pressures during their medical education.

Over the years many senior academic doctors were referred or made self-referrals to the Centre for Occupational Health and Wellbeing, often in significant crisis. These complex cases were reviewed in our clinical team meetings, where one of our senior nurses could sometimes be heard to quietly mutter: 'brains as big as planets but not an iota of common sense when it comes to looking after themselves ... !'

It became increasingly obvious that many of our doctor patients were practising only very limited self-care due to a combination of lack of awareness, knowledge, skills, and time. Our concern about these doctors was one of several factors that led to the creation of our 'What's Up Doc?' occupational health and wellbeing programme for doctors in the hospital. This included a session at the monthly doctors' induction (which every new doctor attended), lectures and workshops for foundation year doctors (interns), doctors in training (residents) and consultants (senior specialists) including slots on the medical and surgical grand rounds. Where possible the programme was linked to training programme competencies e.g. the foundation training programme curriculum (UK Foundation Programme, 2015). The training programmes were regularly updated, taking into account the range of problems and difficulties that our doctor patients were grappling with on a daily basis.

A few years ago, I was given the opportunity to use my accumulated knowledge and experience to develop a new health and wellbeing module for first year students at the Technion American Medical School. I was asked to take over a 12-week behavioural science course which had been taught in the first semester of the postgraduate medical programme. The only stipulation was that the last five sessions of the module were to remain as the *Healer's Art* course developed by The Remen Institute for the Study of Health & Illness (Rishi, n.d.) This left seven, two and a half hour sessions available for the new course.

Literature review revealed only limited evidence on content and efficacy of medical school stress management and resilience training interventions. Therefore, after careful consideration, I decided to build the module using a joint lifestyle medicine and occupational health approach instead. Lifestyle medicine involves the therapeutic use of lifestyle to prevent, treat and often reverse the lifestyle related chronic diseases that cause an estimated two-thirds of worldwide non-communicable chronic disease (Chopra et al., 2003). Occupational Health focuses on maintaining the wellbeing of those studying or employed in the university, preventing and removing ill-health and developing solutions to keep students and staff with health issues at study or work (developed from Society Occupational Medicine, n.d.).

The module aims to give students an introduction to lifestyle and occupational medicine, an understanding that doctors are role models for their patients plus a range to tools to create their own health and wellbeing plan for medical school and beyond.

The workshops utilize active learning strategies including flipped classroom model, role play, experiential learning, think-pair-share activities, and self-reflection. The students initially apply the learning to their own health and wellbeing but in the process, acquire a range of tools they can use when looking after patients in the future.

Some aspects of resilience training are woven into the programme, including the Robertson Cooper model which describes four aspects of personality which help to determine resilience: confidence (building self-confidence), adaptability (ability to be flexible to changing situations), purposefulness (clear sense of purpose and direction) and social support (building good relationships with others) (Robertson Cooper, 2015).

The seven experiential workshops cover the following topics:

1. Introduction to the six main pillars of lifestyle medicine: stress management, nutrition, exercise, sleep, tobacco and alcohol use, and management of healthy relationships (Society of Lifestyle Medicine, Israel Association of Family Physicians, 2014).
2. Introduction to occupational health and wellbeing issues for medical students (three-level model of prevention, stressors, perfectionism, barriers to seeking help, delayed gratification, medical student illness behaviour, drugs, and alcohol, overcoming stigma, self-care, where to obtain confidential help, not to self-treat, problems of corridor consultations etc.)

3. Myers Briggs personality type (MBTI) -to help students look at the management of healthy relationships at work and at home, plus understand how different personalities experience and cope with stress. MBTI is one of the few models of personality that describes personality differences in a positive manner. (I included the MBTI as many of the doctors in difficulty that I saw were struggling with stress caused by workplace relationship issues and dysfunctional teams. I found MBTI to be a useful tool in helping the doctors understand personality differences and improve workplace relationships.)

4. CBT skills, particularly learning to manage and challenge negative thoughts.

5. Introduction to mindfulness as a possible stress management skill.

6. Behaviour change skills including an introduction to motivational interviewing and smart goals with particular reference to their own nutrition and exercise stage of change.

7. Nutrition and cooking, including hands on cooking session, buying food, and quick, healthy recipes to feed oneself as a student.

8. Exercise including an introduction to yoga and other exercise ideas.

9. Sleep hygiene for medical school and life.

10. Workstation ergonomics with a plan to set up their own computer workstation, plus yoga exercises for computer users, and the importance of how to take breaks.

In addition, the last five workshops are taken up with *The Healer's Art*, which is run as a compulsory course within the module. The Healer's Art describes itself as 'an innovative discovery model course in values clarification and professionalism for first- and second-year medical students now offered annually at over 100 US medical schools as well as medical schools around the world'. Designed in 1991 by Rachel Naomi Remen, MD, the course offers a safe learning environment for a personal in-depth exploration of the time-honoured values of service, healing relationship, reverence for life and compassionate care (Rishi, n.d.). The Healer's Art creates small group supportive communities for the duration of the course. The students are then encouraged to continue meeting in these small 'Finding Meaning in Medicine' groups on a regular basis throughout the four years of medical school. These groups aim to build an empathetic community and foster good interpersonal relationships (Rabow et al., 2007).

At the end of the module, the students are asked to write a reflective paper on the topics and tools covered in relation to themselves, plus a bullet point personal self-care and lifestyle plan for medical school and beyond. It is made clear that every student is an individual; different strategies work for different people at different times in their lives, and each student needs to build their own personal toolbox. In writing the paper the students need to review and reflect on the topics covered and embed the learning.

The students are also asked to complete an anonymous survey to assess the module after they have written their reflective papers. The response rate is good and indeed, 100% of the students (n = 24) completed the survey in 2022. (Results presented at the Association for Medical Education in Europe, AMEE conference August 2022.)

Answers to the survey showed that all of the students (100%) would recommend the module to fellow medical students. One wrote: 'I especially liked how interactive the course was and the fact that we did hands on work'. All of the students (100%) said the module had given them tools to manage their health and wellbeing, and one commented: 'Challenging these negative emotions has been a complete game changer for me'. In addition, 23 of the students (96%) agreed that their health and wellbeing had improved because of the module, and the other one stated that their health and wellbeing was already in a good place. One student commented: 'I learned a lot about wellbeing and how important it is to care for ourselves. It was great getting a deeper understanding of how to live a balanced healthy life'.

Another wrote: ' ... our health and wellbeing are extremely important and more easily attained than I realized. It's hard to make changes especially when we're in such a stressful time in medical school but the little changes I have made due to this course are ones I had been wanting to change for a while and I'm so happy with them. Not sure where I would've found the motivation to do so without this course ... '

The experience of delivering this module over several years in conjunction with the positive student feedback and survey results, reinforces my belief that student health and wellbeing should be included in the syllabus from day one of medical school. Furthermore, the mixture of experiential and active learning strategies utilized in the module appeared to be effective and were enjoyed and well received by the students. Hopefully we have achieved our aim of providing the students with a personal toolbox to better cope with the stressors of life and work going forwards. However, we appreciate that these are only initial survey results, however promising, and further research is required to ascertain which interventions/tools/pedagogical methods are most effective in achieving positive health and wellbeing outcomes in the longer term.

It is also important to consider which additional health and wellbeing topics, plus top up learning, should be included in the curriculum in other years of medical school. For example, moving to the clinical environment brings many new challenges and situations that can evoke strong emotions, including coming into contact with death and dying for the first time. Students may benefit from discussing these new life experiences in small groups with trained facilitators. In Healer's Art, the students spend several sessions contemplating the issues surrounding grief and loss, including an exercise where they compile a list of behaviours and phrases that can be of help to someone who has suffered a loss, and another list of behaviours and phrases which do not help in this situation. The students also reflect on three unanswered and unanswerable questions on the nature of death, and then write them on a piece of paper which is sealed in an envelope and kept in a safe place—to be opened at some point in the future after their first patient has died (Rishi, n.d.).

Another essential but often neglected area is training students regarding their personal workplace health before they enter the clinical healthcare environment. Occupational health topics include understanding the importance of their workplace immunization programme, prevention and management of needlestick injuries to prevent transmission of blood borne viruses such as HIV, Hepatitis B and Hepatitis C, correct manual handling of patients to prevent musculoskeletal injuries, skin care education to prevent hand dermatitis following repeated hand washing and glove use, evidence-based techniques for managing shift and night work (Wallace & Haber,2020), plus training and working when pregnant and breast feeding. Too many junior doctors start work with limited knowledge of these occupational health issues which have the potential to significantly adversely impact their health and wellbeing. Most of these work-related health problems are preventable with the right training and approach.

Last but not least, faculty members should also receive training on how to optimize their own health and wellbeing as well as that of their students, and this training should include the recognition and management of students in difficulty.

Tertiary Prevention

Tertiary prevention aims to provide timely help and treatment for a disease or injury that has already occurred. The medical school would need to provide early, free, and most importantly, confidential rehabilitation/treatment once mental health problems have arisen in their students.

We know there are many barriers which delay and prevent doctors from reaching out for help, and students can quickly pick up the medical zeitgeist of self-reliance and coping, along with the conviction that they are the ones who will be doing the treating and will never be the patients who will need to be treated. This concept is discussed in Dr Robert Klitzman's 2007 book *When Doctors Become Patients*. Dr Klitzman is a Professor of Clinical Psychiatry at Columbia University who tragically lost his sister in the 9/11 World Trade Centre attacks and afterwards was shocked to find himself suffering from symptoms of significant depression. He decided to interview other doctors who had become seriously ill to understand how they had dealt with 'moving to the dark side' of the therapeutic relationship and these interviews helped him on his own journey to recovery. One of the doctors he interviewed in the book was a middle-aged oncologist with metastatic cancer who movingly explained the issue: 'We doctors wear magic white coats … we destroy disease all the time … how could it ever attack us? (Klitzman, 2008)'

At the end of every talk or workshop I run locally, nationally or internationally, I put up a slide with phone numbers and local resources for doctors and medical students to access support. I always ask the participants to take out their phones and take a photo of the slide, saying 'I know you think you will never need this, but please humour me and have the information on your phones just in case.'

Invariably, after talking at a grand round or running a workshop for consultants I would get a phone call or email from a senior colleague a day or two later, sheepishly asking if they could pop in or see me for a coffee. We would start the conversation sitting in the postgraduate medical centre or at the round table in my office, and gradually agree that we would move into doctor patient consultation mode at my desk. It was always a great feeling of achievement when a doctor felt able to reach out to our team for support after attending a 'What's Up Doc?' talk or workshop.

Another significant barrier to seeking help is the fear of stigma following a mental health diagnosis. A meta-analysis of 195 studies including 129,00 medical students identified that 27.2% of them were suffering from symptoms consistent with a diagnosis of depression with 11.1% experiencing suicidal ideation. However, sadly only 15.7% of the medical students had felt able to reach out for help (Rotenstein et al., 2016).

This percentage of medical students reaching out for help is worryingly even lower than the results of a cross sectional study in surgeons published in 2011. An anonymous survey to assess psychological wellbeing was sent to members of the American College of Surgeons, and 32% of the 25,000 surgeons responded. Of these, 501 surgeons admitted to experiencing suicidal ideation in the previous year but only 26% of them had felt able to seek support (Shanafelt, 2011). It has been estimated that tragically between 300 and 400 doctors commit suicide each year in the United States (Center et al., 2003), with the relative risk of suicide in physicians compared to other professionals being 3.7 to 4.5 in women doctors and 1.5 to 3.8 in their male counterparts (Hawton et al.,2004).

Medical schools have a responsibility to proactively work to overcome the barriers preventing students from seeking help, including the stigma of mental health challenges, and should promote a culture where it is both normal and appropriate for students and Faculty members to access help and support. This should include confidential counselling which should be easy to access, readily available, and ideally free for all students.

The joint GMC and Medical Schools Council report, Supporting Medical Students with Mental Health Conditions has a range of recommendations including normalizing stress and challenging myths about mental health held by medical students, including:

'If I have a mental health condition, it will damage my career prospects'.
'Seeking help is seen as a sign of weakness'.
'I can never take time out from my studies'.
'If I tell my medical school that I have a mental health condition, I will automatically be referred to a fitness to practise committee'.

In order to reduce the stigma associated with accessing help, medical schools need to remind students that mental health conditions are common, and that confidential support is available for them. 'In almost every case, a mental health condition does not prevent a student from completing his or her course and continuing a career in medicine (Supporting medical students with mental health conditions, n.d.).'

Confidentiality is another area that understandably worries students. It is strongly recommended that doctors in the medical school should not be responsible for the clinical care of students if they become less well, with clear boundaries and policies regarding confidentiality. Instead, students with health concerns should be referred to an experienced occupational health service. HEOPS (Higher Education Occupational Practitioners) is the professional association for occupational health professionals working in the UK higher education sector. Their guidance recommends that all universities should have access to at least one specialist physician in occupational medicine and a specialist in occupational health nursing (HEOPS, n.d.). HEOPS has published standards on medical student fitness to train, and their practitioners can perform an assessment of fitness to study including recommendations for any reasonable adjustments, including time out of the course and the option for a flexible reintroduction (Medical Students, Standards of medical fitness to train, n.d.).

Conclusions

I started this chapter writing about the White Coat Ceremony, which is held at the beginning of medical school, so it is only appropriate that I finish it with the Graduation (Commencement) Ceremony, which takes place at the end of medical studies.

For the past three years I have been honoured to be mistress of ceremonies at our TeAMS Graduation Ceremony. (I suspect I was invited to take on this role because the North Americans like my English accent!) It is a wonderful occasion of joy and pride when we celebrate the dedication and achievements of our students as they are awarded their medical degrees. The event includes a Hooding Ceremony when each student is 'hooded' by a nominated faculty or medical family member and is personally welcomed into the medical profession. This was another new experience for me, as although hooding is based on a medieval European academic tradition, I have not personally seen this practised in England. Interestingly the modern hood is separate to the academic robe, but it was originally attached and could be pulled over the head when required as protection against inclement weather. Although our students have to give back their academic dress at the end of the ceremony, I would like them to take their 'metaphorical hood' with them after graduation, to help protect themselves from the storms of work and life they will encounter going forward. As part of the ceremony, I remind the graduating class that if they don't look after themselves first, they won't be able to optimally look after the patients in their care. It is a similar message to the one we hear from cabin crew during the pre-flight safety briefing; you must always put on your personal oxygen mask before helping others do the same. I also remind our students that they will all experience challenging times as doctors in the weeks, months and years ahead, and that there is no shame or stigma in reaching out for help. These are important messages that need to be heard on day one of medical school and be reinforced at every stage of our medical careers.

Although recommendations on medical student health and wellbeing have been published by organizations around the world including the General Medical Council (Supporting medical students with mental health conditions, n.d.), the American Medical Association (edhub. ama-assn.org, n.d.) and a consensus from medical school leads in Australia and New Zealand (Kemp et al., 2019), it is clear that the evidence base on this topic is limited and there is a pressing need for further research to be undertaken.

In the meantime, I hope the framework I have laid out in this chapter will give medical schools some practical tools they can use to implement change and support wellbeing in medical education now, whilst keeping a careful eye on new evidence being published in the future. TeAMS is a small medical school and some of the ideas suggested in this chapter may need to be adapted for use in bigger organizations; each individual medical school will need to carefully consider what will work for them. A health and wellbeing programme could potentially be taught within the behavioural science, lifestyle medicine, occupational medicine, public health, or psychological medicine curricula.

Promoting health and wellbeing in medical schools is only the first step in the long career progression of medical student to senior doctor. As a profession we need to make sure that our health and wellbeing remains a priority at every step of the way in the workplace of the future, both for us and for the patients in our care.

References

Ama-assn.org. (2020). *Establishing a Chief Wellness Officer Position*. [online] Available at: https://edhub. ama-assn.org/steps-forward/module/2767739 [Accessed 2 Aug. 2022].

Bloodgood, R., Short, J., Jackson, J. and Martindale, J., 2009. A Change to Pass/Fail Grading in the First Two Years at One Medical School Results in Improved Psychological Well-Being. *Academic Medicine*, 84(5), pp.655–662.

Boorman, S., 2009. [online] Webarchive.nationalarchives.gov.uk. Available at: <https://webarchive. nationalarchives.gov.uk/ukgwa/20130124052412/http:/www.dh.gov.uk/prod_consum_dh/groups/ dh_digitalassets/documents/digitalasset/dh_108907.pdf> [Accessed 31 July 2022].

Center, C., Davis, M., Detre, T., Ford, D.E., Hansbrough, W., Hendin, H., Laszlo, J., Litts, D.A., Mann, J., Mansky, P.A., Michels, R., Miles, S.H., Proujansky, R., Reynolds III, C.F. and Silverman, M.M. (2003). Confronting Depression and Suicide in Physicians. *JAMA*, 289(23), p.3161. doi:10.1001/ jama.289.23.3161.

Chopra, M., Galbraith, S. and Darnton-Hill, I. (2003). A global response to a global problem: the epidemic of overnutrition. *Bull World Health Ordgan.*, 80(12), pp.952–958.

Dodge, R., Daly, A., Huyton, J. and Sanders, L., 2012. The challenge of defining wellbeing. *International Journal of Wellbeing*, 2(3), pp.222–235.

edhub.ama-assn.org. (n.d.). *Medical Student Well-Being.* [online] Available at: https://edhub.ama-assn.org/steps-forward/module/2757082.

Health and Safety Executive (2019). *Tackling work-related stress using the Management Standards approach - HSE.* [online] Hse.gov.uk. Available at: https://www.hse.gov.uk/pubns/wbk01.htm.

HEOPS. (n.d.). *Guidance on provision of occupational health in HE.* [online] Available at: https://heops.org.uk/guidance/ [Accessed 2 Aug. 2022].

Hill, M.R., Goicochea, S. and Merlo, L.J. (2018). In their own words: stressors facing medical students in the millennial generation. *Medical Education Online*, [online] 23(1), p.1530558. doi:10.1080/10872981.2018.1530558.

Hawton, K., Malmberg, A. and Simkin, S. (2004). Suicide in doctors. *Journal of Psychosomatic Research*, 57(1), pp.1–4. doi:10.1016/s0022-3999(03)00372-6.

Kemp, S., Hu, W., Bishop, J., Forrest, K., Hudson, J.N., Wilson, I., Teodorczuk, A., Rogers, G.D., Roberts, C. and Wearn, A. (2019). Medical student wellbeing – a consensus statement from Australia and New Zealand. *BMC Medical Education* 19, 69 (2019). doi:10.1186/s12909-019-1505-2.

Kinman, G. and Teoh, K. (2018). *What could make a difference to the mental health of UK doctors? A review of the research evidence.* [online] Available at: https://www.som.org.uk/sites/som.org.uk/files/What_could_make_a_difference_to_the_mental_health_of_UK_doctors_LTF_SOM.pdf.

Klitzman, R. (2008). *When doctors become patients.* Oxford; New York: Oxford University Press.

learninghub.leadershipacademy.nhs.uk. (n.d.). *Wellbeing Guardians – Leadership Academy.* [online] Available at: https://learninghub.leadershipacademy.nhs.uk/wp-content/uploads/dlm_uploads/2021/09/B0189-Wellbeing-Guardian-Implementation-Guidance-Final-for-publishing.pdf

lcme.org. (n.d.). *Standards, Publications, & Notification Forms | LCME.* [online] Available at: https://lcme.org/publications/.

Medical Students -Standards of medical fitness to train. (n.d.). [online] Available at: https://heops.org.uk/wp-content/uploads/bsk-pdf-manager/2019/09/1521730794HEOPS_Medical_Students_fitness_standards_2015_v12.pdf [Accessed 2 Aug. 2022].

Milne, A.A. (1928). *The House at Pooh Corner.* London: Methuen & Co. Ltd.

Promoting excellence: standards for medical education and training. (n.d.). [online] Available at: https://www.gmc-uk.org/-/media/documents/promoting-excellence-standards-for-medical-education-and-training-2109_pdf-61939165.pdf

Rabow, M.W., Wrubel, J. and Remen, R.N. (2007). Authentic Community as an Educational Strategy for Advancing Professionalism: A National Evaluation of the Healer's Art Course. *Journal of General Internal Medicine*, 22(10), pp.1422–1428. doi:10.1007/s11606-007-0274-5.

Ramesar, S., Koortzen, P. and Oosthuizen, R., 2009. The relationship between emotional intelligence and stress management. *SA Journal of Industrial Psychology*, 35(1), p. a443.

Reed, D., Shanafelt, T., Satele, D., Power, D., Eacker, A., Harper, W., Moutier, C., Durning, S., Massie, F., Thomas, M., Sloan, J. and Dyrbye, L., 2011. Relationship of Pass/Fail Grading and Curriculum Structure With Well-Being Among Preclinical Medical Students: A Multi-Institutional Study. *Academic Medicine*, 86(11), pp.1367–1373.

Rishi. (n.d.). *Healer's Art Overview.* [online] Available at: https://rishiprograms.org/healers-art/ [Accessed 31 Jul. 2022].

Robertson Cooper. (2015). *What is resilience? | Robertson Cooper.* [online] Available at: https://www.robertsoncooper.com/blog/what-is-resilience/.

Rohe, D.E., Barrier, P.A., Clark, M.M., Cook, D.A., Vickers, K.S. and Decker, P.A. (2006). The Benefits of Pass-Fail Grading on Stress, Mood, and Group Cohesion in Medical Students. *Mayo Clinic Proceedings*, [online] 81(11), pp.1443–1448. doi:10.4065/81.11.1443.

Rotenstein, L.S., Ramos, M.A., Torre, M., Segal, J.B., Peluso, M.J., Guille, C., Sen, S. and Mata, D.A. (2016). Prevalence of Depression, Depressive Symptoms, and Suicidal Ideation Among Medical Students. *JAMA*, [online] 316(21), p.2214. doi:10.1001/jama.2016.17324.

Shanafelt, T.D. (2011). Special Report. *Archives of Surgery*, 146(1), p.54. doi:10.1001/archsurg.2010.292.

Slavin, S., Schindler, D. and Chibnall, J., 2014. Medical Student Mental Health 3.0. *Academic Medicine*, 89(4), pp.573–577.

Society of Lifestyle Medicine, Israel Association of Family Physicians, The Israeli Medical Association. Themes and topics for the study of lifestyle medicine. (2014). [online] Available at: https://cdn.med net.co.il/2015/08/syllabus-lifestyle-medicine.pdf [Accessed 1 Aug. 2022].

Society of Occupational Medicine, n.d. [online] Available at: ttps://www.som.org.uk/work-and-health [Accessed 31 Jul. 2022].

Supporting medical students with mental health conditions. (n.d.). [online] Available at: https://www. gmc-uk.org/-media/documents/ Supporting_students_with_mental_health_conditions_0816.pdf_ 53047904.pdf.

Thorndike, A. (2022). *The roots of burnout start early. See: Applying to medical school.* [online] Available at: https://www.statnews.com/2022/05/03/burnout-starts-early-applying-to-medical-school/ [Accessed 8 Aug. 2022].

UK Foundation Programme. (2019). *Curriculum - UK Foundation Programme.* [online] Available at: https://foundationprogramme.nhs.uk/curriculum/.

Wallace, P.J. and Haber, J.J. (2020). Top 10 evidence-based countermeasures for night shift workers. *Emergency Medicine Journal*, 37(9), pp.562–564. doi:10.1136/emermed-2019-209134.

31

How Can Medical Students Look After Themselves?

Anna Collini and Caroline Elton

Introduction

A number of factors differentiate medicine from other subjects studied at university including the length of training, the heavy assessment and examination load (which will continue for many years after graduation), frequent transitions between learning environments, and the fact that as an integral part of training, students get exposed to disease, distress, disability and death (MacLeod et al., 2003; Wear, 2002). In addition, in some parts of the world, significant financial debt can add to the psychological demands of training for some students (Pisaniello et al., 2019). And of course, medical students can also experience other challenges that are not unique to medicine, including (on undergraduate courses) the difficulties that come with moving away from home for the first time and for both undergraduate and postgraduate students, relationship issues, financial stresses, family bereavement, or illness (Dyrbye et al., 2005).

A systematic review of studies of American and Canadian medical schools suggests a high prevalence of depression and anxiety among medical students with levels of overall psychological distress that are consistently higher than in the general population as well as in age-matched peers (Dyrbye et al., 2006). Similarly, another meta-analysis reported a global prevalence of depression amongst medical students to be 27.2%—a figure which is nearly treble the prevalence of age-matched peers (Rotenstein et al., 2016). These are worrying levels of psychological distress in this student population. Furthermore, not only is there a moral imperative that medical training shouldn't harm those undergoing it—there is also the significant issue of the future wellbeing of the medical workforce. As earlier age of onset of first episode of depression and the number of previous episodes may increase the risk of recurrence (Burcusa & Iacono, 2007)—the elevated rates of depression evident amongst medical students could potentially increase the risk of depression amongst practising doctors.

Who Is Responsible for the Wellbeing of Medical Students?

Often the rhetoric around the wellbeing of qualified doctors focusses on building individual resilience (Howe et al., 2012). However, research evidence clearly demonstrates that lthough individual factors play a part, the primary drivers of occupational wellbeing are

Anna Collini and Caroline Elton, *How Can Medical Students Look After Themselves?* In: *The Mental Health of Medical Students.*
Edited by: Andrew Molodynski, Sarah Marie Farrell, and Dinesh Bhugra, Oxford University Press. © Oxford University Press 2024.
DOI: 10.1093/oso/9780192864871.003.0031

systemic—including having a manageable workload, being adequately trained for the job, and feeling that one is part of a team (Shanafelt & Noseworthy, 2017). The same is likely to hold true for the psychological wellbeing of medical students. Although some studies of this population have focussed on building individual resilience (Seo et al., 2021), others have argued the main problem often originates from the environment in which the students are learning, rather than lack of resilience in the students themselves (Slavin, 2016). Seo et al. have highlighted features of the medical school environment that can have a positive impact on medical student wellbeing such as implementing pass-fail grading systems, reduction of pre-clinical and clinical contact hours, and educating faculty about medical student distress (Seo et al., 2021). However, even if environmental factors, rather than lack of individual resilience are the most significant drivers of medical student wellbeing this doesn't mean that medical students are powerless in this respect—as will be outlined in the rest of this chapter.

Understanding Wellbeing

The first question to consider is what exactly is meant by the term 'wellbeing'. Within the field of physician and medical student wellbeing, this has often been seen as the absence of mental distress—burnout, depression, or other symptoms of mental illness (Brady et al., 2018). However, as emphasized by the positive psychology movement and the World Health Organization (WHO) in their definition of health, wellbeing should not only be seen as an *absence* of mental or physical illness (Sheldon & King, 2001; World Health Organization, 2005). Wellbeing should also encompass the ability to thrive. Brady et al. described four domains in their definition of physician wellness—mental, physical, social, and integrated wellbeing. How students can promote wellbeing in each of these domains will be discussed in this chapter, but it is important to note that these are difficult to separate out entirely from each other due to their inter-related nature. Wellbeing should also be seen as a dynamic state—a balancing act between challenges faced, and the psychological, physical, and social resources an individual has to cope with these (Dodge et al., 2012). Many of the challenges that students face will require systemic changes at an institutional, or even pan-institutional level—for example altering the examination system or the national medical curriculum. Other challenges may require students to become more willing to ask for help and to access pastoral, financial, or psychological support.

Enhancing Mental Wellbeing

It is important to note that mental wellbeing is closely intertwined with all the other aspects of wellbeing described next. Whilst mental wellbeing is often characterized as the lack of psychological distress, such as burnout or symptoms of mental health disorders, it can also encompass positive aspects such as a healthy self-image, self-acceptance, and resilience (Feeney & Collins, 2015).

Throughout medical school, students are forming a professional identity and learning 'to think, act and feel like a physician' (Cruess et al., 2014, p. 1447). Much of this is learnt through observing and modelling the behaviour of others within their social group, which can perpetuate unachievable or sometimes negative ideals (Miles, 2020). Medicine still appears to have a culture of perfectionism where doctors are expected to perform without error, and this may be felt by medical students (Bynum et al., 2021). Historically there was an ideal that doctor's should be immune to feeling anything of the patient's suffering. As an example, William Osler expressed in his essay 'Aequanimitas' an ideal that the doctor should aspire to a form of emotional detachment characterized by—'a callousness which thinks only of the good to be effected' (Osler, 1906, p. 5). Contemporary researchers now advocate that there needs to be a balance between having compassion and empathy for patients without being overwhelmed by the emotional labour inherent in confronting suffering (Miles, 2020).

Students on clinical placements will be exposed to the suffering of others and other potentially traumatic experiences. Such exposure has the potential to be experienced as moral injury if the standards of care that patients receive falls far short of that which the students expect—where the students feel there has been a transgression of their strongly held beliefs about the world (Murray et al., 2018). Moral injury can result in feelings of guilt and shame—with shame in particular being a painful emotion. Where guilt can be seen as feeling bad because of a behaviour, shame is to feel negatively about yourself as a person—'believing we are flawed' (Brown, 2006, p. 45). Moral injury is not the only potential source of shame at medical school. Bynum et al. describe a complex interplay of personal and environmental characteristics that contribute to shame reactions in response to individual triggers (Bynum et al., 2021). Whilst many of these characteristics are outside of students, control, others are able to be modified. They found that some students experienced shame during normal learning processes, for example getting something wrong or receiving negative feedback. This was associated with a fixed mindset—the idea that their ability was innate and unchangeable, and performance-based self esteem—where their self-worth is dependent on the level at which they feel they are performing. Bynum et al. suggest that educators and learners can modify these characteristics through realistic goal setting, seeing struggle as a challenge rather than a threat, and developing self-awareness of shame. Shame is a normal and universal human emotion—we cannot and perhaps should not eliminate it, but it is possible to become more resilient to it. Brené Brown's shame resilience theory emphasizes the importance of interpersonal connection and an empathetic response to an experience of shame (Brown, 2006). This can be challenging, as shame may often cause people to socially withdraw. However, finding somewhere safe to share these experiences is likely to improve wellbeing. This may be with informal support networks such as friends and family, professional support services, or peer support.

Many universities and healthcare providers have recognized the need to create spaces for reflection on the challenges of medical practice—the uncertainties, errors, and particularly the emotional impact of working in healthcare. These take different forms in different places but include Balint groups (Monk et al., 2018), Schwartz rounds (The Schwartz Centre, 2022), and other forms of peer support. Seeing others experiencing these emotional challenges can help normalize them, may reduce shame and create a more realistic ideal professional self. Often these offerings are voluntary, but by participating students help not only themselves but others too. Not all students will feel comfortable talking about their experiences, and for these students expressive writing may be an alternative. It has been shown that talking or writing about emotional experiences can benefit both mental and physical wellbeing (Pennebaker & Chung, 2011).

To conceptualize resilience, we can return to the idea of wellbeing as a balance between challenges and resources. A resilient individual is able to use their resources and maintain their wellbeing despite adversity. Whilst it appears obvious that promoting resilience is a good thing, valid concerns have been raised that focussing on resilience places the responsibility firmly on the individual rather than the flawed systems they work in (Oliver, 2017). This can create a negative bias towards interventions to improve wellbeing such as mindfulness, yoga, or practising gratitude. However, the individual vs. the systemic perspectives are not in fact incompatible—both have the potential to contribute to a student's wellbeing (West et al., 2018).

Mindfulness has evolved from its Buddhist roots into a well-established practice within Western medical and psychological culture, and has been associated with improved psychological wellbeing (Keng et al., 2011). In simple terms it can be described as 'a process of bringing a certain quality of attention to moment-by-moment experience' (Bishop et al., 2004, p. 230). Mindfulness is often taught through meditation, where individuals aim to keep their attention on a specific focus, commonly their own breathing, but sometimes other physical sensations such as points of contact between the body and the floor or chair, or by focussing on sounds in the room. They should notice when their attention naturally wanders away from this focus, and gently bring themselves back to the physical sensations or to the sounds. Bishop et al. describe two aspects to mindfulness—self-regulation of attention and orientation to experience (Bishop et al., 2004). Self-regulation of attention is that part of mindfulness where an individual is able to sustain their attention on a particular focus. Thoughts, feelings, and sensations are noticed and acknowledged but not elaborated on. By bringing the focus back to physical sensations in the body, trains of thought are interrupted, allowing the focus to remain on the current moment. Bishop describes the importance of the orientation an individual takes to their experience and how this should be one of curiosity and openness. This involves noticing where the mind wanders to, accepting the experience for what it is and not trying to change particular thoughts or feelings (Bishop et al., 2004).

How might this help? There is evidence that the skills learned through meditation are likely to be used at other times, which may be how mindfulness leads to its positive psychological effects. It is thought it may prevent negative self-critical ruminations by interrupting these trains of thought and the practice can also promote an open, curious and accepting mindset (McConville et al., 2017). Mindfulness has also been linked to increased empathy in healthcare students (McConville et al., 2017), and has been recognized as important to practising as a doctor (Epstein, 1999). The practice of mindfulness allows more cognitive space to listen and understand, and to become more aware of our own judgements and biases. Living mindfully will be unique to each individual, and students should think about what helps them be 'in the moment'. This may be formal meditation practices, physical activity (particularly yoga and martial arts), activities that provide a sense of 'flow', or just noticing the world around you while out for a walk.

Another practice that has been associated with improved mental wellbeing is practising gratitude—'the appreciation of what is valuable and meaningful to oneself and represents a general state of thankfulness and/or appreciation' (Sansone & Sansone, 2010, p. 18). This can be done in a number of ways, such as keeping a journal, writing down individual things you are grateful for at the end of each week or genuinely thanking people to demonstrate your gratitude. One of the authors (CE) keeps a folder of thank-you notes from former clients and has found it can be helpful to read through the folder when work is particularly challenging.

Enhancing Physical Wellbeing

Physical wellbeing can be described as having a sense of physical fitness—being of a healthy weight, participating in physical activity, and a relative lack of illness or disease (Feeney & Collins, 2015). Looking after our bodies is an act of self-care and can take many forms, depending upon personal preference and fitness levels. Physical activity is beneficial for the body through numerous mechanisms, leading to a reduction in the risk of chronic disease and improved psychological wellbeing (Warburton, 2006). Exercise may also contribute to integrated wellbeing as described next, and if done as part of a team can have social benefits. A good quality diet not only improves physical health, but is also associated with improved mental health (Firth et al., 2020). Many students may be learning how to make their own food for the first time, in addition to the financial and cultural influences that will affect what they eat. A diet that includes healthy fats, fruits, vegetables, and high fibre foods as well as limited 'fast foods' is likely to contribute to physical wellbeing.

Sleep is essential for health, but sleep disturbance appears to be more common in medical students compared to other populations, perhaps due to the academic demands of medical training and out of hours working (Azad et al., 2015). This is likely to impact on wellbeing, as poor sleep is associated with various physical and mental disorders as well as affecting cognition and the ability to learn (Cvejic et al., 2018). There are a number of steps that can be taken to improve sleep quality, the following advice is based on the work of Dr Michael Farquhar, a sleep specialist with an interest in doctors' wellbeing (Farquhar, 2017). The place where one sleeps should be cool, comfortable, and as dark as possible, using blackout blinds or curtains if necessary. In addition to minimizing light, the room needs to be as quiet as possible; white noise machines or ear plugs can help achieve this in noisier environments. A sleep routine is helpful for promoting good-quality sleep and includes going to bed and waking up at similar times each day, winding down beforehand, and avoiding electronics for an hour before sleeping. Exposure to natural light during the daytime, exercise, regular meals (with an evening meal more than two hours before bedtime) and minimizing alcohol and caffeine intake is also beneficial.

Medical students, particularly those who are struggling with their wellbeing, may misuse alcohol or illicit drugs and this can be harmful for wellbeing (World Health Organization, 2022). Significant levels of harmful drinking and cannabis use have been found in medical students, although this unsurprisingly varies between cultures (Molodynski et al., 2021). In addition, misuse of drugs or alcohol runs the risk of a student's fitness to practise being called into question. In turn, this could impact on their ability to finish their studies and qualify as a doctor. In the UK, this would include driving under the influence of alcohol or drugs, or exhibiting a pattern of consumption that impairs performance at medical school (General Medical Council, 2016). Students should get help to cut down or stop drinking alcohol if they find themselves drinking alcohol every day, if their drinking gets them into trouble or other people express concerns about their levels of drinking (NHS, 2022). The General Medical Council (GMC) also considers possession or supply of drugs a fitness to practise issue, even if no legal proceedings result from the incident. Medical students need to be mindful of the potential consequences of being found with even small amounts of illegal drugs; if they find themselves developing a pattern of regular use, they should seek help.

Enhancing Social Wellbeing

Social wellbeing comes from the meaningful relationships we have with others, which can be seen to fulfil two main functions—to act as a source of support in times of stress, and to provide opportunities for personal growth (Feeney & Collins, 2015). Loneliness seems to be a significant factor for psychological distress in students (Brown, 2018) and it appears that having support from friends at university is particularly important for wellbeing (Byrnes et al., 2020; McIntyre et al., 2018). It is not surprising that the transition to university, often involving moving away from home and building a new social network, can be a stressful period for students (Chew-Graham et al., 2003). The recent COVID-19 pandemic has had a significant impact on the ability of students to connect with each other and with faculty (Leal Filho et al., 2021), and the long-term implications of this are still unclear.

Strong social relationships can help students manage the challenges they face during medical training. Feeny and Collins describe how relationships can be seen as a 'safe haven'—a space where negative emotions can be expressed and comfort, understanding and reassurance given (Feeney & Collins, 2015). They also describe how one student can support another to overcome challenges through helping them develop their strengths and abilities, and keeping them motivated (Feeney & Collins, 2015). However, social relationships do more than just provide support during difficult times; such relationships also allow us to thrive by encouraging us to seize opportunities and achieve our goals. Our relationships with others help us to grow through exposure to different perspectives, opinions, and interests. Social media is increasingly used as a way of forming social connections, and can be a positive way to build social capital and a sense of community (Ryan et al., 2017). However, as with most things, it should be used in moderation as it appears that intensive social media use is associated with lower wellbeing (Valkenburg, 2022). Most universities run social events and offer clubs and societies which may allow students to continue with an existing interest or to try something new, helping students to form social connections and build a sense of belonging. Successful relationships need nurturing, an investment in building our side of the bridge. Reaching out to others can sometimes feel risky—what if we are rejected?—but a certain amount of vulnerability is inevitable until a strong bond is formed.

Enhancing Integrated Wellbeing

Integrated wellbeing can be seen to incorporate the following constructs—overall quality of life, spiritual wellbeing, and 'eudaimonic wellbeing' (Brady et al., 2018). Eudaimonic wellbeing can be described as 'having purpose and meaning in life' (Feeney & Collins, 2015, p. 115), with spiritual wellbeing referring to the feeling of being part of something bigger than ourselves. This can be religious, or secular—for example being outside in the natural world (Mayer & Frantz, 2004). The activities that contribute to this sense of wellbeing will be different for each individual, but are likely to be things that allows the student to be themselves authentically (Brady et al., 2018). This could include many of the activities described earlier in this chapter—physical activity, social interaction, or mindfulness as examples. Often it will be activities that provide a sense of control, progression towards a goal, or mastery of a skill. For some students this may be their studies at medical school, for others it may be participating in sports or something creative. Traditionally the scientific nature of the medical degree does not leave much space for creativity, but there has been increasing recognition that the arts and humanities can play an important role within medical education (Dennhardt et al., 2016). These can allow the expression of emotion and forge connections with others (Younie, 2021), as well as increase feelings of autonomy and mastery as described earlier, and should be encouraged in those students who feel they would benefit.

Time management is a key part of successfully managing work life integration (Picton, 2021). Students should be advised to consider what their priorities are, and to make time for activities that give them a sense of wellbeing. These priorities will be dynamic—there will be times when workload is heavier, for example around exam time, when studying may take precedence over other activities for a short period. Seeking support to manage these competing priorities may be beneficial—from friends, family, or the university support services. Often universities offer free advice to help students to work more efficiently, maximizing their study skills. Creating boundaries can also be helpful, these may be temporal in nature—where a specific time is dedicated to a specific activity, or environmental—where work is done in a separate environment (for example on campus) from other aspects of life (Picton, 2021). Maintaining these boundaries has been particularly challenging during the COVID-19 pandemic, with the move for many to online learning from home rather than on campus. However, there are creative ways to separate work and home life even if these all take place in the same environment—for example, a short 5-minute walk after finishing work for the day.

Making space for activities beyond students' formal studies will not always be easy, and students will typically have other demands on their time, energy, and financial resources. It is also worth recognizing that within medicine there has been a culture of altruism, where the needs of others are seen to come before your own (Bishop & Rees, 2007), and this may act as a psychological barrier to setting aside time to prioritize one's own wellbeing. From the outset of their studies it should therefore be stressed to students that making time for activities that enhance their quality of life is not only critical for their own wellbeing, but ultimately may contribute to improved patient safety when they are practising as doctors (Hall et al., 2016).

Asking for Help

Although this chapter has focussed on how medical students can best look after themselves, it is important to point out that often the best way for students to maximize their own wellbeing is to seek help from others. Universities often offer a range of services and opportunities to promote wellbeing, which may go beyond academic and mental health support. Both the universities where the authors work (King's College London and Norwich Medical School, respectively) have initiatives to promote physical health and social wellbeing, one-to-one academic and pastoral support through personal tutoring, and offer general study skills advice. In addition, students in both universities have access to personal counselling and mental health services. Asking for help is not always easy, and with medical students there appear to be additional barriers preventing them from doing so. The body of literature examining this phenomenon mainly focusses on barriers to accessing support for mental wellbeing, but it appears that students may be reluctant to seek help for academic issues too (Cleland et al., 2005; Stegers-Jager et al., 2011).

Stigma appears to be a considerable barrier to seeking help for mental health problems (Chew-Graham et al., 2003; Clement et al., 2015; Gulliver et al., 2010; Shahaf-Oren et al., 2021). Often this is due to a dissonance between how people see themselves and their beliefs about people with mental health issues (Clement et al., 2015). These beliefs may include that people who struggle with their mental health are weak or a failure, which is in particular contrast to the 'ideal' medical student as someone who is strong, healthy and high achieving (Shahaf-Oren et al., 2021). Healthcare professionals have an identity as a healer, not as someone who becomes unwell. In addition to this self-stigma, there are also often concerns about confidentiality and whether disclosing a mental health issue will impact on their career prospects, particularly in relation to fitness to practice decisions (Chew-Graham et al., 2003; Shahaf-Oren et al., 2021). In the UK, the GMC has made it clear that they support doctors with mental health conditions to continue practising as long as they are able to care for patients safely. This involves having insight into their condition, asking for help, receiving treatment if required, and taking time off if needed (General Medical Council, 2021). However, not all licencing bodies take this approach. There is concern in the USA that medical licensure boards are asking inappropriate questions about doctors' mental health, and this discourages them from seeking help (Jones et al., 2018). It is important to reframe how we see the 'ideal' medical student or doctor. Rather than someone who is able to manage everything alone, the ideal should be presented as someone who is self-aware and asks for help when they need it.

Other barriers to seeking help appear to be difficulties with identifying symptoms of poor mental health and knowing when to seek help for these (Gulliver et al., 2010; Shahaf-Oren et al., 2021; Velasco et al., 2020). It may be that poor wellbeing is normalized in medical training—students expect it to be difficult (Winter et al., 2017). We need to be able to challenge this narrative without pathologizing the normal challenges faced during medical school. If students are unsure whether they need help, speaking to a trusted friend, family member, or someone at the medical school is a good first step to think through the options and services that may be available to them. Students should be encouraged to seek help if they are often feeling worried, struggling to get enjoyment from things, or having thoughts and feelings that are problematic and affecting their studies and/or their personal lives (MIND).

Conclusion

Medical students face significant challenges to their wellbeing, and there is a need for systemic change to address these. However, students are able to influence their own wellbeing through living mindfully, practising gratitude, exercising, eating well, sleeping well, and making connections with others. Making time for this, and any other activities that bring enjoyment, is not easy whilst at medical school or when working as a doctor. However, students should be encouraged and supported to practise self-care, and to keep this habit when working as doctors—we must look after ourselves to be able to look after others. This includes asking for help, something that many of us (including both authors) find challenging, but ultimately hugely beneficial.

References

Azad, M.C. *et al.* (2015) 'Sleep Disturbances among Medical Students: A Global Perspective', *Journal of Clinical Sleep Medicine*, 11(01), pp. 69–74.

Bishop, J.P. and Rees, C.E. (2007) 'Hero or has-been: Is there a future for altruism in medical education?', *Advances in Health Sciences Education*, 12(3), pp. 391–399.

Bishop, S.R. *et al.* (2004) 'Mindfulness: A proposed operational definition', *Clinical Psychology: Science and Practice*, 11(3), pp. 230–241.

Brady, K.J.S. *et al.* (2018) 'What Do We Mean by Physician Wellness? A Systematic Review of Its Definition and Measurement', *Academic Psychiatry*, 42(1), pp. 94–108.

Brown, B. (2006) 'Shame Resilience Theory: A Grounded Theory Study on Women and Shame', *Families in Society: The Journal of Contemporary Social Services*, 87(1), pp. 43–52.

Brown, J.S.L. (2018) 'Student mental health: some answers and more questions', *Journal of Mental Health*, 27(3), pp. 193–196.

Burcusa, S.L. and Iacono, W.G. (2007) 'Risk for recurrence in depression', *Clinical Psychology Review*, 27(8), pp. 959–985.

Bynum, W.E. *et al.* (2021) '"I'm unworthy of being in this space": The origins of shame in medical students', *Medical Education*, 55(2), pp. 185–197.

Byrnes, C. *et al.* (2020) 'Medical student perceptions of curricular influences on their wellbeing: a qualitative study', *BMC Medical Education*, 20(1), p. 288.

Chew-Graham, C.A., Rogers, A. and Yassin, N. (2003) '"I wouldn't want it on my CV or their records": medical students' experiences of help-seeking for mental health problems', *Medical Education*, 37(10), pp. 873–880.

Cleland, J., Arnold, R. and Chesser, A. (2005) 'Failing finals is often a surprise for the student but not the teacher: identifying difficulties and', *Medical Teacher*, 27(6), pp. 504–508.

Clement, S. *et al.* (2015) 'What is the impact of mental health-related stigma on help-seeking? A systematic review of quantitative and qualitative studies', *Psychological Medicine*, 45, pp. 11–27.

Cruess, R.L. *et al.* (2014) 'Reframing medical education to support professional identity formation', *Academic Medicine*, 89(11), pp. 1446–1451.

Cvejic, E., Huang, S. and Vollmer-Conna, U. (2018) 'Can you snooze your way to an "A"? Exploring the complex relationship between sleep, autonomic activity, wellbeing and performance in medical students', *Australian & New Zealand Journal of Psychiatry*, 52(1), pp. 39–46.

Dennhardt, S. *et al.* (2016) 'Rethinking research in the medical humanities: a scoping review and narrative synthesis of quantitative outcome studies', *Medical Education*, 50(3), pp. 285–299.

Dodge, R. *et al.* (2012) 'The challenge of defining wellbeing', *International Journal of Wellbeing*, 2(3), pp. 222–235.

Dyrbye, L.N., Thomas, M.R. and Shanafelt, T.D. (2005) 'Medical Student Distress: Causes, Consequences, and Proposed Solutions', *Mayo Clinic Proceedings*, 80(12), pp. 1613–1622.

Dyrbye, L.N., Thomas, M.R. and Shanafelt, T.D. (2006) 'Systematic Review of Depression, Anxiety, and Other Indicators of Psychological Distress Among U.S. and Canadian Medical Students':, *Academic Medicine*, 81(4), pp. 354–373.

Epstein, R.M. (1999) 'Mindful Practice', *JAMA*, 282(9), pp. 833–839.

Farquhar, M. (2017) 'Fifteen-minute consultation: problems in the healthy paediatrician—managing the effects of shift work on your health', *Archives of disease in childhood - Education & practice edition*, 102(3), pp. 127–132.

Feeney, B.C. and Collins, N.L. (2015) 'A New Look at Social Support: A Theoretical Perspective on Thriving Through Relationships', *Personality and Social Psychology Review*, 19(2), pp. 113–147.

Firth, J. *et al.* (2020) 'Food and mood: how do diet and nutrition affect mental wellbeing?', *BMJ*, 369, p. m2382.

General Medical Council (2016) *Professional behaviour and fitness to practice: guidance for medical schools and their students*. London: General Medical Council.

General Medical Council (2021) *When does the regulator get involved in a doctor's mental health?*, *General Medical Council*. Available at: https://gmcuk.wordpress.com/2021/10/11/when-does-the-regulator-get-involved-in-a-doctors-mental-health/ (Accessed: 24 March 2022).

Gulliver, A., Griffiths, K.M. and Christensen, H. (2010) 'Perceived barriers and facilitators to mental health help-seeking in young people: a systematic review', *BMC Psychiatry*, 10(1), p. 113.

Hall, L.H. *et al.* (2016) 'Healthcare Staff Wellbeing, Burnout, and Patient Safety: A Systematic Review', *PLOS ONE*, 11(7), p. e0159015.

Howe, A., Smajdor, A. and Stöckl, A. (2012) 'Towards an understanding of resilience and its relevance to medical training: Resilience and its relevance to medical training', *Medical Education*, 46(4), pp. 349–356.

Jones, J.T.R. *et al.* (2018) 'Medical Licensure Questions About Mental Illness and Compliance with the Americans With Disabilities Act', *The Journal of the American Academy of Psychiatry and the Law*, 46(4), p. 14.

Keng, S.-L., Smoski, M.J. and Robins, C.J. (2011) 'Effects of mindfulness on psychological health: A review of empirical studies', *Clinical Psychology Review*, 31(6), pp. 1041–1056.

Leal Filho, W. *et al.* (2021) 'Impacts of COVID-19 and social isolation on academic staff and students at universities: a cross-sectional study', *BMC Public Health*, 21(1), p. 1213.

MacLeod, R.D. *et al.* (2003) 'Early clinical exposure to people who are dying: learning to care at the end of life', *Medical Education*, 37(1), pp. 51–58.

Mayer, F.S. and Frantz, C.M. (2004) 'The connectedness to nature scale: A measure of individuals' feeling in community with nature', *Journal of Environmental Psychology*, 24(4), pp. 503–515.

McConville, J., McAleer, R. and Hahne, A. (2017) 'Mindfulness Training for Health Profession Students—The Effect of Mindfulness Training on Psychological Well-Being, Learning and Clinical Performance of Health Professional Students: A Systematic Review of Randomized and Non-randomized Controlled Trials', *EXPLORE*, 13(1), pp. 26–45.

McIntyre, J.C. *et al.* (2018) 'Academic and non-academic predictors of student psychological distress: the role of social identity and loneliness', *Journal of Mental Health*, 27(3), pp. 230–239.

Miles, S. (2020) 'Addressing shame: what role does shame play in the formation of a modern medical professional identity?', *BJPsych Bulletin*, 44(1), pp. 1–5.

MIND *Seeking help for a mental health problem*. Available at: https://www.mind.org.uk/information-support/guides-to-support-and-services/seeking-help-for-a-mental-health-problem/where-to-start/ (Accessed: 24 March 2022).

Molodynski, A. *et al.* (2021) 'Cultural variations in wellbeing, burnout and substance use amongst medical students in twelve countries', *International Review of Psychiatry*, 33(1–2), pp. 37–42.

Monk, A., Hind, D. and Crimlisk, H. (2018) 'Balint groups in undergraduate medical education: a systematic review', *Psychoanalytic Psychotherapy*, 32(1), pp. 61–86.

Murray, E., Krahé, C. and Goodsman, D. (2018) 'Are medical students in prehospital care at risk of moral injury?', *Emergency Medicine Journal*, 35(10), pp. 590–594.

NHS (2022) *NHS Live Well Alcohol Support, NHS Live Well*. Available at: https://www.nhs.uk/live-well/alcohol-advice/alcohol-support/ (Accessed: 7 April 2022).

Oliver, D. (2017) 'David Oliver: When "resilience" becomes a dirty word', *BMJ*, 358, p. j3604.

Osler, W. (1906) *Aequanimitas : with other addresses to medical students, nurses and practitioners of medicine*. 2nd ed. London: H. K. Lewis and Company.

Pennebaker, J.W. and Chung, C.K. (2011) 'Expressive Writing: Connections to Physical and Mental Health', in *The Oxford Handbook of Health Psychology*. Oxford University Press. Available at: https://doi.org/10.1093/oxfordhb/9780195342819.013.0018.

Picton, A. (2021) 'Work-life balance in medical students: self-care in a culture of self-sacrifice', *BMC Medical Education*, 21(1), p. 8.

Pisaniello, M.S. *et al.* (2019) 'Effect of medical student debt on mental health, academic performance and specialty choice: a systematic review', *BMJ Open*, 9(7), p. e029980.

Rotenstein, L.S. *et al.* (2016) 'Prevalence of Depression, Depressive Symptoms, and Suicidal Ideation Among Medical Students: A Systematic Review and Meta-Analysis', *JAMA*, 316(21), p. 2214.

Ryan, T. *et al.* (2017) 'How Social Are Social Media? A Review of Online Social Behaviour and Connectedness', *Journal of Relationships Research*, 8, p. e8.

Sansone, R.A. and Sansone, L.A. (2010) 'Gratitude and well being: the benefits of appreciation', *Psychiatry (Edgmont)*, 7(11), pp. 18–22.

Seo, C. *et al.* (2021) 'Addressing the physician burnout epidemic with resilience curricula in medical education: a systematic review', *BMC Medical Education*, 21(1), p. 80.

Shahaf-Oren, B., Madan, I. and Henderson, C. (2021) '"A lot of medical students, their biggest fear is failing at being seen to be a functional human": disclosure and help-seeking decisions by medical students with health problems', *BMC Medical Education*, 21(1), p. 599.

Shanafelt, T.D. and Noseworthy, J.H. (2017) 'Executive Leadership and Physician Well-being', *Mayo Clinic Proceedings*, 92(1), pp. 129–146.

Sheldon, K.M. and King, L. (2001) 'Why positive psychology is necessary', *American Psychologist*, 56(3), pp. 216–217.

Slavin, S.J. (2016) 'Medical Student Mental Health: Culture, Environment, and the Need for Change', *JAMA*, 316(21), p. 2195.

Stegers-Jager, K.M. *et al.* (2011) 'Academic dismissal policy for medical students: effect on study progress and help seeking behaviour', *Medical Education*, 45, pp. 987–994.

The Schwartz Centre (2022) *Schwartz Rounds*. Available at: https://www.theschwartzcenter.org/progr ams/schwartz-rounds/ (Accessed: 21 March 2022).

Valkenburg, P.M. (2022) 'Social media use and well-being: What we know and what we need to know', *Current Opinion in Psychology*, 45, p. 101294.

Velasco, A.A. *et al.* (2020) 'What are the barriers, facilitators and interventions targeting help-seeking behaviours for common mental health problems in adolescents? A systematic review', *BMC Psychiatry*, 20, p. 293.

Warburton, D.E.R. (2006) 'Health benefits of physical activity: the evidence', *Canadian Medical Association Journal*, 174(6), pp. 801–809.

Wear, D. (2002) '"Face-to-face with It": Medical Students' Narratives about Their End-of-life Education', *Academic Medicine*, 77(4), pp. 271–277.

West, C.P., Dyrbye, L.N. and Shanafelt, T.D. (2018) 'Physician burnout: contributors, consequences and solutions', *Journal of Internal Medicine*, 283(6), pp. 516–529.

Winter, R.I., Patel, R. and Norman, R.I. (2017) 'A Qualitative Exploration of the Help-Seeking Behaviors of Students Who Experience Psychological Distress Around Assessment at Medical School', *Academic Psychiatry*, 41(4), pp. 477–485.

World Health Organization (2005) *WHO Constitution*. Available at: https://www.who.int/about/gov ernance/constitution (Accessed: 17 January 2022).

World Health Organization (2022) *Global Information System on Alcohol and Health*, World Health Organisation. Available at: https://www.who.int/data/gho/data/themes/global-information-system-on-alcohol-and-health (Accessed: 7 April 2022).

Younie, L. (2021) 'What Does Creative Enquiry Have to Contribute to Flourishing in Medical Education', in E. Murray and J. Brown (eds) *The mental health and wellbeing of healthcare practitioners: research and practice*. First edition. Hoboken, NJ: Wiley, pp 14–27.

32
Aiming for Fulfilment

Grace W. Gengoux, Yamilka Alsina Martin, and Isheeta Zalpuri

Aiming for Fulfilment

Professional fulfilment is a key determinant of clinical success and career longevity for physicians. Enhancing professional fulfilment requires a deep understanding of the intrinsic motivators that drive so many diverse individuals to pursue a career in medicine. Many individuals choose a career in medicine because of a desire to help others, and often these individuals have naturally high levels of empathy and strong personal resilience (Akgün et al., 2020; West et al., 2020). Personal characteristics such as empathy and resilience can contribute to clinical success, especially when it comes to patient satisfaction. However, systemic factors in modern healthcare and pressures during training experiences can place even the most resilient and empathic medical students at risk for burnout—and these challenges are amplified for individuals from underrepresented minority backgrounds (Ahmad et al., 2021). The growing recognition of barriers to professional fulfilment has led to innovative changes in medical school curricula, which have been proposed in order to simultaneously mitigate risk for burnout among medical students, support the mental health of the increasingly diverse population of medical trainees, and harness the medical school period overall as a forum for teaching and implementing wellness practices that will lead to more fulfilling medical careers for graduates. This chapter begins by describing several foundational considerations related to professional fulfilment for medical trainees, including common motivations for pursuing a career in medicine, the structures that encourage medical students to make early, meaningful contributions to their field, and the role of resilience and self-valuation in preventing physician burnout. Next, there is a discussion of the importance of professional fulfilment for physicians in both the short and long-term and some of the particular fulfilment challenges and opportunities during the medical school years. Finally, the chapter concludes with a brief overview of some of the individually focused, as well as systems-focused, programmes that have been piloted to support medical student wellbeing and professional fulfilment.

Professional Motivation and Fulfilment

The stronger a physician's internal motivation to practice medicine, the better they may be able to handle the challenging demands of their profession. Motivating factors can be classified as extrinsic to the work, such as salary and schedule autonomy, or intrinsic to the work (Ratanawongsa et al., 2006) (see Figure 32.1). For instance, there is evidence that job demands, job control, electronic medical record, income, and other incentives, collegial

Grace W. Gengoux, Yamilka Alsina Martin, and Isheeta Zalpuri, *Aiming for Fulfilment* In: *The Mental Health of Medical Students*. Edited by: Andrew Molodynski, Sarah Marie Farrell, and Dinesh Bhugra, Oxford University Press. © Oxford University Press 2024. DOI: 10.1093/oso/9780192864871.003.0032

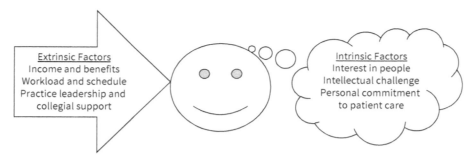

Figure 32.1 Extrinsic and intrinsic factors both influence professional fulfilment.

support, and practice leadership are all pertinent extrinsic mediating factors for physician career satisfaction (Friedberg et al., 2013; Scheurer et al., 2009). Intrinsic variables, such as self-expression and intellectual challenge, also play a crucial role in physician wellbeing and productivity. For instance, a survey conducted over the past three decades with a cohort of Finnish junior physicians indicated that 'interest in people' was a primary motive for studying medicine (Heikkilä et al., 2015). Strong intrinsic motivation seems to predict a satisfying career long-term (Schrijver et al., 2016). A national representative survey of 2000 US physicians measured wellbeing by five variables: career satisfaction, life satisfaction, meaning in life, commitment to direct patient care, and clinical commitment (Tak et al., 2017). Intrinsic motivators were associated with each measure of physician wellbeing, while extrinsic motivators were not associated with meaning in life or clinical commitment (Romero et al., 2020). Ratanawongsa and colleagues (2006) argue that career resilience hinges on physicians reflecting on and defining the sources of their intrinsic motivation (Ratanawongsa et al., 2006). Self-awareness of one's motivations can help physicians structure their work in a way that maximizes meaning and fulfilment in the long run.

While physicians as a group derive fulfilment from following their intrinsic motivation to help others, personal and demographic characteristics, such as gender differences, contribute to variability. Heikkilä and colleagues (2015) found that good salary and professional prestige were stronger motives for men, while vocation and interest in people were stronger motives for women. Additionally, emerging evidence suggests that younger generations of physicians value work-life balance more highly than older physicians (Cribari et al., 2019).

A strong understanding of the factors that motivate medical school applicants will help medical education programmes tailor their curricula and clinical clerkships to support long-term career satisfaction. Programmes that teach technical skills and teach students how to connect their work with the intrinsic values that inspired them to enter medicine in the first place will be helping these students derive a sense of meaning from their experiences.

Making Meaning in One's Profession

Search for meaning is a long-recognized human need. Aristotle argued that when humans strive to reach their potential, this effort gives their lives meaning and purpose. In her book, *The Power of Meaning,* author Emily Esfahani Smith notes that using your skills to help others is an important pillar of a meaningful life (Smith, 2017). Despite being a challenging profession, healthcare possesses a lot of inherent meaning. In fact, there are few professions with as much potential for meaning as a career in medicine. When clinicians can offer meaningful professional contributions, the benefits can be great, not only for the clinician's own wellbeing, but also for society as a whole.

While many aspects of medical practice can trigger physical and emotional exhaustion, an individual's sense that their work is meaningful can shield them from burnout and increase engagement and fulfilment (Shanafelt et al., 2009). This is one reason that it is important for professionals to feel valued and to feel that they are contributing to their field. In a study by Tak and colleagues, satisfaction with having found meaning in one's life and commitment to direct patient care were positively associated with a strong sense of calling (Tak, Curlin and Yoon, 2017), suggesting that clinicians are likely to thrive best in systems where they can do the work that brings them a sense of meaning.

Meaning making will inevitably be different for each individual. The fit between an individual's professional aspirations, values, strengths and the nature of their work will have a large impact on their professional and personal fulfilment in the long run (see Figure 32.2). In a study of 465 internal medicine physicians, Shanafelt and colleagues reported a strong inverse relationship between burnout and the amount of time these physicians spent in a given week doing the type of work they reported was most personally meaningful (Shanafelt et al., 2009). That is, rates of burnout were approximately doubled for doctors who spent less than 20% time in their most meaningful activity, compared to doctors who were spending more than 20% of their time engaged in the types of work they rated as most meaningful (whether clinical, research, education, or administration). A strong sense of meaning can also be actively cultivated by reflecting on one's underlying values and deliberately recalling how aspects of one's work relate to these values. Individuals who are able to mentally connect their daily tasks with outcomes they care about are likely to feel more engaged and satisfied at work (Gengoux et al., 2020).

At the start of their training, medical students are learning a vast amount of new content at a rapid pace. Increasingly, however, there is a recognition that contributing in innovative ways will enhance the medical student's engagement, learning, and sense of meaning, setting them up for a more fulfilling career (Jolly, 2009). For some medical students, the most meaningful work will be the chance to contribute to clinical care of a disease that has affected a loved one. For others, the chance to contribute to novel scientific discoveries or dissemination of research findings at conferences or through writing papers may be meaningful.

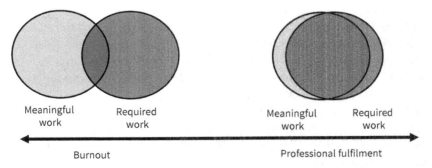

Figure 32.2 More overlap between meaningful work and required work leads to stronger professional fulfilment and prevents burnout.

For many, meaning may come from helping an underserved population access care. While medical students must receive broad and comprehensive training, connecting their work to a sense of personal meaning will help to buffer against burnout in the long-term. Instructors and clinical attendings can help medical students discover personal meaning in their work and can customize mentorship opportunities in order to help students discover a clinical specialty or role that resonates with them personally.

What professional fulfilment means to an individual may vary depending on cultural values. Disparities in health are already closely linked to class and race; wellness programming designed primarily for those who are already in positions of privilege will not adequately address the unique needs of minority groups (Kirkland, 2014). For first-generation physicians and those from ethnic and racial groups historically underrepresented in medicine (URM), visibility, support, and recognition will be even more important to achieving long-term professional fulfilment.

Resilience and Self-valuation

Burnout is a serious barrier to professional fulfilment. Burnout is typically described as a state of emotional exhaustion, depersonalization, and low personal accomplishment (Romani and Ashkar, 2014). Studies of practising physicians provide important clues about behaviours, cognitions, and coping strategies that might be critical to enhance during the medical school years, in order to increase the likelihood of long-term career satisfaction and resilience against burnout. While physician burnout is increasingly acknowledged as a major problem in healthcare (Shanafelt, Goh and Sinsky, 2017) and recent studies have shown that over 40% of physicians may experience burnout at some point in their careers (Yates, 2020), resilience and self-compassion have an inverse correlation to burnout (Atkinson et al., 2017). In addition, personal resources such as optimism and self-efficacy have been identified as key as buffers against perceived stress (Heinen, Bullinger and Kocalevent, 2017).

A cross-sectional national study of 5,445 US physicians found that they demonstrated higher levels of resilience than the general working population (West et al., 2020). However, burnout rates were considerable even among physicians with the highest levels of resilience. In other words, while maintaining or strengthening resilience is essential, there should also be an emphasis on alternative and complementary efforts, specifically those which address practice-related characteristics and external factors (e.g. regulatory requirements) that contribute to burnout (West et al., 2020).

In order to explore factors that lead to burnout in otherwise highly resilient populations, such as physicians, researchers at Stanford University have devised a self-valuation scale (Trockel et al., 2019). The scale was developed to try to better understand predictors of burnout. The concept of self-valuation is comprised of two components: 1) appropriate prioritization of self-care as opposed to deferring self-care and 2) growth mindset rather than self-condemnation. Physicians are likely to have difficulty with self-valuation due to aspects of clinical practice and medical culture. In order to value oneself, one must take an introspective approach, acknowledging one's own human limitations and prioritizing self-care even when rigid cultural norms prioritize caretaking of others (Trockel et al., 2021).

Compared to other workers, physicians have a lower sense of self-valuation. In a study of 250 physicians from five academic institutions, low self-valuation was associated with burnout and sleep-related impairment. Adjusting for self-valuation eliminated the association between being a physician and a higher chance of burnout (Trockel et al., 2021). It has been argued that understanding these factors and methods for enhancing resilience can serve as an antidote to help ameliorate burnout symptoms for doctors at every level of training (Shanafelt et al., 2022). To prevent and treat physician burnout and improve physician wellbeing, the authors argue that interventions to enhance physician self-valuation should be developed and tested. Such interventions could potentially address either harsh reactions to personal errors and imperfections or deferred self-care or both.

Self-valuation has not yet been investigated directly in medical students, but similar to physicians later in their careers, medical students show higher rates of psychological distress than age-matched peers (Baker & Sen, 2016a; Brazeau et al., 2014; Dyrbye et al., 2006). In fact, 28% of medical students show signs of depression (Dyrbye et al., 2006; Puthran et al., 2016), while anxiety, suicidal thoughts, and substance abuse are also present among students (Dyrbye et al., 2005). Despite these troubling statistics, individuals who choose to enter medical school as a group have many strengths and high potential for success. These individuals may have lower rates of burnout and depression than the general population before entering medical school. Unfortunately, studies show that many students may experience a decline in mental health during their enrollment in medical school. It is hypothesized that perceptions of stigma contribute to this lack of care-seeking behaviour (Thompson et al., 2016). Stress from academic demands, major stressful life events, harassment, or discrimination, low social support, and suboptimal learning environments contribute to the high prevalence of distress among medical students (Brazeau et al., 2014).

It will be critical for future studies to evaluate the role of self-valuation for medical students and to explore interventions that can help sustain their resilience during training.

Importance of Professional Fulfilment for Medical Students and Physicians

Professional fulfilment is a sign of optimal engagement in work over the long-term, and can be considered the opposite of burnout. Bohman and colleagues have developed a helpful model of professional fulfilment for physicians, which can also be informative when considering the goal of enhancing fulfilment for medical trainees (Bohman et al., 2017). In their model, the key drivers of fulfilment are 1) efficiency of practice, 2) culture of wellness, and 3) personal resilience. That is, an individual's own acts of self-care, which enhance their capacity for resilience in the face of stress, are critical but not sufficient for professional fulfilment. In addition, system supports must be in place that allow work to be completed in a timely and organized manner and that promote an overall culture of clinician wellbeing. For medical trainees, this model suggests that in addition to cultivating personal capacity to cope with stressful experiences, there is also a need to ensure that organizational aspects of the training environment, including both day-to-day training requirements and values expressed by interactions with supervisors, support the health and wellbeing of students. Enhancing professional fulfilment for medical students is important, given evidence that this type of positive engagement enhances learning in the short-term, and contributes to quality patient care and to career satisfaction for physicians in the long-term.

Fulfilment is associated with engagement and learning effectiveness (Ramalho et al., 2020). In a study of elective courses for medical students, the more satisfied students were with their educational experience, the greater their engagement was in learning. In contrast, medical students with higher levels of stress tend to have lower academic scores due to the negative effect of stress on working memory and decision-making (Waechter et al., 2021). Studies have shown that over time, medical students reduce their use of active coping strategies and increase use of emotional strategies. Emotional strategies are associated with poor academic performance in clinical years. These shifts in coping methods may be detrimental to student performance and learning. Therefore, improving students' ability to cope with stress and providing other forms of support should be an educational priority (Schiller et al., 2018). Access to elective programmes tailored to an individual's unique professional interests is a promising way to support student autonomy and enhance engagement in learning (Wiskin et al., 2018).

Strong professional fulfilment is also related to high quality patient care. For instance, researchers have documented a correlation between physician satisfaction and patient satisfaction (Shanafelt et al., 2017). Furthermore, there is a dose-response relationship between burnout and medical errors among residents and practising physicians (Trockel et al., 2018) and researchers have found links between burnout and suboptimal patient care behaviours, including not fully explaining treatment options or not adequately answering patient questions. There is a connection between physician job satisfaction and suboptimal prescribing habits, ordering of tests, and patient compliance with their physicians' advice (Shanafelt et al., 2017).

In the long-term, strong professional fulfilment will also contribute to career longevity. Data show that burnout and excessive workload are often the reason for physicians' early retirement (Silver et al., 2016). When physicians experience low job satisfaction, low job control, low morale, or feel undervalued, they may lose interest in their work and seek a career change. A Stanford University study on burnout published in 2018 showed high rates of turnover due to burnout: 26% of physicians surveyed reported burnout at baseline, and 28% said they planned to leave within two years. Two years later, 13% of the physicians surveyed had left the organization (Hamidi et al., 2018). In decades of research, diversity among healthcare students and physicians has been associated with better educational experiences, better patient care outcomes, and more culturally competent healthcare (Mason et al., 2022).

Challenges to Professional Fulfilment in Medical School

Medical professionals face serious risks during their training. First, there are obvious risks, such as long working hours, sleep deprivation, financial strain, and potential for mistreatment by authority figures. Working excessively long hours during residency may contribute to developing a deferred self-care habit (Trockel et al., 2019). Trainees may avoid or neglect their basic medical care (Dunn et al. 2009; Gross et al. 2000), perhaps under time pressure (Ey et al., 2013) or concerns about confidentiality or stigma (Roberts et al. 2005; Roberts et al. 2011). Academic pressures, heavy workload, and the need to apply classroom learning to *in vivo* clinical scenarios can be highly stressful for medical trainees (Dyrbye et al., 2006; Matheson et al., 2016). The hidden curriculum (Hafferty & Franks, 1994) may also expose trainees to an unrealistic ideal of perfectionism and self-sacrifice.

Moral distress is an additional facet of the psychological burden that clinicians face in patient care. As the term suggests, moral distress refers to the suffering that is caused by the moral subjectivity of care decisions or by acting in a way that violates one's professional or personal values due to a barrier or constraint (Kherbache et al., 2022). A clinician's wellbeing can be negatively impacted by repeated exposure to morally distressing situations. In a highly competitive environment, trainees are often taught that struggling is a normal part of their training process and that admitting to distress is a sign of weakness. Medical students may even be encouraged not to seek help when they are struggling (Baker & Sen, 2016a).

Finally, challenges associated with the COVID-19 pandemic have further exacerbated medical student mental health risk (Papapanou et al., 2022). Extensive use of online communication and learning solutions may negatively affect student wellbeing, causing increased isolation and conditions such as Zoom fatigue (Chakladar et al., 2022). In addition, insufficient in-person training and decreased clinical experience are perceived as obstacles by students, lowering trainee confidence when applying to residency positions. These additional barriers must be considered in the design of programmes to support professional fulfilment for the generation of students who completed portions of their training during the acute phases of the pandemic.

While medical students are a vulnerable group as a whole, throughout their training, URM medical students and LGBTQ + trainees experience higher rates of discrimination, isolation, and mental illness than their white, heterosexual, cisgender peers (Orom et al., 2013; Przedworski et al., 2015). Evidence shows that students from racial/ethnic minority groups and LGBTQ+ students are at substantial risk for depression (Hunt et al., 2015; Lapinski & Sexton, 2014; Przedworski et al., 2015). According to Dyrbye and colleagues (2019), non-white students had significantly higher rates of depression compared to white students enrolled in 49 medical schools. URM students experience unique burdens due to lack of support, discrimination, and lack of representation (Osseo-Asare et al., 2018). Medical students feel devalued by microaggressions and identify microaggressions as affecting their academic performance and personal wellbeing (Ackerman-Barger et al., 2020).

For those individuals who may be the first in their family to pursue higher education, starting a career can also be incredibly challenging. A trainee's vital social support network may be strained by time pressure and geographical separation from family (Irving et al. 2009). Whether or not they belong to a racial/ethnic or gender minority group, first-generation students suffer from a higher level of stress, physical and emotional fatigue, lower perceived social support, and are less likely to practice self-care (Gallegos et al., 2022). Along with lower grade point averages, first-generation students report less social and academic satisfaction (Mehta et al., 2011). First-generation students are also less involved, lack financial and social support, and do not prefer active coping strategies (Heinen, Bullinger and Kocalevent, 2017). There are fewer educational and administrative initiatives to support first-generation students. Many undergraduate colleges across the country have launched initiatives on university culture readiness, financial wellness, stereotype threat, imposter syndrome, psychological family stressors, and lack of professional-social networks in medical school. Unfortunately, medical schools do not typically offer similar programming (Gallegos et al., 2022).

In cultivating a culture of recognition, support, and inclusion in medical education, increasing awareness of the first-generation and underrepresented minorities experience is important. Diversity in medical education has been known to enrich discussions and better support students for providing culturally competent care. Communicating with diverse peers is also known to enhance students' educational experience (Whitla et al., 2003). URM students often go on to serve underrepresented minority communities (Thurmond & Kirch, 1998). The role of medical educators and leaders is critical to maximizing the potential of first-generation medical students. With more inclusive practices and culturally informed supports, medical trainees from historically marginalized and underserved populations will be uniquely poised to join and lead efforts combating structural injustices in medicine that result in countless health disparities and poor-quality healthcare. Diversity, inclusion, and equity are critical for improving the future state of healthcare delivery for all patients (Gallegos et al., 2022).

Enhancing Professional Fulfilment in Medical School

Interventions to improve wellbeing and reduce burnout risk for medical students have ranged widely in type (Jordan et al., 2019). Systematic reviews of interventions to decrease burnout and stress in medical students have indicated that a wide range of behavioural, cognitive, and mindfulness interventions may be useful to medical students (Williams et al., 2015). In addition, improvements in interpersonal communication and systemic supports can be critical for mitigating burnout (Baker & Sen, 2016). For example, many medical schools have developed programmes to assist medical students in accessing mental health resources (e.g. confidential counselling programmes) and didactic sessions focused on mental health (Thompson et al., 2010). Some programmes have provided access to elective programmes like Mindfulness Based Stress Reduction (Rosenzweig et al., 2003; Saunders et al., 2007; Slavin et al., 2014). While access to mental health treatment and wellness programming is critical, any successful intervention must be tailored to the busy schedules of medical students. Many authors have referenced the challenges of ensuring robust utilization of wellness programming (Waechter et al., 2021).

Increasingly, medical school programmes are also endeavouring to re-design educational programming and clinical experiences to better assist medical students in balancing life responsibilities during their training in preparation for a sustainable and fulfilling medical career (Waechter et al., 2021). Growing recognition of the pervasive wellbeing challenges experienced by medical students has led to a shift from primarily individually focused interventions to treat medical student distress to systemic modifications to training programmes for prevention of these challenges so that the experience of training does less harm to students (Moir et al., 2018; Slavin et al., 2014). In their article titled 'Medical Student Mental Health 3.0', Slavin et al. discuss how addressing root causes of stress within the curriculum and training experiences themselves is important (Slavin et al., 2014b). Consistent with the finding that system-focused interventions may be more effective than physician-focused interventions for burnout prevention in practising doctors (Panagioti et al., 2017), there is now increased acknowledgement of the need for multitiered approaches that can address both individual needs and institutional systems in medical education (Baker & Sen, 2016).

A number of medical schools have implemented targeted programmes supporting medical student wellness. For example:

1) Vanderbilt University School of Medicine developed a programme in 2005 (Drolet & Rodgers, 2010) with mentoring and advising, student leadership, and personal growth as core priorities.

2) UC Davis School of Medicine Office of Student Wellness started a programme that focused on principles related to ease of access, confidentiality and cultural humility, and transparency, and trust as they launched an educational campaign and platform for assessment and intervention related to medical student mental health. The authors reported that leadership commitment to student wellness has allowed for policy changes (e.g. more flexible student absence policy) and that utilization of mental health supports has increased along with student assessment of mental health (Seritan et al., 2015).

3) University of Hawaii John A. Burns School of Medicine maintains a programme focused on reducing symptoms of depression and suicidal ideation in medical students through improved access to confidential counselling, a curriculum for students (i.e. lectures and handbook), and faculty education.

4) Saint Louis University School of Medicine has implemented interventions including pass/fail grading, engagement with learning communities, reducing class time, and free time for longitudinal elective activities, which together have led to significant reductions in anxiety and depression experienced by first and second-year medical students relative to prior cohorts (Slavin et al., 2014).

While methodological limitations such as small sample size, lack of control groups, and heterogeneity across training year and rotation type make it difficult at present to definitively conclude from the existing literature which interventions are most effective (Baker & Sen, 2016; Shiralkar et al., 2013; Williams et al., 2015), preliminary results from these models suggest good potential for improving wellbeing for medical students through targeted interventions. In the next section, we review a range of the intervention types that have been tried to support medical student wellbeing generally, and which have particular promise for improving professional fulfilment during and after medical education.

Individual Interventions

Encouraging Self-Care and Providing Access to Wellness Programming

Medical students are human beings at different life stages with many different personal needs. Some medical students will themselves need medical care or disability accommodations during their training. Importantly, these diverse life experiences may also enhance a trainee's empathy as a future doctor. If a student's personal circumstances can be handled with compassion during training, this experience can ideally contribute to student learning. There is increasing recognition that patterns and habits established in medical school can either help or hinder a student's long-term health prospects (Dunn et al., 2008; Dyrbye et al., 2017). To effectively practice self-care, however, medical students also need role models who can demonstrate that self-care is consistent with excellent patient care.

The Liaison Committee in Medical Education requires medical schools to provide education on topics such as stress management and wellbeing to students and to provide access to activities to support mental and physical health during training. Access to counselling resources is a routine benefit offered by many medical schools. There is growing recognition of the need for special arrangements with off-site community providers not involved in the training programme, for reasons of confidentiality and ethical separation of roles (Roberts, 2016; Roberts & Termuehlen, 2022).

Evidence that self-compassion and mindfulness are associated with lower risk for burnout and greater resilience in medical trainees suggests that these may be promising targets for intervention during medical school (Dunn et al., 2008; Dyrbye et al., 2017). It has been suggested that wellness programming can be embedded directly into the medical education curriculum as a proactive way to enhance mental health during training (Drolet & Rodgers 2010; West et al., 2014). A number of studies have investigated the potential benefits of practices such as narrative medicine, stress-management instruction, and mindfulness courses. For instance, Wild and colleagues studied the effects of teaching relaxation techniques to mitigate anxiety and burnout symptoms expected to affect many medical students, given the inherent stresses introduced during medical training. The authors argue that integration of these practices into medical curricula should be considered (Wild et al., 2014). Waechter and colleagues evaluated random assignment to one of several mandatory wellness interventions (i.e. yoga, mindfulness, and walking programmes) and concluded that participation was associated with reduced anxiety and appeared to protect participants from increased stress observed in the control group. Overall satisfaction with the programme was positive (Waechter et al., 2021), supporting the argument that medical education programmes should increase support and offer programmes designed specifically to reduce distress during medical training.

The process of medical training may negatively affect the natural empathy of students. Some medical schools have designed programmes to help medical students sustain and deliberately cultivate empathy while they refine their technical skills. For instance, a wide variety of interventions have been explored and have demonstrated positive short-term impact on self-reported empathy, including programmes incorporating creative arts, writing, drama, interpersonal and communication skills training, as well as patient narratives, interviews, and experiential learning opportunities (Batt-Rawden et al., 2013).

Digital interventions may be helpful supplements to in-person programmes. The initial phase of response to the COVID-19 pandemic necessitated innovation regarding virtual opportunities for medical students to connect with each other and receive support for their mental health. In a programme at Vanderbilt University School of Medicine, Virtual Wellness and Learning Communities were initiated to provide support over a period of several months while medical students had to complete all of their learning online (Ahlers et al., 2021). Participating medical students reported increased peer connectivity (79% agreed) and improved wellness (61%). Over half of participants (55%) reported that they would like the events to continue to supplement in-person programming.

System Interventions: Changing the Learning Environment

The most common types of changes to the learning environment have been curricular changes like introduction of pass/fail grading systems and duty hour restrictions. Studies of duty hour restrictions have yielded mixed results regarding burnout prevention for medical trainees (Williams et al., 2015). Pass/fail grading systems have had more consistent positive reviews (Bloodgood et al., 2009; Robins et al., 1995; Rohe et al., 2006). While these changes may not directly impact fulfilment, they can mitigate burnout and negative mental health effects of training.

Slavin argues that modifications to the clinical environment, including manageable workload, fairness, and opportunities for mastery and control, as well as connection to community and meaning are also critical to consider in the design of clinical practice environments for medical students (Slavin, 2019). In a cross-sectional study of 400 students across three medical education programmes, one in Israel, one in Malaysia, and one in China, results indicated that students' favourable perception of the learning environment was related to their subjective wellbeing (Tackett et al., 2017). Having a community of peers was particularly important for quality of life and associated with reduced emotional exhaustion and lower levels of depersonalization.

Access to a wide range of electives during medical education has long been a core component of enhancing professional fulfilment for medical students. Allowing students to select aspects of their training experience is a way to individualize the curriculum and potentially tap into some of the intrinsic motivation that led the student to pursue medicine as a career (Mihalynuk et al., 2006). Students are likely to find experiences that they choose for themselves to be more satisfying. Students also gain valuable experience taking responsibility for their own professional education, a lifelong skill relevant for physicians. Compared to other aspects of medical education, there is limited published literature about optimal organizational structures and guidance related to design of elective opportunities (Jolly, 2009; Wiskin et al., 2018). In a study of 229 medical students in Portugal, agreement with teaching methodology and agreement with assessment methodology were strongly associated with overall satisfaction (Ramalho et al., 2020) supporting a student-centred approach. Students appreciate being continuously engaged in an elective, but satisfaction drops when there is an extensive workload outside of the designated elective time.

Regular assessment is critical for evaluating the impact of changes to a programme. The ACGME has formalized a requirement for training programmes to monitor fatigue and burnout in medical trainees, as part of the Clinical Learning Environment Review. In addition, having structures in place for iterative student feedback is critical to make sure curricular changes are enhancing meaning and delivering the promised benefits without undue burden on students.

The Role of Professional Networks

Mentorship.   Formal mentorship programmes are another important way schools can promote both career exploration and wellbeing. Mentors are role models who help shape their mentees' personal and professional development over time. Mentors provide input and guidance on research and clinical work, as well as career development and advancement. Mentors build the confidence, credibility, and competence needed to reach career milestones. A mentorship relationship is successful when the mentor acts as a coach who gives technical advice and works with the mentee to help them understand how to do something, while also creating psychological safety for the mentee and offering emotional support.

The traditional dyad model of mentorship is most frequently used in programmes, followed by a combination of group and dyad mentorship. Faculty time and salary support can be barriers to mentorships. A proposed solution is to use a combination of mentorship models. Group mentorship may be led by residents, as this may reduce the faculty time commitment and associated costs by improving the efficiency of individual meetings with faculty members (Farkas et al., 2019). In a successful mentorship relationship, mentees benefit from career advice, professional development, and individualized support, Simultaneously, mentors experience professional fulfilment by building meaningful relationships with students and providing support. Professional development has been identified as a strategy for resilience in medicine (Zwack).

Mentors who are willing to be vulnerable, self-reflect, and disclose some of their personal struggles with their mentees are able to encourage a growth mindset. Vulnerable students are often not adequately recognized or supported in the current medical education system. The culture of medicine makes it difficult for trainees to make mistakes or face their own shortcomings. In fact, the hidden curriculum in medicine tends to equate mistakes with failure. Luckily, mentors are able to identify students under distress early on. Mentors can destigmatize help seeking for mental health and model growth and acceptance of imperfection. An interesting study by Martin et al. found that having exposure to senior physicians who openly shared their lived experiences with mental illness had a measurable impact on medical students' attitudes about psychiatry in general and about individuals with mental illness. This intervention consisted not only of physicians' disclosures, but also facilitated discussions in small break-out groups, during which students could process and generalize their feelings (Martin et al., 2020).

Sponsorship.   While mentorship has its value, there is growing awareness that it may not be sufficient for career advancement, particularly for women and URM medical students. Women of colour are often implicitly asked to work harder for recognition than their peers who are white men and women of colour are also less likely to have supervisors promote their work contributions to others. Sponsorship is defined as active support by someone appropriately placed in the organization who has significant influence on decision-making processes or structures and who is advocating for, protecting, and fighting for the career advancement of an early career individual. For a medical student, a sponsor might be a resident, fellow, attending or someone in a position of leadership at the school of medicine. A sponsor might provide advice, make important connections to influential people, or provide opportunities such as collaborating on a presentation or co-authoring a manuscript. A sponsor can also publicly advocate for students in settings where they are not able to advocate for themselves. While mentorship is described as addressing one's overall longitudinal career development, sponsorship is characterized as episodic and focused on specific high-visibility opportunities. Mentors support through discussions about building skills and confidence, while sponsors promote proteges directly using influence and networks. Mentors help mentees to craft their career vision, whereas sponsors help drive their protege's career vision.

Coaching.   Coaching is a concept from the business world that is increasingly being recognized in the context of career development in medicine. Coaches are complementary to, but distinct from, mentors and advisors. Coaching uses inquiry, encouragement, accountability, and reflection to increase self-awareness, motivation, and the capacity to take effective action. Informal coaching, which is often buried within the hidden curriculum, can heavily impact students' career choices. Formal coaching programmes can help students to develop a comprehensive self-understanding of their aptitudes, interests, and personality traits (Farkas et al., 2019); explore possible career choices and decide on a career path (Martin et al., 2020); and develop the competencies needed to prepare for their future careers (Hur et al., 2018).

Given the unique challenges faced by URM medical students, intentional mentorship, sponsorship, and coaching opportunities for this group are essential. Ensuring 1:1 peer mentorship and faculty mentors for URM students can be crucial for their career development and wellbeing. Near-peer mentoring has been found to be beneficial for URM students (Youmans et al., 2020). One study found that mentored clerkships for URM medical students increased interest in applying to otolaryngology–head and neck surgery residency training programmes, hence also contributing to enhanced physician diversity in the field (Nellis et al., 2016).

Some examples of mentorship programmes that have been developed with the aim to promote career development, professional development, and wellbeing among medical students include:

1. The Johns Hopkins Department of Otolaryngology–Head and Neck Surgery a created a clerkship programme for underrepresented minority medical students. The programme included regular mentorship opportunities, where the mentor and student met to discuss clerkship goals, career goals, feedback, concerns, possible research interests, teaching, and career mentorship (Nellis et al., 2016).
2. Authors at Harbor-UCLA Medical Center and Mount Sinai Hospital evaluated the impact of a mentorship programme on burnout in fourth-year medical students during their emergency medicine (EM) subinternship, and found that the programme provided career guidance and professional fulfilment, positively impacted personal and professional development, and reduced stress for students (Jordan et al., 2019).
3. The Stanford Clinical Opportunity for Residency Experience (SCORE) brings fourth-year medical students from diverse backgrounds (underrepresented in medicine, socially, economically, or educationally disadvantaged) to Stanford for a four-week residential clinical training programme. SCORE students are matched with faculty and resident mentors who share similar clinical interests. The students participate in mentorship activities with a clinical advisor, as well as clinical rotations, programmes, and activities with Stanford medical students or a research advisor. In the year 2022, 25% (n = 17) of SCORE students matched at various residency programmes at Stanford.
4. Another mentorship programme that paired first year medical students in primary care with primary care mentors found that more students who participated in the mentoring programme had more fulfilling experiences and also were more likely to match into primary care specialties compared to non-participating students from the same medical school graduating class (Indyk et al., 2011).

Conclusion

The medical school experience provides a critical opportunity to prepare students for both the challenges and rewards of their future medical career. There is increasing recognition that substantive changes to medical education are needed in order to prevent burnout and encourage professional fulfilment. Many promising pilot programmes are emerging to serve as models. Attention during the training years to enhancing fulfilment and providing meaningful opportunities to contribute to the field will set students up for career success. Healthcare systems now face the challenge of providing extrinsic workplace conditions that allow physicians to practice in ways consistent with their values and intrinsic motivations (Bodenheimer and Sinsky, 2014; Shanafelt et al., 2022). More research is needed to explore how medical education programmes can best harness the full range of potential motivators driving clinical commitment and life satisfaction to help early career physicians build satisfying professional careers.

References

Ackerman-Barger, K. *et al.* (2020) 'Seeking Inclusion Excellence: Understanding Racial Microaggressions as Experienced by Underrepresented Medical and Nursing Students', *Academic Medicine: Journal of the Association of American Medical Colleges*, 95(5), pp. 758–763.

Ahlers, C.G. *et al.* (2021) 'A Virtual Wellness and Learning Communities Program for Medical Students during the COVID-19 Pandemic', *Southern Medical Journal*, 114(12), pp. 807–811.

Ahmad, H.S. *et al.* (2021) 'Improving Access to Medical Education for Underrepresented and Low-Income Students', *Academic Medicine*, 96(8), pp. 1077–1078.

Akgün, Ö. *et al.* (2020) 'Medical Students' Empathy Level Differences by Medical Year, Gender, and Specialty Interest in Akdeniz University', *Journal of Medical Education and Curricular Development*, 7, p. 2382120520940658.

Atkinson, D.M. *et al.* (2017) 'Examining Burnout, Depression, and Self-Compassion in Veterans Affairs Mental Health Staff', *The Journal of Alternative and Complementary Medicine*, 23(7), pp. 551–557.

Baker, K. and Sen, S. (2016) 'Healing Medicine's Future: Prioritizing Physician Trainee Mental Health', *AMA Journal of Ethics*, 18(6), pp. 604–613.

Batt-Rawden, S.A. *et al.* (2013) 'Teaching Empathy to Medical Students: An Updated, Systematic Review', *Academic Medicine*, 88(8), pp. 1171–1177.

Bloodgood, R.A. *et al.* (2009) 'A change to pass/fail grading in the first two years at one medical school results in improved psychological well-being', *Academic Medicine: Journal of the Association of American Medical Colleges*, 84(5), pp. 655–662.

Bodenheimer, T. and Sinsky, C. (2014) 'From Triple to Quadruple Aim: Care of the Patient Requires Care of the Provider', *The Annals of Family Medicine*, 12(6), pp. 573–576.

Bohman, B. *et al.* (2017) 'Physician Well-Being: The Reciprocity of Practice Efficiency, Culture of Wellness, and Personal Resilience', *NEJM Catalyst* [Preprint]. Available at: http://catalyst.nejm.org/doi/full/10.1056/CAT.17.0429 (Accessed: 16 May 2022).

Brazeau, C.M.L.R. *et al.* (2014) 'Distress Among Matriculating Medical Students Relative to the General Population', *Academic Medicine*, 89(11), pp. 1520–1525.

Chakladar, J. *et al.* (2022) 'Medical student's perception of the COVID-19 pandemic effect on their education and well-being: a cross-sectional survey in the United States', *BMC Medical Education*, 22(1), p. 149.

Cribari, M. *et al.* (2019) 'What makes internal medicine attractive for the millennial generation? A survey of residents in internal medicine in Switzerland', *Swiss Medical Weekly* [Preprint], (49).

Drolet, B.C. and Rodgers, S. (2010) 'A comprehensive medical student wellness program--design and implementation at Vanderbilt School of Medicine', *Academic Medicine: Journal of the Association of American Medical Colleges*, 85(1), pp. 103–110.

Dunn, L.B., Green Hammond, K.A. and Roberts, L.W. (2009) 'Delaying care, avoiding stigma: residents' attitudes toward obtaining personal health care', *Academic Medicine: Journal of the Association of American Medical Colleges*, 84(2), pp. 242–250.

Dunn, L.B., Iglewicz, A. and Moutier, C. (2008) 'A Conceptual Model of Medical Student Well-Being: Promoting Resilience and Preventing Burnout', *Academic Psychiatry*, 32(1), pp. 44–53.

Dyrbye, L.N. *et al.* (2019) 'A Prognostic Index to Identify the Risk of Developing Depression Symptoms Among U.S. Medical Students Derived From a National, Four-Year Longitudinal Study', *Academic Medicine: Journal of the Association of American Medical Colleges*, 94(2), pp. 217–226.

Dyrbye, L.N., Satele, D. and Shanafelt, T.D. (2017) 'Healthy Exercise Habits Are Associated With Lower Risk of Burnout and Higher Quality of Life Among U.S. Medical Students':, *Academic Medicine*, 92(7), pp. 1006–1011.

Dyrbye, L.N., Thomas, M.R. and Shanafelt, T.D. (2005) 'Medical student distress: causes, consequences, and proposed solutions', *Mayo Clinic Proceedings*, 80(12), pp. 1613–1622.

Dyrbye, L.N., Thomas, M.R. and Shanafelt, T.D. (2006) 'Systematic review of depression, anxiety, and other indicators of psychological distress among U.S. and Canadian medical students', *Academic Medicine: Journal of the Association of American Medical Colleges*, 81(4), pp. 354–373.

Ey, S. *et al.* (2013) '"If You Build It, They Will Come": Attitudes of Medical Residents and Fellows About Seeking Services in a Resident Wellness Program', *Journal of Graduate Medical Education*, 5(3), pp. 486–492.

Farkas, A.H. *et al.* (2019) 'Mentorship of US Medical Students: a Systematic Review', *Journal of General Internal Medicine*, 34(11), pp. 2602–2609.

Friedberg, M.W. *et al.* (2013) *Factors Affecting Physician Professional Satisfaction and Their Implications for Patient Care, Health Systems, and Health Policy*. RAND Corporation. Available at: https://www.rand.org/pubs/research_reports/RR439.html (Accessed: 21 April 2022).

Gallegos, A. *et al.* (2022) 'Visibility & support for first generation college graduates in medicine', *Medical Education Online*, 27(1), p. 2011605.

Gengoux, G.W. *et al.* (2020) *Professional Well-being: Enhancing Wellness Among Psychiatrists, Psychologists, and Mental Health Clinicians*. APA Publishing.

Gross, C.P. *et al.* (2000) 'Physician, heal Thyself? Regular source of care and use of preventive health services among physicians', *Archives of Internal Medicine*, 160(21), pp. 3209–3214.

Hafferty, F.W. and Franks, R. (1994) 'The hidden curriculum, ethics teaching, and the structure of medical education', *Academic Medicine: Journal of the Association of American Medical Colleges*, 69(11), pp. 861–871.

Hamidi, M.S. *et al.* (2018) 'Estimating institutional physician turnover attributable to self-reported burnout and associated financial burden: a case study', *BMC Health Services Research*, 18(1), p. 851.

Heikkilä, T.J. *et al.* (2015) 'Factors important in the choice of a medical career: a Finnish national study', *BMC Medical Education*, 15, p. 169.

Heinen, I., Bullinger, M. and Kocalevent, R.D. (2017) 'Perceived stress in first year medical students - associations with personal resources and emotional distress', *BMC Medical Education*, 17(1), p. 4. doi:10.1186/s12909-016-0841-8. PMID: 28056972; PMCID: PMC5216588.

Hunt, J.B. *et al.* (2015) 'Racial/Ethnic Disparities in Mental Health Care Utilization among U.S. College Students: Applying the Institution of Medicine Definition of Health Care Disparities', *Academic Psychiatry: The Journal of the American Association of Directors of Psychiatric Residency Training and the Association for Academic Psychiatry*, 39(5), pp. 520–526.

Hur, Y., Cho, A.R. and Kwon, M. (2018) 'Development of a systematic career coaching program for medical students', *Korean Journal of Medical Education*, 30(1), pp. 41–50.

Indyk, D. *et al.* (2011) 'The influence of longitudinal mentoring on medical student selection of primary care residencies', *BMC Medical Education*, 11(27), p. 1–7.

Irving, J.A., Dobkin, P.L. and Park, J. (2009) 'Cultivating mindfulness in health care professionals: a review of empirical studies of mindfulness-based stress reduction (MBSR)', *Complementary Therapies in Clinical Practice*, 15(2), pp. 61–66. doi: 10.1016/j.ctcp.2009.01.002. Epub 2009 Feb 28. PMID: 19341981.

Jolly, B. (2009) 'A missed opportunity', *Medical Education*, 43(2), pp. 104–105.

Jordan, J. *et al.* (2019) 'Impact of a Mentorship Program on Medical Student Burnout', *AEM Education and Training*. Edited by S.J. Cico, 3(3), pp. 218–225.

Kherbache, A., Mertens, E. and Denier, Y. (2022) 'Moral distress in medicine: An ethical analysis', *Journal of Health Psychology*, 27(8), pp. 1971–1990. doi:10.1177/13591053211014586. Epub 2021 May 2. PMID: 33938314.

Kirkland, A. (2014) 'Critical Perspectives on Wellness', *Journal of Health Politics, Policy and Law*, 39(5), pp. 971–988.

Lapinski, J. and Sexton, P. (2014) 'Still in the closet: the invisible minority in medical education', *BMC medical education*, 14, p. 171.

Martin, A. *et al.* (2020) 'Physician Self-disclosure of Lived Experience Improves Mental Health Attitudes Among Medical Students: A Randomized Study', *Journal of Medical Education and Curricular Development*, 7, p. 238212051988935.

Mason, H.R.C. *et al.* (2022) 'First-generation and continuing-generation college graduates' application, acceptance, and matriculation to U.S. medical schools: a national cohort study', *Medical Education Online*, 27(1), p. 2010291.

Matheson, K.M. *et al.* (2016) 'Experiences of Psychological Distress and Sources of Stress and Support During Medical Training: a Survey of Medical Students', *Academic Psychiatry: The Journal of the American Association of Directors of Psychiatric Residency Training and the Association for Academic Psychiatry*, 40(1), pp. 63–68.

Mehta, S.S. *et al.* (2011) 'Why do first-generation students fail?', *College Student Journal*, 45(1), pp. 20–36.

Mihalynuk, T. *et al.* (2006) 'Free choice and career choice: Clerkship electives in medical education', *Medical Education*, 40(11), pp. 1065–1071.

Moir, F. *et al.* (2018) 'Depression in medical students: current insights', *Advances in Medical Education and Practice*, Volume 9, pp. 323–333.

Nellis, J.C. *et al.* (2016) 'Impact of a mentored student clerkship on underrepresented minority diversity in otolaryngology-head and neck surgery', *The Laryngoscope*, 126(12), pp. 2684–2688.

Orom, H., Semalulu, T. and Underwood, W. (2013) 'The social and learning environments experienced by underrepresented minority medical students: a narrative review', *Academic Medicine: Journal of the Association of American Medical Colleges*, 88(11), pp. 1765–1777.

Osseo-Asare, A. *et al.* (2018) 'Minority Resident Physicians' Views on the Role of Race/Ethnicity in Their Training Experiences in the Workplace', *JAMA network open*, 1(5), p. e182723.

Panagioti, M. *et al.* (2017) 'Controlled Interventions to Reduce Burnout in Physicians: A Systematic Review and Meta-analysis', *JAMA Internal Medicine*, 177(2), p. 195.

Papapanou, M., Routsi, E., Tsamakis, K., Fotis, L., Marinos, G., Lidoriki, I., Karamanou, M., Papaioannou, T.G., Tsiptsios, D., Smyrnis, N., Rizos, E. and Schizas, D. (2022) 'Medical education challenges and innovations during COVID-19 pandemic', *Postgrad Med J.* 98(1159), pp. 321–327. doi: 10.1136/postgradmedj-2021-140032. Epub 2021 Mar 29. PMID: 33782202.

Przedworski, J.M. *et al.* (2015) 'A Comparison of the Mental Health and Well-Being of Sexual Minority and Heterosexual First-Year Medical Students: A Report From the Medical Student CHANGE Study', *Academic Medicine: Journal of the Association of American Medical Colleges*, 90(5), pp. 652–659.

Puthran, R. *et al.* (2016) 'Prevalence of depression amongst medical students: a meta-analysis', *Medical Education*, 50(4), pp. 456–468.

Ramalho, A.R. *et al.* (2020) 'Electives in the medical curriculum – an opportunity to achieve students' satisfaction?', *BMC Medical Education*, 20(1), p. 449.

Ratanawongsa, N., Howell, E.E. and Wright, S.M. (2006) 'What motivates physicians throughout their careers in medicine?', *Comprehensive Therapy*, 32(4), pp. 210–217.

Regehr, C. *et al.* (2014) 'Interventions to reduce the consequences of stress in physicians: a review and meta-analysis', *The Journal of Nervous and Mental Disease*, 202(5), pp. 353–359.

Roberts, L.W. (2016) *A Clinical Guide to Psychiatric Ethics*. American Psychiatric Association Publishing.

Roberts, L.W. and Termuehlen, G. (2022) *Professionalism and Eithcs: Q&A Self Study Guide for Mental Health Professionals, Second Edition*. American Psychiatric Association Publishing.

Roberts, L.W. *et al.* (2005) 'Medical student illness and impairment: a vignette-based survey study involving 955 students at 9 medical schools', *Comprehensive Psychiatry*, 46(3), pp. 229–237.

Roberts, L.W. *et al.* (2011) 'Medical students as patients: implications of their dual role as explored in a vignette-based survey study of 1027 medical students at nine medical schools', *Comprehensive Psychiatry*, 52(4), pp. 405–412.

Robins, L.S. *et al.* (1995) 'The effect of pass/fail grading and weekly quizzes on first-year students' performances and satisfaction', *Academic Medicine: Journal of the Association of American Medical Colleges*, 70(4), pp. 327–329.

Rohe, D.E. *et al.* (2006) 'The benefits of pass-fail grading on stress, mood, and group cohesion in medical students', *Mayo Clinic Proceedings*, 81(11), pp. 1443–1448.

Romani, M. and Ashkar, K. (2014) 'Burnout among physicians', *The Libyan Journal of Medicine*, 9, p. 10.3402/ljm.v9.23556.

Romero, R. *et al.* (2020) 'Understanding the Experiences of First-Generation Medical Students: Implications for a Diverse Physician Workforce', *Academic Psychiatry: The Journal of the American Association of Directors of Psychiatric Residency Training and the Association for Academic Psychiatry*, 44(4), pp. 467–470.

Rosenzweig, S. *et al.* (2003) 'Mindfulness-based stress reduction lowers psychological distress in medical students', *Teaching and Learning in Medicine*, 15(2), pp. 88–92.

Saunders, P.A. *et al.* (2007) 'Promoting self-awareness and reflection through an experiential mind-body skills course for first year medical students', *Medical Teacher*, 29(8), pp. 778–784.

Scheurer, D. *et al.* (2009) 'U.S. physician satisfaction: a systematic review', *Journal of Hospital Medicine*, 4(9), pp. 560–568.

Schiller, J. H. *et al.* (2018) 'Medical Students' Use of Different Coping Strategies and Relationship With Academic Performance in Preclinical and Clinical Years', *Teaching and Learning in Medicine*, 30(1), pp. 15–21.

Schrijver, I., Brady, K.J.S. and Trockel, M. (2016) 'An exploration of key issues and potential solutions that impact physician wellbeing and professional fulfilment at an academic center', *PeerJ*, 4, p. e1783.

Seritan, A.L. *et al.* (2015) 'The Office of Student Wellness: Innovating to Improve Student Mental Health', *Academic Psychiatry*, 39(1), pp. 80–84.

Shanafelt, T., Goh, J. and Sinsky, C. (2017) 'The Business Case for Investing in Physician Well-being', *JAMA Internal Medicine*, 177(12), pp. 1826–1832.

Shanafelt, T.D. *et al.* (2009) 'Career Fit and Burnout Among Academic Faculty', *Archives of Internal Medicine*, 169(10), p. 990.

Shanafelt, T.D. *et al.* (2022) 'Changes in Burnout and Satisfaction With Work-Life Integration in Physicians and the General US Working Population Between 2011 and 2020', *Mayo Clinic Proceedings*, 97(3), pp. 491–506.

Shiralkar, M.T. *et al.* (2013) 'A systematic review of stress-management programs for medical students', *Academic Psychiatry: The Journal of the American Association of Directors of Psychiatric Residency Training and the Association for Academic Psychiatry*, 37(3), pp. 158–164.

Silver, M.P. *et al.* (2016) 'A systematic review of physician retirement planning', *Human Resources for Health*, 14(1), p. 67.

Slavin, S. (2019) 'Reflections on a Decade Leading a Medical Student Well-Being Initiative', *Academic Medicine*, 94(6), pp. 771–774.

Slavin, S.J., Schindler, D.L. and Chibnall, J.T. (2014) 'Medical student mental health 3.0: improving student wellness through curricular changes', *Academic Medicine: Journal of the Association of American Medical Colleges*, 89(4), pp. 573–577.

Smith, E.E. (2017) *The Power of Meaning: Finding Fulfilment in a World Obsessed with Happiness*. Broadway Books.

Tackett, S. *et al.* (2017) 'International study of medical school learning environments and their relationship with student well-being and empathy', *Medical Education*, 51(3), pp. 280–289.

Tak, H.J., Curlin, F.A. and Yoon, J.D. (2017) 'Association of Intrinsic Motivating Factors and Markers of Physician Well-Being: A National Physician Survey', *Journal of General Internal Medicine*, 32(7), pp. 739–746.

Thompson, D., Goebert, D. and Takeshita, J. (2010) 'A program for reducing depressive symptoms and suicidal ideation in medical students', *Academic Medicine: Journal of the Association of American Medical Colleges*, 85(10), pp. 1635–1639.

Thompson, G. *et al.* (2016) 'Resilience Among Medical Students: The Role of Coping Style and Social Support', *Teaching and Learning in Medicine*, 28(2), pp. 174–182.

Thurmond, V.B. and Kirch, D.G. (1998) 'Impact of minority physicians on health care', *Southern Medical Journal*, 91(11), pp. 1009–1013.

Trockel, M. *et al.* (2021) 'Self-Valuation Challenges in the Culture and Practice of Medicine and Physician Well-being', *Mayo Clinic Proceedings*, 96(8), pp. 2123–2132.

Trockel, M.T. *et al.* (2019) 'Self-valuation: Attending to the Most Important Instrument in the Practice of Medicine', *Mayo Clinic Proceedings*, 94(10), pp. 2022–2031.

Trockel, M., *et al.* (2018) 'A Brief Instrument to Assess Both Burnout and Professional Fulfilment in Physicians: Reliability and Validity, Including Correlation with Self-Reported Medical Errors, in a Sample of Resident and Practicing Physicians', *Academic Psychiatry: The Journal of the American Association of Directors of Psychiatric Residency Training and the Association for Academic Psychiatry*, 42(1), pp. 11–24.

Waechter, R. *et al.* (2021) 'Mitigating medical student stress and anxiety: Should schools mandate participation in wellness intervention programs?', *Medical Teacher*, 43(8), pp. 945–955.

West, C.P. *et al.* (2014) 'Intervention to Promote Physician Well-being, Job Satisfaction, and Professionalism: A Randomized Clinical Trial', *JAMA Internal Medicine*, 174(4), pp. 527–533.

West, C.P. *et al.* (2020) 'Resilience and Burnout Among Physicians and the General US Working Population', *JAMA Network Open*, 3(7), p. e209385.

Whitla, D.K. *et al.* (2003) 'Educational benefits of diversity in medical school: a survey of students', *Academic Medicine: Journal of the Association of American Medical Colleges*, 78(5), pp. 460–466.

Wild, K. et al. (2014) 'Strategies against Burnout and Anxiety in Medical Education – Implementation and Evaluation of a New Course on Relaxation Techniques (Relacs) for Medical Students', *PLoS ONE*. Edited by D.S. Courvoisier, 9(12), p. e114967.

Williams, D. *et al.* (2015) 'Efficacy of Burnout Interventions in the Medical Education Pipeline', *Academic Psychiatry*, 39(1), pp. 47–54.

Wiskin, C. et al. (2018) 'Recommendations for undergraduate medical electives: a UK consensus statement', *Medical Education*, 52(1), pp. 14–23.

Yates, S.W. (2020) 'Physician Stress and Burnout', *The American Journal of Medicine*, 133(2), pp. 160–164.

Youmans, Q.R. et al. (2020) 'The STRIVE Initiative: A Resident-Led Mentorship Framework for Underrepresented Minority Medical Students', *Journal of Graduate Medical Education*, 12(1), pp. 74–79.

33
What is Being Done, and Does It Work?

Jay Kaplan

Background

Being a physician in modern society has never been easy. Multiple surveys over the past 15 years have shown that physicians in all specialties suffer from chronic stress, with a far greater prevalence of depression, substance use, and suicide than the general population. Burnout, classically defined as emotional exhaustion, loss of work fulfilment, and depersonalization (negativity/cynicism), is rampant. Medical students are not immune to these same stresses. Distress during medical school can lead to burnout, with significant consequences, particularly if burnout continues into residency and beyond. A systematic review of burnout in medical students published in 2013 (Ishak et al., 2013) revealed that burnout is prevalent during medical school, with major US multi-institutional studies estimating that at least half of all medical students may be affected by burnout during their medical education. This literature review showed that a variety of personal and professional characteristics correlate well with burnout, and hence potential interventions could include school-based and individual-based activities to increase overall student wellbeing.

Another study from the United Kingdom found that 54.8% of medical students reported high levels of emotional exhaustion (EE), 34% reported high levels of depersonalization (DP), and 46.6% reported low levels of personal accomplishment (PA). Linear regression analysis revealed that year of study, physical activity, and smoking status significantly predicted EE whilst gender, year of study, and institution significantly predicted DP. PA was significantly predicted by alcohol binge score, year of study, gender, and physical activity (Cecil et al., 2014).

The global pandemic since 2020 has clearly added to the stresses of being a medical student. Concerns for one's patients, for oneself and one's family have magnified the difficulties faced by learners in the hospital and outpatient settings.

> *You don't know if your patient will be next*
> *as death can be seen wherever you gaze*
> *old and young*
> *chronically ill or previously well*
> *it doesn't seem to much matter*
> *you search for those facts which put your patient at risk*
> *hoping to ease your own fears*
> *to reassure yourself that you are safe*

Jay Kaplan, *What is Being Done, and Does It Work?* In: *The Mental Health of Medical Students.* Edited by: Andrew Molodynski, Sarah Marie Farrell, and Dinesh Bhugra, Oxford University Press. © Oxford University Press 2024. DOI: 10.1093/oso/9780192864871.003.0033

> but there is no such relief
> you don't know if you will be next
>   and so
>   you worry for your patients
>   and you worry for your family
>   and you worry for yourself (Kaplan, 2020)

Isolation due to the need to move from in-person learning to the virtual environment has complicated the wellbeing of medical students by denying them the social interaction and sharing opportunities which have been so important to handling the stresses and insecurities of being learners in highly charged life-and-death situations.

On top of their educational concerns, medical students have faced the same stressors that all people are experiencing during this pandemic. It is no wonder that many are functioning on the high arousal (overload) end of the Yerkes-Dodson Human Performance and Stress Curve where anxiety, panic, and anger dominate (Gino, 2016). These external stressors are likely to continue as this pandemic lingers and society faces periods of community cohesion, disillusionment, setbacks, and finally, rebuilding. The typical disaster response curve is in Figure 33.1 (CCP, 2016).

Figure 33.2 is a graph of hospitalizations in the state of Louisiana from March 2020 to July of 2022, and it is a clear illustration of the rollercoaster that healthcare professionals, including medical students, have been on, obstructing the usual climb out of disillusionment and to recovery:

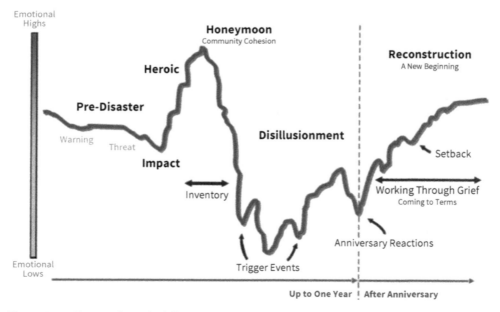

Figure 33.1 Phases of a typical disaster response.

Reproduced from Substance Abuse and Mental Health Services Administration: Crisis Counseling Assistance and Training Program Guidance. CCP Application Toolkit, Version 5.0, July 2016, p. 7. Available at https://www. samhsa.gov/sites/default/files/images/fema-ccp-guidance.pdf

Number of COVID Patients in Hospital in the State of Louisiana March 2020 - March 2022

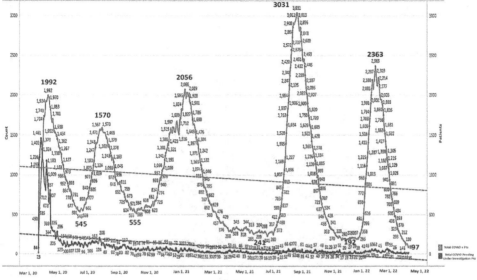

Figure 33.2 Hospitalizations in the state of Louisiana of COVID-19-positive patients and patients under investigation for COVID, from March 2020 to July 2022.
Source: Reproduced from Louisiana Department of Health.

Clinician Wellbeing Conceptual Model

In 2017 the National Academy of Medicine created the Action Collaborative on Clinician Wellbeing and Resilience. The Action Collaborative on Clinician Wellbeing and Resilience is a network of more than 50 organizations committed to reversing trends in clinician burnout. Goals for the Action Collaborative include:

(1) Improve baseline understanding of challenges to clinician wellbeing
(2) Raise the visibility of clinician stress and burnout
(3) Elevate evidence-based, multidisciplinary solutions that will improve patient care by caring for the caregiver.

The Clinician Wellbeing Knowledge Hub is a website intended to provide an easy-to-navigate repository of helpful resources for those seeking information and guidance on how to combat clinician burnout in their organizations and in their personal lives. The conceptual model working group of the National Academy of Medicine's Action Collaborative on Clinician Wellbeing and Resilience set out to create a model that could be used by individuals and organizations to understand the causes and effects of burnout, identify strategies to prevent and treat burnout and promote wellbeing, and improve healthcare delivery and patient outcomes. The model in Figure 33.3 depicts the domains and factors associated with burnout and wellbeing, and applies them across all healthcare professions and career stages, including

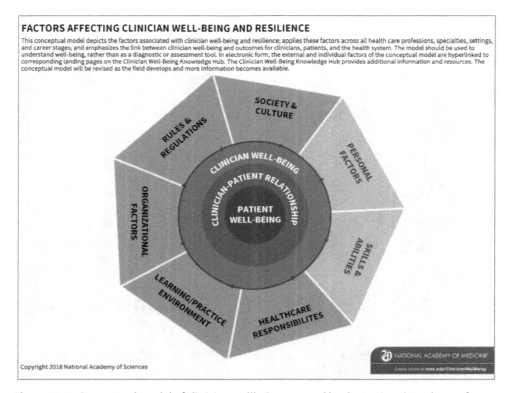

FACTORS AFFECTING CLINICIAN WELL-BEING AND RESILIENCE

This conceptual model depicts the factors associated with clinician well-being and resilience; applies these factors across all health care professions, specialties, settings, and career stages; and emphasizes the link between clinician well-being and outcomes for clinicians, patients, and the health system. The model should be used to understand well-being, rather than as a diagnostic or assessment tool. In electronic form, the external and individual factors of the conceptual model are hyperlinked to corresponding landing pages on the Clinician Well-Being Knowledge Hub. The Clinician Well-Being Knowledge Hub provides additional information and resources. The conceptual model will be revised as the field develops and more information becomes available.

Copyright 2018 National Academy of Sciences

Figure 33.3 Conceptual model of clinician wellbeing, created by the National Academy of Medicine Action Collaborative on Clinician Wellbeing and Resilience.

Brigham, T., C. Barden, A. L. Dopp, A. Hengerer, J. Kaplan, B. Malone, C. Martin, M. McHugh, and L. M. Nora. 2018. A Journey to Construct an All-Encompassing Conceptual Model of Factors Affecting Clinician Wellbeing and Resilience. NAM Perspectives. Discussion Paper, National Academy of Medicine, Washington, DC. https://doi.org/10.31478/201801b. Reproduced with permission from the National Academy of Sciences, Courtesy of the National Academies Press, Washington, D.C.

that of the student, and clearly identifies the link between clinician wellbeing and outcomes for clinicians, patients, and the health system (Brigham et al., 2020).

What is clear from this conceptual model is that most of the causes of burnout, and hence much of the support for wellbeing, must come from environmental factors rather than from the personal skills and abilities of the individual medical student. A simpler model is the Stanford Professional Model of Fulfilment that has the premise that promoting professional fulfillment and mitigating burnout requires organization-wide change and that wellbeing is driven not only by individual personal resilience but also through an organization's dedication to fostering a Culture of Wellness and Efficiency of Practice (Figure 33.4).

These conceptual models are important in guiding any discussion of supporting wellbeing in medical education.

Medical students tend to begin their studies with mental health profiles that are better than their peers in other fields. But for many students that profile progressively worsens due to a myriad of factors: large workloads, increased competition for residency slots, competitiveness, and first-time exposure to human suffering and death. Medical schools play an enormous role in addressing the mental health of students, but teaching students resilience

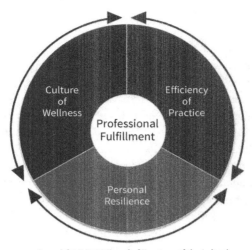

Figure 33.4 Stanford medicine model of professional fulfilment.
Reproduced with permission from Stanford Medicine. Available at https://wellmd.stanford.edu/
about/model-external.html. © 2016 Board of Trustees of the Leland Stanford Junior University.
All rights reserved.

and self-care skills can only be a part of the solution. Medical schools themselves have to look at their organizational contribution to medical student mental health and attempt to improve the learning environment by fostering wellness practices and decreasing, where possible, the environmental stressors.

Actions to Reduce Medical Student Burnout—What is Being Done

So what have medical schools and organizations like the Association of American Medical Colleges and the American Medical Association been doing to address burnout and support the mental health of its learners? Initiatives may be categorized into organizational and personal approaches.

Change the Grading System

Many academic medical centres have switched to a pass/fail grading system for the first two years of medical school, with the intention of reducing student competition and isolation and fostering collaboration. In 2017–2018, 108 medical schools in the US used pass/fail grading in the pre-clerkship years, while only 14 utilized that system for the clinical years. Liselotte N. Dyrbye, MD, MHPE, now Senior Associate Dean for Faculty and Chief Wellbeing Officer for the University of Colorado, studied factors which affected medical student burnout, including grading scale, how many hours of small group education, how many exams, and how much vacation. 'The only thing that mattered was whether or not they were in a pass-fail curriculum. Students who were not in a pass-fail curriculum had more burnout, more stress and were more likely to think about dropping out' (Reed et al., 2011). Dyrbye and others also published an article on 'Medical School Strategies to Address Student Wellbeing: A National Survey' in 2019 (Dyrbye et al., 2019). They found 59% of responding medical schools had a student wellbeing curriculum, with content scheduled during regular curricular hours at most (81%). These sessions were held at least monthly (75%), and there was a combination of optional and mandatory attendance (56%). Most responding schools offered a variety of emotional/spiritual, physical, financial, and social wellbeing activities. Nearly one-quarter had a specific wellbeing competency (22%), and most schools relied on participation rates (96%) and student satisfaction (81%) to evaluate effectiveness. 59% assessed student wellbeing from survey data, and 26% offered students access to self-assessment tools. Other common elements included an individual dedicated to overseeing student wellbeing (82%), a student wellbeing committee (82%), pass/fail grading in preclinical courses (74%), and the presence of learning communities (81%). Their conclusion was 'Schools have implemented a broad range of wellbeing curricula and activities intended to promote self-care, reduce stress, and build social support for medical students, with variable resources, infrastructure, and evaluation. Implementing dedicated wellbeing competencies and rigorously evaluating their impact would help ensure appropriate allocation of time and resources and determine if wellbeing strategies are making a difference. Strengthening evaluation is an important next step in alleviating learner distress and ultimately improving student wellbeing'.

Addressing Faculty Burnout—The Importance of the Role Model

Recognizing the degree to which the burnout and the relative wellbeing of faculty play in the mental health of students, some schools have focused on modifying the stressors and reducing burnout in the faculty. It has become clear that teaching personal resilience skills to students is hampered if there is not a simultaneous effort to decease burnout in their teachers. The American Medical Association has created its Steps Forward modules and Practice Transformation effort, which includes tools and playbooks to support innovative approaches to changing the practice environment (https://www.ama-assn.org/practice-management/ama-steps-forward/practice-innovation-strategies-physician-burnout?gclid=CjwKCAjwkaSaBhA4EiwALBgQaF7o5r4QMBMakQGhFHdSIc_kobQ2ssvL1LGJE1ZJLj1605t_49Z5HxoC4gsQAvD_BwE):

- Taming the EHR Playbook
- Creating the Organizational Foundation for Joy in Medicine™
- Scholars of Wellness
- Stress First Aid for Health Care Professionals
- Caring for the Healthcare Workforce During Crisis
- Establishing a Chief Wellness Officer Position
- Chief Wellness Officer Road Map
- Peer Support Programmes for Physicians
- Medical Student Wellbeing
- Preventing Physician Suicide
- Resident and Fellow Burnout
- Physician Burnout
- Physician Wellbeing

- Hospitalist Wellbeing
- Caring for the Healthcare Workforce During Crisis
- Chief Wellness Officer Road Map
- Creating the Organizational Foundation for Joy in Medicine™
- Establishing a Chief Wellness Officer Position
- Hospitalist Wellbeing
- Listening Campaign: Engage Physicians to Uncover Sources of Burnout
- Medical Student Wellbeing
- Peer Support Programmes for Physicians
- Physician Burnout
- Physician Wellbeing
- Preventing Physician Suicide
- Resident and Fellow Burnout
- Scholars of Wellness
- Stress First Aid for Healthcare Professionals
- Taming the EHR Playbook

As this helps faculty respond better to the stresses of the work environment, it will support the capability of those clinicians to create a more optimal learning environment for students.

Strategies Created by Medical Students

The Association of American Medical Colleges has been a leader in the US in promoting medical student wellbeing (https://students-residents.aamc.org/medical-student-well-being/medical-student-well-being). Their webpage is robust with testimonials and strategies shared by medical students to assist their fellow students (Figure 33.5):

Wellness Medical Student Curricula

The AAMC also has resources including medical student wellness curricula from multiple sources with links to the following topics:

- AAMC Financial Wellness: https://www.aamc.org/about-us/mission-areas/medical-education/wellbeing#financial
- Addressing Guilt and Moral Distress: https://www.aamc.org/about-us/mission-areas/medical-education/wellbeing#guilt
- Health Boundary Setting in Order to Maintain Wellness: https://www.aamc.org/about-us/mission-areas/medical-education/wellbeing#boundary
- Impostor experience: https://www.aamc.org/about-us/mission-areas/medical-education/wellbeing#impostor
- Meditation 101—Simple Practices for Maintaining Wellbeing and Fostering Resilience: https://www.aamc.org/about-us/mission-areas/medical-education/wellbeing#meditation
- Mental Health and Suicide Awareness: https://www.aamc.org/about-us/mission-areas/medical-education/wellbeing#mental-health
- Overcoming Procrastination: https://www.aamc.org/about-us/mission-areas/medical-education/wellbeing#procrastination

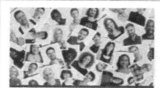

Reclaiming Your Identity

But one of the lessons I learned is easily accessible: we are not solely defined by how we have spent our time.

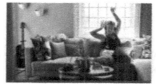

Understanding your Mental Health

A big red flag telling me that my mental health is declining is the food that I'm eating. During high-stress periods, I'll notice that all my meals come from the freezer or from takeout. These options have their place, they're quick, tasty, and sometimes necessary for long days.

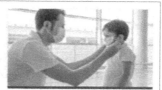

Caring for Yourself Before You Care for Others

Sometimes it feels like medical school has made me an amplified version of myself, for better and for worse.

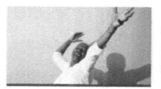

Graduating Out of My Self-Sacrifice

With vaccinations still rolling out, social distancing and masks are unquestionable accessories to our caps and gowns.

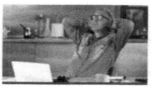

From Desperation to Freedom

FREE. I was so happy and wanted to be there; my patients could tell. BELIEVE. What matters is that I know I am doing my best. KNOW. I am capable and have the spirit and humility to improve every day. HARD WORK. Helping the most incredible women I know - my patients.

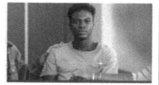

3 Subtle Signs of Burnout and 3 Not-so-Subtle Ways of Reclaiming Your Well-being

My hope is that by raising awareness of the subtle signs of burnout, physicians will not only be introspective of their own "internal battery", but also unfaltering advocates for the mental and physical health of their colleagues. Without further delay, here are three subtle signs of burnout I have recognized throughout my medical training.

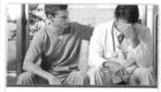

Courage and Mental Health: Physicians and Physicians-in-Training Sharing Their Personal Narratives

An editorial that examines the potential value of self-disclosure about mental distress and illness.

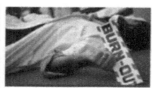

We Burn Out, We Break, We Die: Medical Schools Must Change Their Culture to Preserve Medical Student Health

The author explores medical student depression and suicide through the lens of personal struggles.

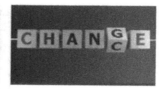

Transition to residency (and beyond) with kindness

"Are you satisfied with your scores?" This question tends to cause distress for many of us. But the intention of this article is not to cause distress nor to provide bullet-proof science defending a thesis.

Figure 33.5 Association of American Medical Colleges Medical Student Wellbeing Webpage. Reproduced with permission from AAMC. Available at https://students-residents.aamc.org/medical-student-well-being/medical-student-well-being (accessed 2023)

- Overview of Medical Student Wellness: https://www.aamc.org/about-us/mission-areas/medical-education/wellbeing#overview
- Positive Medicine: https://www.aamc.org/about-us/mission-areas/medical-education/wellbeing#positive
- Religion and Spirituality in Healthcare: https://www.aamc.org/about-us/mission-areas/medical-education/wellbeing#religion
- Smarter, Not Harder—Optimizing Your Personal Resources: https://www.aamc.org/about-us/mission-areas/medical-education/wellbeing#smarter
- The Power of Social Connections: https://www.aamc.org/about-us/mission-areas/medical-education/wellbeing#social

The AAMC GSA Committee on Student Affairs provides guidance on issues related to student support and services, including personal advising, career advising; the health and wellbeing of medical students; the ethical and professional development of students; academic support and resources, and the preparation of students for the transition from medical school to residency.

Strategies Focused on the Elements of Medical Student Wellbeing

Another strategy to promote medical student wellbeing is to identify the elements of that wellbeing. The American Medical Association defines those elements as:

Physical—maintaining a nutritional diet, regular exercise, and sleep hygiene—striving for seven to nine hours of sleep per night. Students should also be sure to get regular check-ups with a physician and work to manage any known pre-existing health conditions.

Emotional—Negative emotions and reactions are natural, but having awareness of them can help students change them. It can also help to speak to friends and family in their support system about their problems and how they might find solutions to them.

Social—Having an outlet and speaking to others in their support system can help a student identify their problems and come up with potential solutions.

Sense of purpose—Those pursuing a career in medicine are likely altruistic individuals. Having a student understand their core values and how they align with their career can be invaluable.

Initiatives that specifically support these concepts include: (1) connecting students with a primary care physician where there is no concern for loss of confidentiality, creating easy-to-access and safe exercise facilities at any hour of the day or night, and teaching nutrition; (2) Breaking down the stigma of seeking help by normalizing reaching out for help and emphasizing that 'it's okay to not be okay', as well as ensuring that off-site mental health support is existing and that time is made available for that support; (3) Creating a peer-to-peer support programme—training students to develop the skills necessary to provide one-on-one support to their peers, obviating the fear of impact on their careers from faculty services and decreasing the belief that the services would not be helpful (Mongrain et al., 2022); and (4) Assisting students in identifying their personal mission statement and recommending the identification of a daily Gratitude Moment ('What is one thing that you are grateful for today?') and a daily Legacy Moment ('What is one way that you have made a difference in someone's life today?').

In its Steps Forward education module, the AMA discusses eight strategies to decrease medical student burnout (https://edhub.ama-assn.org/steps-forward/module/2757082).

The module, titled *Medical Student Wellbeing: Minimize Burnout and Improve Mental Health Among Medical Students* includes the following actions:

- **Recognize shared responsibility.** Individual medical students do have responsibility for self-care that includes participating in healthy activities such as maintaining a nutritious diet and getting adequate sleep. Still, within the demanding schedules students face, institutions and faculty must put in place wellbeing related strategies and the personnel to carry them out. That means having faculty, such as a director of student wellbeing who is able to carry out school-level changes and collaborating with clinical rotation sites to create a supportive learning environment.
- **Measure student wellbeing.** What you don't measure you cannot manage. Schools should routinely perform wellbeing checks using a standardized assessment. Aggregate student body results should be compared with national benchmarks to get a sense of how students are doing locally versus nationally.
- **Optimize the curriculum.** While a number of curriculum-related factors and their influence on wellbeing have been studied, the only tangible evidence of a curricular intervention that has a positive effect on wellbeing is pass-fail grading. 'Medical students not in a pass-fail curriculum have nearly double rates of burnout, higher stress levels, and were 60% more likely to consider dropping out' (Rohe et al., 2006).
- **Help control student-loan debt.** Three out of four medical students graduate with debt related to their training, and according to the Association of American Medical Colleges, the average debt load 2017 medical school graduates carried upon completion of training was $192,000. Schools are required by accreditors to provide counselling for students on debt management and to have measures in place to minimize direct educational expenses.
- **Optimize the learning environment and cultivate community.** Learning environment, rather than workload, seems to be the culprit when looking for the roots of medical student burnout. Students need to be learning in an organized supportive environment that promotes their development. It is incumbent on the institution, the module says, to build a community between students and students and faculty. That can include the creation of study groups that create comradery and reduce stress and anxiety.
- **Promote self-care and resiliency.** Knowing that students have a very limited schedule, the module calls for students to be 'educated to strive for healthy self-improvement and to avoid the self-destructive and exhausting road of perfectionism'. Some institutions are offering students personal days during their clerkship year, as an intervention to promote self-care.
- **Provide adequate services for those already affected by burnout and distress.** While efforts are being made to address student wellbeing, the module cites the facts that about half of medical students experience symptoms of burnout and nearly a third show symptoms of depression. A proactive approach, the module says, requires medical schools to offer barrier-free access to mental healthcare. To avoid stigma, 'health professionals providing any services, including psychiatric or psychological counselling, should not be involved in the academic assessment or promotion of students in a medical school programme'.

- **Fund organizational science around wellbeing.** To identify solutions, it's imperative, the module states, to understand systems-level factors that contribute to medical student distress. Well-designed studies that can ultimately offer solutions require institutional investment.

Additional Online Resources—the National Academy of Medicine

Finally, it is worthwhile to refer back to the National Academy of Medicine Action Collaborative on Clinician Wellbeing and Resilience. Its website contains tools and case studies that can amplify what has worked and what has not, and can be instructive for any reader to refer to. The website is https://nam.edu/clinicianwellbeing/. The case studies, including several related specifically to wellbeing programmes for medical students, can be reached at https://nam.edu/clinicianwellbeing/case-studies/.

Conclusion

Burnout is rampant among medical professionals and it begins in medical school, especially as medical students enter their clinical years. The time to prevent burnout by addressing the environmental contributors and building resilience skills must be early during the education and training of those wanting to pursue medicine as a profession. Medical schools and large national organizations are taking specific action steps and defining approaches to improving medical student wellbeing that give hope that the epidemic of burnout can be treated before it becomes just a part of being a physician.

References

Brigham, T., Huffman, C.S., Connor, C.D., Swick, M., Danhauer, S.C., & Gibbs, M.A. (2020). 'A journey to construct an all-encompassing conceptual model of factors affecting clinician well-being and resilience'. National Academy of Medicine. https://nam.edu/journey-construct-encompassing-conceptual-model-factors-affecting-clinician-well-resilience/

Cecil, J., McHale, C., Hart, J., & Laidlaw, A. (2014). 'Behaviour and burnout in medical students'. *Med Educ Online* 19(1): 25209.

Dyrbye, L.N., Sciolla, A.F., Dekhtyar, M., Rajasekaran, S., Allgood, J.A., Rea, M., Knight, A.P., Haywood, A., Smith, S., & Stephens, M.B. (2019). 'Medical school strategies to address student well-being'. *Acad Med* 94(6): 861–868.

Gino, F. (April 14, 2016). 'Are you too stressed to be productive? Or not stressed enough?' *Harvard Business Review*. https://hbr.org/2016/04/are-you-too-stressed-to-be-productive-or-not-stressed-enough

IsHak, W., Nikravesh, R., Lederer, S., Perry, R., Ogunyemi, D., & Bernstein, C. (2013) 'Burnout in medical students: a systematic review'. *Clin Teach* 10(4): 242–245.

Kaplan, J. (2020). *Present Moment*. Unpublished poem, 1st stanza.

Mongrain, K., Simmons, A., Shore, I., Prinja, X., & Reaume, M. (2022). 'Side-by-side: A one-on-one peer support program for medical students'. *Acad Med* 97(8): 1170–1174.

Reed, D.A., Shanafelt, T.D., Satele, D.W., Power, D.V., Eacker, A., Harper, W., Moutier, C., Durning, S., Massie, F.S. Jr, Thomas, M.R., Sloan, J.A., & Dyrbye, L.N. (2011). 'Relationship of pass/fail grading and curriculum structure with well-being among preclinical medical students: a multi-institutional study'. *Acad Med* **86**(11): 1367–1373.

Rohe, D.E., Barrier, P.A., Clark, M.M., Cook, D.A., Vickers, K.S., & Decker, P.A. (2006) 'The benefits of pass-fail grading on stress, mood, and group cohesion in medical students'. *Mayo Clin Proc* **81**(11): 1443–1448.

Substance Abuse and Mental Health Services Administration. https://www.samhsa.gov/dtac

Substance Abuse and Mental Health Services Administration (2016). *Crisis Counseling Assistance and Training Program Guidance*. CCP Application Toolkit, Version 5.0, July 2016, p. 11.

34
Conclusions

Andrew Molodynski, Sarah Marie Farrell, and Dinesh Bhugra

Introduction

As is clear from the chapters in this volume, the mental health and wellbeing of medical students has emerged as a major issue across the globe. It is heartening to see that a large number of individuals, including contributors to this volume, are keen to take this forward. In many countries, not only was it difficult to collect data but there appeared to be a degree of risk, in spite of which authors delivered their contributions on time. The openness of colleagues in many countries and students wherever we found them strongly contrasted with a number of institutions in the United Kingdom and in the United States of America, who were resistant to allowing their students to have this freedom of expression. In the same way we admire and honour those above, we ask of these (often famed) institutions—'*you know who you are*'- We wonder what you were so afraid of finding out and why?

The combination of wide-ranging discourse on the history and development of training, the measurement of burnout, and the challenges faced by different systems around the world should provide a point of reference in a developing field. The reports from an unprecedented 21 countries, containing data regarding the extent of 'the problem' followed by initiatives taken, give an unrivalled richness of detail that the interested reader can pick their way through and hopefully discover useful things they can implement in their own lives and/ or for their own training schemes. The same applies to the sections regarding the needs of particular groups such as medical students with additional challenges, those studying outside their country of birth, and those with substance misuse issues. The very final chapters of the book offer potential solutions, both theoretical and those already being utilized, to try to improve matters on various levels. Wellbeing programmes are outlined alongside individual interventions. The crucial topic of fulfilment, so much thought about, and so little vocalized in medical education and further training, gives the possibility of a new framework for medical education and careers.

Challenges

There are several geo-political challenges that fundamentally affect medical training and remind us of its importance. The world's population continues to both grow and age. Multimorbidity is increasingly common and brings with it huge challenges around medical specialization and the need to be able to look after the whole person rather than them having numerous people looking after different 'bits' of somebody. Many health systems across the

Andrew Molodynski, Sarah Marie Farrell, and Dinesh Bhugra, *Conclusions* In: *The Mental Health of Medical Students*.
Edited by: Andrew Molodynski, Sarah Marie Farrell, and Dinesh Bhugra, Oxford University Press. © Oxford University Press 2024.
DOI: 10.1093/oso/9780192864871.003.0034

world are under intolerable pressure and there are long waits for treatments and unnecessarily poor outcomes. Increases in life expectancy in High Income Group (HIG) countries are slowing and in some have begun to stagnate. Given the pressure on services, there has been a noticeable shift towards prevention and public health. This is obviously welcome— much better to prevent someone from becoming ill than letting it happen and then trying to treat them, often at great expense and with undesired consequences for them. It does bring with it however a need to significantly adjust a model of medical training that remains overwhelmingly focused on the identification and treatment of disease.

Globalization and the increased movement of people and ideas over recent decades have enhanced the lives of many citizens and most would argue have brought us closer together. The events of late 2019 and early 2020 however brought home the downside. Who can forget watching the spread of a respiratory virus from China across the whole world, aided by cruise ships, airplanes, cars, and other forms of transport with hotspots cropping up In Italy, Iran, and other countries before every country ended up being affected? The opposite of globalization then occurred, national and local lockdowns as in *The Plague* by Camus. Some restrictions even persist to time of writing in late 2022. The medical profession was immediately at the forefront of the global effort and the need for doctors to be flexible, multilingual, and able to absorb data and clinical information from other contexts became paramount to save millions of lives. More for medical schools and their crowded schedules to fit in!

Recent decades have also brought an increased realization of the effects of climate change upon our lives, our communities, and our physical and mental health. These are already being seen in so called 'natural disasters' such as the floods in Nigeria and Pakistan this year (2022). Changes in weather will bring changes in illness distribution and extreme events will bring worry, anxiety, and post-traumatic stress symptoms (not to mention low mood and substance misuse) for many. Again, we need our next generation of doctors to be ready and prepared for this challenge in terms of their training and their wellbeing.

Welcome changes include a greater focus on mental healthcare globally. In many countries however, mental healthcare is still barely acknowledged in medical training and this needs to change. Other welcome changes in medical care such as the increasing use of technology, artificial intelligence, ever more sophisticated scanning techniques, and the computerization and roboticization of some medical care also call for huge changes in what medical students learn *and* in the way they learn it. Development of other specialist support roles such as nurse specialists and physician associates adds another dimension to the changing role of the future workforce which will impact upon training.

These bring us on to the challenge posed by the internet (including social media), possibly the most multifaceted change of all. We all know that, for better or worse (or a bit of both generally!), the internet has transformed our existence in the last 20 years. In medicine, the effects have been profound. There are new conditions linked solely to the internet and many conditions that are exacerbated by internet use, especially in terms of our mental health. The internet has allowed for electronic records systems and accounting systems across healthcare, and these are frequently held up as simultaneously an advance for patient care and a source of added burden for healthcare staff. On the other hand, without the internet the covid response would have taken months if not years longer to materialize fully, with many more lives lost. Evidence can now be transferred and made freely available in the click of a button. It is no longer possible for a doctor or medical student to be familiar with all or even most of the empirical evidence. There is also much 'evidence' out there now that is poorly peer reviewed and not in line with good, safe practice. These things are new, and it is common now that our patients have read what we have- or often more! This then leads to a fundamental shift in the doctor–patient relationship, with doctor as guide and interpreter rather than as an expert holder of privileged information. While most of us will regard this as a positive change, it calls for substantial shifts in medical education to allow the necessary skills to develop and the associated anxieties to dissipate. It also calls for substantial shifts in the expectations of societies, a very difficult outcome to achieve.

The Current Situation of Medical Students

For a multitude of reasons outlined throughout this book, medical students are under great pressure, and many are showing signs of distress. With rates of burnout of between 61% and 99% (weighted average of 84% for disengagement and 86% for exhaustion), up to 95% meeting caseness on the GHQ12 (weighted average 69%) screening tool for having a mental disorder, and with high rates of substance misuse in most countries, this group is showing clear signs of distress. Levels are in excess of age-matched peers, both those on other university courses and those in the general population. There is evidence that these measures of distress worsen as courses continue and that progressively more students seek help. What is happening to this cohort of young people who are amongst the brightest and most motivated in their society, often from families with high levels of social capital—a well-known protection against many of the vagaries of life?

We can only conclude that being at medical school, in the widest sense, can be both pressurizing and toxic. Our surveys asked about different stressors and demonstrated these to be high across the board. Financial, family, and relationship worries competed with those directly related to work. While reported sources of stress vary significantly across countries, levels are high everywhere. Interventions have begun in recent years in many places, but the impact of these has yet to be evaluated over time. Indeed, even as they are introduced, the pressures above are causing courses to warp and flex to meet ever-new demands and with that come ever-new challenges. More worryingly, many places have made minimal or no changes to support their students. This is perhaps understandable in countries and institutions where resources are extremely scarce, but it is unforgivable in many wealthier countries where it appears to be a result of those in positions of authority not being able to recognize the problem and begin to grapple with it. High-profile individual tragedies of students taking their own lives are now creating the pressure needed for urgent change.

The Future

Until recently, most attempts to address the poor levels of wellbeing and high levels of psychiatric symptoms, burnout, and substance misuse amongst medical students have generally focused on the students themselves. There have been notable exceptions as described in several chapters, but overwhelmingly the focus has been on the treatment of those who present as 'cases' by being in distress, self-harming, or coming to the attention of schools in other ways such as with poor performance or disciplinary problems. Increasingly educators are recognizing that they must adopt a preventative model as outlined in Chapter 30 (Kemp), strongly rooted in an occupational health background and using those principles. The importance for individuals of psychological, physical, and social wellbeing ultimately leading to integrative wellbeing as in Chapter 31 (Collini/Elton) complements this institutional approach and strengthens it. Moving further forwards with integrating wellbeing come the concepts of fulfilment and satisfaction, that in turn lead on to better patient care and careers that are more sustainable—a real 'win-win-win' situation for patient, employee, and employer alike. Embedding these factors in medical school can only be the right thing to do.

We have seen in this book the scale of the problem laid bare—a generation of medical students struggling with poor mental health and burnout. We have at the same time seen great causes for hope in the reports of initiatives for change from individual countries and in the chapters just described. It is clear that a triple approach of institutional reform to support students and reduce distress is needed alongside well-resourced and available supports for wellbeing and accessible care and support for those who need it. Crucially though, all these things must happen, as so eloquently put in Chapter 3 with its farming analogy, in 'good soil' free of toxins and containing enough nutrients for necessary growth. We have tried to capture the essence of this book and the existing evidence around the world to make a useful and practical charter that can be utilized by policy makers and funders, educators, and students alike. It is deliberately broad to allow for its use in different cultures and economies but its key themes are relevant everywhere—please use them!.

Appendix: Medical Student Wellbeing Charter

Introduction

It is widely recognized that medical students are a vulnerable group of people with high levels of stress, burnout, mental health problems, and substance misuse (Drybe & Shanafelt, 2016). Medical students in general are at a vulnerable stage in life and also have higher than base population levels of burnout and symptoms of mental ill-health.

There is thus an important responsibility on health professionals to ensure the wellbeing of the next generation of doctors, for the students' own sake and also because they will come to make up a crucial part of both the healthcare workforce and of their society.

There has traditionally been a focus on resilience and individual factors alongside treating those whose difficulties become manifest, but it is important to recognize that most stressors are system based. They are therefore amenable to intervention at institutional level and the institutions concerned have a clear responsibility to look after their students. The evidence base for interventions is still evolving and any guidance will necessarily evolve also. However, we endeavour here to provide a charter of basic steps that all institutions should take to safeguard their students and to reassure funders and students alike (indeed the two overlap enormously!) that they provide a safe and supportive environment for learning. Although there is clearly variation of approach internationally, levels of distress are high, and the charter is broad enough to be applicable regardless of geography.

This charter stands unashamedly on the shoulders of giants (British Medical Association 2022; Kemp et al., 2019; General Medical Council, 2015).

1. All medical schools should explicitly include student wellbeing in their core documentation.
2. Induction programmes should include sessions around stress, wellbeing, and in person introductions to those who provide support services (not just information giving).
3. The early part of medical training should have a strong focus on self-care and the physical and psychological effects of stress.
4. Peer mentoring arrangements should be routine and attract protected time.
5. Curricula should be designed to minimize 'pinch points' of high stress while maintaining rigour. A pass/ fail approach will be appropriate in most (if not all) exams.
6. Curricula should allow students protected time to take part in wellbeing activities individually and in groups
7. Placements that rotate geographically need to be managed to reduce disruption and allow for access to support for students. Ideally, they should also allow for flexibility, taking into account student preferences and need.
8. Clear arrangements and support for subsequent job finding must be made available to final-year students, preferably as part of a coordinated matching scheme by the institution.
9. All medical schools should have a wellbeing department for students that is adequately resourced, well signposted, and supported at the very highest level by a wellbeing responsible officer ensuring confidentiality and privacy.
10. Funding for student support and wellbeing must be clearly identified and spent transparently. There should be student representation on committees that make decisions regarding the amount of funding and how it is spent.
11. The responsible officer for wellbeing is a legally accountable board member of the medical school council or appropriate body for the purposes of reporting, quality control and health and safety investigations.

References

British Medical Association (2022). Medical student wellbeing checklist. med-students-wellbeing-checklist.pdf (bma.org.uk)

Dyrbye, L. & Shanafelt, T. (2016). 'A narrative review on burnout experienced by medical students and residents'. *Med Educ* **50**(1): 132–149.

General Medical Council (2015). 'Supporting medical students with mental health conditions. Supporting medical students with mental health conditions' (gmc-uk.org)

Kemp, S., Hu, W., Bishop, J., Forrest, K., Hudson, J.N., Wilson, I., Teodorczuk, A., Rogers, G.D., Roberts, C., & Wearn, A. (2019). 'Medical student wellbeing–a consensus statement from Australia and New Zealand'. *BMC Med Educ* **19**(1): 1–8.

Index